Diagnosis and Treatment of Human Mycoses

Infectious Disease

SERIES EDITOR: *Vassil St. Georgiev*

National Institute of Allergy and Infectious Diseases
National Institutes of Health

Diagnosis and Treatment of Human Mycoses, edited by ***Duane R. Hospenthal, MD, PhD and Michael G. Rinaldi, PhD, 2008***

Foodborne Diseases, edited by ***Shabbir Simjee, PhD, 2007***

Reverse Transcriptase Inhibitors in HIV/AIDS Therapy, edited by ***Gail Skowron, MD and Richard Ogden, PhD, 2006***

Vaccine Adjuvants: Immunological and Clinical Principles, edited by ***Charles J. Hackett, PhD and Donald A. Harn, Jr., PhD, 2006***

Congenital and Perinatal Infections: A Concise Guide to Diagnosis, edited by ***Cecelia Hutto, MD, 2006***

Drug Interactions in Infectious Diseases: Second Edition, edited by ***Stephen C. Piscitelli, PharmD and Keith A. Rodvold, PharmD, 2005***

Biological Weapons Defense: Infectious Disease and Counterbioterrorism, edited by ***Luther E. Lindler, PhD, Frank J. Lebeda, PhD, and George W. Korch, PhD, 2005***

Microbial Genomes, edited by ***Claire M. Fraser, PhD, Timothy D. Read, PhD, and Karen E. Nelson, PhD, 2004***

Management of Multiple Drug-Resistant Infections, edited by ***Stephen H. Gillespie, MD, 2004***

Aging, Immunity, and Infection, by ***Joseph F. Albright, PhD and Julia W. Albright, PhD, 2003***

Handbook of Cytokines and Chemokines in Infectious Diseases, edited by ***Malak Kotb, PhD and Thierry Calandra, MD, PhD, 2003***

Opportunistic Infections: *Treatment and Prophylaxis,* ***Vassil St. Georgiev, PhD, 2003***

Innate Immunity, edited by ***R. Alan B. Ezekowitz, MBChB, DPhil, FAAP, and Jules A. Hoffmann, PhD, 2003***

Pathogen Genomics: *Impact on Human Health,* edited by ***Karen Joy Shaw, PhD, 2002***

Immunotherapy for Infectious Diseases, edited by ***Jeffrey M. Jacobson, MD, 2002***

Retroviral Immunology: *Immune Response and Restoration,* edited by ***Giuseppe Pantaleo, MD and Bruce D. Walker, MD, 2001***

Infectious Disease

Diagnosis and Treatment of Human Mycoses

Edited by

Duane R. Hospenthal, MD, PhD

Infectious Disease Service, Department of Medicine, Brooke Army Medical Center, Fort Sam Houston, TX; F. Edward Hébert School of Medicine, Uniformed Services University of Health Sciences, Bethesda, MD

Michael G. Rinaldi, PhD

Fungus Testing Laboratory, Department of Pathology, University of Texas Health Science Center at San Antonio, San Antonio, TX

HUMANA PRESS ✻ TOTOWA, NEW JERSEY

999 Riverview Drive, Suite 208
Totowa, New Jersey 07512

www.humanapress.com

This publication is printed on acid-free paper. ∞

ANSI Z39.48-1984 (American Standards Institute) Permanence of Paper for Printed Library Materials

Cover design by Karen Schulz

Cover illustration: Septate, uniform hyphae of *Aspergillus fumigatus* (*see* Color plate 1, following p. 48).

For additional copies, pricing for bulk purchases, and/or information about other Humana titles, contact Humana at the above address or at any of the following numbers: Tel.: 973-256-1699; Fax: 973-256-8341; or visit our Website: www.humanapress.com

Additional material to this book can be downloaded from http://extras.springer.com.

e-ISBN 978-1-59745-325-7

Printed in the United States of America. 10 9 8 7 6 5 4 3 2 1

Library of Congress Control Number: 2007929353

Preface

With the rapid expansion of medical technologies and treatments over the past several decades fungi have emerged as important causative agents of human infection (mycosis). Improved survival afforded by cancer and human immunodeficiency virus (HIV) therapies, intensive care units, and broad-spectrum antibacterial agents continue to increase the population at risk for these infections. Fortunately, our understanding of the fungi, and ability to diagnose and treat fungal infections, has also progressed over this time. *Diagnosis and Treatment of Human Mycoses* brings together globally recognized mycoses experts to guide readers in the use of the current knowledge in the field of medical mycology to manage those who suffer from fungal infections (mycoses).

Diagnostic strategies and tests, including basic and directed culturing techniques, histopathology with standard and special stains, serological methods, and radiological studies, often all need to be considered and commonly combined to make the diagnosis of fungal infection. This book introduces and reviews these tools first separately and later as they pertain to specific infections or groups of diseases.

The antifungal armamentarium has almost exponentially expanded over the past decade alone. In addition to amphotericin B, multiple systemically active triazole and echinocandin antifungal agents are now available. Selecting which drug to use has now progressed beyond amphotericin B or no amphotericin B, allowing many options for therapy, but also increasing the complexity of choosing which agent to employ. With the differing spectrums of these agents, diagnosis to species level has become more necessary to provide the best care to those infected. This expansion and increases in disease also raises questions of prophylactic therapy and preemptive and combination use of these drugs. The development of standardized antifungal susceptibility testing promises to help with questions of selecting the best antifungal for individual patients, but has also introduced questions of how and when to best use this still emerging technology.

Diagnosis and Treatment of Human Mycoses is meant to be a concise text that will provide the busy infectious disease, hematology–oncology, pulmonology, or critical care specialist a practical tool to diagnose and manage fungal infections. In addition, the depth of the material in the text will provide these and other medical specialists and trainees an excellent reference and learning resource.

The text is divided into four parts to guide the reader. Part I gives a general introduction with epidemiology and presents practical approaches for using patient risk factors, exposures, and site of infection to direct diagnostic evaluations. Part II introduces the science of mycology and the current tools available to diagnose fungal infections, in the clinical mycology laboratory, using histopathology and diagnostic immunology, and with radiological technologies. Part III provides an in-depth review of the available antifungal drugs, their use, and discussion of resistance and antifungal susceptibility testing. After the reader is provided with the overview of diagnostic and therapeutic tools in Parts I to III, Part IV presents the human mycoses in 15 uniform, easy to read chapters, with accompanying tables and figures. At the end of the text are 18 instructive cases that provide the reader a review of many of the important concepts presented in the book. Each case is presented as an unknown to test the knowledge obtained or to emphasize an important or complex subject in the field.

Duane R. Hospenthal, MD, PhD
Michael G. Rinaldi, PhD

Contents

Contributors

CARLOS A. AGUDELO, MD • *Facultad de Medicina, Universidad Pontificia Bolivariana, Medellín, Colombia*

ELIAS J. ANAISSIE, MD • *Myeloma Institute for Research and Therapy, Division of Cancer Supportive Care, University of Arkansas for Medical Sciences, Little Rock, AR*

CHARALAMPOS ANTACHOPOULOS, MD • *Immunocompromised Host Section, Pediatric Oncology Branch, National Cancer Institute, National Institutes of Health, Bethesda, MD*

SHEHLA BAQI, MD • *Division of Infectious Diseases, Department of Medicine, David Geffen School of Medicine at the University of California at Los Angeles; and Department of Medicine, Kern Medical Center, Bakersfield, CA*

HELEN W. BOUCHER, MD • *Division of Infectious Diseases, Department of Medicine, Tufts University–New England Medical Center, Boston, MA*

STANLEY W. CHAPMAN, MD • *Division of Infectious Diseases, Department of Medicine, University of Mississippi Medical Center, Jackson, MS*

METHEE CHAYAKULKEEREE, MD • *Division of Infectious Diseases, Department of Medicine, Duke University Medical Center, Durham, NC*

NICHOLAS G. CONGER, MD • *Division of Infectious Diseases, Landstuhl Regional Medical Center, Landstuhl Germany*

ELIZABETH A. COOPER, HBSc • *Mediprobe Research Inc., London, Ontario, Canada*

SAMIT S. DESAI, MD • *Infectious Diseases Section, Yale University School of Medicine, New Haven; and Infectious Diseases Section, Veterans Affairs Connecticut Healthcare System, West Haven, CT*

RHONDA V. FLEMING, MD • *Division of Infectious Diseases, Department of Internal Medicine, Texas Tech University Health Sciences Center, El Paso, TX*

ANNETTE W. FOTHERGILL, MA, MBA • *Fungus Testing Laboratory, Department of Pathology, University of Texas Health Science Center at San Antonio, San Antonio, TX*

JUAN C. GEA-BANACLOCHE, MD • *Experimental Immunology Branch, National Cancer Institute, National Institutes of Health, Bethesda, MD*

FRANCIS GIGLIOTTI, MD • *Division of Infectious Diseases, Department of Pediatrics; and Department of Microbiology and Immunology, University of Rochester School of Medicine and Dentistry, Rochester, NY*

ADITYA K. GUPTA, MD, PhD • *Division of Dermatology, Department of Medicine, Sunnybrook Health Sciences Center, Toronto; University of Toronto, Toronto; and Mediprobe Research, Inc., London, Ontario, Canada*

CONSTANZA J. GUTIERREZ, MD • *Department of Radiology, University of Texas Health Science Center at San Antonio, San Antonio, TX*

DUANE R. HOSPENTHAL, MD, PhD • *Infectious Disease Service, Department of Medicine, Brooke Army Medical Center, Fort Sam Houston, TX; F. Edward Hébert School of Medicine, Uniformed Services University of Health Sciences, Bethesda, MD*

MARIA ANGELA C. HOSPENTHAL, MD • *Division of Pulmonary/Critical Care Medicine, Department of Medicine, University of Texas Health Science Center at San Antonio, San Antonio, TX*

ROYCE H. JOHNSON, MD • *Division of Infectious Diseases, Department of Medicine, David Geffen School of Medicine at the University of California at Los Angeles; and Department of Medicine, Kern Medical Center, Bakersfield, CA*

CAROL A. KAUFFMAN, MD • *Division of Infectious Diseases, University of Michigan Medical School and Veterans Affairs Ann Arbor Healthcare System, Ann Arbor, MI*

RUSSELL E. LEWIS, PharmD • *University of Houston College of Pharmacy, Houston, TX*

MICHAEL R. MCGINNIS, PhD • *Department of Pathology; and Medical Mycology Research Center, University of Texas Medical Branch, Galveston, TX*

CLINTON K. MURRAY, MD • *Infectious Disease Service, Department of Medicine, Brooke Army Medical Center, Fort Sam Houston, TX; F. Edward Hébert School of Medicine, Uniformed Services University of Health Sciences, Bethesda, MD*

THOMAS F. PATTERSON, MD • *Division of Infectious Diseases, Department of Medicine, University of Texas Health Science Center at San Antonio; and Audie L. Murphy Division, South Texas Veterans Health Care System, San Antonio, TX*

JOHN R. PERFECT, MD • *Division of Infectious Diseases, Department of Medicine, Duke University Medical Center, Durham, NC*

ANGELA RESTREPO, PhD • *Corporación para Investigaciones Biológicas (CIB), Medellín, Colombia*

SANJAY G. REVANKAR, MD • *Division of Infectious Diseases, Wayne State University School of Medicine, Detroit, MI*

MICHAEL G. RINALDI, PhD • *Fungus Testing Laboratory, Department of Pathology, University of Texas Health Science Center at San Antonio, San Antonio, TX*

MICHAEL B. SMITH, MD • *Department of Pathology, University of Texas Medical Branch, Galveston, TX*

JACK D. SOBEL, MD • *Division of Infectious Diseases, Wayne State University School of Medicine, Detroit, MI*

DONNA C. SULLIVAN, PhD • *Division of Infectious Diseases, Department of Medicine, University of Mississippi Medical Center, Jackson, MS*

DEANNA A. SUTTON, PhD • *Fungus Testing Laboratory, Department of Pathology, University of Texas Health Science Center at San Antonio, San Antonio, TX*

ANGELA M. TOBÓN, MD • *Corporación para Investigaciones Biológicas (CIB); Facultad de Medicina, Universidad Pontificia Bolivariana; and Hospital La María, Medellín, Colombia*

JOSE A. VAZQUEZ, MD • *Division of Infectious Diseases, Henry Ford Hospital; and Division of Infectious Diseases, Wayne State University School of Medicine, Detroit, MI*

THOMAS J. WALSH, MD • *Immunocompromised Host Section, Pediatric Oncology Branch, National Cancer Institute, National Institutes of Health, Bethesda, MD*

L. JOSEPH WHEAT, MD • *MiraVista Diagnostics and Mirabella Technologies, Indianapolis, IN*

BRIAN WONG, MD • *Division of Infectious Diseases, Department of Medicine, Oregon Health and Science University, Portland, OR*

TERRY W. WRIGHT, PhD • *Division of Infectious Diseases, Department of Pediatrics; and Department of Microbiology and Immunology, University of Rochester School of Medicine and Dentistry, Rochester, NY*

Color Plates

Color Plates follow p. 48

Companion CD

Color versions of illustrations listed here may be found on the Companion CD attached to the inside back cover. The image files are organized into folders by chapter number and are viewable in most Web browsers. The number following "f" at the end of the file name identifies the corresponding figure in the text. The CD is compatible with both Mac and PC operating systems.

Chapter 2	Figs. 1–16
Chapter 3	Figs. 1–12
Chapter 6	Figs. 2–4 and 6
Chapter 8	Fig. 1
Chapter 9	Figs. 1 and 2
Chapter 10	Fig. 1
Chapter 11	Figs. 2 and 3
Chapter 12	Figs. 1, 2 and 3
Chapter 13	Fig. 1
Chapter 14	Figs. 4–7
Chapter 15	Figs. 1, 7 and 8
Chapter 16	Figs. 6–9
Chapter 17	Figs. 1, 2 and 6
Chapter 18	Figs. 1, 2 and 4–6
Chapter 19	Figs. 1–5
Chapter 20	Figs. 1–12
Chapter 21	Figs. 1–4

Instructive Case: Figs. 1–5, 7, 10, 12–14 and 17

I

Approach to Patients

1
Approach to Patients with Suspected Fungal Infections

Clinton K. Murray, MD and Duane R. Hospenthal, MD, PhD

1. INTRODUCTION

The incidence of fungal infections (mycoses) is increasing throughout the world as a result of modern medical advances that use immunosuppressive therapies, broad-spectrum antibiotics, and central venous access devices, as well as a rise in the population of individuals at risk. Technology has led to the improved survival of persons with malignancies, transplanted organs, and human immunodeficiency virus (HIV) infection; those who have experienced trauma; and persons at the extremes of age. The medical community has met this challenge with the introduction of new antifungal agents, often with less toxicity and improved spectrums of activity. In addition, newer, more sensitive and specific diagnostic strategies such as improved radiographic imaging and serological tests have provided clinicians with better tools to detect fungal infections earlier, potentially influencing disease outcomes. Despite these advances, the approach to the diagnosis and management of fungal infections still relies on recognizing the interaction of the pathogen and the host. Although some fungal diseases have classic presentations, many of these occur so rarely that clinicians may not initially include them in their differential diagnoses. In the setting of immunosuppression, mycoses may produce nonspecific signs and symptoms, making their diagnosis a challenge. Early recognition and treatment are fundamental to modifying disease outcomes in many fungal infections, especially those in immunocompromised individuals. Increased awareness of key risk factors and clinical presentations of the human mycoses may enable clinicians to develop an inclusive approach to the diagnosis of these diseases.

From: *Infectious Disease: Diagnosis and Treatment of Human Mycoses*
Edited by: D. R. Hospenthal and M. G. Rinaldi © Humana Press Inc., Totowa, NJ

2. EPIDEMIOLOGY

Deaths associated with mycoses have increased in the United States, advancing from the 10th most common infectious disease cause of death in 1980 to the 7th in 1997 *(1)*. Sepsis due to fungal infection increased more than 200% in the United States between 1979 and 2000 *(2)*. Fungal sepsis is chiefly secondary to infection with *Candida*, which continues to be the fourth most common organism recovered from bloodstream infections in the United States, associated with an estimated mortality of about 40% *(3,4)*. Candidemia and disseminated (also termed systemic or invasive) candidiasis continue to be the most common nosocomial fungal infections, responsible for more than 80% of these infections and up to 15% of nosocomial infections overall. Infections with *Candida* have declined in patients with cancer and in those undergoing hematopoietic stem cell transplantation (HSCT), likely in association with antifungal prophylaxis. The incidence of candidemia, after surging in the 1980s, appears to have declined, at least in the intensive care setting *(5)*. This overall decline is chiefly due to fewer infections with *C. albicans*, as non-*albicans Candida* (NAC) candidemia has increased over this same period, 1989–1999.

The range of hosts who develop opportunistic mould infections, most commonly caused by the *Aspergillus* species, continues to expand from severely neutropenic cancer patients to patients with other risk factors, including persons with prolonged immunosuppressive therapies with corticosteroids and newer agents, including those that inhibit tumor necrosis factor-alpha (TNF-α) *(6)*. *Aspergillus* is the second most common cause of nosocomial fungal infection and the most common mould to cause invasive mycosis. Other rare opportunistic moulds (e.g., the zygomycetes, *Fusarium*, and *Scedosporium*) and yeasts (e.g., *Trichosporon* and *Malassezia*) have emerged as more frequent causes of disease in patients with a wide range of risks *(7–13)*.

Outbreaks of endemic mycoses, including coccidioidomycosis in association with the growing urbanization of the US Southwest, and on a smaller scale, histoplasmosis, continue to be reported more frequently, often affecting greater numbers of persons. Outbreaks of endemic disease are occasionally diagnosed outside their known geographical areas, occurring in travelers to those locales. A localized outbreak of infection with the non-*neoformans Cryptococcus*, *C. gattii*, in immunocompetent patients has recently been reported in southwest Canada (Vancouver Island) *(14)*.

3. SUSPICION BASED ON RISK FACTORS

The risks for fungal infections are highly dependent on the combination of host immune competency and the specific exposures people have both within the healthcare system and in their communities.

3.1. Immunocompromise

Host immune status is probably the most important underlying factor determining whether people develop life-threatening, self-limiting, or no infection after exposure to fungi in their environment. Defense against invasive mycoses depends chiefly on intact mucosal barriers, the innate immunity provided by phagocytic cells, and cell-mediated immunity (CMI). The impact of humoral immunity appears limited and remains poorly defined in defense against the fungi.

3.1.1. Neutropenia and Altered Phagocytic Function

Classically, neutropenia has been associated with candidemia and invasive candidiasis. With prolonged neutropenia, *Aspergillus* species become more common causes of infection. Infection with the zygomycetes, *Fusarium*, *Scedosporium*, *Trichosporon*, and other rare species can also been seen with prolonged loss of neutrophils. The incidence of candidiasis in the highest risk populations appears to have declined over the past decade in association with antifungal prophylaxis of these patients. This decrease has been associated with an increase in aspergillosis and other invasive mould infections. In addition to insufficient numbers of neutrophils, decline in phagocytic function also raises the risk of mycoses. The phagocytic dysfunction seen in chronic granulomatous disease (CGD) is associated with fungal infections, especially aspergillosis.

3.1.2. Impaired Cell-Mediated Immunity

Impaired CMI occurs in patients infected with HIV and in those receiving many of the currently used immunosuppressive therapies. Impairment of CMI is associated with mucocutaneous candidiasis, *Pneumocystis* pneumonia, infection with *Cryptococcus*, and more severe and/or disseminated endemic mycoses. The specific mycoses associated with $CD4^+$ T lymphocyte decline as seen in HIV/AIDS have been carefully documented, allowing the clinician to increase the level of suspicion for particular fungal infections based on $CD4^+$ T lymphocyte counts of their patients (Table 1.1).

3.1.3. Organ Transplantation

Solid organ and HSCT recipients are at great risk for fungal infections *(15–17)*. In addition to immunosuppressive therapies, the mucosal damage and intensive therapy associated with these procedures place the persons who receive them at risk for the entire spectrum of fungal disease. Transplant medicine has seen substantial advancements in tailoring regimens to minimize the duration of neutropenia and to reduce immunosuppressive treatments used to control rejection. Unfortunately, most of these still place patients at a substantial risk for opportunistic infections. In solid organ transplantation, the risk of fungal infection is associated with risk surrounding the initial surgery and the use of immunosuppression to prevent rejection. This risk varies greatly based on the organ transplanted and underlying condition of the recipient. As

Table 1.1
Mycoses commonly associated with HIV infection

$CD4^+$ T lymphocyte cell count (cells/μl)	Fungal infections
>500	Candidal vaginitis
200–500	Thrush (oropharyngeal candidiasis)
<200	PCP, disseminated histoplasmosis, disseminated coccidioidomycosis
<100	Cryptococcosis, candidal esophagitis, penicilliosis

PCP, *Pneumocystis* pneumonia.

an example, in liver transplantation the substantial risk of *Candida* infection in the first month is associated mostly with surgical manipulation of the gastrointestinal tract and need for intensive care monitoring, as well as initial immunosuppressive agents given to control rejection (Table 1.2). Lung transplants are at high risk for invasive pulmonary aspergillosis, likely secondary to the route of inoculation and immunosuppression. Although a similar sequence of occurrence of fungal infection is seen in HSCT, the underlying factors creating risk differ from those of solid organ transplant (Table 1.3). In HSCT, initial conditioning commonly leads to neutropenia and breakdown of the mucosal surfaces. This neutropenia can be prolonged and associated with life-threatening mould infections. In allogeneic HSCT, graft versus host disease (GvHD) and its treatment may put the patient at risk for fungal infection for a prolonged period of time after engraftment.

3.2. Healthcare Exposure (Nosocomial)

A multitude of risk factors for nosocomial fungal infections have been identified (Table 1.4) *(6,18,19)*. Unfortunately, many of these healthcare-associated risk factors overlap with those associated with bacterial infections or are risks that are common to many or most hospitalized patients. This is especially true for patients hospitalized in intensive care units, the majority of whom have central venous catheters and are receiving broad-spectrum antibiotics *(20,21)*. In addition to the use of vascular catheters, other procedures including urinary catheterization and intubation establish portals of entry for fungal pathogens. Other risk factors include immunosuppression seen with the use of corticosteroids and chemotherapy, malnutrition and malignancy.

Table 1.2
Fungi associated with solid organ transplantation

Time period	Common fungi	Other fungi
First month	*Candida*	
1–6 months	*Aspergillus*, *Pneumocystis*, *Cryptococcus*	Endemic fungi[a]
>6 months	Endemic fungi[a]	*Cryptococcus*

[a]Chiefly, *Coccidioides* and *Histoplasma*.
Table produced from data in ref. 16.

Table 1.3
Fungi associated with hematopoietic stem cell transplantation

Time period	Common fungi	Other fungi
Preengraftment (<30 days)	*Candida*	*Aspergillus*
Postengraphment (30–100 days)	*Aspergillus*,*Candida*, *Pneumocystis*	Zygomycetes, *Fusarium*, *Pseudallescheria* (*Scedosporium*)
Late (>100 days)	*Aspergillus*, *Pneumocystis*	

Table produced from data in ref. 15.

Table 1.4
Risk factors commonly associated with healthcare-associated invasive mycoses

Mycosis	Risk factors
Candidiasis	*Candida* colonization, surgery (especially abdominal), acute renal failure, parenteral nutrition, central venous catheters, neutropenia, broad spectrum antibacterial antimicrobials, mucosal surface disruption
Aspergillosis	Prolonged neutropenia, corticosteroids, neutrophil dysfunction, hematologic malignancy, cytotoxic drugs, AIDS, HSCT (highest in allogeneic), solid organ transplantation (highest heart-lung), underlying lung disease, GvHD, GvHD therapies (TNF-α blockers)

HSCT, hematopoietic stem cell transplantation; GvHD, graft versus host disease; TNF-α, tumor necrosis factor alpha.

Infusion of contaminated infusates, inclusion of lipids in parenteral nutrition, and construction within the hospital are additional exposures that can lead to fungal infections. A few specific risks allow the clinician to suspect certain fungi. Ketoacidosis and deferoxamine therapy has been clearly shown to be a risk for zygomycosis (mucormycosis). Unfortunately, given the overlapping nature of most of these risk factors with those associated with bacterial infections, it is often difficult to apply these risk factors to differentiate patients at higher risk of fungal versus bacterial infection.

3.3. *Community Exposure*

The fungi that cause community-acquired infections commonly originate in the environment and are "true pathogens," that is, cause disease in persons with normal immune status. Most are restricted to certain geographic environments or exposure risks (Table 1.5). The sources of disease include inhalation, ingestion, or traumatic inoculation of the fungi. Diseases most commonly afflict the lungs, paranasal sinuses, skin, and soft tissues. Rarely, disseminated, central nervous system, or osteoarticular disease occurs. The most commonly recognized community-acquired infections are the endemic mycoses, each with their limited geographical areas of exposure. With the extensive use of antibiotics, corticosteroids, and other immune modulators in the community, as well as the increased number of elderly and populations of immunocompromised persons receiving their care outside of the hospital, the boundaries between community-acquired and healthcare-associated infection have become blurred.

3.4. *Other Risks*

Other risks or probable risks associated with immune competency or genetic disposition include gender and race. The role of gender, and potentially inhibitory effect of estrogen, has been postulated to be important in the risk of clinical paracoccidioidomycosis. A clear risk for disseminated coccidioidomycosis has been seen in women when disease is acquired in pregnancy. Disseminated and severe coccidioidomycosis has also been associated with Filipino and African descent.

Table 1.5
Geographic areas in which the endemic mycoses reside

Mycosis	Region	Specific countries/areas with increased prevalence	Associated exposure risks[a]
Blastomycosis	North America[b]	Southeastern and south central United States, Canada	Soil exposure near fresh water (fishing, hunting, farming, construction)
Coccidioidomycosis	Western Hemisphere	Southwestern United States, Central and South America	Soil/dust exposure (construction, archeology)
Histoplasmosis	Worldwide	Mississippi and Ohio River valleys, Western Africa	Soil or organic material associated with bird or bat guano (construction, demolition, spelunking)
Paracoccidioidomycosis	Latin America	Brazil, Columbia, Venezuela, Ecuador, Argentina	Farming or other outdoor employment
Penicilliosis[c]	Southeast Asia	China, Northeast India, Taiwan, Thailand, Vietnam	Rice farming, rodent burrows
Sporotrichosis	Worldwide	North America, Japan	Gardening, sphagnum moss, hay, roses/thorns

[a]Not all well-proven.
[b]Rare reports from Africa, Central and South America, India, and the Middle East.
[c]Restricted almost exclusively to persons with AIDS.

Table 1.6
Mycosis by organ system chiefly affected

Focus of disease on presentation	Community-associated fungi	Healthcare-associated fungi
Pulmonary	*Blastomyces*, *Coccidioides*, *Histoplasma*, *Paracoccidioides*	*Aspergillus*, zygomycetes, *Pseudallescheria* (*Scedosporium*),*Fusarium*, *Cryptococcus*, *Pneumocystis*
Superficial/cutaneous/subcutaneous	Dermatophytes (*Trichophyton*, *Microsporum*, *Epidermophyton*), *Candida*, *Malassezia*, agents of mycetoma, agents of chromblastomycosis, *Blastomyces*, *Paracoccidioides*, *Cryptococcus*, *Sporothrix*, zygomycetes, phaeohyphomycetes, *Lacazia*	*Candida*, *Fusarium*, *Trichosporon*
Bone and joint	*Blastomyces*, *Coccidioides*, *Histoplasma*, *Paracoccidioides*, *Sporothrix*	*Candida*, *Cryptococcus*
Central nervous system	*Cryptococcus*, *Coccidioides*, *Blastomyces*, *Histoplasma*, phaeohyphomycetes, *Pseudallescheria* (*Scedosporium*)	*Aspergillus*, *Candida*
Genitourinary	*Blastomyces*, *Coccidioides*, *Histoplasma*	*Candida*, *Trichosporon*
Oral	*Histoplasma*, *Paracoccidioides*, *Candida*	*Candida*
Eye	Keratitis—*Candida*, *Aspergillus*, *Fusarium*, phaeohyphomycetes, other hyalohyphomycetes	Endophthalmitis/retinitis—*Candida*
Disseminated disease	*Coccidioides*, *Histoplasma*, *Paracoccidioides*, *Penicillium marneffei*	*Candida*, *Aspergillus*, *Fusarium*, zygomycetes, *Cryptococcus*, *Trichosporon* and other rare yeasts

The use of antifungal therapy or prophylaxis in populations at risk should also be kept in mind when evaluating patients for potential fungal infections. The last decade has seen an emergence of NAC, non-*fumigatus Aspergillus* infections, and increased numbers of infections with the more rare yeasts and moulds. This shift appears to reflect our greater use of antifungals and the newer agents. Included in this change in epidemiology is the emergence of fluconazole-resistant *Candida* (i.e., *C. krusei*) and the recent increase in non-*Aspergillus* moulds (e.g., the zygomycetes, *Fusarium*, and *Scedosporium*) that have decreased susceptibility or resistance to many of the currently available antifungal agents.

4. SUSPICION BASED ON ORGANS INVOLVED

Although the fungi may and often do cause disease in more than one organ system, many of these are associated with certain organ system infections. The presentation of disease (e.g., prolonged or chronic pneumonia with lymphadenopathy on chest radiography) can guide the clinician to the diagnosis. Disease localization and presentation can be altered based on the host immune system, route of pathogen inoculation (e.g., inhalation, cutaneous inoculation, ingestion), and quantity of inoculum. The most common presentations are pulmonary, cutaneous/subcutaneous, and disseminated diseases (Table 1.6). Other presentations include those localized or involving the central nervous system, bones, joints, genitourinary tract, oral cavity, eyes, or gastrointestinal tract. Fungal infection can affect any organ or system, often after asymptomatic respiratory system colonization and dissemination. The fungus recovered at a specific site may portend varying diagnoses based on the combination of fungus and site, often modified by patient immune status. Oral lesions in histoplasmosis or paracoccidioidomycosis typically indicate the presence of disseminated disease. Oral lesions from *Candida* in a patient recently given a short course of corticosteroids likely only indicate mild, transient, localized disease.

REFERENCES

1. McNeil MM, Nash SL, Hajjeh RA, et al. Trends in the mortality due to invasive mycotic diseases in the United States, 1980–1997. Clin Infect Dis 2001;33:641–647.
2. Martin GS, Mannino DM, Eaton S, Moss M. The epidemiology of sepsis in the United States from 1979 through 2000. N Engl J Med 2003;348:1546–1554.
3. Edmund MB, Wallace SE, McClish DK, Pfaller MA, Jones RN, Wenzel RP. Nosocomial bloodstream infections in United States hospitals: a three-year analysis. Clin Infect Dis 1999;29:239–244.
4. Wisplinghoff H, Bischoff T, Tallent SM, Seifert H, Wenzel RP, Edmond MB. Nosocomial bloodstream infections in US hospitals: analysis of 24,179 cases from a prospective nationwide surveillance study. Clin Infect Dis 2004;39:309–317.
5. Trick WE, Fridkin SK, Edwards JR, Hajjeh RA, Gaynes RP, National Nosocomial Infections Surveillance System hospitals. Secular trends in hospital-acquired candidemia among intensive care unit patients in the United States during 1989–1999. Clin Infect Dis 2002;35:627–630.
6. Cornillet A, Camus C, Nimubona S, et al. Comparison of epidemiological, clinical, and biological features in invasive aspergillosis in neutropenic and nonneutropenic patients: a 6-year survey. Clin Infect Dis 2006;43:577–584.

7. Chamilos G, Luna M, Lewis RE, et al. Invasive fungal infections in patients with hematologic malignancies in a tertiary care cancer center: an autopsy study over a 15-year period (1989–2003). Haematologica 2006;91:986–989.
8. Husain S, Alexander BD, Munoz P, et al. Opportunistic mycelial fungal infections in organ transplant recipients: emerging importance of non-*Aspergillus* mycelial fungi. Clin Infect Dis 2003;37:221–229.
9. Jahagirdar BN, Morrison VA. Emerging fungal pathogens in patients with hematologic malignancies and marrow/stem-cell transplant recipients. Semin Respir Infect 2002;17: 113–120.
10. Marr KA, Carter RA, Crippa F, Wald A, Corey L. Epidemiology and outcome of mould infections in hematopoietic stem cell transplant recipients. Clin Infect Dis 2002;34:909–917.
11. Nucci M, Marr KA. Emerging fungal diseases. Clin Infect Dis 2005;41:521–526.
12. Patterson TF. Advances and challenges in management of invasive mycoses. Lancet 2005;366:1013–1025.
13. Walsh TJ, Groll A, Hiemenz J, Fleming R, Roilides E, Anaissie E. Infection due to emerging and uncommon MEDICALLY important fungal pathogens. Clin Microbiol Infect 2004;10 (Suppl 1): 48–66.
14. Hoang LMN, Maguire JA, Doyle P, Fyfe M, Roscoe DL. *Cryptococcus neoformans* infections at Vancouver Hospital and Health Sciences Centre (1997–2002): epidemiology, microbiology and histopathology. J Med Microbiol 2004;53:935–940.
15. Centers for Disease Control and Prevention. Guidelines for preventing opportunistic infections among hematopoietic stem cell transplant recipients. MMWR 2000;49(RR-10):1–125.
16. Fishman JA, Rubin RH. Infection in organ-transplant recipients. New Engl J Med 1998–338:1741–1751.
17. Singh N. Fungal infections in the recipients of solid organ transplantation. Infect Dis N Am 2003;17:113–134.
18. Enoch DA, Ludlam HA, Brown NM. Invasive fungal infections: a review of epidemiology and management options. J Med Microbiol 2006;55:809–818.
19. Fridkin SK. The changing face of fungal infections in health care settings. Clin Infect Dis 2005;41:1455–1460.
20. Eggimann P, Garbino J, Pittet D. Epidemiology of *Candida* species infections in critically ill non-immunosuppressed patients. Lancet Infect Dis 2003;3:685–702.
21. Blumberg HM, Jarvis WR, Soucie JM, et al. Risk factors for candidal bloodstream infections in surgical intensive care unit patients: the NEMIS prospective multicenter study. Clin Infect Dis 2001;33:177–186.

SUGGESTED READINGS

Clark TA, Hajjeh RA. Recent trends in the epidemiology of invasive mycoses. Curr Opin Infect Dis 2002;15:569–574.

Enoch DA, Ludlam HA, Brown NM. Invasive fungal infections: a review of epidemiology and management options. J Med Microbiol 2006;55:809–818.

Fridkin SK. The changing face of fungal infections in health care settings. Clin Infect Dis 2005;41:1455–1460.

Husain S, Alexander BD, Munoz P, et al. Opportunistic mycelial fungal infections in organ transplant recipients: emerging importance of non-*Aspergillus* mycelial fungi. Clin Infect Dis 2003;37:221–229.

Walsh TJ, Groll A, Hiemenz J, Fleming R, Roilides E, Anaissie E. Infection due to emerging and uncommon medically important fungal pathogens. Clin Microbiol Infect 2004;10 (Suppl 1): 48–66.

OTHER KEY RESOURCES

Anaissie EJ, McGinnis MR, Pfaller MA, eds. Clinical mycology. Philadelphia: Churchill Livingstone, 2003:1–608.

Dismukes WE, Pappas PG, Sobel JD, eds. Clinical mycology. New York: Oxford University Press, 2003:1–519.

Kwon-Chung KJ, Bennett JE. Medical mycology. Malvern, PA: Lea & Febiger, 1992:1–866.

Section G. Mycoses. In: Mandell GL, Bennett JE, Dolin R, eds. Mandell, Douglas, and Bennett's principles and practice of infectious diseases. 6th ed. Philadelphia: Elsevier Churchill Livingstone, 2005:2935–3094.

www.doctorfungus.org is an excellent Internet resource for information about current taxonomy and other quick reference material.

II
Laboratory and Radiological Diagnosis

2
Basic Mycology

Deanna A. Sutton, PhD

1. INTRODUCTION

The mycology laboratory plays a vital role in the diagnosis of fungal infections by recovery of the etiologic agent. Specimen collection from appropriate sites is critical, as is the proper transport, storage, and processing of samples. Fungal elements seen via direct microscopy often provide the first clues to a fungal infection, and are the basis on which empiric therapy is initiated. To ensure recovery of the fungus, a sufficient number and type of media should be utilized for primary isolation based on the clinical history and any possible organisms being expected. Accurate fungal identification, in combination with antifungal susceptibility testing, provides the basis for appropriate organism-directed antifungal therapy and is essential for conducting epidemiologic investigations.

Human and/or animal pathogens historically considered to be fungal are now placed in three kingdoms: Fungi, Straminipila, and Protoctista, with the bulk of the human pathogens in the kingdom Fungi *(1)*. Organisms within this kingdom are eukaryotic (have cells containing a membrane-bound nucleus); heterotrophic (lack chlorophyll or other pigments capable of photosynthesis for making food and therefore must obtain nourishment from an external food source); may be unicellular or filamentous; and have cells surrounded by cell walls containing glucan, chitin, or both. Unlike animals, fungi possess cell walls, but unlike in plants, the major cell wall component is not cellulose. In the past, medical problems attributed to these organisms, in comparison to those caused by the bacteria, viruses, and parasites, have been relatively few, and included allergic symptoms, mushroom poisoning, mycotoxicoses from ingested fungal toxins, and occasional fungal infections *(2)*. Fungal infections (mycoses) have increased over the past decades, with the advent of modern medical advances utilizing immunosuppressive regimens, and with an increase in diseases/underlying conditions significantly altering the human immune system. The recovery of these organisms from host tissue and their identification is often critical to the diagnosis and treatment of mycotic disease and is the classic method for documentation of pathogenicity. Histopathology, and other adjunctive tools such as antigen or antibody assays and molecular techniques, addressed elsewhere in this text, may also be relied on for empiric/preemptive therapeutic decisions, when cultures are either not available or fail to provide unequivocal

From: *Infectious Disease: Diagnosis and Treatment of Human Mycoses*
Edited by: D. R. Hospenthal and M. G. Rinaldi © Humana Press Inc., Totowa, NJ

information. The proper collection, transport, and processing of specimens; selection of fungal stains and preliminary direct microscopy techniques; and use of appropriate media and incubation conditions are all important to the accurate identification of fungal infection. This chapter provides a cursory review of the laboratory fundamentals as they relate to medical mycology. It also reviews basic taxonomy, classification, and nomenclature regarding the kingdom Fungi, and a description of mycologic terms/features common to the most frequently recovered etiologic agents in the teleomorphic (sexual) phyla Ascomycota, Basidiomycota, Zygomycota, and in the anamorphic (asexual) fungi. Fungi without known sexual states are referred to as "mitosporic" (based on their reproductive mitotic processes). The mitosporic fungi are the most common etiologic agents of human and animal disease.

2. SPECIMEN COLLECTION, TRANSPORT, AND PROCESSING

The likelihood of recovering a fungal etiologic agent is directly proportional to the quality of methods employed in the collection, transport, and processing of clinical specimens. For all disease processes, recovery is highest from an active site of infection. Common (but not all-inclusive) specimen types include those from the respiratory tract *(3)*, draining sites, aspirated abscess fluids, normally sterile body fluids, urine *(4)*, vaginal secretions *(5)*, corneal scrapings *(6)*, surgical tissue specimens, intravenous catheter tips (obtained by the Maki roll method *(7)*), and various surgically removed medical devices *(8)*. Although tissue may be homogenized for the recovery of *Histoplasma capsulatum*, when the patient history suggests infection with a zygomycete or other filamentous fungi, tissue grinding should be avoided because it may be deleterious to the growth in culture of fragile fungal hyphae *(8)*. Specimens peripheral to the site of infection, such as blood or bone marrow, may be diagnostic in disseminated disease or when foci are not easily accessible. Several blood culture systems reliably recover yeast pathogens. If manual blood cultures are used, a broth/agar biphasic system in which an agar paddle it attached to the bottle (Septi-Chek, BD Diagnostic Systems, Sparks, MD) may be preferred. Several automated, continuously monitored blood culture systems are available for higher volume laboratories. These include the ESP (Trek Diagnostics, Inc., Cleveland, Ohio), BacT/Alert (bio Mérieux, Durham, NC), and BACTEC (BD Diagnostic Systems, Sparks, MD) systems *(9–15)*. Always follow the manufacturer's recommendations for the specific system, using the maximum amount of blood samples recommended. The ratio of blood to broth is the most critical factor in fungal recovery, and should be near 1:5 in most systems *(16)*. Lysis centrifugation methods, either commercially available as the Isolator™ system (Wampole Laboratories, Princeton, NJ) or manual methods *(17,18)*, are recommended for dimorphic fungal pathogens and filamentous fungi *(19,20)*. Intravascular catheter tips are also frequently submitted, and should be cultured according to the semiquantitative method of Maki *(8)*. Blood cultures should also be drawn at the time of catheter removal to correlate catheter colony counts and organisms recovered with catheter-related septicemia. Catheter colony counts of less than 15 are less likely to forewarn of septicemia. Specimens should be transported, at room temperature, to the laboratory as soon as possible, ideally within 2 hours. Exceptions include storage of central nervous system specimens at 30°C, and 4°C extended storage for specimens likely to have bacterial contamination. Hair, skin, and nails may be transported in clean paper envelopes. Several sources provide specific guidelines for the collection, transport, and processing of various types of specimens for fungal culture *(8,21,22)*. See Table 2.1 for common collection sites.

Table 2.1
Common specimen collection sites for fungal cultures[a]

Collection site	Comments
Abscesses, subcutaneous sites	Aspirate abscess; sample base of subcutaneous lesions
Blood	Use maximum amount of blood recommended for the system being used
Bone marrow	Pediatric Isolator™ recommended[b]
CSF	Do not refrigerate
Draining sinus tracts	Search for granules of eumycotic mycetoma; wash several times with saline containing antibiotics
Ear	Rotate swab firmly in outer ear
Eye	Inoculate corneal scrapings directly only plates in a "C" shape
Hair	Use forceps to collect several hairs with shaft intact and sample any active lesions
Intravenous catheters	Use Maki method
Lower respiratory	Process promptly for dimorphic pathogens (BAL, brush, aspirate, wash, sputum)
Medical devices (valves, hardware, etc.)	Dislodge any biofilms before inoculation into liquid medium
Nails	For dermatophytes, agents of dermatomycoses, and *Candida* spp.; clean with 70% alcohol; collect subungual debris and clip affected nails
Nasal sinus	Surgical collection, commonly ethmoid and maxillary sinuses
Open wound	Aspirate or swab vigorously
Prostatic fluid	Primarily for blastomycosis
Skin	For dermatophytes; clean with 70% alcohol and scrape vigorously
Sterile body fluids	May be concentrated by centrifugation or syringe filtration
Tissue	Surgical collection; use punch biopsies for skin lesions
Urine	Early morning midstream collection
Vagina	Primarily for refractory vaginal candidiasis
Vitreous fluid	Needle aspiration
Upper respiratory (oral)	Swab lesions, use selective media for yeasts

[a]This list is not all inclusive.
[b]Wampole Laboratories, Princeton, NJ.

Before receipt in the mycology laboratory, a portion of all tissue samples submitted for culture should also be placed in formalin for submission to the histology laboratory. Histopathologic examination with appropriate stains is usually necessary to document fungal invasion. These may include the routine hematoxylin and eosin stain (H&E), Gomori methenamine silver stain (GMS), periodic acid-Schiff stain (PAS), and others. A discussion of the use of histopathology and of mycological stains is provided in Chapter 3 of this book. As part of routine processing, the mycology laboratory should also examine a portion of the specimen directly via microscopy, typically with the use of a potassium hydroxide (KOH) preparation, Gram stain, calcofluor white fluorescent stain, India ink stain (limited to cerebrospinal fluid examination for *Cryptococcus neoformans*), or some other method (Table 2.2). Observation of fungal structures via direct microscopy and/or histopathology is essential to corroborate organism recovery in culture (rule out contamination).

The media used for primary isolation may vary according to personal preference; however, certain basic tenets apply to all media used for primary recovery. Material from nonsterile sites should be cultured on media that will support fungal growth but also inhibit bacteria. Antibacterial agents, alone or in combination, are added for this purpose. Common choices include chloramphenicol (<16 μg/ml), gentamicin (5 to 100 μg/ml), penicillin (20 U/ml), streptomycin (40 μg/ml), and ciprofloxacin (5 μg/ml). These agents should not be included, however, when actinomycetes are suspected. Media may also be made selective by the addition of the eukaryotic protein synthesis inhibitor cycloheximide at 0.5 μg/ml. This may be useful in the detection of dimorphic fungi and dermatophytes; however, many clinically significant, saprobic fungi may be suppressed, leading to failure in recovering opportunistic etiologic agents in compromised hosts. Therefore, media with and without this agent should routinely be employed. Enriched

Table 2.2
Useful direct microscopy methods for the routine mycology laboratory[a]

Method	Comments
Calcofluor white	Requires fluorescence microscope; can be used with KOH to detect all fungi, including *Pneumocystis*
Gram stain	Detects most fungi present, however *Cryptococcus* spp. may exhibit only faint staining
Giemsa stain	Several modifications; detects intracellular *Histoplasma capsulatum* and intracystic bodies and trophozoites of *Pneumocystis*
India Ink stain	Commonly used from demonstration of capsular material of *Cryptococcus neoformans* in CSF
Potassium hydroxide	Clears debris so fungi more readily observed; stains may be added for better visualization of fungal elements
Wright stain	Useful to detect intracellular *Histoplasma capsulatum* in bone marrow and peripheral smears

[a]Additional fungal stains are available through the histopathology laboratory. This list is not all inclusive.

media with 5% to 10% sheep erythrocytes may be incorporated into the battery for fastidious thermally dimorphic fungi such as *Histoplasma capsulatum* and *Blastomyces dermatitidis*. Peptone-based versus plant-based media may also be a consideration. Many of the opportunistic filamentous fungi prefer plant-based media, producing more typical colony morphologies and more diagnostic structures, thus increasing the potential to make identification possible from primary plates. Plant-based media may also be made selective with antibacterial agents or cycloheximide. Table 2.3 lists several commercially available media that may be used for both primary isolation and identification. The choice of tubed versus plated media is made based on space constraints, personal preference, and safety. The greater surface area provided by plates is preferred by many laboratorians (and always preferred by the fungi!), as manipulation of cultures, isolation procedures, and so forth is more easily performed on plates. When used, plate lids should be firmly attached with an air-permeable material or plates sealed in air-permeable bags to avoid cross-contamination or laboratory worker exposure.

Optimally, cultures should be incubated at 30°C (± 1°C). If this temperature is not available, room temperature near 25°C should be used. A 7-day incubation is generally adequate when screening for yeasts from oropharyngeal or vaginal sites. Although

Table 2.3
Media useful for primary isolation and identification[a]

Medium	Uses/comments
Sabouraud dextrose agar (SDA)	For yeasts Usually adequate for aspergilli Poor color and conidiation for black moulds Classic morphologic descriptions for dermatophytes
CHROMagar Candida[b]	Contains chromogenic substrates and antimicrobial agents; for isolation and identification of yeasts
Albicans ID[c]	As above
Potato dextrose agar (PDA) Potato flakes agar (PFA) Brain heart infusion agar (BHI) Inhibitory mould agar (IMA) Yeast extract phosphate medium Sabhi agar	Useful for all mould recovery/identification
Mycosel agar™[d] or Mycobiotic agar Dermatophyte test medium (DTM) Dermatophyte identification medium (DIM)	SDA with chloramphenicol and cycloheximide

[a]This list is not all-inclusive. All are commercially available.
[b]CHROMagar Microbiology, Paris, France.
[c]bioMérieux, Marcy l'Etoile, France.
[d]BD Diagnostic Systems, Sparks, MD.

4-week incubation times have traditionally recommended, recent studies suggest that 3 weeks is adequate to detect growth of a fungi from most other specimens, excluding those from skin, hair, and nails, and in cultures requested specifically to attempt to recover dimorphic pathogens *(23)*. The time required for development of diagnostic structures, particularly for some coelomycetes and ascomycetes, may be considerably longer, up to several weeks *(24)*.

3. EXAMINING CULTURES

Cultures should be examined every day for the first 3 days and preferably twice a week thereafter. Cultures of yeasts are typically creamy to waxy, while moulds appear velvety to woolly to cottony. Some safety precautions common to both yeasts and moulds include the careful handling of plates and tubes so as not to create aerosols of infectious material and the prevention of contamination of patient cultures with ubiquitous fungi from the work surroundings.

3.1. Yeast and Yeast-like Organism Identification

One may handle yeast cultures, consisting of unicellular organisms that replicate by budding, on the open bench, adhering to the same safety precautions as for bacteria. Yeast and yeast-like fungi should be examined for their colony color (white to cream to pink; brownish-black for the yeast synanamorph of *Exophiala* species when observed on Sabouraud dextrose agar; blue to green to pink for *Candida* species on CHROMagar Candida™ [CHROMagar Microbiology, Paris, France]), growth rate, temperature requirements (or preferences), macroscopic morphology (smooth, wrinkled, glabrous, moist, dry, etc.), and microscopic morphology (size and shape, presence of blastoconidia, capsules, germ tubes, pseudohyphae, true hyphae, chlamydoconidia, etc.). Yeast morphology is most reliably observed on a cornmeal agar plate via the Dalmau method *(25)*. This technique involves streaking a very small amount of yeast onto a plate in two parallel lines, streaking back and forth over these lines for better isolation, and covering the area with a flame-sterilized coverslip. The plate is incubated at room temperature for 18 to 24 hours and then examined microscopically for diagnostic structures. Tease mounts may also provide useful information. Additional procedures that may be required for identification of yeast include the reduction of nitrate to nitrite, urease activity, the ability of the organism to grow on media containing cycloheximide, and assimilation and fermentation patterns. Many commercial systems, both manual and automated, are available to assist in yeast identification.

3.2. mould Identification

Any filamentous organisms recovered on culture should be examined and manipulated in a biological safety cabinet. While moulds can be recovered on a variety of media, conidiation/sporulation is generally enhanced on plant-based media. If not used in primary isolation, plant-based media should be employed in identification schema. moulds should be examined for their growth rate, temperature requirements, and macroscopic morphology to include color (hyaline to brightly colored or phaeoid [brownish to blackish]), texture (velvety, woolly, granular, cottony, etc.), and the observation of any diagnostic features visible to the naked eye. The microscopic detail may be studied using tease mounts or temporary tape mounts (clear tape only) in lactophenol cotton blue. The preferred technique to demonstrate diagnostic structures and methods of conidiogenesis for most filamentous fungi is the slide culture method. This method also provides a permanent mount that can be preserved in a slide collection for future studies and is extremely useful for comparison with other similar isolates or atypical strains. Slide cultures should not, however, be set up on moulds in which the clinical history suggests a dimorphic pathogen such as *Histoplasma capsulatum*, *Blastomyces dermatitidis*, *Coccidioides* species, *Paracoccidioides brasiliensis* (not commonly seen in the United States), or *Penicillium marneffei* (usually restricted to human immunodeficiency virus [HIV]-infected individuals from endemic areas of Southeast Asia). Tease mounts should be prepared for these isolates in a mounting fluid known to kill the fungus, such as lactophenol cotton blue. *Sporothrix schenckii*, another dimorphic organism, poses less of an exposure risk, and may be examined via slide culture. *Histoplasma capsulatum*, *B. dermatitidis*, and *Coccidioides* species may be definitively identified using DNA GenProbe® (AccuProbe, San Diego, CA) methodology. Zygomycetes may rapidly overgrow slide cultures, making the method less than optimal for studying this group of fungi.

4. TAXONOMY, CLASSIFICATION, AND NOMENCLATURE

Many volumes have been dedicated to the taxonomy, classification, and nomenclature of clinically significant fungi. Herein, this work highlights only some of the basic concepts. The classification scheme accepted by most authorities is presented for the kingdom Fungi. The term classification, in the fungal sense, refers to the application of names for the categories into which the taxa (taxonomic groups) may be grouped, with some subdivisions regarding their relative order. "Taxonomy" refers to this classification in a very systematic way, and nomenclature is the assigning of names to fungi that must abide by the rules of the International Code of Botanical Nomenclature (ICBN). The following is an abbreviated classification scheme for the kingdom Fungi:

Group	Group Ending
Kingdom	none
Phylum	-mycota
Class	-mycetes
Order	-ales
Family	-aceae
Genus	-no specific ending
Species	-no specific ending
Variety	-no specific ending

The phyla in which the sexual or teleomorph forms of the majority of human/animal pathogens reside are the Ascomycota, Basidiomycota, and Zygomycota *(1)*. An example of this classification scheme for the ascomycete *Microascus cinereus*, an etiologic agent of nail infections, maxillary sinusitis, endocarditis, and brain abscess would look like this:

Kingdom: Fungi
Phylum: Ascomycota
Order: Microascales
Family: Microascaceae
Genus: *Microascus*
Species: *Microascus cinereus*

Microascus cinereus, a sexual fungus (or the teleomorph) that produces perithecia, asci, and ascospores in culture, also simultaneously produces an asexual form (the anamorph) that is microscopically quite different. Asexual fungi, previously given the prefix "Form-" in the classification scheme, such as Form-Class, Form-Order, etc., are now commonly known as "mitosporic" fungi, or those reproducing my mitosis rather than meiosis. The anamorphic form of *Microascus cinereus* is the phaeoid fungus *Scopulariopsis cinereus.* Anamorphic fungi are identified mostly on the basis of their method of conidiogenesis (how they form their reproductive structures). Asexual reproductive propagules are referred to as conidia, hence the term conidiogenesis. Sexual fungi are identified mostly based on the method they use to form their sexual reproductive propagules (ascospores, basidiospores, or zygospores). Not all taxonomists agree that we should apply different names to the anamorph and teleomorph of the same fungus, the holomorph, or "whole fungus"; however, this is the current practice. Adding to this confusion, some fungi produce multiple anamorph forms, such as is seen with the fungus *Pseudallescheria boydii. Pseudallescheria boydii* is the teleomorph, *Scedosporium apiospermum* is the anamorph, and *Graphium eumorphum* is the synanamorph, or other anamorphic form of the "whole fungus." Practically speaking, most etiologic agents are identified in the laboratory on the basis of structures formed by the anamorphic form of the fungus. Although many mitosporic fungi have known teleomorphs, most require two mating strains to produce the sexual form. These are referred to as heterothallic. A few clinically significant fungi require only one strain to produce the teleomorph, and these are considered homothallic. *Microascus cinereus* and *Pseudallescheria boydii,* cited in the preceding text, are examples of homothallic fungi.

5. FUNGAL IDENTIFICATION

Yeast identification is performed in a manner similar to that for bacterial identification, and easily lends itself to various compartmentalized and automated methods that measure various physiologic characteristics. Mould identification, however, currently relies more on the observation of macroscopic morphologies, such as color and colonial features, growth rate, temperature maximums and minimums, and microscopic structures. Some of these more common identifying characteristics are exemplified in the organisms chosen in the thumbnail sketch of the kingdom Fungi as illustrated in Table 2.4.

5.1. Ascomycota

Under the phylum Ascomycota, the ascomycetous yeasts are usually identified by yeast methods, while the moulds are identified based on the structures they produce. Some of the filamentous homothallic ascomycetes produce ascomata known as cleistothecia, perithecia, or gymnothecia in which the asci and ascospores are contained (Figs. 2.1 to 2.4).

Table 2.4
Simplified schematic of the kingdom Fungi for *most* human/animal pathogens

Phylum Ascomycota
- Class Hemiascomycetes—yeasts
- Class Euascomycetes—moulds; produce ascospores in a variety of sexual structures known as ascomata (*pl.*), ascoma (*sing.*)
  - Cleistothecium—round, closed ascoma
    - Example: *Pseudallescheria boydii*, Fig. 2.1
  - Perithecium—pear-shaped ascoma, with an opening or ostiole
    - Example: *Microascus cirrosus*, Fig. 2.2
  - Gymnothecium—ascoma with a loose network of hyphae
    - Example: *Myxotrichum deflexum*, Fig. 2.3
  - Asci (*pl.*), ascus (*sing.*)—within the ascoma and containing ascospores
  - Ascospores, various sizes, shapes, colors, ornamentation
    - Example: *Sporomiella* sp., Fig. 2.4

Phylum Basidiomycota
- Class Urediniomycetes—contains a few red yeasts
- Class Ustilaginomycetes—contains yeast-like members of smut fungi
- Class Hymenomycetes—contains mushrooms (basidiocarps) producing yeast anamorphs (*Cryptococcus* species) and filamentous anamorphs that are frequently sterile or may produce arthroconidia
  - Example: *Schizophyllum commune*, a human etiologic agent, produces spicules (small protrusions) along the hyphae, Fig. 2.5
    - Basidiospores sometimes seen from basidiocarps of *S. commune*, Fig. 2.6

Phylum Zygomycota
- Class Zygomycetes
  - Order Mucorales—asexual reproduction by multispored or few- (to one) spored sporangia (sporangiola)
    - Heterothallic genera (require two mating strains) include some spp. of *Rhizopus, Absidia, Mucor,* and others; produce sporangiospores
      - Example: *Rhizopus microsporus* var *rhizopodiformis,* Fig. 2.7
    - Homothallic genera/species (one mating strain required) produce zygospores
      - Example: *Cokeromyces recurvatus,* Fig. 2.8
  - Order Entomophthorales—characterized by forcibly discharged conidia.
    - Produce asexual primary conidia and smaller secondary conidia
    - Example: *Conidiobolus incongruus,* Fig. 2.9
    - Example: *Basidiobolus ranarum*, produces zygospores

Mitosporic Fungi (formerly Fungi Imperfecti)
- Methods of conidiogenesis
  - Blasticconidia blown out
    - Phialidic conidiogenous cell—often have discernible collarettes and produce phialoconidia
      - Example: *Phialophora americana,* Fig. 2.10, and *Aspergillus flavus,* Fig. 2.11
    - Annellidic conidiogenous cells—have rings or annellations and become longer and narrower with production of annelloconidia
      - Example: *Scopulariopsis cirrosus,* Fig. 2.12

(Continued)

Table 2.4
(Continued)

Some species blow out conidia through pores on geniculate conidiophores
Example: *Bipolaris hawaiiensis,* Fig. 2.13
Thallic—conidia formed from preexisting hypha
Arthroconidia produced that may or may not have intervening disjunctor cells
Example: *Coccidioides* species, Fig. 2.14, and dematiaceous arthroconidia of *Scytalidium dimidiatum,* Fig. 2.15
Hyphomycetes—bear their conidia free and display various colors, methods of conidiogenesis, growth rates, etc.
Example: *Aspergillus flavus*, Fig. 2.11
Coelomycetes—bear their conidia within some type of asexual structure known as a conidioma (*sing.*) [conidiomata (*pl.*)] and display various colors, methods of conidiogenesis,, growth rates, etc.
Pycnidium—round conidioma with an opening (ostiole) and contained within;
Example: *Phoma* species, Fig. 2.16
Acervulus—flat, cup-shaped conidioma, with conidia more or less exposed
Example: *Colletotrichum* species

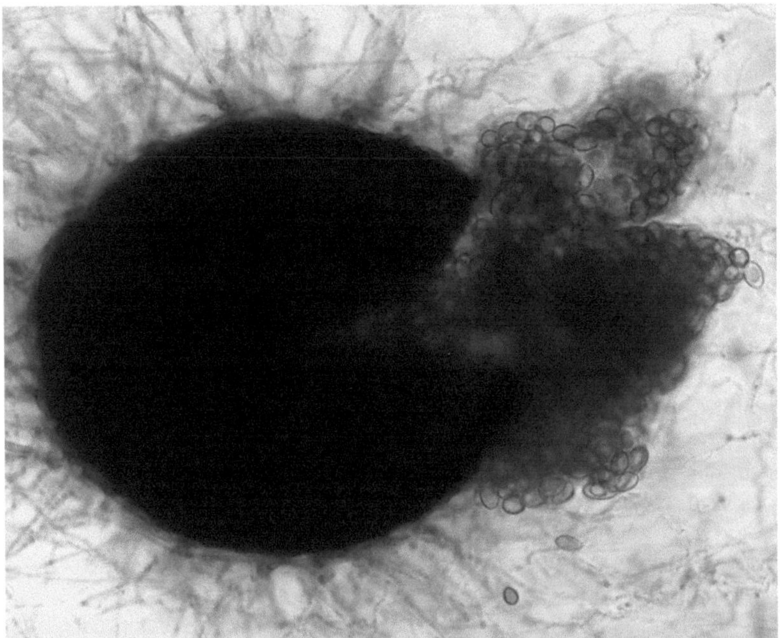

Fig. 2.1. Globose ascoma (closed cleistothecium) of *Pseudallescheria boydii*. [Figure in color on CD-ROM].

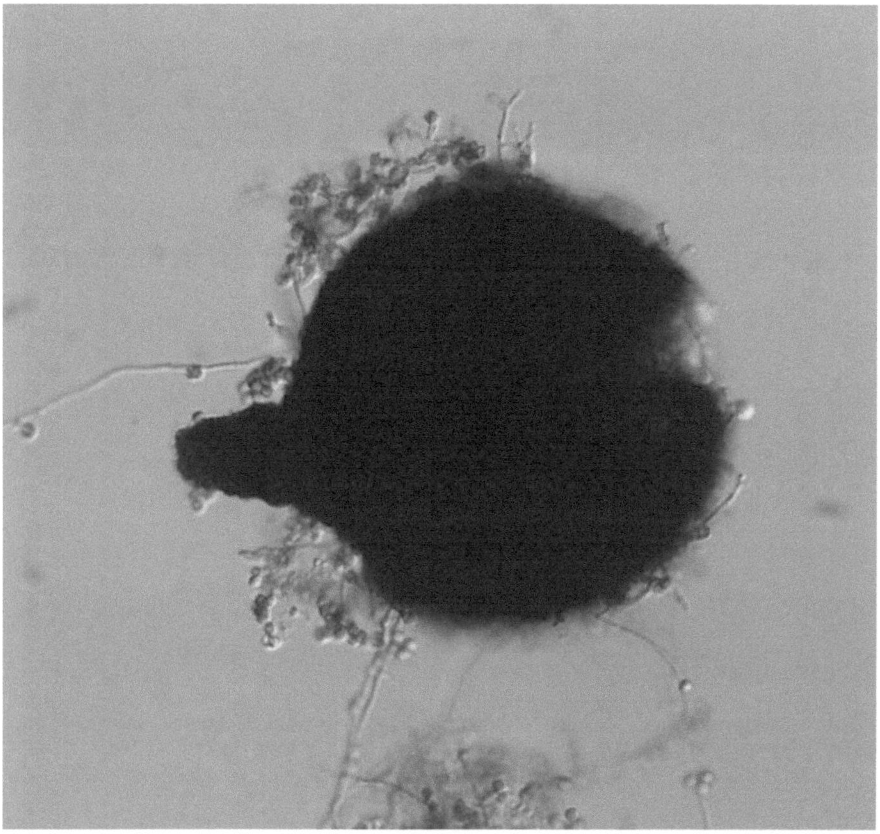

Fig. 2.2. Pear-shaped ascoma (perithecium with an opening or ostiole) of *Microascus cirrosus*. [Figure in color on CD-ROM].

5.2. *Basidiomycota*

Similarly, the red and white yeasts within the phylum Basidiomycota are commonly identified via yeast methodologies. The filamentous basidiomycetes pose identification dilemmas, as they frequently remain sterile in culture, producing no unique reproductive structures. *Schizophyllum commune* is one of the few that may sometimes be tentatively identified by its production of spicules along the sides of the hyphae, and occasionally by clamp connections (Fig. 2.5), basidiocarps, and basidiospores (Fig. 2.6) when dikaryons (compartments of a hypha that contain two nuclei, each derived from a different parent) are present.

5.3. *Zygomycota*

Human and animal pathogens of the phylum Zygomycota are contained within two orders in the class Zygomycetes; the Mucorales and the Entomophthorales. The Mucorales contain the most common zygomycete genera such as *Absidia, Rhizopus* (Fig. 2.7)*, Mucor, Rhizomucor, Cunninghamella,* and *Cokeromyces* (Fig. 2.8), while the

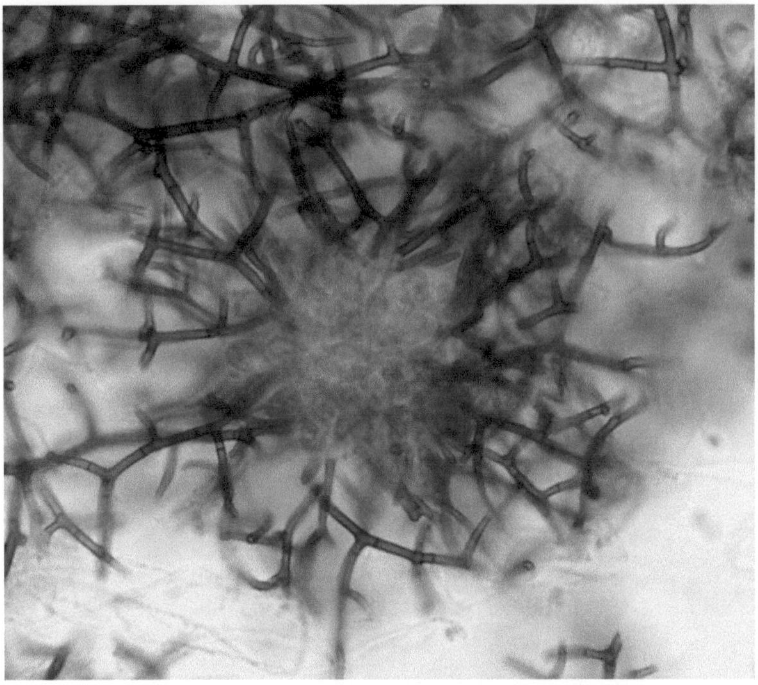

Fig. 2.3. Gymnothecium (ascoma with a loose hyphal network surrounding central ascospores) of *Myxotrichum deflexum*. [Figure in color on CD-ROM].

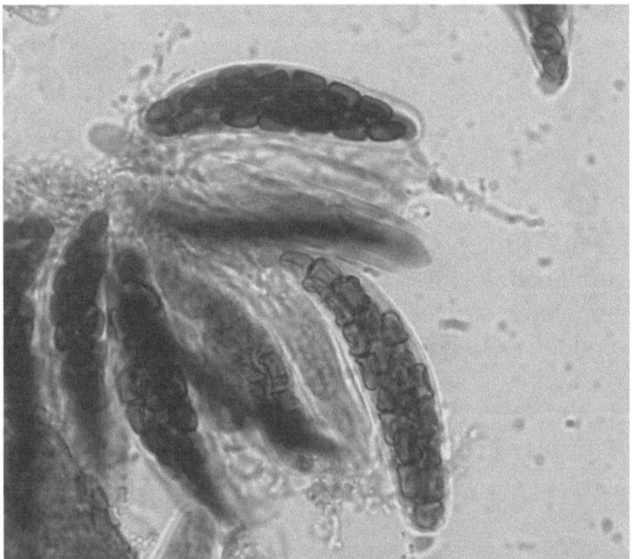

Fig. 2.4. Asci containing dark ascospores of a *Sporomiella* species. [Figure in color on CD-ROM].

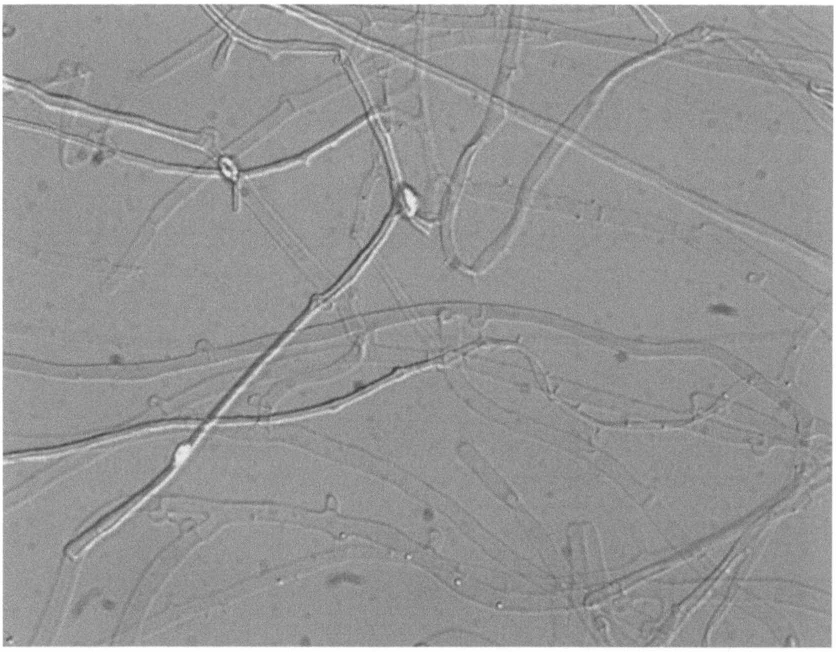

Fig. 2.5. Spicules and clamp connections on hyphae of *Schizophyllum commune*. [Figure in color on CD-ROM].

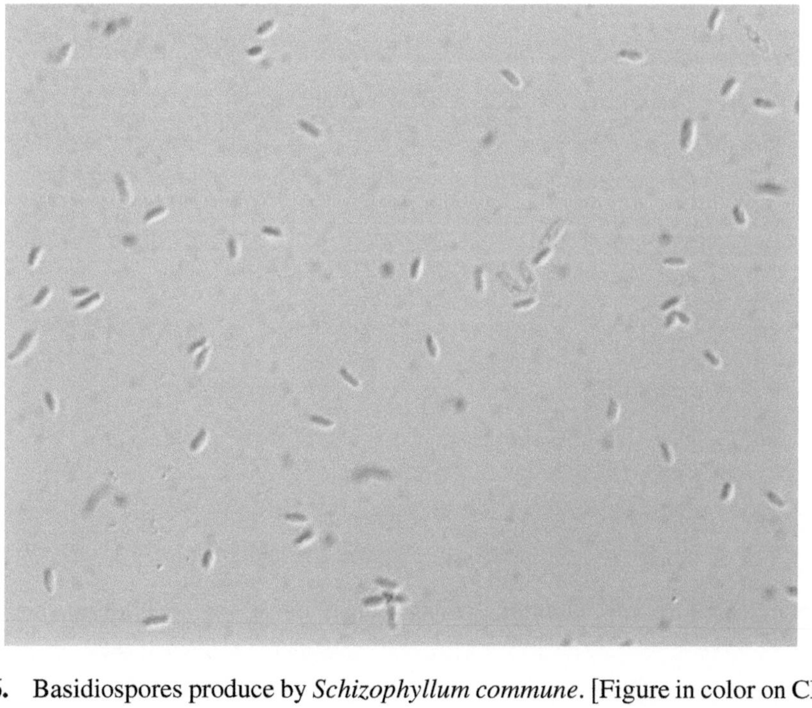

Fig. 2.6. Basidiospores produce by *Schizophyllum commune*. [Figure in color on CD-ROM].

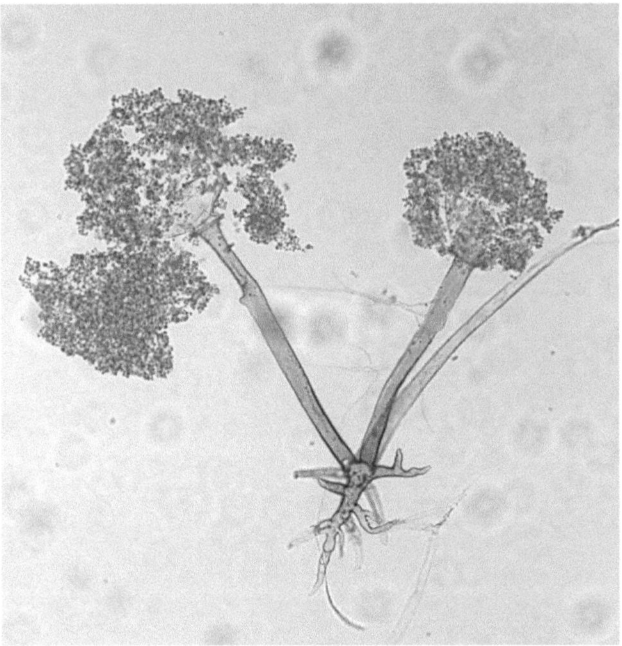

Fig. 2.7. Ramified rhizoids, short, dark sporangiophores, collapsed columellae, and sporangiospores of *Rhizopus microsporus* var. *rhizopodiformis*. [Figure in color on CD-ROM].

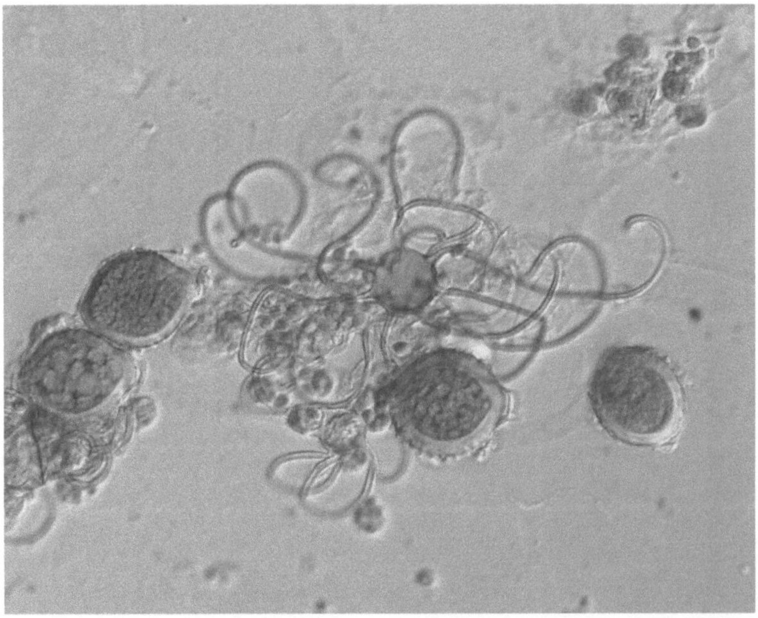

Fig. 2.8. Central vesicle, recurving stalks with terminal sporangioles containing sporangiospores, and thick-walled zygospores of *Cokeromyces recurvatus*. [Figure in color on CD-ROM].

Entomophthorales encompass the less frequently seen genera *Conidiobolus* (Fig. 2.9) and *Basidiobolus* (both characterized by forcibly discharged conidia).

5.4. Mitosporic Fungi

The group that contains the most human etiologic agents, by far, is one known as the "Mitosporic Fungi," or previously, the "Fungi Imperfecti." While these fungi may by related to various sexual phyla, these associations have not been yet demonstrated, and therefore these fungi are identified on the basis of their asexual rather than sexual reproductive propagules (method of conidial formation or conidiogenesis). Two main groups exist within the mitosporic fungi. The hyphomycetes bear their conidia free to the air, whereas the conidia of the coelomycetes are contained within some type of enclosed to semi-enclosed structure. The hyphomycetes contain numerous common moniliaceous (hyaline) and phaeoid or dematiaceous (dark) genera and generally produce their conidia by either blastic or thallic methods. Blastic conidia arc "blown out" of somc type of conidiogenous cell. These include those produced from phialides, as in *Phialophora* species (Fig. 2.10) or *Aspergillus* species such as *A. flavus* (Fig. 2.11), or from annellides, as in *Scopulariopsis cirrosus* (Fig. 2.12). Some species blow out their conidia through pores, such as in *Bipolaris hawaiiensis* (Fig. 2.13). Thallic conidia are formed from preexisting hyphae, as in *Coccidioides* species (Fig. 2.14), *Malbranchea* species, and *Scytalidium*

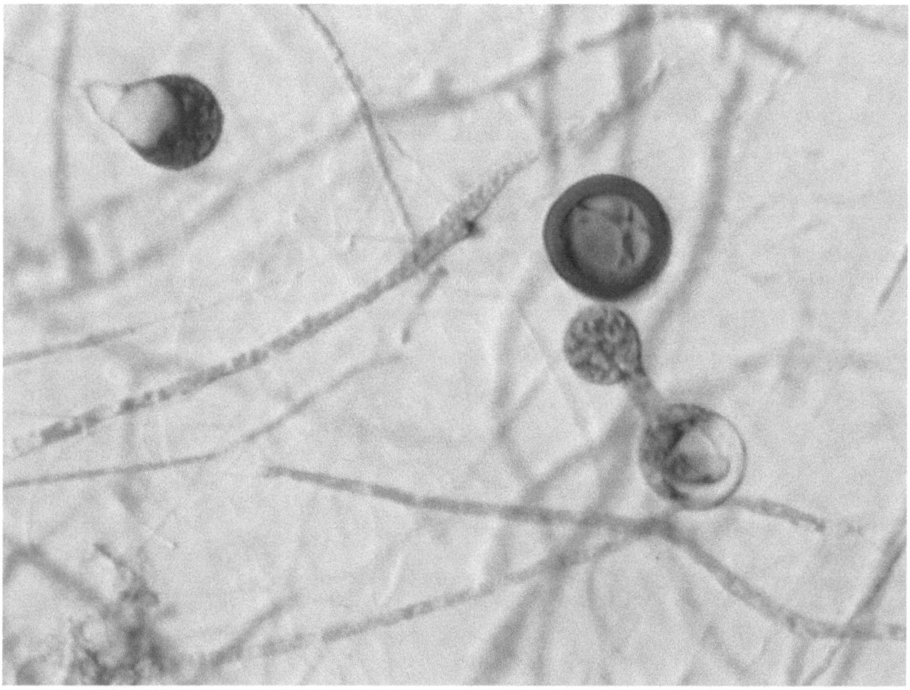

Fig. 2.9. Primary sporangiole giving rise to secondary sporangiole of *Conidiobolus coronatus*. [Figure in color on CD-ROM].

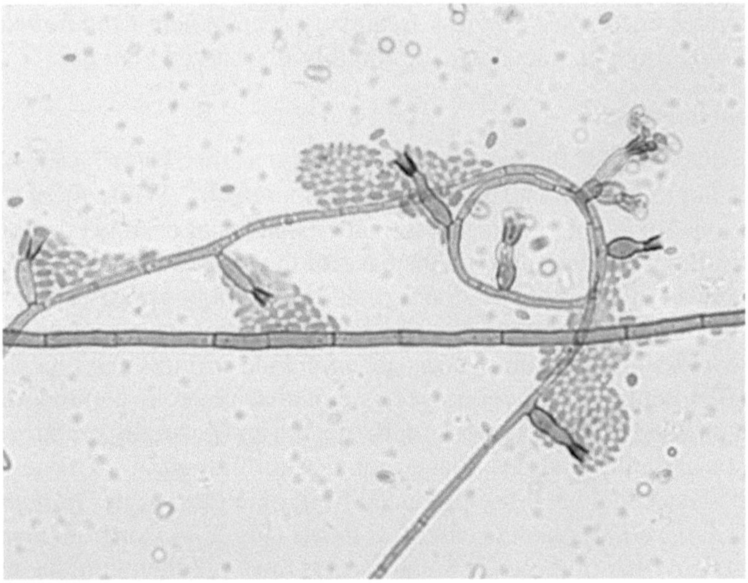

Fig. 2.10. Phialides of *Phialophora americana* with deep collarettes producing phialoconidia. [Figure in color on CD-ROM].

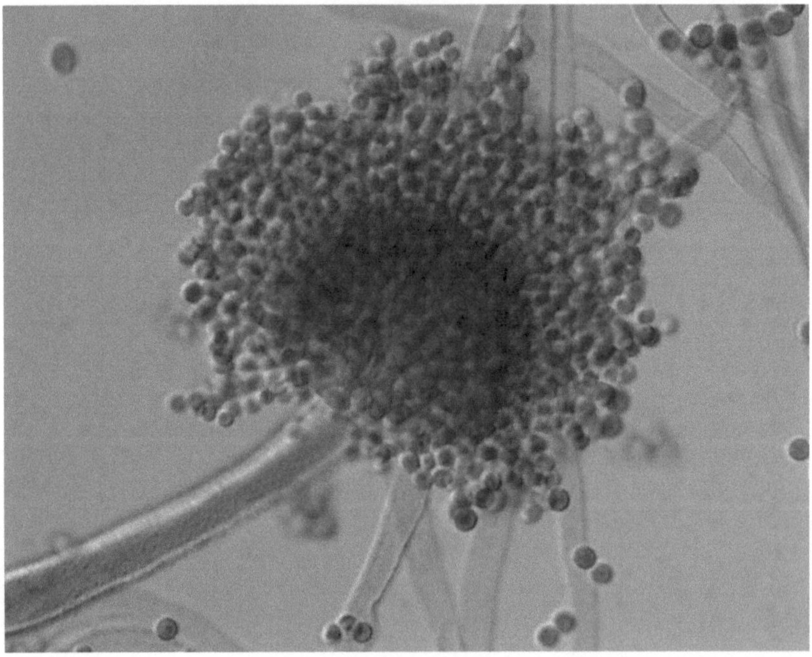

Fig. 2.11. Rough conidiophore and biseriate fruiting head of *Aspergillus flavus*. [Figure in color on CD-ROM].

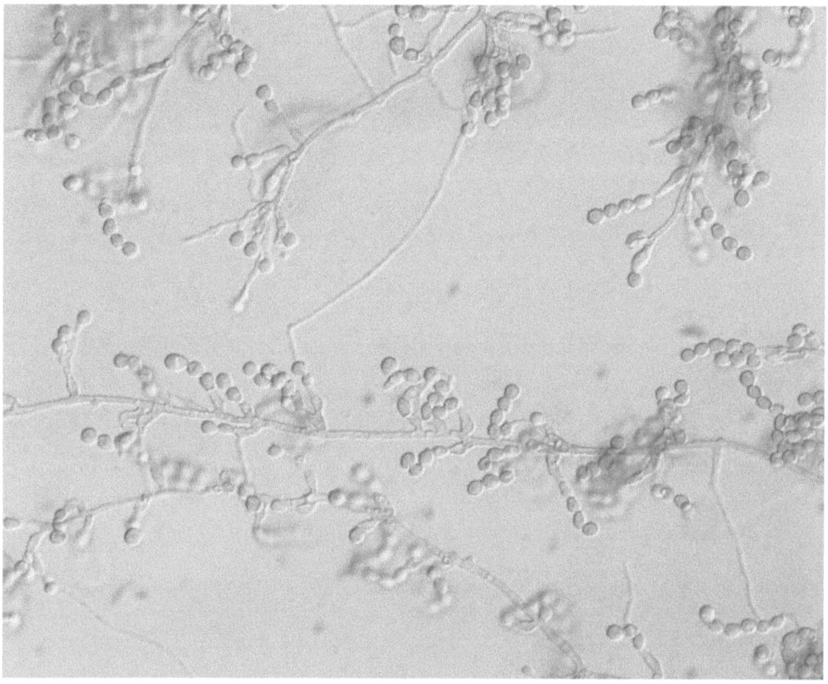

Fig. 2.12. Annellides and chains of annelloconidia produced by *Scopulariopsis cirrosus*. [Figure in color on CD-ROM].

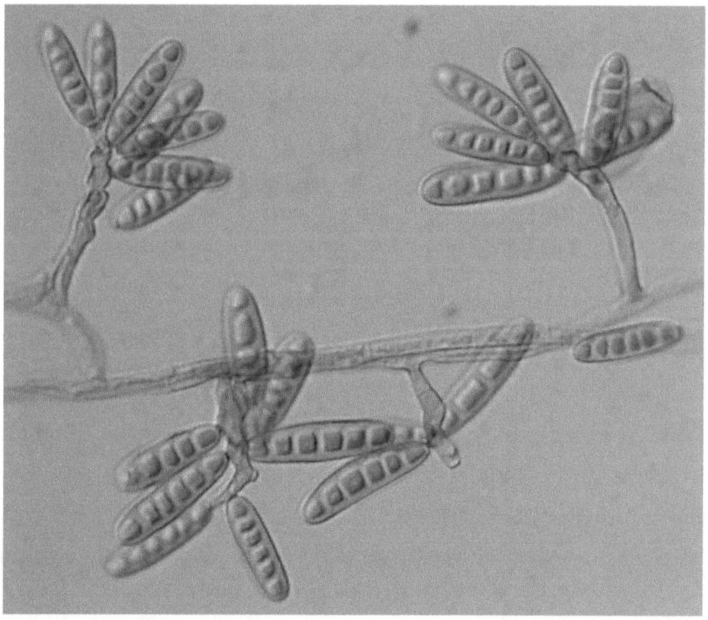

Fig. 2.13. Geniculate conidiophores with pores through which the conidia of *Bipolaris hawaiiensis* are blown out. [Figure in color on CD-ROM].

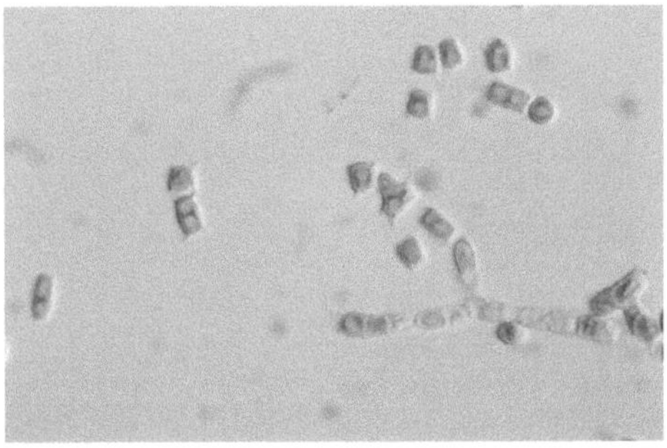

Fig. 2.14. Hyphae and arthroconidia with disjunctor cells of *Coccidioides* species. [Figure in color on CD-ROM].

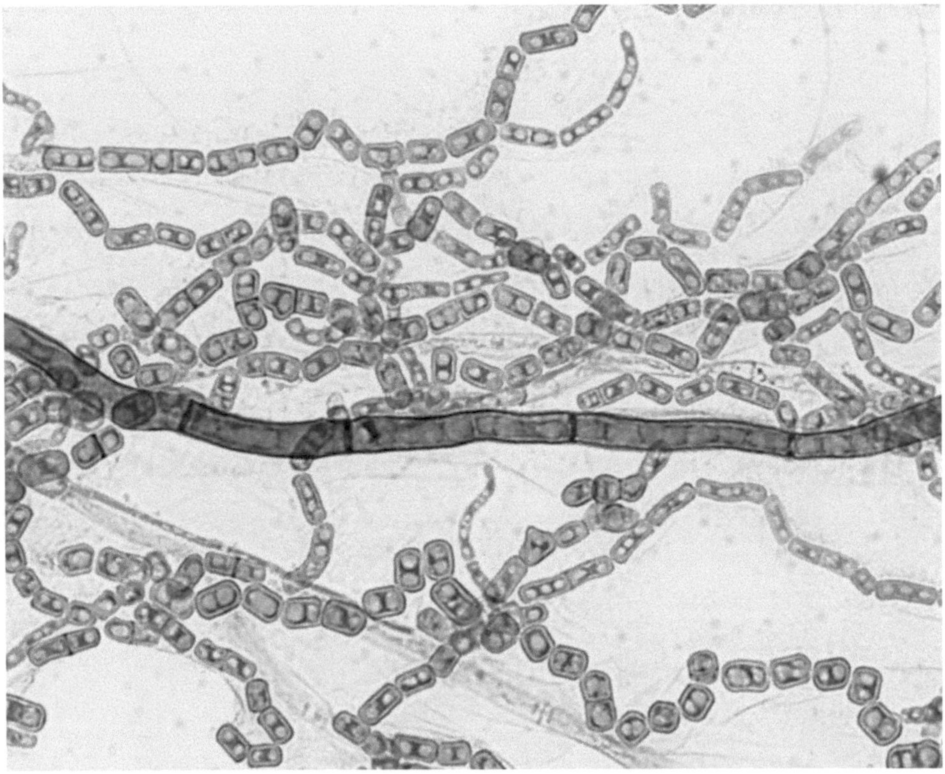

Fig. 2.15. Dematiaceous hyphae and arthroconidia of *Scytalidium dimidiatum* which lack disjunctor cells. [Figure in color on CD-ROM].

dimidiatum (Fig. 2.15). The structures produced by coelomycetes to contain their conidia are known as conidioma (*sing.*) or conidiomata (*pl.*). They may be round structures with an opening or ostiole known as a pycnidium, as in *Phoma* species (Fig. 2.16), or a flat, cup-shaped, semi-enclosed structure known as an acervulus. The conidiogenous cells within both of these conidiomata may be either phialidic or annellidic.

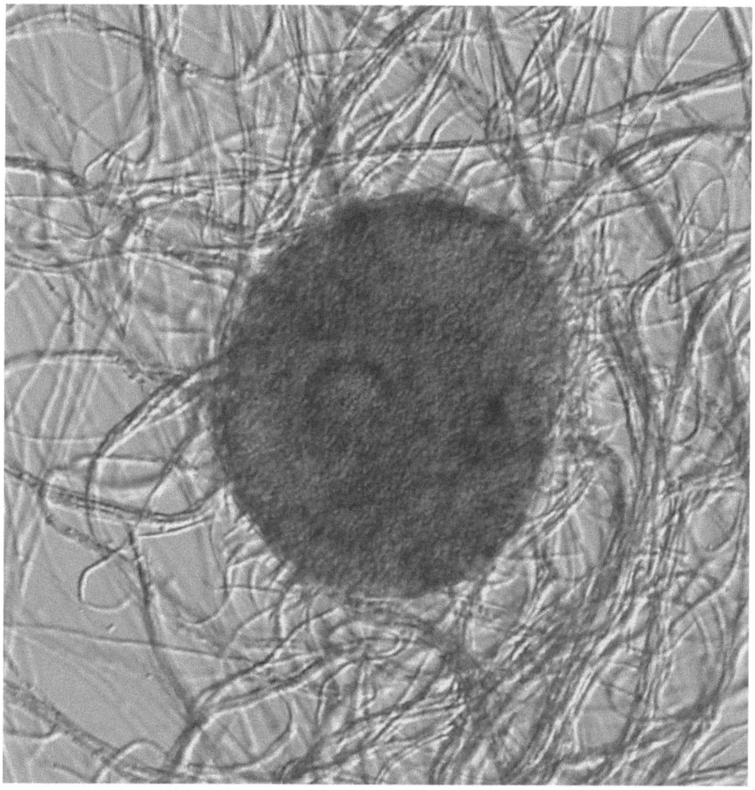

Fig. 2.16. Conidioma of a *Phoma* species containing a large central ostiole or opening. [Figure in color on CD-ROM].

REFERENCES

1. Howard DH. An introduction to the taxonomy of zoopathogenic fungi. In: Howard DH, ed. Pathogenic fungi in humans and animals. 2nd ed. Vol 16. New York: Marcel Dekker, 2003:1–16.
2. Sutton DA, Fothergill AW, Rinaldi MG. Guide to clinically significant fungi. Baltimore: Lippincott Williams & Wilkins, 1998.
3. Bartlett JG, Ryan KJ, Smith TF, Wilson WR. Cumitech 7A, Laboratory diagnosis of lower respiratory tract infections. Washington II JA, Coordinating ed. Washington, DC: American Society of Microbiology, 1987.
4. Clarridge Je, Pezzlo MT, Vosti KL. Cumitech 2A. Laboratory diagnosis of urinary tract infections. Weissfeld AW, coordinating ed. Washington, DC: American Society for Microbiology, 1987.
5. Eschenbach D, Pollock HM, Schacter J. Cumitech 17. Laboratory diagnosis of female genital tracts infections. Rubin SJ, coordinating ed. Washington, DC: American Society for Microbiology, 1983.
6. Jones DB, Liesegang TJ, Robinson NM. Cumitech 13. Laboratory diagnosis of ocular infections. Washington JA, coordinating ed. Washington, DC: American Society for Microbiology, 1981.

7. Maki DG, Weise CD, Sarafin HW. A semiquantitative culture method for identifying intravenous-catheter-related infection. N Engl J Med 1977;296:1303–1309.
8. Sutton DA. Specimen collection, transport, and processing: mycology. In: Murray PR, Baron EJ, Jorgensen JH, Landry ML, MA Pfaller MA, eds. Manual of clinical microbiology. 9th ed. Washington, DC: American Society for Microbiology, 2007;1728–1736.
9. Jorgensen JH, Mirrett S, McDonald LC, et al. Controlled clinical laboratory comparison of BACTEC Plus Aerobic/F resin medium with BacT/Alert aerobic FAM medium for detection of bacteremia and fungemia. J Clin Microbiol 1997;35:53–58.
10. Mattia AR. FDA review criteria for blood culture systems. Clin Microbiol Newsl 1993;15:132–136.
11. Horvath LL, George BJ, Murray CK, Harrison LS, Hospenthal DR. Direct comparison of the BACTEC 9240 and BacT/ALERT 3D automated blood culture systems for *Candida* growth detection. J Clin Microbiol 2004;42:115–118.
12. Horvath LL, Hospenthal DR, Murray CK, Dooley DP. Detection of simulated candidemia by the BACTEC 9240 SYSTEM WITH plus Aerobic/F and Anaerobic/F blood culture bottles. J Clin Microbiol 2003;41:4714–4717.
13. Horvath LL, Hospenthal DR, Murray CK, Dooley DP. Direct isolation of *Candida* spp. from blood cultures on the chromogenic medium CHROMagar Candida. J Clin Microbiol 2003;41:2629–2632.
14. McDonald LC, Weinstein MP, Fune J, Mirrett S, Reimer LG, Reller LB. Controlled comparison of BacT/ALERT FAN aerobic medium and BACTEC fungal blood culture medium for detection of fungemia. J Clin Microbiol 2004;39:622–624.
15. Meyer M-H, Letscher-Bru V, Jaulhac B, Waller J, Candolfi E. Comparison of Mycosis IC/F and Plus Aerobic/F Media for diagnosis of fungemia by the BACTEC 9240 system. J Clin Microbiol 2004;42:773–777.
16. Auckenthaler R, Ilstrup DM, Washington II JA. Comparison of recovery of organisms from blood cultures diluted 10% (volume/volume) and 20% (volume/volume). J Clin Microbiol 1982;15:860–864.
17. Billi J, Stockman L, Roberts GD, Horstmeier CD, Istrup DM. Evaluation of a lysis-centrifugation system for recovery of yeasts and filamentous fungi from blood. J Clin Microbiol 1983;18:469–471.
18. Bille J, Edson RS, Roberts GD. Clinical evaluation of the lysis-centrifugation blood culture system for detection of fungemia and comparison with a conventional biphasic broth blood culture system. J Clin Microbiol 1984;19:126–128.
19. Guerra-Romero L, Edson RC, Dockerill FR, Horstmeier CD, Roberts GD. Comparison of Dupont Isolator and Roche Septi-check for detection of fungemia. J Clin Microbial 1987;25:1623–1625.
20. Lyon R, Woods G. Comparison of the BacT/Alert and ISOLATOR blood culture systems for recovery of fungi. Am J Clin Pathol 1995;103:660–662.
21. Hazen KC. Section 6. Mycology and aerobic actinomycetes. In: Isenberg HD, ed. Essential procedures for clinical microbiology. Washington, DC: American Society for Microbiology, 1998:255–283.
22. Miller JM. A guide to specimen management in clinical microbiology. 2nd ed. Washington, DC: American Society for Microbiology Press, 1999.
23. Labarca JAI, Wagar EA, Grasmick AE, Kokkinos HM, Bruckner DA. Critical evaluation of a 4-week incubation for fungal cultures: is the fourth week useful? J Clin Microbiol 1998; 36:3686–3685.
24. Sutton DA. Coelomycetous fungi in human disease. A review: clinical entities, pathogenesis, identification and therapy. Rev Iberoam Micol 1999;16:171–179.
25. McGinnis MR. Laboratory handbook of medical mycology. New York: Academic Press, 1980.

SUGGESTED READINGS

Chandler FW, Watts JC. Pathologic diagnosis of fungal infections. Chicago: American Society of Clinical Pathologists Press, 1987.

deHoog GS, Guarro J, Gene J, Figueras MJ. Atlas of clinical fungi. 2nd ed. Utrecht, The Netherlands: Centraalbureau voor Schimmelcultures, 2000.

Larone DH. Medically important fungi: a guide to identification. 4th ed. Washington, DC: American Society for Microbiology Press, 2002.

Mandell GL, ed. in Chief, Diamond RD, ed. Atlas of infectious diseases. Fungal infections. Philadelphia: Current Medicine, 2000.

Miller JM. A guide to specimen management in clinical microbiology. 2nd ed. Washington, DC: American Society for Microbiology Press, 1999.

Sutton DA. Specimen collection, transport, and processing: mycology. In: Murray PR, Baron EJ, Jorgensen JH, Landry ML, Pfaller MA, eds. Manual of clinical microbiology. 9th Ed. Washington, DC: American Society for Microbiology, 2007;1728–1736.

Sutton DA, Fothergill AW, Rinaldi MG. Guide to clinically significant fungi. Baltimore: Lippincott Williams & Wilkins, 1998.

www.doctorfungus.org is an excellent source for current names and morphology of fungi of medical importance.

3
Diagnostic Histopathology

Michael B. Smith, MD and Michael R. McGinnis, PhD

1. INTRODUCTION

Fungal infections can be diagnosed on the basis of mycologic, immunologic, clinical, and histopathologic information. Of these procedures, histopathology can provide important diagnostic information in a relatively short period of time, but is limited in that much of the information obtained from the examination of tissue sections can provide only tentative fungal identification, unless specialized techniques such as immunofluorescence are used or when the etiologic agent has distinctly unique structures (such as spherules containing endospores). These limitations are particularly evident in the case of filamentous fungi, as many of the opportunistic filamentous pathogens have similar tissue morphology (Fig. 3.1). Although this often makes identification of these organisms from tissue sections essentially impossible, examination of tissue sections is critical in determining whether fungi are involved in invasion, colonization, or simply have been recovered in culture as contaminants. The technique is rapid, inexpensive, and accurate, and the information it provides can have enormous and immediate patient care implications.

Even though the most specific method in identifying a fungus is to recover it in culture so that it can be properly and accurately identified, cultures may not be submitted for various reasons. In addition, some organisms, such as *Lacazia loboi* (Fig. 3.2) and *Rhinosporidium seeberi* (Fig. 3.3), have not yet been grown in vitro. In the absence of culture recovery, the diagnosis of fungal infection via histology rests on the size, morphology, and staining properties of fungal elements in tissue along with the assessment of invasion of normally sterile tissue and body fluids.

2. STAINS

A number of specific stains are available that can assist in visualizing fungi in tissue (Table 3.1). With the exception of immunofluorescence using species-specific antibodies, all stains are nonspecific and serve only to demonstrate the morphological structures of the fungus, which usually allows categorization in most cases, or definitive identification to species in some cases. A good example is the ability of mucicarmine to stain the polysaccharide capsule of *Cryptococcus neoformans* (Fig. 3.4). Although not completely specific, with the appropriate morphology of the yeast cells, the staining

From: *Infectious Disease: Diagnosis and Treatment of Human Mycoses*
Edited by: D. R. Hospenthal and M. G. Rinaldi © Humana Press Inc., Totowa, NJ

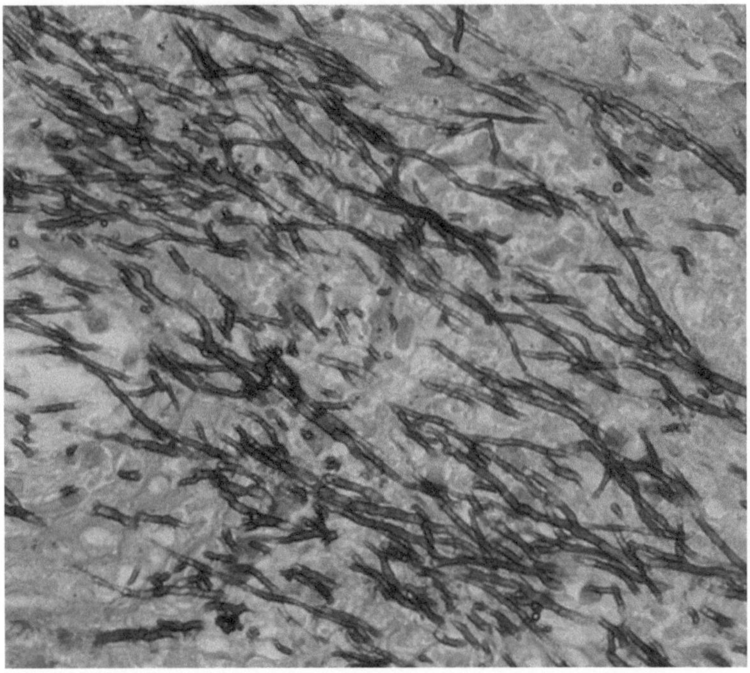

Fig. 3.1. Septate, uniform hyphae of *Aspergillus fumigatus*. Hyphae morphology is characteristic but not specific. GMS. [*See* color plate 1, following p. 48]. [Figure in color on CD-ROM].

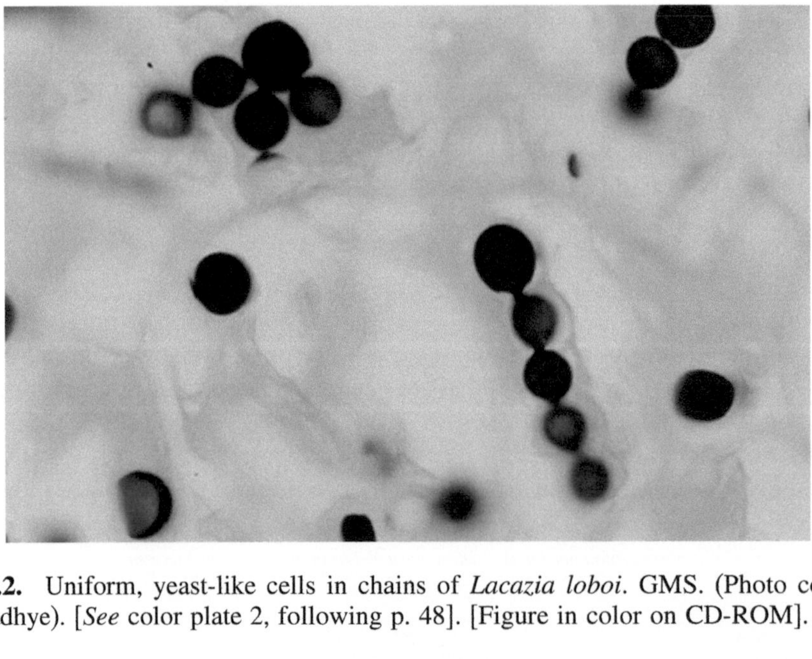

Fig. 3.2. Uniform, yeast-like cells in chains of *Lacazia loboi*. GMS. (Photo courtesy of Dr. A. Padhye). [*See* color plate 2, following p. 48]. [Figure in color on CD-ROM].

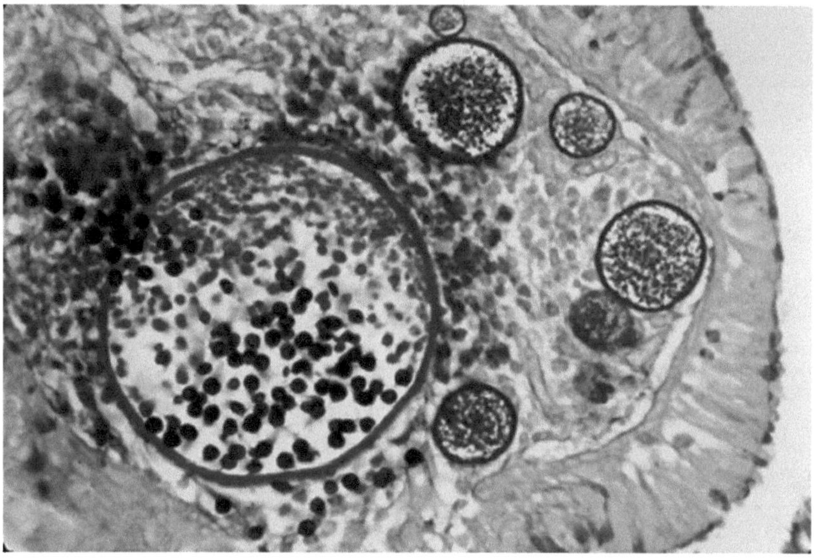

Fig. 3.3. Large sporangium containing sporangiospores and smaller trophocytes of *Rhinosporidium seeberi*. PAS. [*See* color plate 3, following p. 48]. [Figure in color on CD-ROM].

Table 3.1
Stains useful in the diagnosis of fungal infection

Stain	Reaction	Comments
Fontana-Masson	Chromaffin reaction that oxidizes melanin or melanin precursor as it reduces silver. Fungal cell walls are black. Background is pale pink.	Useful for staining cell walls of suspected dematiaceous fungi when the nature of their cell wall is not evident. Useful for staining *Cryptococcus neoformans*. Natural color of cell walls masked by this staining technique. Tissue response cannot be studied.
Gomori methenamine silver (Grocott's modification) (GMS)	Chromic acid oxidizes cell wall polysaccharides to aldehydes. Aldehyde products reduce methenamine silver nitrate to metallic silver. Erythrocytes and fungal cell walls are brown-to-black. Background is pale green.	Enhances visualization of fungi and their morphology. Natural color of cell walls masked by the staining. Tissue response cannot be studied. Ideal special fungal stain to evaluate fungal structures. Cell nuclei can mimic yeasts.

(Continued)

Table 3.1
Continued

Stain	Reaction	Comments
Gridley's Fungus	Chromic acid oxidizes adjacent hydroxyl groups of cell wall polysaccharides to aldehydes. Aldehyde groups combine with Schiff reagent. Aldehyde fuchsin occupies uninvolved linkages of the Schiff reagent. Fungal cell walls are rose to purple and the background is yellow.	Enhances visualization of fungi and their morphology. Natural color of cell walls masked. Tissue response cannot be studied.
Hematoxylin and eosin (H&E)	Hematein-mordant stains DNA in the nucleus and nuclear proteins. Nuclei blue, cartilage and calcium deposits blue; cytoplasm and other components shades of red and erythrocytes bright red.	Visualizes host tissue response to the fungus. *Aspergillus* and zygomycetes stain well. Difficult to see some fungi in tissue, especially if they are present in small numbers. Dematiaceous nature of fungal cell wall can often be seen.
Immunofluorescence	Direct technique: Specific fluorescein-labeled antibody reacts with fungal cell wall antigens. Indirect technique: Unlabeled antibody complexes with fungal antigens. Fluorescein-labeled conjugate reacts with globulins attached to fungal antigens. Cell walls fluoresce yellow-green.	Specific and highly sensitive. Some use immunoperoxidase technique. Can be used to detect and measure antibodies. Reagents often available only in specialized laboratories.
Mayer's Mucicarmine	Aluminum binds acid groups of the mucopolysaccharides of the capsule where carmine is attached as a complex. Capsule stains deep rose to red. Background is yellow.	Alcian blue may also be used as capsular stain. Not specific for *Cryptococcus neoformans*. *Rhinosporidium seeberi* and *Blastomyces dermatitidis* cells are occasionally stained.
Periodic acid-Schiff (Hotchkiss-McManus technique) (PAS)	Periodic acid oxidizes adjacent hydroxyl groups of cell wall polysaccharides to aldehydes. Aldehyde combines with Schiff reagent. Fungi are red-purple. Background is green.	Enhances visualization of fungi and their morphology. Natural color of cell walls is masked. Tissue response cannot be studied.

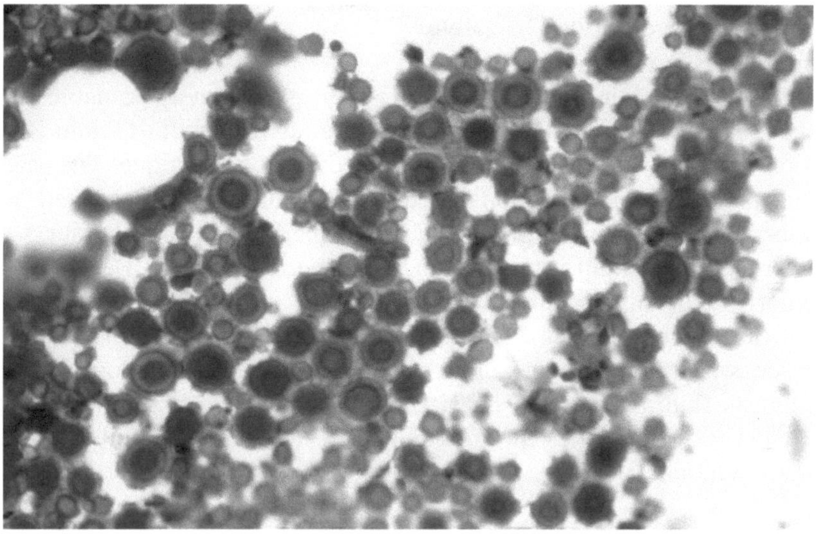

Fig. 3.4. Mucicarmine stain demonstrating positive staining of capsule of *Cryptococcus neoformans*. Mayer's mucicarmine. [*See* color plate 4, following p. 48]. [Figure in color on CD-ROM].

allows a presumptive diagnosis of *C. neoformans*. The ability of these fungal stains to highlight the appearance of the organisms does, however, come with some disadvantages, as the stains mask the presence of pigment in the walls of the pigmented fungi (Fig. 3.5), and neither the host inflammatory reaction nor the viability of the tissue in

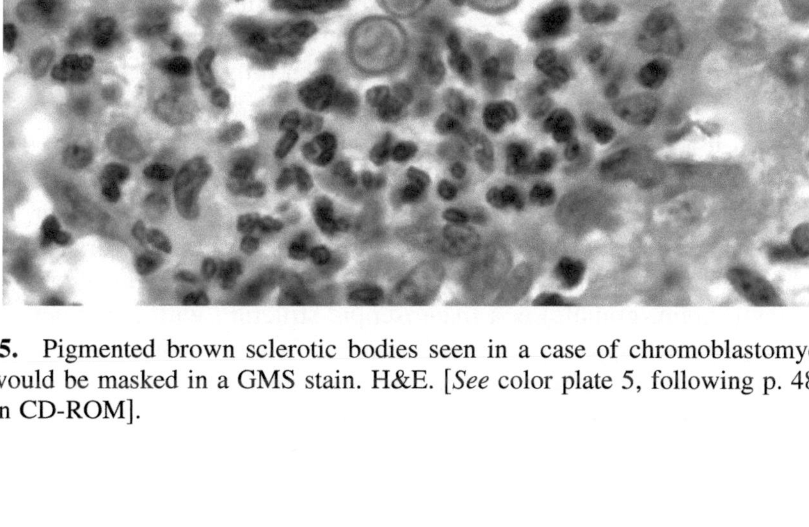

Fig. 3.5. Pigmented brown sclerotic bodies seen in a case of chromoblastomycosis. The pigment would be masked in a GMS stain. H&E. [*See* color plate 5, following p. 48]. [Figure in color on CD-ROM].

which the fungus is present can be assessed. The latter may be crucial in determining whether the fungus is invasive.

The routine hematoxylin and eosin (H&E) stain is extremely valuable for studying the host's response to the fungus. Frequently, fungi are difficult to see in H&E stained tissue sections because they are not readily stained by this technique. The aspergilli and zygomycetes tend to be an exception because they usually stain very well. In addition to difficulties in recognizing fungi in tissue, especially when their numbers within the pathologic process are small, their presence can be overlooked. Because stains such as the Gomori methenamine silver (GMS), Gridley fungus, and periodic acid-Schiff (PAS) stain the fungus, they provide the advantage of allowing the histopathologist to clearly see small numbers of fungi as well as their morphology. A number of histopathologists find a combined H&E and GMS stain to be an excellent technique because it clearly distinguishes the fungus and at the same time allows visualization of the tissue reaction.

3. FUNGAL MORPHOLOGY

Confusion may result from tissue components associated with pathologic processes that resemble fungi. These include Russell bodies, karyorrhectic debris, calcified bodies, elastic fibers, small blood vessels, and other host components. Care must always be exercised when examining tissue. Multiple fields should always be examined microscopically before reaching a diagnosis. When determining whether a structure represents a fungus, and if so, which species it represents, the morphology of structures in tissue must always be carefully evaluated.

3.1. *Yeasts in Tissue*

Yeast cells are characterized by their size, budding (location and attachment of daughter cells), color (hyaline or dematiaceous), presence or absence of a capsule, number of nuclei, and thickness of their cell walls. Other associated forms, such as pseudohyphae (well developed or rudimentary), hyphae, and arthroconidia, are helpful in identifying the etiologic agents. Dimorphic fungi, yeasts such as *Candida albicans*, and several other fungi may produce yeast cells in tissue. The location of yeast cells can provide valuable data. For example, *H. capsulatum* forms solitary, budding 2 to 5 μm cells that are intracellular (Fig. 3.6). Care must be taken to avoid confusing *H. capsulatum* with *Penicillium marneffei*, another intracellular dimorphic fungus (Fig. 3.7). The yeast cells of *P. marneffei* divide by fission, and not by budding as in *H. capsulatum*. Geographically, infection with *P. marneffei* is limited to Southeast Asia.

3.2. *Hyphae in Tissue*

Hyphae are filaments that are characterized by their diameter, branching pattern, septation, color, consistency of shape, cell wall contour, and organizational pattern. A sclerotium (syn. grain, granule) is a macroscopic structure with a distinct, organized, hyphal architecture, whereas a fungus ball consists of a mass of disorganized hyphae. The fungus ball overall can be organized as repeating zones of hyphae and necrotic tissue. Additional structures such as arthroconidia, blastoconidia, vesicles, chlamydo-

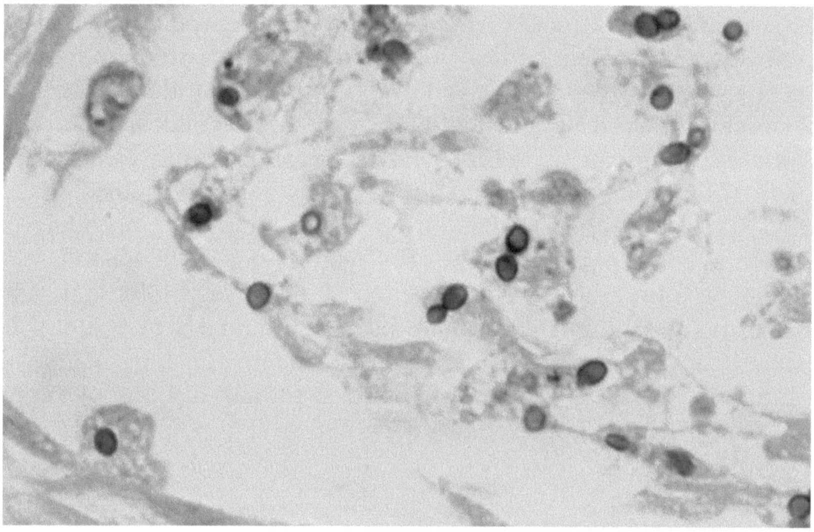

Fig. 3.6. Small intracellular yeast with budding, characteristic of *Histoplasma capsulatum*. GMS. [*See* color plate 6, following p. 48]. [Figure in color on CD-ROM].

conidia, and others are helpful for the recognition of different fungi and fungus-like pathogens.

3.3. Other Structures in Tissue

A definitive diagnosis can be made when the number of organisms present is adequate and they are typical of the etiologic agent. For example, a spherule containing

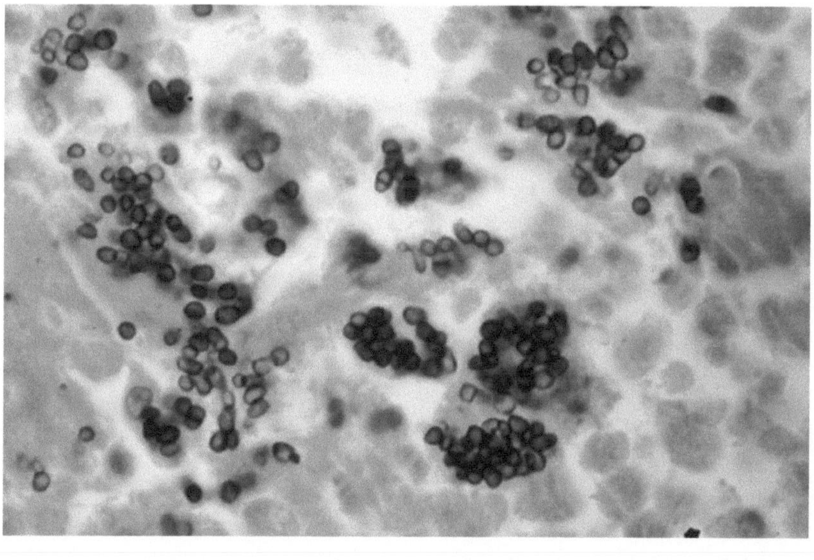

Fig. 3.7. *Penicillium marneffei*. Yeast showing occasional transverse septa (center). Note absence of budding. GMS. [*See* color plate 7, following p. 48]. [Figure in color on CD-ROM].

endospores is characteristic of *Coccidioides*. To an inexperienced person, spherules could be confused with "parent bodies" that contain small, 5- to 7-μm round structures (which appear to represent altered erythrocytes) in myospherulosis. The sporangia of *Prototheca* species, Russell bodies, and closely appressed endospores may resemble the yeast form of *B. dermatitidis*. *Chlorella* species, which are green algae, may be confused with *Coccidioides* and *Prototheca* species in H&E stained tissue sections because their chlorophyll is destroyed during the fixation and embedding process. A green color due to chlorophyll can be readily seen in smears of fresh tissue. Because *Coccidioides* may form hyphae that develop into arthroconidia, and subsequently spherules, transition forms might be confused with a number of hyalohyphomycetes when spherules containing endospores are not evident. The type of etiologic agent present, the quality of the staining, the stains selected, and the skill of the pathologist contribute to the quality of the tissue diagnosis.

4. HOST RESPONSE

Although there is no specific inflammatory tissue reaction associated with a particular fungus, some have characteristic inflammatory infiltrates or produce characteristic effects on tissue. For example, *Blastomyces dermatitidis* characteristically is seen with a mixed suppurative–granulomatous inflammatory infiltrate (Fig. 3.8). Several of the other thermally dimorphic pathogens, such as *Coccidioides* (Fig. 3.9) and *Sporothrix schenckii* (Fig. 3.10), can show similar reactions. Infections due to *Fusarium* species are usually seen with a suppurative inflammatory infiltrate, and often show angioinvasion with associated tissue infarction. A number of other opportunistic filamentous fungi will produce these identical findings in tissue. The inflammatory

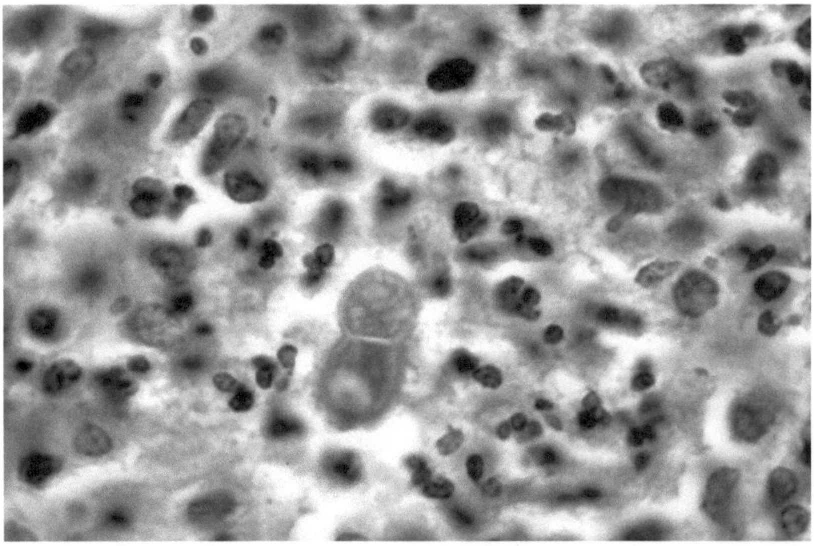

Fig. 3.8. Broad-based budding of *Blastomyces dermatitidis* in a background of neutrophils and histiocytes. H&E. [*See* color plate 8, following p. 48]. [Figure in color on CD-ROM].

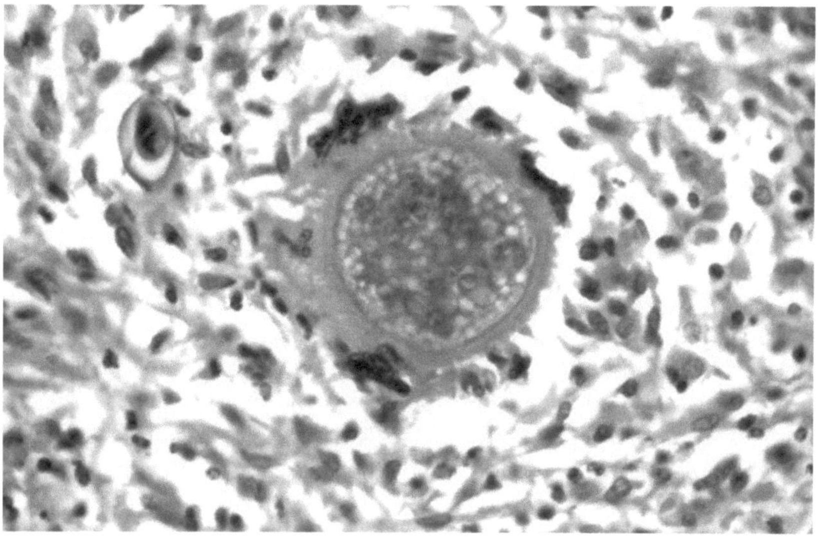

Fig. 3.9. Large spherule containing endospores of *Coccidioides* species. H&E. [*See* color plate 9, following p. 48]. [Figure in color on CD-ROM].

infiltrate associated with an infection is influenced not only by the infecting organism, but also by the immune status of the patient. A characteristic inflammatory infiltrate, seen with infection by a given organism in an immunocompetent patient, may not be present or may be altered in a severely immunocompromised individual.

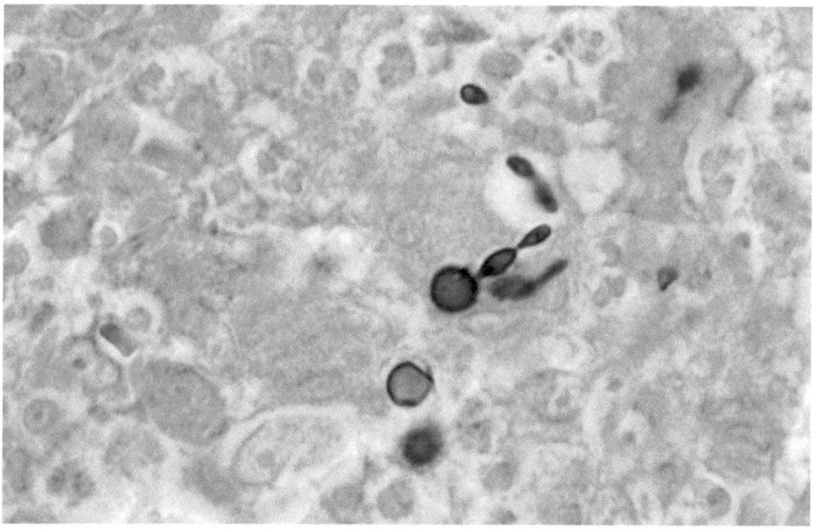

Fig. 3.10. *Sporothrix schenckii* with characteristic "cigar-shaped" buds attached by narrow base to the parent cell. GMS. [*See* color plate 10, following p. 48]. [Figure in color on CD-ROM].

Pyogenic inflammation, abscess formation, suppurative necrosis, and a propensity to invade blood vessels associated with hyaline, sparsely septate hyphae with irregular branching and large diameter are characteristic of Zygomycetes hyphae, such as *Absidia, Mucor, Rhizomucor*, and others (Fig. 3.11). Rarely, chlamydoconidia may be formed by species such as *Rhizopus arrhizus*. Occasionally Zygomycetes hyphae will stain positive with the Fontana–Masson stain. In contrast, a mixed purulent necrotizing inflammation with hyaline septate, dichotomously branching hyphae having a consistent and uniform diameter is associated with *Aspergillus* species. If a cavity is present, the aspergilli often form conidial heads that allow for the identification of the *Aspergillus* to species. Some species such as *A. terreus* form lateral one-celled aleurioconidia along their hyphae in tissue (Fig. 3.12). When calcium oxalate crystals that originated from fungal oxalic acid are present near hyphae in necrotic tissue, *A. niger* should be considered. *Aspergillus* and *Pseudallescheria boydii* resemble each other in tissue, and often cannot be differentiated histologically. When conidial heads of *Aspergillus* species are seen in tissue, which usually occurs only in lesions exposed to air, such as in a lung cavity, a specific histopathologic diagnosis of aspergillosis can be rendered.

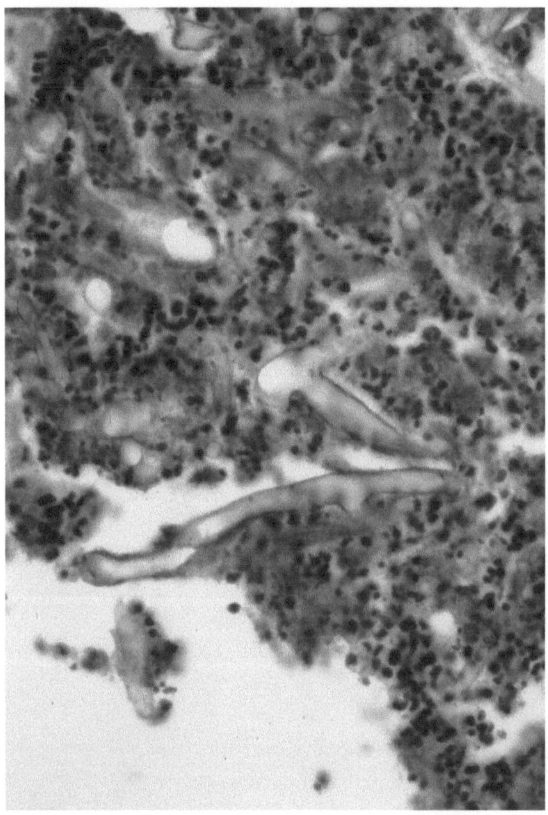

Fig. 3.11. Hyphae of a Zygomycete. H&E. [*See* color plate 11, following p. 48]. [Figure in color on CD-ROM].

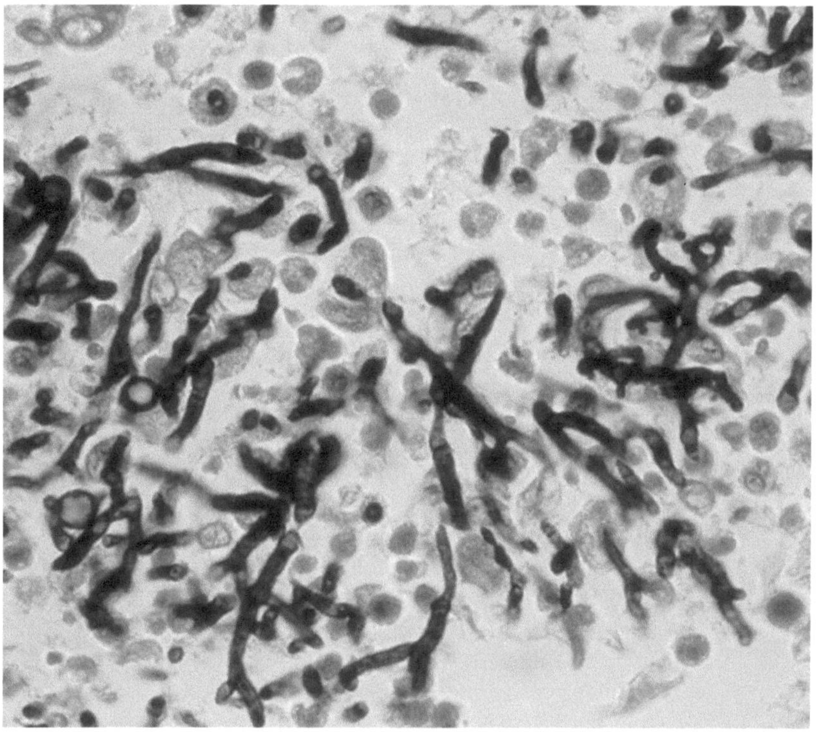

Fig. 3.12. Hyphae of *Aspergillus terreus* with small, lateral aleurioconidia. GMS. [*See* color plate 12, following p. 48]. [Figure in color on CD-ROM].

5. OTHER IMPORTANT CONSIDERATIONS

The accuracy of a histopathologic examination of tissue sections is also impacted by a number of parameters that are out of the control of the histopathologist. The selection of the sample by the clinician or surgeon is crucial. The central portion, as well as the periphery of the lesion, is important because some fungi tend to be predominantly in one portion rather than the other. *H. capsulatum* tends to be in the central portion of lesions, whereas *Blastomyces dermatitidis* appears at the edge. Because fixatives used in histology kill fungi, a portion of the specimen must be concurrently sent to the mycology laboratory, where the fungi causing the infectious disease process can be isolated and identified. Important fungal pathogens and their morphology in tissue are summarized in Table 3.2.

Often, presumptive identifications are made first via histopathology, with the definitive identification being delayed until the isolated fungus is identified in the laboratory (Fig. 3.13). Even if the etiologic agent cannot be identified, the tissue forms seen may result in the recognition of the disease and allow initiation of treatment. For example, granules are associated with mycetoma, muriform cells with chromoblastomycosis, and oval yeast cells and pseudohyphae with candidiasis. The fungal forms seen in tissue are extremely important in diagnosing the disease, even if they cannot be used to identify the specific fungus causing the disease. Simply determining the presence or

Table 3.2
Typical characteristics of fungal structures found in human tissue

Infection	Fungal morphology	Differential diagnosis
Adiaspiromycosis	Solitary cells, 200–400 μm, cell wall 10–80 μm, hyaline. Endosporulation, budding cells, and hyphae absent.	NA
Aspergillosis	Hyphae, 2.5–6 μm, swollen cells up to 12 μm, dichotomous branching, septate, parallel walls, hyaline. Calcium oxalate crystals maybe present. Conidial heads may form within cavities.	Candidiasis (hyphae), hyalohyphomycosis (hyaline hyphae), phaeohyphomycosis (phaeoid hyphae), *Pseudallescheria boydii*, occasionally zygomycetes.
Blastomycosis	Small yeast cells, 2–4 μm. Typical cells, 6–15 μm. Large yeast cells, 20–30 μm. Single blastoconidia, broad base between parent and daughter cells, thick cell wall, consistent size, hyaline. Extracellular, more than one nucleus may be present. Pseudohyphae and hyphae may be present in areas of body with lower temperature (ears, upper airway). Yeast tends to be at edge of lesions.	Coccidioidomycosis (endospores), cryptococcosis (small capsule form), histoplasmosis.
Candidiasis	Yeast 2.5–6 μm, globose to ovoid. Pseudohyphae. Hyphae may be present, hyaline.	Aspergillosis (hyphae), blastomycosis (small yeast form), cryptococcosis (small capsule), phaeohyphomycosis (pseudohyphae).
Chromoblasto-mycosis	Muriform cells, 5–12 μm, chestnut brown, crust-like material may be present on cells. Septate, branching, dematiaceous hyphae in epidermis.	Phaeohyphomycosis.
Coccidioidomycosis	Spherules, 20–200 μm, endospores 2–5 μm. Hyphae, arthroconidia, and developing spherules may be present, hyaline. Portions of spherule wall often present.	Blastomycosis, cryptococcosis (small capsule form), protothecosis.
Cryptococcosis	Yeast, 2–20 μm, globose, ovoid, elliptical to crescent shaped, variable in size, capsule. Narrow neck between parent and daughter cells. Melanin in cell wall stains with Fontana-Masson stain.	Blastomycosis (small yeast form),candidiasis, histoplasmosis.

(*Continued*)

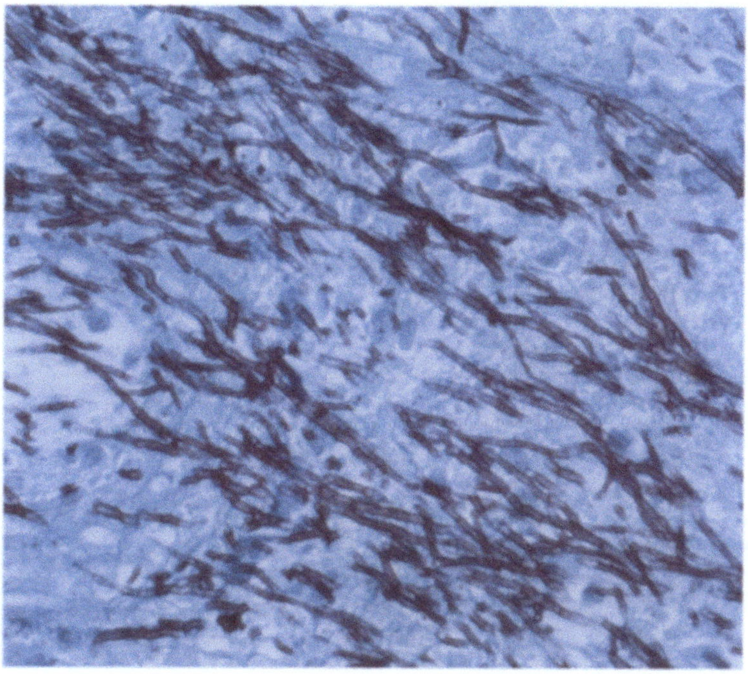

Color Plate 1. Septate, uniform hyphae of *Aspergillus fumigatus*. Hyphae morphology is characteristic but not specific. GMS. *See* discussion on p. 37.

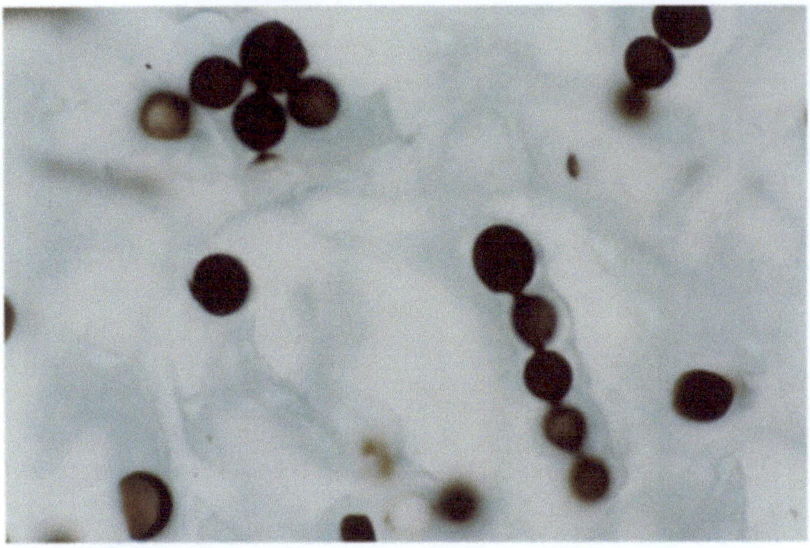

Color Plate 2. Uniform, yeast-like cells in chains of *Lacazia loboi*. GMS. (Photo courtesy of Dr. A. Padhye). *See* discussion on p. 37.

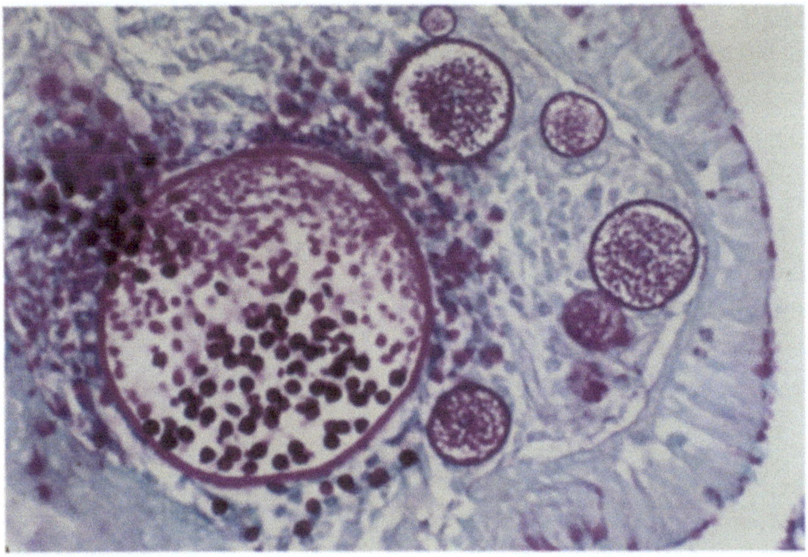

Color Plate 3. Large sporangium containing sporangiospores and smaller trophocytes of *Rhinosporidium seeberi*. PAS. *See* discussion on p. 37.

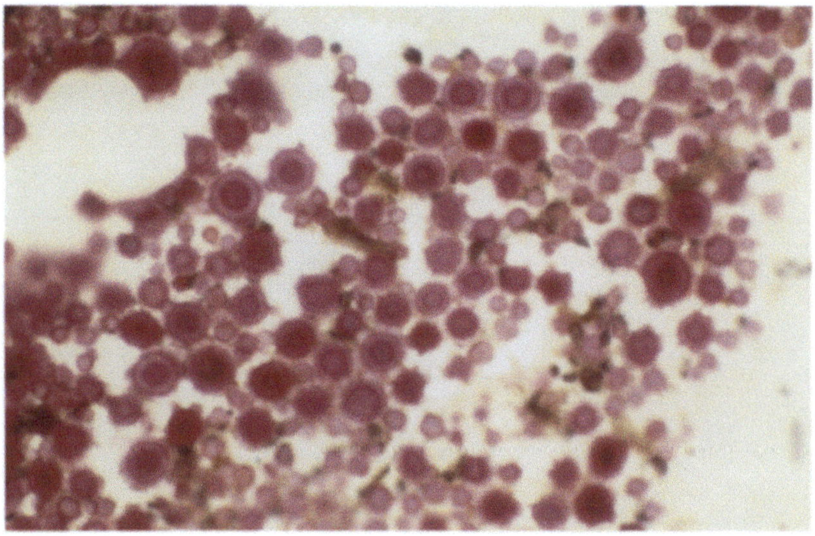

Color Plate 4. Mucicarmine stain demonstrating positive staining of capsule of *Cryptococcus neoformans*. Mayer's mucicarmine. *See* discussion on pp. 37, 41.

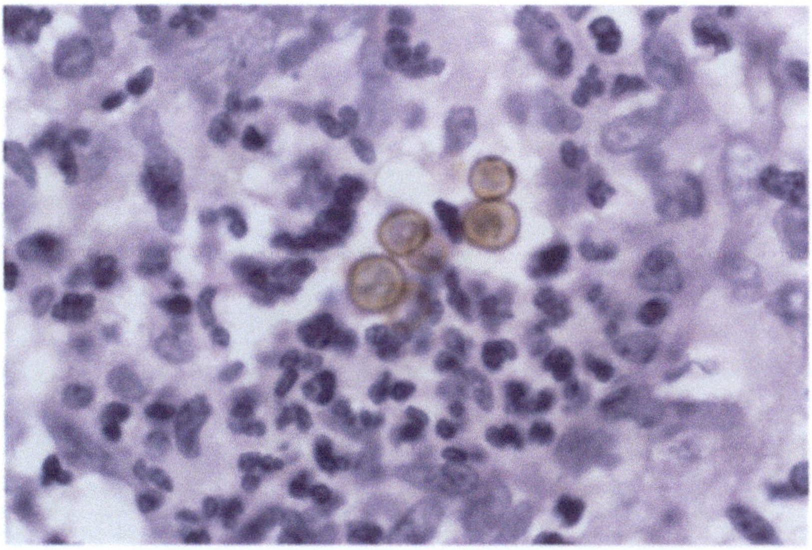

Color Plate 5. Pigmented brown sclerotic bodies seen in a case of chromoblastomycosis. The pigment would be masked in a GMS stain. H&E. *See* discussion on p. 41.

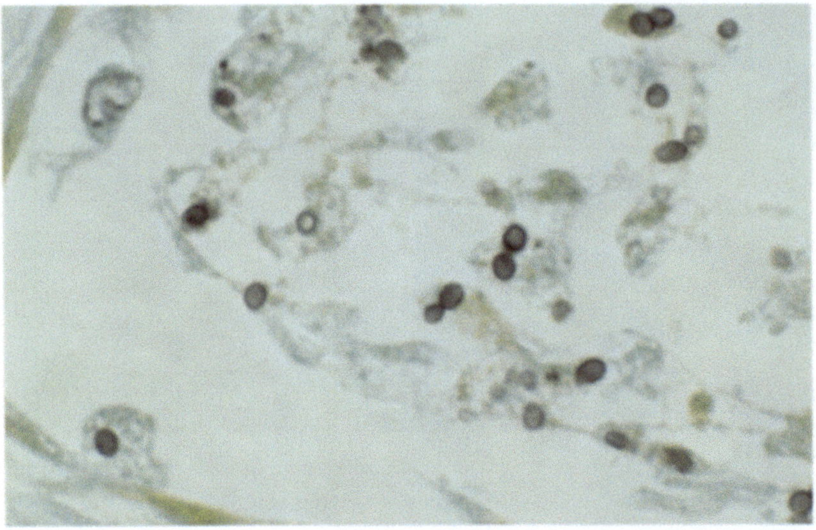

Color Plate 6. Small intracellular yeast with budding, characteristic of *Histoplasma capsulatum*. GMS. *See* discussion on p. 42.

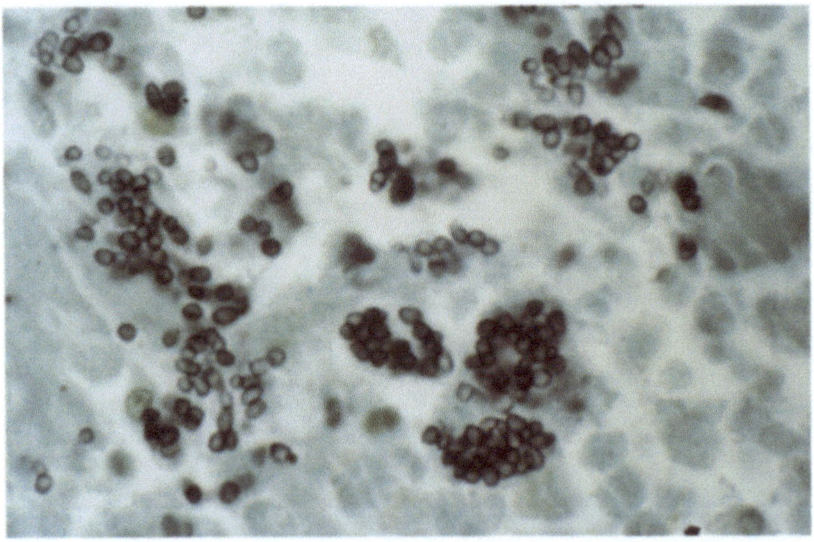

Color Plate 7. *Penicillium marneffei*. Yeast showing occasional transverse septa (center). Note absence of budding. GMS. *See* discussion on p. 42.

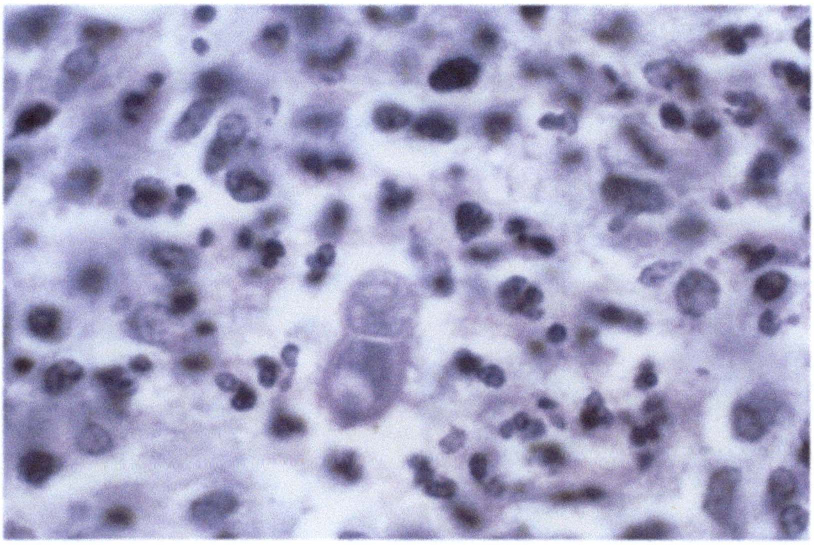

Color Plate 8. Broad-based budding of *Blastomyces dermatitidis* in a background of neutrophils and histiocytes. H&E. *See* discussion on p. 44.

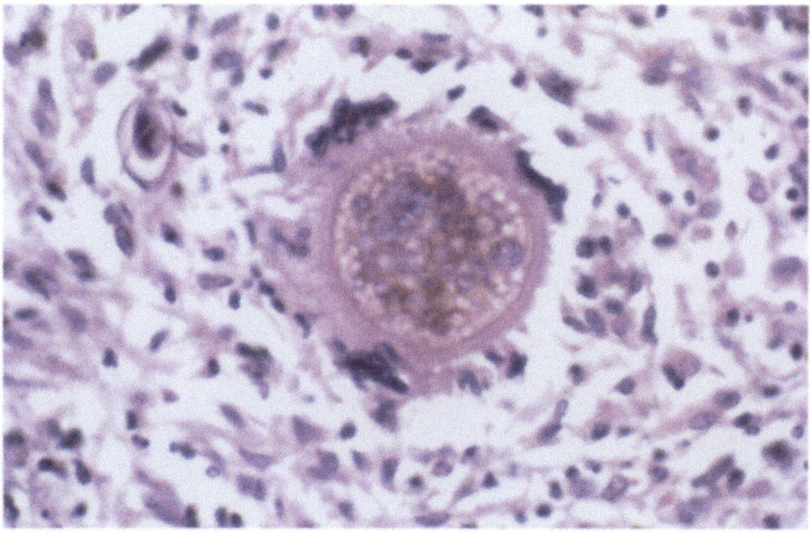

Color Plate 9. Large spherule containing endospores of *Coccidioides* species. H&E. *See* discussion on p. 44.

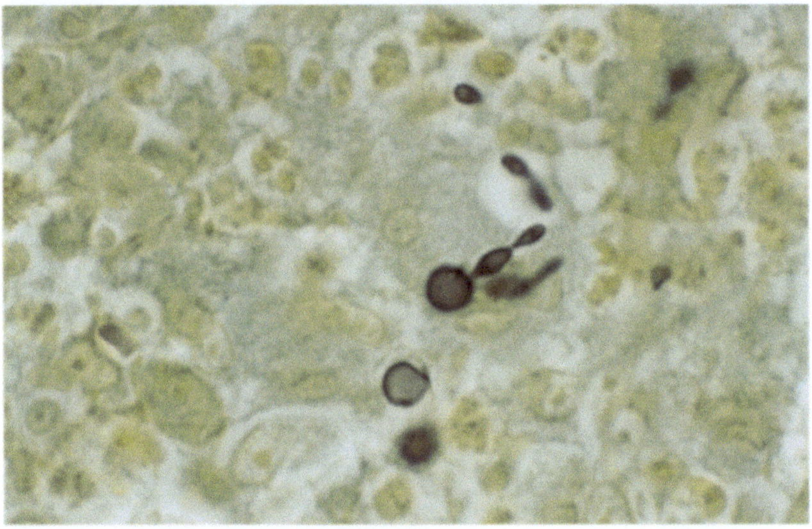

Color Plate 10. *Sporothrix schenckii* with characteristic "cigar-shaped" buds attached by narrow base to the parent cell. GMS. *See* discussion on pp. 44, 45.

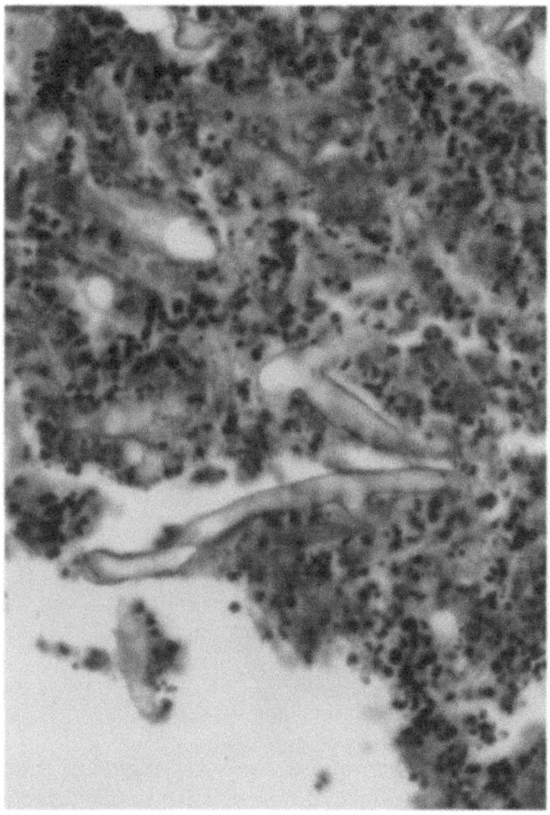

Color Plate 11. Hyphae of a Zygomycete. H&E. *See* discussion on p. 46.

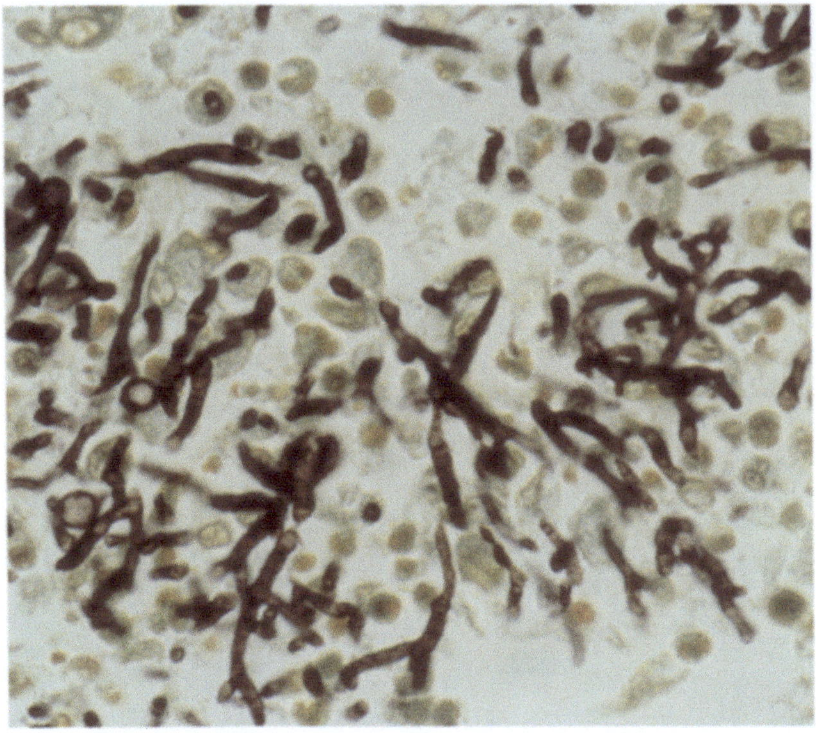

Color Plate 12. Hyphae of *Aspergillus terreus* with small, lateral aleurioconidia. GMS. *See* discussion on p. 46.

Table 3.2 ***(Continued)***
Typical characteristics of fungal structures found in human tissue

Infection	Fungal morphology	Differential diagnosis
Histoplasmosis	Yeast 2–5 μm, globose to ovoid, single blastoconidium, intracellular, single nucleus, hyaline. Halo between cell wall and fungal cytoplasm in H&E stained sections. Poorly stained cell walls in calcified lesions (coin lesions). Yeast tends to be in center of lesions.	Candidiasis, cryptococcosis (yeast in histiocytes), *Penicillium marneffei*.
Histoplasmosis (African variety)	Yeast 8–15 μm, globose to ovoid, single blastoconidium, intracellular, single nucleus, hyaline. Halo between cell wall and fungal cytoplasm in H&E stained sections.	Blastomycosis (especially large yeast form).
Hyalohyphomycosis	Hyphae 2.5–7 μm, septate, branching, may have swollen cells, hyaline. This is the non-pigmented counter part to phaeohyphomycosis.	Phaeohyphomycosis.
Lobomycosis	Series of globose cells, 5–12 μm, thick walls, narrow tubular connections, hyaline. Hyphae absent. Melanin in cell wall stains with Fontana-Masson stain. Typically in cutaneous-subcutaneous tissue. Paracoccidioidomycosis and lobomycosis often occur together in some geographic regions.	Paracoccidioidomycosis.
Mycetoma	Sclerotia (syn. grains, granules) 1–4 mm, organized masses of hyphae. Hyphae 2–6 μm, often with swollen cells. Variable in color.	Actinomycotic mycetoma, botryomycosis.
Paracoccidioido-mycosis	Yeast 5–60 μm, globose to oval, multiple blastoconidia, attached by narrow tubular connections; budded cells remain attached, hyaline. Cell wall thick, especially central cells. Does not stain with Fontana-Masson stain.	Blastomycosis, cryptococcosis (small capsule form), histoplasmosis, lobomycosis.
Penicilliosis (*Penicillium marneffei*)	Yeast 2.5–4.5 μm, some cells 1–2 × 3 to 6 μm, globose to ovoid, division by fission, hyaline. Blastoconidia absent. Intracellular.	Histoplasmosis
Phaeohyphomycosis	Yeast, pseudohyphae, hyphae, or any combination. Hyphae 2.5–6 μm, often with swollen cells up to 25 μm, pale brown to hyaline. Morphology extremely variable.	Hyalohyphomycosis

(Continued)

Table 3.2
Continued

Infection	Fungal morphology	Differential diagnosis
Protothecosis (algae)	Sporangia 2–2.5 μm, 2–8 sporangiospores, often with one central spore, hyaline. Hyphae and blastoconidia absent.	*Chlorella* species, coccidioidomycosis.
Rhinosporidiosis (protozoan)	Sporangia, 6 to >300 μm, mature sporangiospores 6–7 μm, sporangial wall approximately 5 μm thick, hyaline.	Adiaspiromycosis, coccidioidomycosis.
Sporotrichosis	Yeast 2–6 μm, rarely up to 20 μm, globose to ovoid ("cigar-shaped"), hyphae rare, hyaline.	Candidiasis, histoplasmosis.
Zygomycosis	Hyphae, 3–25 μm, sparsely septate, irregular diameter, irregular branching, nonparallel walls, often distorted. Tend to invade blood vessels.	Aspergillosis, hyalohyphomycosis, pythiosis.

absence of invasion of fungal pathogens by histopathology can influence a patient's course tremendously. With close cooperation and communication between a patient's physician, surgeon, and histopathologist, the microscopic assessment of fungi in tissue can make an important if not crucial contribution to a patient's treatment and clinical course.

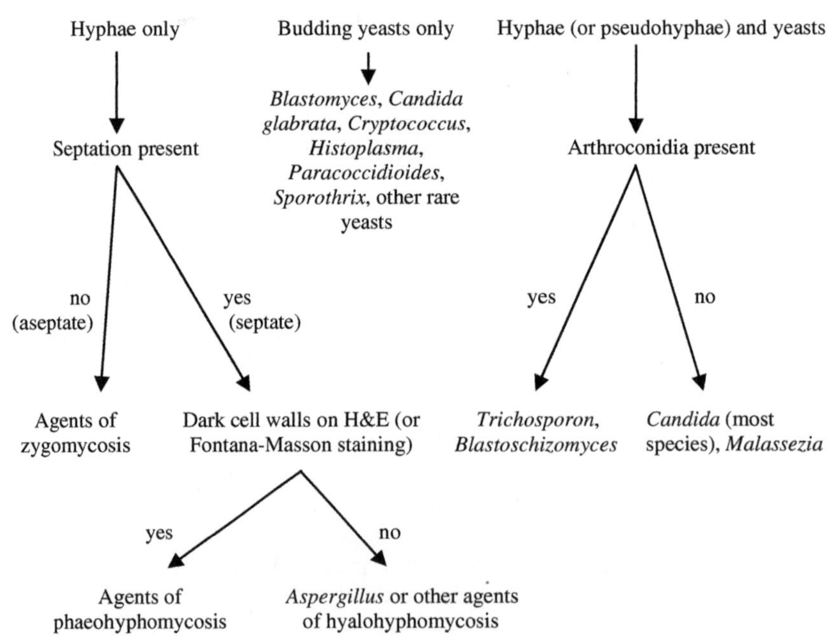

Fig. 3.13. Simple flow algorithm for diagnosis of fungal infection by histopathology.

SUGGESTED READINGS

Chandler FW, Kaplan W, Ajello L. A colour atlas and textbook of the histopathology of mycotic diseases. London: Wolfe Medical Publications, 1980.

Chandler FW, Watts JC. Pathologic diagnosis of fungal infections. Chicago: ASCP Press, 1987.

Salfelder K. Atlas of fungal pathology. Boston: Kluwer Academic Publishers, 1990.

Sheehan DC, Hrapchak BB. Theory and practice of histotechnology. 2nd ed. St Louis, MO: CV Mosby, 1980.

4
Diagnostic Immunology

Samit S. Desai, MD and Brian Wong, MD

1. INTRODUCTION

The frequency of invasive fungal infections has risen dramatically in recent years, primarily because of a larger population of at-risk patients who are immunocompromised, neutropenic, or critically ill. For clinicians evaluating these patients, it has become increasingly important to make the diagnosis early so that timely antifungal therapy can be instituted. Although culture of body fluids or tissue for the causative fungus continues to be the gold standard for definitive diagnosis, it may sometimes take several weeks to obtain results and the process often lacks sufficient sensitivity. For example, blood cultures are positive in only approximately 50% of cases of invasive candidiasis (IC) and in fewer than 10% of cases of invasive aspergillosis (IA) *(1)*. A presumptive diagnosis can also be made on the basis of characteristic histopathology and special tissue stains. However, obtaining adequate samples from protected anatomical sites is often not feasible in the populations at highest risk for such infections. Non-culture-based diagnostic tests are classified into four groups according to which component of the invading pathogen or host immune response they target. These include detection of host antibody, fungal antigen, fungal metabolites, or fungal nucleic acid. Overall, despite these multiple potential targets and extensive efforts toward development, only a handful of non-culture-based tests have proven clinically useful, and even fewer have reached commercial availability. As current diagnostic techniques are less than ideal, development of new methods is a priority in medical mycology. This chapter outlines the available tests according to the component of the invading pathogen or host immune response they target and provides some discussion of their strengths and weaknesses. Given the growing interest in this field, an introduction to newer assays that are currently being investigated is included. Specific recommendations for utilizing the currently available tests in conjunction with the culture and histopathology are discussed for individual fungal species and specific disease manifestations.

From: *Infectious Disease: Diagnosis and Treatment of Human Mycoses*
Edited by: D. R. Hospenthal and M. G. Rinaldi © Humana Press Inc., Totowa, NJ

1.1. Antibody Testing

Many tests in current use have been developed to detect host antibodies against specific fungal antigens. These require identification of one or more distinctive antigens to which host antibodies are directed, sufficient immunocompetence on the part of the host to mount a specific antibody response, and the use of a variety of techniques to detect the antibody, such as tube precipitin (TP) assays, immunodiffusion (ID) assays, complement fixation (CF) assays, radioimmunoassays (RIA), and enzyme-linked immunosorbent assays (ELISA/EIA). The major limitation of this general approach is that immunocompromised patients have impaired abilities to mount specific antibody responses. Moreover, these responses may be delayed and antibodies do not necessarily distinguish acute infection from chronic infection or colonization.

1.2. Antigen Testing

A second common method to diagnose fungal infection includes tests that use immunologic reagents to identify antigenic components of the fungus. These require the presence of circulating antigenemia with unique antigens and use of a variety of techniques to detect the antigens, including latex agglutination (LA) assays, dot immunobinding assays, ELISA, and RIA. Monoclonal or polyclonal antibody is often needed in these assays to help detect the antigen of interest. The major limitations of this general approach are the low level and transient nature of antigenemia in some hosts, occasional cross-reactions between antigens derived from different fungal species, and lack of specificity for a particular antigen when polyclonal antibodies are used.

1.3. Metabolite Testing

Another methodology includes the direct detection of fungal metabolites in patient serum or other samples. They are usually by-products of a specific fungus that are detected via gas chromatography, mass spectrometry, or an enzymatic reaction. One limitation of these tests is that the metabolic products are not unique to individual fungal species and may be present in small amounts in uninfected individuals. Further, the level of metabolite may not be present in sufficient quantity outside of the local tissue being invaded, making detection difficult.

1.4. Nucleic Acid Testing

Most recently, tests that use nucleic acid amplification techniques to identify specific fungal nucleic acid sequences have been explored. The basic steps required are sample preparation, nucleic acid target selection, amplification, and detection of the amplified products. There is still significant debate among researchers as to how best to accomplish each of these steps; however, there is consensus that this general approach has numerous advantages. First, fungal DNA or RNA may be amplified and detected even if viable fungal cells are not present. Second, the results can be generated within 4 to 8 hours of sample collection and even faster with some newer methods. Finally, the results may correlate well with disease burden and subsequent clinical outcome. Potential limitations of the technique include its possible inability to distinguish colonization from true infection and its potential false-positive results due to cross-contamination.

2. PAN-FUNGAL (1,3-β-D-GLUCAN) TESTING

1,3-β-D-glucan (BG) is a major component of the cell walls of many different fungi. The ability of fungal BG to activate an enzyme in the clotting cascade of the horseshoe crab has led to the development of assays capable of detecting very small amounts of BG. Two separate assays, Fungitec-G test (Seikagaku Corp., Tokyo, Japan) and Fungitell™ assay (Cape Cod Assoc., East Falmouth, MA), have been developed for this purpose. The Fungitec-G test has shown high sensitivity and specificity when used prospectively to predict a fungal etiology for fever in high-risk populations *(2)* and also when tested retrospectively in patients with known invasive aspergillosis *(3)*. The Fungitell assay has also shown good correlation when used retrospectively in patients with proven or probable fungal infections *(4)*, but it has not been prospectively studied for its ability to predict or diagnose fungal infections. The major limitation of these tests is their inability to differentiate between different species of fungi, because BG is a component of the cell walls of *Candida*, *Aspergillus*, *Trichosporon*, *Fusarium*, and *Saccharomyces* species, though not of *Cryptococcus* or the agents of zygomycosis. False-positive results occur in patients exposed to other sources of BG such as dialysis membranes and filters, cotton gauze and sponges used in surgery, and some medications.

3. CANDIDIASIS

Candida species are now the fourth most common microorganism isolated from the bloodstream of hospitalized patients in the United States and the sixth most common nosocomial pathogen overall *(5)*. Rapid detection of IC is critical and warrants the development of nonculture diagnostic approaches. This goal has drawn much attention, but owing to limited results still requires further investigation.

3.1. Antibody Detection

Antibody detection assays were the area of earliest interest but yielded tests with poor sensitivity and specificity. These tests have since fallen out of favor and are not recommended for routine use.

3.2. Antigen Detection

Several tests that target a variety of cell-wall and cytoplasmic components have been developed to detect macromolecular *Candida* antigens (Table 4.1). Some of these are no longer available, such as an assay to detect enolase antigen. Of the available tests, the earliest was the Cand-Tec LA assay (Ramco Laboratories, Stafford, TX), which was designed to detect circulating *Candida* antigen in patients with serious, disseminated infection. Unfortunately, there are conflicting reports *(6,7)* on its overall sensitivity and specificity, especially in patients with renal failure or rheumatoid factor positivity, making it difficult to confirm the diagnosis of candidiasis by the Cand-Tec assay alone.

The mannan component of the *Candida* cell wall is a major antigen and the target of many serum detection assays. These assays vary in the laboratory method and type of antibody used for detection. Two tests that use the same monoclonal antibody are the Pastorex *Candida* LA test (Bio-Rad, Marnes-la-Coquette, France) and the Platelia

Table 4.1
Studies of immunological assays for *Candida* infection

Target	Assay	Population tested	Sensitivity	Specificity	Comments	Ref.
			Antigen tests			
Unknown	Cand-Tec LA[a]	Retrospective analysis of patients with candidemia and controlpatients with superficial candidal colonization, other deep mycosesand healthy subjects	30/39 (77%)	35/40 (88%)	Titer of 1:4 considered positive	*(6)*
			16/39 (41%)	38/40 (95%)	Titer of 1:8 considered positive	
		Prospective analysis of patients at-risk for disseminated candidiasis	16/23 (70%)	123/179 (69%)	Titer of 1:4 considered positive	*(7)*
			7/23 (30%)	159/179 (89%)	Titer of 1:8 considered positive	
Mannan	Pastorex LA[b]	As above	10/39 (26%)	40/40 (100%)		*(6)*
	Pastorex LA	Retrospective analysis of patients with proven invasive candidiasis and control patients that included hospitalized, ICU patients, patients with other deep mycoses and healthy subjects.	8/23 (35%)	150/150 (100%)	Candidemia patients	*(8)*
			4/20 (20%)		*Candida* infection of other sterile sites	
	Platelia EIA[c]	As above	11/23 (42%) 7/20 (35%)	147/150 (98%)	Candidemia patients *Candida* infection of other sterile sites	*(8)*

	Platelia Ag/Ab EIA[b]	As above	19/23 (83%)	140/150 (93%)	Candidemia patients	
			17/20 (85%)		*Candida* infection of other sterile sites	*(8)*
	Fungitec-G test[d]	Prospective analysis of febrile mostly hematology-oncology patients and a small population of patients with other chronic illnesses (unable to differentiate *Candida* sub-group information)	6/7 (86%)	59/59 (100%)	Autopsy proven invasive deep mycosis	*(2)*
			23/24 (96)		Fungemia patients	
			1/2 (50%)		Fungal catheter-related infection	
			2/2 (100%)		Fungal meningitis	
			5/6 (83%)		Other fungal infections	
1,3-β-D-glucan	Fungitell[e]	Retrospective analysis of patients with proven or probable invasive fungal infections and healthy controls (only proven *Candida* infection data shown here)	76/92 (83%)	148/170 (87%)	Candidemia pts. at BG cut-off of 60 pg/ml	*(4)*
			11/15 (73%)	157/170 (92%)	Other *Candida* infections at BG cut-off 60 pg/ml	
			72/92 (78%)		Candidemia pts. at BG cut-off of 80 pg/ml	
			11/15 (73%)		Other *Candida* infections at BG cut-off 80 pg/ml	

(Continued)

Table 4.1 *(Continued)*

Target	Assay	Population tested	Sensitivity	Specificity	Comments	Ref.
			Metabolic tests			
D-arabinitol	Enzymatic-chromogenic	Prospective analysis of high risk oncology patients and control patients that included those with fever, neutropenia, and mucosal colonization with *Candida* but no culture evidence of IC, and those without these and also without culture evidence of IC.	31/42 (74%)	178/206 (86%)	Candidemia patients	*(9)*
			25/30 (83%)		Persistent candidemia patients	
			4/10 (40%)		Invasive tissue candidiasis w/o candidemia	
			7/16 (44%)		Deep mucosal candidiasis patients	
	Enzymatic-fluorometric	Retrospective evaluation of patients with candidemia and healthy control patients	63/83 (76%)	89/100 (89%)	Candidemia patients	*(10)*
			25/30 (83%)		Persistent candidemia patients	

BG, 1,3-β-D-glucan.
[a]Ramco Laboratories, Stafford, TX.
[b]Bio-Rad, Marnes-la-Coquette, France.
[c]Bio-Rad, Munich, Germany.
[d]Seikagaku Corp., Tokyo, Japan.
[e]Cape Cod Assoc., East Falmouth, MA.

Candida EIA test (Bio-Rad, Munich, Germany). Although the EIA test is more sensitive than the LA test, they are both limited by the rapid clearance of mannan antigenemia. In an effort to overcome this, a combination EIA test was developed to detect mannan antigen and anti-mannan antibodies simultaneously, marketed as the Platelia *Candida* Antibody and Antigen test (Bio-Rad, Marnes-la-Coquette, France). When this test was used retrospectively in high-risk patients with proven invasive candidiasis and control patients who included hospitalized patients without *Candida* infections, patients with other deep-seated mycoses and normal healthy patients, this combination test showed a sensitivity of 80% and specificity of 93% *(8)*.

3.3. Detection of Fungal Metabolites

D-Arabinitol (DA) is a five-carbon polyol metabolite that is produced by several pathogenic *Candida* species (except for *C. krusei* and *C. glabrata*). It has been shown to be present in higher serum concentrations in humans and animals with IC than in uninfected or colonized controls, making it potentially useful as a diagnostic marker for IC. There are two general methods to measure DA: gas chromatography or an enzymatic method. The former is labor intensive and not readily available in most hospital labs, while the latter is more suited to a commercial test kit, as is currently marketed in Japan as Arabinitec-Auto (Marukin Diagnostics, Osaka, Japan). This assay is also available for DA testing on urine samples. Several studies have shown that DA can be detected earlier than *Candida* in blood cultures and that serial measurements correlate well with clinical response to therapy *(9,10)*.

3.4. Nucleic Acid Detection

Many different methods have been developed and studied with promising results, but each has different limitations, such as sensitivity, specificity, reproducibility, cost, or commercial availability.

3.5. Conclusions and Recommendations

Tests being investigated are promising as additional diagnostic strategies in the detection of IC. In general, there does seem to be utility in the tests for mannan antigen/antibody, serum BG, and serum DA as adjunctive tests in combination with cultures, histopathology, and radiology. As yet, no single test has been demonstrated to have optimal sensitivity and specificity. Several studies have compared these tests with one another, with variable results, differences in methodology, and small sample populations making it difficult to draw any conclusions. Their greatest value appears to be in serial testing of high-risk populations in which the trend (rather than a single value) will improve sensitivity, help make an earlier diagnosis, and monitor the effectiveness of empirically instituted antifungal therapy. A potential strategy would be the use of two or more of these tests in combination to further improve accuracy in making the correct diagnosis. For now, these modalities can only be recommended as supplements and cannot be relied on as sole diagnostic methods. Further, rigorous, prospective clinical trials are needed to determine which will offer the greatest clinical utility.

4. ASPERGILLOSIS

There are a variety of clinical manifestations of *Aspergillus* infection including aspergillomas, allergic bronchopulmonary aspergillosis (ABPA), chronic invasive aspergillosis, and IA. Different types of immunologic tests have shown different utility for this spectrum of disease.

4.1. Antibody Detection

The diagnosis of aspergilloma is made by combined radiologic and serologic testing, where immunoglobulin G (IgG) antibodies are usually positive. Similarly, for ABPA, a combination of routine blood tests, radiographic findings, skin testing for *Aspergillus* sensitivity, and both IgG and IgE antibody positivity are used for diagnosis. Conversely, antibody detection is less useful and not recommended for invasive disease because the immunocompromised patients most at risk are less likely to mount a sufficient response.

4.2. Antigen Detection

Galactomannan (GM) is a polysaccharide component of the *Aspergillus* cell wall. It has been demonstrated in the sera of patients with IA and thus has been the target of several serum detection assays. These assays vary in the laboratory method and antibody type used for detection. An earlier test called the Pastorex *Aspergillus* (Bio-Rad, Hercules, CA) utilized an LA method with a monoclonal antibody. It yielded disappointing results with low sensitivity unless multiple samples were used and false-positive reactions from cross-reactivity of the antibody with several other fungal species *(11,12)*. A newer, commercially available test is the Platelia *Aspergillus* (Bio-Rad, Hercules, CA). This sandwich ELISA uses the same monoclonal antibody but has the ability to detect GM at much lower limits, thereby improving the test's sensitivity and allowing earlier detection of IA. In a retrospective review of stored specimens on bone marrow transplant and leukemia patients, the study leading to its FDA approval, this assay had a sensitivity of 81% and specificity of 89% *(13)*. Several prospective studies have tested it on a variety of patients, from those with hematopoietic stem cell transplants to those with neutropenic fevers, with variable results *(14,15)*. False-negative results can occur due to limited angioinvasion, low fungal load, high antibody titers, or the use of prophylactic or preemptive antifungals. Alternatively, false positives occur due to cross-reactivity of the assay with other fungal species, certain bacterial exoantigens, or several fungal-derived antibiotics. Although it can be detected in other body fluids, the GM assay is validated only for serum samples at this time (Table 4.2).

4.3. Detection of Fungal Metabolites

Mannitol, a six-carbon acyclic polyol, is produced in large amounts by many different fungi, including several *Aspergillus* species in culture. Unfortunately, available data do not support the usefulness of mannitol as a diagnostic marker.

4.4. Nucleic Acid Detection

While DNA detection assays for *Aspergillus* have had mixed results, mRNA detection assays have shown more promise but still need further evaluation *(17)*.

Table 4.2
Studies of *Aspergillus* galactomannan antigen detection

Assay	Population tested	Sensitivity	Specificity	Comments	Ref.
Pastorex LA[a]	Retrospective analysis of at-risk neutropenic patients	Prov/Prob 7/10 (70%)	44/51 (86%)	Single positive test was considered true positive	*(11)*
Platelia ELISA[a]	As above	Prov/Prob 9/10 (90%)	36/51 (71%)	ELISA was able to detect IA earlier then LA	*(11)*
Pastorex LA	Retrospective analysis of bone marrow transplant recipients	Prov 4/25 (16%) Prob 7/15 (47%) Poss 0/8 (0%)	169/169 (100%)	Single positive test was considered true positive	*(12)*
Platelia ELISA	As above	Prov 19/25 (76%) Prob 14/15 (93%) Poss 8/8 (100%)	138/169 (82%)	ELISA was able to detect IA earlier than LA earlier than LA	*(12)*
Platelia ELISA	Prospective monitoring of hematopoietic stem cell transplant patients	Prov 17/18 (94%) Prob 0/0 (0%) Poss 0/6 (0%)	72/73 (99%)	ELISA was able to detect IA earlier than by other means. Consecutive positives were considered true positive	*(14)*
Platelia ELISA	Retrospective analysis of orthotopic liver transplant recipients	Prov/Prob 5/9 (56)	31/33 (94%)	Consecutive positive were considered true positive	*(16)*

(*Continued*)

Table 4.2 *(Continued)*

Assay	Population tested	Sensitivity	Specificity	Comments	Ref.
Platelia ELISA	Prospective monitoring of hematology- oncology and intensive care unit patients	Prov 0/3 (0%) Prob 17/31 (55%) Poss 14/22 (64%)	748/751 (100%)	Consecutive positive were considered true positive	*(15)*
Platelia ELISA	Retrospective analysis of bone marrow transplant and leukemia patients (including children)	Prov/Prob 25/31 (81%)	132/148 (89%)		*(13)*

Prov, proven; Prob, probable; Poss, possible.
[a]Bio-Rad, Hercules, CA.

4.5. Conclusions and Recommendations

Despite the broad spectrum of disease caused by *Aspergillus* organisms, it is the invasive disease that is most important and most challenging diagnostically. While nucleic acid detection assays seem to hold some promise, only the Platelia *Aspergillus* GM assay can currently be recommended to support a diagnosis of IA in the appropriate clinical setting. This test has shown increased specificity with serial sampling and can be used to screen patients on a twice weekly basis during periods of severe immunosuppression or to monitor patients once or twice weekly while they are on therapy. All clinicians should keep in mind the potential for false-positive and false-negative results and incorporate the GM results into the general clinical assessment of the patient, rather than as the sole basis on which to change management. For instance, a change in the assay from negative to positive in an immunosuppressed patient under surveillance should prompt a more thorough investigation for IA, while a change from positive to negative should lend support to other evidence that proper therapy has been instituted. In addition, it is important to remember that the positive predictive value of this test is highest in populations with a high pretest probability; using it for routine diagnosis in lower risk populations will likely increase the chance that a positive result is a false positive. Despite its limitations, this assay is a suitable, noninvasive adjunct for diagnosing and managing IA (Box 4.1).

Box 4.1. Recommendations for using *Aspergillus* galactomannan antigen assay

1. Twice weekly monitoring of patients during periods of severe immunosuppression
2. Retesting of any positive results during this time period to improve specificity
3. For patients presenting with compatible clinical findings, use it as an adjunct in making a diagnosis
4. Once treatment is initiated, use it to monitor response to treatment (usually once a week)
5. Always interpret the results in the context of other clinical and laboratory findings

5. CRYPTOCOCCOSIS

Culture and histopathology remain the gold standards for diagnosing cryptococcal disease. An alternate method is serologic tests, which have the advantage of more rapidly establishing a diagnosis and allowing initiation of treatment.

5.1. Antibody Detection

Tests for cryptococcal antibodies are not useful and are not widely available for clinical use because they have high false-positive and false-negative rates.

5.2. Antigen Detection

Some of the most important and rapid serodiagnostic tests available for any fungi are those used to detect the cryptococcal capsular polysaccharide antigen (Table 4.3). These tests utilize a variety of different laboratory techniques for antigen detection. In a comparison study of four LA assays and one ELISA assay, they all performed

Table 4.3
Studies of *Cryptococcus* antigen detection

Assay	Population tested	Sensitivity	Specificity	Comments	Ref.
Crypto LA[a]	182 CSF/90 serum samples. 19 CSF/30 serum positive by culture (48 from HIV patients).	CSF 100% Serum 83%	CSF 98% Serum 98%		*(18)*
Myco-Immune LA[b]	Risk factors of patients with negative results not noted	CSF 100% Serum 83%	CSF 97% Serum 100%		
Immy Latex-Crypto Antigen[c]		CSF 93% Serum 97%	CSF 93% Serum 93%	Uses pronase on CSF/serum	*(18)*
Calas Latex-Crypto Antigen[d]		CSF 100% Serum 97%	CSF 96% Serum 95%	Uses pronase on serum	
Premier EIA[d]		CSF 100% Serum 93%	CSF 98% Serum 96%		
Unknown assay	Case report—2 patients with *Cryptococcus* in pleural fluid and analysis of pleural effusions in a group of controls for cryptococcal antigen	2/2 (100%)	12/12 (100%)		*(20)*

Crypto-LA[a] or Crypto-Test[e]	Retrospective review—multiple samples, 9 immunocompetent/4 immunocompromised patients with cryptococcal meningitis and a large group of uninfected patients	CSF 9/9 (100%)	2997/3000 (100%)(Of 3 positives—1 immune compromised, 2 immune competent)	Immunocompromised patients	(21)
		CSF 3/13 (23%)		Immunocompetent patients	
Unknown assay	Retrospective review—42 HIV-negative patients with pulmonary Cryptococcus (6 patients with disseminated infection)	CSF 3/12 (25%) Serum 7/15 (47%)		Immunocompromised patients	(22)
		CSF 0/3 (0%) Serum 0/3 (0%)		Immunocompetent patients	

[a]International Biological Labs, Cranbury, NJ.
[b]American MicroScan, Mahwah, NJ. [c]Immuno-Mycologics, Norman, OK.
[d]Meridian Diagnostics, Cincinnati, OH.
[e]Bioproducts, Walkersville, MD.

well when used to analyze cerebrospinal fluid (CSF) samples of predominantly human immunodeficiency virus (HIV)-positive patients *(18)*. The same study also showed good results for antigen detection in serum samples, but only with the ELISA and the two pronase pretreated LA assays. It is well known, however, that all of these assays are less sensitive when used in immunocompetent patients. One advantage in either patient population is the quantitative nature of the antigen tests, with higher titers generally indicating a higher burden of organisms. This also gives prognostic information such that titers of 1:32 or greater are found in 90% of patients with ultimately fatal infections, but in only 10% of those who are eventually cured of their infection; and titers of 1:8 or greater at the end of treatment are associated with a higher incidence of relapse *(19)*. These tests can also be used to analyze pleural fluid samples in patients with suspected cryptococcal pneumonia *(20)*. The only limitation of these assays is occasional false-positive results, generally in low titers, in patients with disseminated trichosporonosis, *Capnocytophaga canimorsus* sepsis, and *Stomatococcus* infection.

5.3. Detection of Fungal Metabolites

Cryptococcus species, like *Aspergillus* species, also produce large amounts of mannitol, but it has not proven useful as a diagnostic marker for this disease either.

5.4. Nucleic Acid Detection

Several studies have shown the feasibility of using polymerase chain reaction (PCR) technology to diagnose *Cryptococcus* infections *(23,24)*. Although these findings are encouraging, they have not been fully evaluated to establish sensitivity, specificity, and role in clinical management of patients with suspected cryptococcal disease.

5.5. Conclusions and Recommendations

Cryptococcal infection is the rare condition in which a serodiagnostic test has proven not only to have sufficient sensitivity and specificity, but also to have good clinical correlation. Several kits are commercially available. Although a positive cryptococcal antigen result is highly suggestive of infection and can be the sole basis for initiating targeted therapy, definitive proof of disease still does require culture or histopathology and efforts to prove the diagnosis by these means are always warranted. The clinical utility of these antigen tests is different for acquired immunodeficiency syndrome (AIDS) patients and immunocompetent patients. For AIDS patients with suspected meningeal disease who are able to undergo a lumbar puncture (LP), the CSF antigen test should be used to make a rapid, accurate diagnosis. In patients unable to undergo an LP or with vague central nervous system symptoms not warranting an LP, a serum antigen test may be used as a substitute for screening because it has sensitivity comparable to that of a CSF test in this setting. If the serum test is positive, indicating disseminated disease, the CSF opening pressure should be checked (if no other contraindications exist), as this has implications for management. A pleural fluid antigen titer can also be checked if pneumonia is suspected. In addition, the baseline and end treatment antigen titers are helpful for prognostic purposes. However, serial measurement of antigen titers during therapy is not recommended in this patient population, in whom these fluctuations do not accurately correlate with clinical response. This is especially true for serum specimens.

In immunocompetent patients, because both the CSF and serum assays have a lower sensitivity, both tests should be utilized if meningitis is suspected; pleural fluid can also be tested if pneumonia is suspected. Further, because this population is more capable of clearing antigenemia, serial measurement of antigen titers while on therapy (generally at 2-week intervals) may be useful for documenting therapeutic response and predicting relapse. As is the case for AIDS patients, the baseline and end treatment antigen titers provide useful prognostic information. In both patient populations, care must be taken not to compare titers derived from different kits given the lack of standardization among manufacturers (Box 4.2).

Box 4.2. Recommendations for using cryptococcal antigen tests in different populations AIDS patients

1. For meningeal symptoms, check a cerebrospinal fluid antigen. If unable to do lumbar puncture, can check serum antigen
2. For non-meningeal symptoms, check a serum or site-specific antigen (i.e., pleural fluid)
3. A positive serum antigen suggests disseminated disease (including meningeal involvement) and a lumbar puncture should be done to measure opening pressure, which is important for management
4. Antigen titers correlate with disease burden and provide prognostic information, but should not be followed serially during therapy

NON-IMMUNOSUPPRESSED PATIENTS

1. For meningeal symptoms, check both CSF and serum antigens
2. For non-meningeal symptoms, check a serum or site-specific antigen (i.e., pleural fluid)
3. Antigen titers correlate with disease burden, provide prognostic information, and can be followed at 2- week intervals during therapy to document therapeutic response and predict relapse

6. HISTOPLASMOSIS

The standard method for the diagnosis of histoplasmosis remains isolation and specific identification of the causative organism. The process can take 2 to 4 weeks and the necessary specimens can be difficult to obtain. Immunologic tests offer a more rapid alternative, and in some manifestations of the disease are the preferred means of establishing a diagnosis.

6.1. Antibody Detection

The two *Histoplasma capsulatum* species-specific antigens against which host antibodies are made are the H and M antigens. Antibodies against H antigen form during active histoplasmosis, while antibodies against M antigen may be formed in active or chronic histoplasmosis and are usually the first to arise on seroconversion (Table 4.4). These antibodies can be detected via either ID or CF assays, where ID is

Table 4.4
Studies of *Histoplasma* antigen and antibody detection

Assay	Patients with AIDS and DH	Patients without AIDS with DH	Patients without DH(limited disease)	Controls	Specimen	Ref.
			Antigen			
RIA[a]	19/27 (70)[b]	2/4 (50)		0/122 (0)	BAL fluid	
	25/27 (93)			0/122 (0)	Urine	(26)
	23/26 (89)			0/122 (0)	Serum	
	3/4 (75)	2/10 (20)		1/28 (4)	CSF	
	3/4 (75)	4/10 (40)			Urine	(27)
	2/4 (50)	2/10 (20)			Serum	
	75/79 (95)	22/27 (82)	24/82 (29)		Urine	(28)
	54/63 (86)	7/11 (64)	6/26 (23)		Serum	
	38/40 (95)	12/16 (75)	11/30 (37)	1/96 (1)	Urine	(25)
EIA[a]	38/40 (95)	12/16 (75)	11/30 (37)	1/96 (1)	Urine	(25)
			Antibody			
ID[c]	32/52 (62)	14/21 (67)	65/81(80)		Serum	(28)
		17/21 (81)	210/255 (82)	4/767 (1)	Serum	(29)
CF[d]	29/46 (63)	14/22 (64)	75/83 (90)		Serum	(28)
	0/3 (0)	7/10 (70)			CSF	(27)
	0/3 (0)	8/9 (89)			Serum	
		12/21 (57)	212/255 (83)	15/357 (4)	Serum[e]	(29)
		17/21 (81)	197/255 (77)	8/357 (2)	Serum[f]	

DH, disseminated histoplasmosis; RIA, radioimmunoassay; EIA, enzyme immunoassay; ID, immunodiffusion; CF, complement fixation.
[a]Mira Vista Diagnostics, Indianapolis, IN.
[b]Number of positive tests/total number of subjects (%).
[c]Meridian Diagnostics, Cincinnati, OH.
[d]Immuno-Mycologics, Norman, OK; 1:8 or greater titer considered positive for CF testing.
[e]Antibody to yeast phase antigen.
[f]Antibody to mycelial phase antigen.

more specific and CF is more sensitive. Antibodies against M antigen are detected 6 to 8 weeks after exposure in 50% to 80% of patients, but can persist for years in patients who have recovered from infection; therefore their presence does not distinguish remote infection from current disease. On the other hand, antibodies against H antigen are detected in only 10% to 20% of exposed patients, but their presence signifies an active infection. In general, asymptomatic patients are less likely to have detectable antibody levels, and if present, they are usually in lower titers. This is evidenced by the low levels of antibody detected in approximately 10% of healthy patients residing in an endemic area. Antibody titers generally decline over several months after exposure, but may remain positive for years in some chronic forms of the disease. False-negative results can occur in immunocompromised patients approximately 50% of the time and less frequently in other patients during the early stages of infection. False-positive results occur in approximately 15% of patients, mainly due to cross-reaction with the agents of coccidioidomycosis or blastomycosis.

6.2. Antigen Detection

One of the major developments in diagnostic strategies for histoplasmosis was the introduction of antigen detection assays that could recognize a histoplasmosis polysaccharide antigen (Table 4.4). Depending on the disease manifestation, this antigen can be present in urine, serum, CSF, or bronchoalveolar lavage (BAL) fluid. The original assay was an RIA that was costly and posed a risk to laboratory personnel because of its radioactivity. The newer assay is an EIA test (Mira Vista Diagnostics, Indianapolis, IN) that uses a monoclonal antibody and has shown results similar to the RIA test *(25)*. Antigen detection assays are especially useful for establishing a diagnosis in immunosuppressed patients and patients with acute disseminated forms of disease. Further, these tests are useful for monitoring antigen levels during treatment, where levels decrease with appropriate therapy and increase with disease relapse. Some cross-reactivity of the assay can be seen with penicilliosis, paracoccidioidomycosis, or blastomycosis. False-negative results can also occur depending on the population tested and the severity of illness.

6.3. Detection of Fungal Metabolites

No tests of this nature are currently available.

6.4. Nucleic Acid Detection

Preliminary studies support the feasibility of molecular approaches to the diagnosis of histoplasmosis and suggest that PCR and DNA probes might improve the accuracy for identifying *H. capsulatum* in tissues or body fluids. But these methodologies have not been validated by comparison with culture or antigen detection tests *(30)*.

6.5. Skin Testing

Skin testing with histoplasmin antigen is a useful epidemiologic tool to document past exposure and to investigate histoplasmosis outbreaks. It is of little use in the diagnosis of individual cases. Prior skin test positivity can be lost with disseminated disease or immunosuppression.

6.6. Conclusions and Recommendations

Immunodiagnostic tests for histoplasmosis are a proven adjunct to the usual diagnostic methods of culture and histopathology (Table 4.5). Because of the wide spectrum of disease with histoplasmosis, there are different recommendations to help

Table 4.5
Immunologic tests in different nondisseminated clinical manifestations of histoplasmosis

Disease manifestations	Antigen sensitivity	Antibody sensitivity	Recommendations
1. Acute localized pulmonary histoplasmosis (with possible sequelae of mediastinal granuloma, pericarditis, and rheumatologic syndromes)	<40% overall	>80% when both IDand CF tests are done (at 4–6 weeks)	Antibody testing is preferred method. Send both ID and CF antibody tests.
2. Acute diffuse reticulonodular or miliary pulmonary histoplasmosis	~90% in urine, ~70% in serum, less frequently in other sterile body fluids	60–80%	Antigen testing of serum and urine is preferred method. Antibody testing will identify remaining cases. In routine clinical practice, should send both to speed the diagnostic process.
3. Chronic pulmonary histoplasmosis	~20%	90–100%	Sputum or BAL fluid for culture are preferred. Can use antibody test for remaining cases.
4. Fibrosing mediastinitis, broncholithiasis, asymptomatic lung granulomas, and chronic mediastinal lymphadenopathy	Antigen test is usually negative	50–65%	Antibody testing is preferred method. Send both ID and CF antibody tests.
5. *Histoplasma* meningitis	~20–70% in CSF, ~40–70% in urine, ~20–50% in serum	0–70% in CSF, 0–80% in serum	Antigen testing in CSF, serum, and urine plus antibody testing in serum and CSF (use CF assay).

Data and recommendations from refs. 24–29.

guide the appropriate use of immunologic tests. Patients with acute localized disease and a low burden of organisms or patients with chronic sequelae of a prior histoplasmosis infection should be diagnosed predominantly via antibody testing. Conversely, patients with acute diffuse disease and a high burden of organisms are most amenable to antigen testing. Although urinary antigen detection is the most sensitive for these patients as a whole, CSF and BAL fluid testing may prove more valuable in patients with disease at those specific sites. A third category of patients, those with chronic pulmonary histoplasmosis, can usually be diagnosed by routine cultures of sputum or BAL fluid. Antibody tests can be used if these cultures are negative. Clinicians should use caution when using serial antigen testing to follow disease progression; concurrent testing of both the prior and the current specimens is essential to counter the assay-to-assay variability.

7. BLASTOMYCOSIS

A high level of suspicion for *Blastomyces* infection is important to its successful diagnosis because no clinical syndrome is characteristic for infection with this organism. While definitive diagnosis requires the growth of the organism from clinical specimens, a presumptive diagnosis can be made by histological characteristics and further supportive evidence can be gained from immunologic tests.

7.1. Antibody Detection

Early serologic tests for blastomycosis were directed toward detecting host antibodies against *B. dermatitidis* A antigen. These tests utilized different laboratory techniques including ID, CF, and ELISA. The ID test has the most specificity and the ELISA test has the most sensitivity. However, all the tests have limited sensitivity for diagnosing acute disease because the mean peak seroprevalence of antibody occurs 50 to 70 days after the onset of symptoms *(31)*. An additional limitation is the presence of detectable antibodies for 1 year or more even after successful treatment. Antibody detection assays directed against the WI-1 antigen of the outer cell wall of *B. dermatitidis* have also been explored with promising results, but are not currently available commercially *(32)*.

7.2. Antigen Detection

An antigen detection assay for use on urine specimens of patients with suspected blastomycosis is also available (Mira Vista Diagnostics, Indianapolis, IN). This assay targets a glycoprotein antigen that unfortunately is not genus specific. Although it has a sensitivity of 93%, the specificity is only 79% owing to significant cross-reactivity of the assay with histoplasmosis, paracoccidioidomycosis, and penicilliosis *(33)*.

7.3. Detection of Fungal Metabolites

No tests of this nature are currently available.

7.4. Nucleic Acid Detection

While nucleic acid detection assays have been examined in epidemiologic studies of blastomycosis, they have not been evaluated in clinical specimens of such cases.

7.5. *Conclusions and Recommendations*

Several clinical features of blastomycosis make serodiagnosis relatively less important. Unlike histoplasmosis or coccidioidomycosis, in which many of the recognized cases are acute pulmonary infections with negative sputum smears and cultures, identified blastomycosis cases are usually chronic pulmonary infections or disseminated infections of the skin and bones. In both of these conditions, histopathology and cultures are usually positive and easy to acquire. Further, despite the availability of multiple assays to detect *Blastomyces* antibodies or antigens, their sensitivities and specificities vary significantly and they are generally not helpful for diagnosing blastomycosis. Therefore, a negative test should never be used to rule out disease, nor should a positive test be an indication to start treatment.

8. COCCIDIOIDOMYCOSIS

Culture and histopathology are the gold standards for diagnosing coccidioidomycosis, but have several limitations. First, although *Coccidioides* species are readily cultured, the culture needs to be performed under Biosafety Level 2 conditions and poses a certain degree of risk to laboratory personnel. Second, because *Coccidioides* species are listed by the Centers for Disease Control (CDC) as potential bioterrorism threats, laboratories working with these fungi must follow extensive security practices (and work under Biosafety Level 3 practices). Third, direct examination of clinical specimens is an insensitive test because of the small number of *Coccidioides* organisms present in most clinical specimens. Finally, the mycelial form of growth rarely allows microscopic identification of *Coccidioides* species, requiring further testing to detect coccidioidal antigen in the fungal extract or a specific ribosomal RNA sequence using a DNA probe. This often has to be carried out by a reference laboratory. Given these limitations, immunologic tests are an important adjunct in helping to establish a diagnosis of coccidioidomycosis.

8.1. *Antibody Detection*

Serologic diagnosis of coccidioidomycosis is based on the detection of anti-coccidioidal antibodies via one of several different laboratory methods (Table 4.6). One such method, the tube precipitin (TP) assay, detects IgM antibodies directed against a heat-stable carbohydrate antigen of the fungal cell wall. These antibodies form relatively early during infection, with approximately 90% of patients developing them in the first 3 weeks of symptomatic disease. For patients with a self-limited illness, these antibodies decline to less than 5 percent within 7 months. A second method, the CF assay, detects IgG antibodies to the chitinase antigen, an enzyme of the fungal cell wall. These antibodies are detected later and persist longer. This assay can also be applied to body fluids other than serum; for example, it detects antibodies in CSF specimens of approximately 60% of patients with coccidioidal meningitis *(34–36)*. The antibody concentrations measured by CF are expressed as titers and generally reflect the extent of infection. As variation between testing results from facility to facility exists, it is suggested that serial measurements be conducted using the same

Table 4.6
Studies of *Coccidioides* antibody detection

Assay	Population tested	Sensitivity	Specificity	Comments	Ref.
TP	Retrospective analysis of antibody detection in serum of a large group of patients with various forms of coccidioidal infection	2524/3219 (78%)		Pulmonary disease	*(37)*
		89/226 (39%)		Disseminated disease	
		33/73 (45%)		Meningeal disease	
	Retrospective analysis of HIV patients with coccidioidal infection	3/7 (43%)			*(38)*
CF	As above	1790/3219 (56%)		Pulmonary disease	*(37)*
		222/226 (98%)		Disseminated disease	
		69/73 (95%)		Meningeal disease	
	As above	5/7 (71%)			*(38)*
	Retrospective analysis of patients with chronic renal failure	5/6 (83%)		Dialysis patients	*(39)*
		14/18 (78%)		Renal transplant patients	
	Retrospective analysis of patients with coccidioidal meningitis	29/30 (97%)		Serum samples	*(34)*
		25/30 (83%)		CSF samples	
	Retrospective analysis of HIV patients with disseminated coccidioidal infection	6/8 (75%)		Serum samples	*(35)*
		4/6 (67%)		CSF samples	

(Continued)

Table 4.6 ***(Continued)***

Assay	Population tested	Sensitivity	Specificity	Comments	Ref.
	Retrospective analysis of antibody detection in CSF of a group of patients with various forms of coccidioidal infection and control patients without coccidioidomycosis	0/9 (0%)	13/13 (100%)	Pulmonary disease	*(36)*
		0/2 (0%)		Disseminated disease	
		14/33 (42%)		Meningeal disease	
IDCF[a]	As above	0/9 (0%)	13/13 (100%)	Pulmonary disease	*(36)*
		1/3 (33%)		Disseminated disease	
		10/19 (53%)		Meningeal disease	
	Retrospective analysis of patients with proven coccidioidomycosis infection and control patients with non-coccidioidal pulmonary illness, other fungal illness, HIV disease and no illness.	47/47 (100%)	362/362 (100%)		*(40)*
EIA[b]	As above	43/47 (92%)	352/362 (97%)	IgG alone	*(40)*
		36/47 (77%)	354/362 (98%)	IgM alone	
		47/47 (100%)	347/362 (96%)	IgG and IgM together	
LA	As above	8/9 (89%)	0/13 (0%)	Pulmonary disease	*(36)*
		3/3 (100%)		Disseminated disease	
		31/33 (94%)		Meningeal disease	

TP, tube precipitin; CF, complement fixation; ID CF, immunodiffusion using complement fixation antigen; EIA, enzyme immunoassay; LA, latex agglutination.

[a]Immuno-Mycologics, Norman, OK.

[b]Meridian Diagnostics, Cincinnati, OH.

laboratory to allow comparison. Use of serial testing can help the clinician gauge disease progression, remission, or cure.

Newer assays involve ID, ELISA, and LA techniques. The commercially available IDTP and IDCF tests (Meridian Diagnostics, Newtown, OH and Immuno-Mycologics, Norman, OK) can use a single prepared specimen to detect (with greater sensitivity) the same IgM and IgG antibodies previously detected by the individual TP and CF assays. The ELISA assay (Meridian Diagnostics, Cincinnati, OH) is highly sensitive for detecting IgM and IgG antibodies in serum or CSF, but its specificity is compromised by some false-positive reactions on CSF specimens and with IgM detection. The LA assay is commercially available, easy to use, and provides rapid results, but is limited by a higher number of false-positive reactions compared to the other assays.

8.2. Antigen Detection

Research laboratories have demonstrated the ability to detect coccidioidomycosis antigen in both acute and chronic disease *(41)*. Currently these tests remain a research interest rather than a clinically applicable procedure.

8.3. Detection of Fungal Metabolites

No tests of this nature are currently available.

8.4. Nucleic Acid Detection

Although studies have demonstrated the feasibility of DNA or RNA detection via PCR techniques in the diagnosis of coccidioidomycosis, this is still of limited utility as PCR positivity appears to be transient *(42)*.

8.5. Skin Testing

Skin testing with coccidioidin antigen or spherulin antigen is a useful epidemiologic tool to document past exposure. It may also be useful in patients in whom pulmonary coccidioidomycosis has already been proven by other means. A negative skin test in such a patient may be a bad prognostic sign, suggesting current or impending dissemination. Standardized, FDA-approved antigen is not currently available.

8.6. Conclusions and Recommendations

The manifestations of most early coccidioidal infections overlap with those of other respiratory infections; therefore, specific laboratory testing is usually required to establish a diagnosis of coccidioidomycosis. Serologic tests are important in the diagnosis of these diseases as specific anti-coccidioidal antibodies develop in many, if not most, patients; though they are often not detectable in the first few weeks or even months after disease onset or in severely immunocompromised hosts. For this reason, the absence of detectable anti-coccidioidal antibodies does not generally exclude the diagnosis of coccidioidomycosis. For most patients who resolve their infection, the antibody concentrations decrease to undetectable levels during the course of illness, so measurable antibodies are more likely to represent a recent or active illness. In general, the commercial ID kit is the most often used assay while the old CF assay is generally reserved for specimens other than serum, such as CSF, pleural fluid, peritoneal fluid, or joint fluid. In any assay, repeat testing will improve the diagnostic yield.

9. PARACOCCIDIOIDOMYCOSIS

A definitive diagnosis of paracoccidioidomycosis requires either direct visualization of the organism in body fluids or tissues or its isolation and growth in culture. Immunologic assays are useful and rapid adjuncts for diagnosing this infection, but unfortunately they are not available in the United States.

9.1. Antibody Detection

Initial efforts at antibody detection utilized cytoplasmic extracts and cell wall components as antigen targets. But these antigens caused significant cross-reactivity with other fungal pathogens, leading to the discovery of more specific *P. brasiliensis* antigens. Using these newer antigens, many antibody detection assays have been developed. The major limitation of these different assays is that antibodies can be detected for years after apparent successful therapy, so their presence does not help determine disease activity. In addition, there is still some cross-reactivity with *H. capsulatum* antigens, and antibody responses are difficult to detect in AIDS patients.

9.2. Antigen Detection

The same cell wall and cytoplasmic components were also used as targets in antigen detection assays. Unfortunately, these assays were also limited because of significant cross-reactivity in sera from patients with other mycoses (i.e., aspergillosis and histoplasmosis). To improve on this, a new target was sought, the 43-kDa glycoprotein (gp43) from culture filtrates; now believed to be a dominant antigen in this disease. An immunoblotting assay, performed on urine specimens, has demonstrated good sensitivity and excellent specificity for the detection of this antigen *(43)*. An ELISA technique with a monoclonal antibody has successfully detected this antigen in serum, CSF, and BAL fluid of patients with confirmed acute and chronic disease states *(44)*. Further, these antigen levels can be followed as a marker of treatment response *(45)*.

9.3. Detection of Fungal Metabolites

No tests of this nature are currently available.

9.4. Nucleic Acid Detection

Despite some early studies using PCR on clinical specimens to detect sequences of the gene that codes for gp43 antigen, no tests of this nature are currently available *(46)*.

Conclusions and Recommendations

Immunologic tests are useful for rapid diagnosis in suspected cases of paracoccidioidomycosis, as approximately 90% of patients with clinical disease have specific antibodies at the time of diagnosis. Further, in disseminated disease, antibody production is elevated and titers are high, providing useful prognostic information. Antibody testing is limited, though, as the presence of antibodies does not differentiate disease activity and their absence does not rule out disease, especially in patients with early disease or those who are severely immunocompromised. These are the populations in whom antigenemia may be detectable, before the development of immune complexes. It is currently advisable to use more than one test for the diagnosis of paracoccidioidomycosis. Serum antibody and serum, urine, or site-specific antigen tests should both be ordered and any positive results should be monitored while the patient is on treatment. There is a concern that the assays may be detecting infection with other mycoses, so the results should be evaluated in the context of the entire clinical picture.

10. OTHER MYCOSES

Immunodiagnostic tests have also been investigated for several other fungal infections, namely mycetoma, zygomycosis (mucormycosis), penicilliosis, sporotrichosis, dermatophytoses, and pneumocystosis. While they target a variety of antigens, antibodies, and nucleic acids, they are unfortunately still limited by a lack of prospective trials and commercial availability and cannot yet be recommended for routine clinical use.

REFERENCES

1. Horvath JA, Dummer S. The use of respiratory tract cultures in the diagnosis of invasive pulmonary aspergillosis. Am J Med 1996;100:171–178.
2. Obayashi T, Yoshida M, Mori T, et al. Plasma (1,3)-beta-D-glucan determination in the diagnosis of invasive deep mycosis and fungal febrile episodes. Lancet 1995;345:17–20.
3. Yuasa K, Goto H, Iguchi M, Okamura T, Ieki R. Evaluation of the diagnostic value of the measurement of (1,3)-beta-D-glucan in patients with pulmonary aspergillosis. Respiration 1996;63:78–83.
4. Ostrosky-Zeichner L, Alexander BD, Kett DH, et al. Multicenter clinical evaluation of the (1,3)-beta-D-glucan assay as an aid to diagnosis of fungal infections in humans. Clin Infect Dis 2005;41:654–659.
5. Walsh TJ, Chanock SJ. Diagnosis of invasive fungal infections: advances in nonculture systems. Curr Clin Top Infect Dis 1998;18:101–153.
6. Mitsutake K, Miyazaki T, Tashiro T, et al. Enolase antigen, mannan antigen, Cand-Tec antigen, and beta-glucan in patients with candidemia. J Clin Microbiol 1996;34:1918–1921.
7. Sanchez ML, Pfaller MA, Cabezudo I, Bale M, Buschelman B. Diagnosis of disseminated candidiasis in hospitalized patients using the Cand-Tec latex agglutination assay. Mycopathologia 1992;118:153–162.
8. Sendid B, Tabouret M, Poirot JL, Mathieu D, Fruit J, Poulain D. New enzyme immunoassays for sensitive detection of circulating *Candida albicans* mannan and antimannan antibodies: useful combined test for diagnosis of systemic candidiasis. J Clin Microbiol 1999;37: 1510–1517.
9. Walsh TJ, Merz WG, Lee JW, et al. Diagnosis and therapeutic monitoring of invasive candidiasis by rapid enzymatic detection of serum D-arabinitol. Am J Med 1995;99: 164–172.
10. Yeo SF, Huie S, Sofair A, Campbell S, Durante A, Wong B. Measurement of serum D-arabinitol/creatinine ratios for initial diagnosis and for predicting outcomes in an unselected, population-based sample of patients with *Candida* fungemia. J Clin Microbiol 2006;44:3894–3899.
11. Verweij PE, Stynen D, Rijs AJ, de Pauw BE, Hoogkamp-Korstanje JA, Meis JF. Sandwich enzyme-linked immunosorbent assay compared with Pastorex latex agglutination test

for diagnosing invasive aspergillosis in immunocompromised patients. J Clin Microbiol 1995;33:1912–1914.
12. Sulahian A, Tabouret M, Ribaud P, et al. Comparison of an enzyme immunoassay and latex agglutination test for detection of galactomannan in the diagnosis of invasive aspergillosis. Eur J Clin Microbiol Infect Dis 1996;15:139–145.
13. Wheat LJ. Rapid diagnosis of invasive aspergillosis by antigen detection. Transpl Infect Dis 2003;5:158–166.
14. Maertens J, Van Eldere J, Verhaegen J, Verbeken E, Verschakelen J, Boogaerts M. Use of circulating galactomannan screening for early diagnosis of invasive aspergillosis in allogeneic stem cell transplant recipients. J Infect Dis 2002;186:1297–1306.
15. Pinel C, Fricker-Hidalgo H, Lebeau B, et al. Detection of circulating *Aspergillus fumigatus* galactomannan: value and limits of the Platelia test for diagnosing invasive aspergillosis. J Clin Microbiol 2003;41:2184–2186.
16. Fortun J, Martin-Davila P, Alvarez ME, et al. *Aspergillus* antigenemia sandwich-enzyme immunoassay test as a serodiagnostic method for invasive aspergillosis in liver transplant recipients. Transplantation 2001;71:145–149.
17. Yoo JH, Choi JH, Choi SM, et al. Application of nucleic acid sequence-based amplification for diagnosis of and monitoring the clinical course of invasive aspergillosis in patients with hematologic diseases. Clin Infect Dis 2005;40:392–398.
18. Tanner DC, Weinstein MP, Fedorciw B, Joho KL, Thorpe JJ, Reller L. Comparison of commercial kits for detection of cryptococcal antigen. J Clin Microbiol 1994;32:1680–1684.
19. Davies SF, Sarosi GA. Role of serodiagnostic tests and skin tests in the diagnosis of fungal disease. Clin Chest Med 1987;8:135–146.
20. Young EJ, Hirsh DD, Fainstein V, Williams TW. Pleural effusions due to *Cryptococcus neoformans*: a review of the literature and report of two cases with cryptococcal antigen determinations. Am Rev Respir Dis 1980;121:743–747.
21. Berlin L, Pincus JH. Cryptococcal meningitis: false-negative antigen test results and cultures in nonimmunosuppressed patients. Arch Neurol 1989;46:1312–1316.
22. Aberg JA, Mundy LM, Powderly WG. Pulmonary cryptococcosis in patients without HIV infection. Chest 1999;115:734–740.
23. Bialek R, Weiss M, Bekure-Nemariam K, et al. Detection of *Cryptococcus neoformans* DNA in tissue samples by nested and real-time PCR assays. Clin Diagn Lab Immunol 2002;9:461–469.
24. Rappelli P, Are R, Casu G, Fiori PL, Cappuccinelli P, Aceti A. Development of a nested PCR for detection of *Cryptococcus neoformans* in cerebrospinal fluid. J Clin Microbiol 1998;36:3438–3440.
25. Durkin MM, Connolly PA, Wheat LJ. Comparison of radioimmunoassay and enzyme-linked immunoassay methods for detection of *Histoplasma capsulatum* var. *capsulatum* antigen. J Clin Microbiol 1997;35:2252–2255.
26. Wheat LJ, Connolly-Stringfield P, Williams B et al. Diagnosis of histoplasmosis in patients with the acquired immunodeficiency syndrome by detection of *Histoplasma capsulatum* polysaccharide antigen in bronchoalveolar lavage fluid. Am Rev Respir Dis 1992;145: 1421–1424.
27. Wheat LJ, Kohler RB, Tewari RP, Garten M, French ML. Significance of *Histoplasma* antigen in the cerebrospinal fluid of patients with meningitis. Arch Intern Med 1989;149:302–304.
28. Williams B, Fojtasek M, Connolly-Stringfield P, Wheat J. Diagnosis of histoplasmosis by antigen detection during an outbreak in Indianapolis, Ind. Arch Pathol Lab Med 1994;118:1205–1208.

29. Wheat J, French ML, Kohler RB, et al. The diagnostic laboratory tests for histoplasmosis. Ann Intern Med 1982;97:680–685.
30. Wheat LJ. Current diagnosis of histoplasmosis. Trends Microbiol 2003;11:488–494.
31. Klein BS, Vergeront JM, Kaufman L, et al. Serological tests for blastomycosis: assessments during a large point-source outbreak in Wisconsin. J Infect Dis 1987;155:262–268.
32. Soufleris AJ, Klein BS, Courtney BT, Proctor ME, Jones JM. Utility of anti-WI-1 serological testing in the diagnosis of blastomycosis in Wisconsin residents. Clin Infect Dis 1994; 19:87–92.
33. Durkin M, Witt J, LeMonte A, Wheat B, Connolly P. Antigen assay with the potential to aid in diagnosis of blastomycosis. J Clin Microbiol 2004;42:4873–4875.
34. Bouza E, Dreyer JS, Hewitt WL, Meyer RD. Coccidioidal meningitis: an analysis of thirty-one cases and review of the literature. Medicine 1981;60:139–172.
35. Antoniskis D, Larsen RA, Akil B, Rarick MU, Leedom JM. Seronegative disseminated coccidioidomycosis in patients with HIV infection. AIDS 1990;4:691–693.
36. Pappagianis D, Krasnow RI, Beall S. False-positive reactions of cerebrospinal fluid and diluted sera with the coccidioidal latex-agglutination test. Am J Clin Pathol 1976;66: 916–921.
37. Smith CE, Saito MT, Beard RR, Kepp RM, Clark RW, Eddie BU. Serological tests in the diagnosis and prognosis of coccidioidomycosis. Am J Hyg 1950;52:1–21.
38. Bronnimann DA, Adam RD, Galgiani JN, et al. Coccidioidomycosis in the acquired immunodeficiency syndrome. Ann Intern Med 1987;106:372–379.
39. Cohen IM, Galgiani JN, Potter D, Ogden DA. Coccidioidomycosis in renal replacement therapy. Arch Intern Med 1982;142:489–494.
40. Kaufman L, Sekhon AS, Moledina N, Jalbert M, Pappagianis D. Comparative evaluation of commercial Premier EIA and microimmunodiffusion and complement fixation tests for *Coccidioides immitis* antibodies. J Clin Microbiol 1995;33:618–619.
41. Galgiani JN, Grace GM, Lundergen LL. New serologic tests for early detection of coccidioidomycosis. J Infect Dis 1991;163:671–674.
42. Johnson SM, Simmons KA, Pappagianis D. Amplification of coccidioidal DNA in clinical specimens by PCR. J Clin Microbiol 2004;42:1982–1985.
43. Salina MA, Shikanai-Yasuda MA, Mendes RP, Barraviera B, Mendes-Giannini MJ. Detection of circulating *Paracoccidioides brasiliensis* antigen in urine of paracoccidioidomycosis patients before and during treatment. J Clin Microbiol 1998;36: 1723–1728.
44. Marques da Silva SH, Colombo AL, Blotta MH, Lopes JD, Queiroz-Telles F, Pires de Camargo Z. Detection of circulating gp43 antigen in serum, cerebrospinal fluid and bronchoalveolar lavage of patients with paracoccidioidomycosis. J Clin Microbiol 2003;41:3675–3680.
45. Marques da Silva SH, Queiroz-Telles F, Colombo AL, Blotta MH, Lopes JD, Pires De Camargo Z. Monitoring gp43 antigenemia in paracoccidioidomycosis patients during therapy. J Clin Microbiol 2004;42:2419–2424.
46. Bialek R, Ibricevic A, Aepinus C, et al. Detection of *Paracoccidioides brasiliensis* in tissue samples by a nested PCR assay. J Clin Microbiol 2000;38:2940–2942.

SUGGESTED READINGS

Galgiani J. Laboratory diagnosis of coccidioidomycosis. UpToDate; www.uptodate.com.
Pappagianis D, Zimmer BL. Serology of coccidioidomycosis. Clin Microbiol Rev 1990;3: 247–268.

Powderly WG, Cloud GA, Dismukes WE, Saag MS. Measurement of cryptococcal antigen in serum and cerebrospinal fluid: value in the management of AIDS-associated cryptococcal meningitis. Clin Infect Dis 1994;18:789–792.
Wheat LJ. Rapid diagnosis of invasive aspergillosis by antigen detection. Transpl Infect Dis 2003;5:158–166.
Yeo SF, Wong B. Current status of nonculture methods for diagnosis of invasive fungal infections. Clin Microbiol Rev 2002;15:465–484.

5
Diagnostic Radiology

Maria Angela C. Hospenthal, MD
and Constanza J. Gutierrez, MD

1. INTRODUCTION

Although there are no pathognomonic radiological findings associated with human mycoses, use of diagnostic imaging is integral to the diagnosis and management of most fungal infections. In conjunction with clinical data, including patient symptoms, duration of illness, underlying immune function, and other risk factors (including endemic exposures, invasive devices, coexisting disease, surgeries, and other therapies), radiographic diagnosis can be directed to enhance its sensitivity and thus usefulness. In human fungal infections, imaging of the central nervous system (CNS), upper and lower respiratory tract, abdomen, and musculoskeletal system is generally the focus of these diagnostic studies.

2. CENTRAL NERVOUS SYSTEM IMAGING

Magnetic resonance imaging (MRI) is superior to computed tomography (CT) in evaluating fungal infections of the brain and has been shown to be more sensitive than CT for detecting abnormalities. MRI is especially helpful in the early phases of disease when the brain CT may be nondiagnostic. MRI takes advantage of the inherent properties of molecules, especially hydrogen, and manipulates their behavior in an electromagnetic field to generate an image. The composition of tissues and their differences when pathology is present can therefore be distinguished by altering parameters of the electromagnetic field to see the effect on the molecules of the tissue being evaluated. Terminology to include longitudinal relaxation time (T1) and transverse relaxation time (T2) relate to signal intensities that offer details on specific tissue characteristics. Findings on MRI, such as edema and contrast enhancement, are affected by the inflammatory response, which itself is highly dependent on the competence of the immune system. Nevertheless, noncircumscribed, ill-defined areas with little or no contrast enhancement should raise the suspicion for fungal infection *(1)*. CT of the brain with contrast may be normal initially and thus is more helpful

From: *Infectious Disease: Diagnosis and Treatment of Human Mycoses*
Edited by: D. R. Hospenthal and M. G. Rinaldi © Humana Press Inc., Totowa, NJ

in assessing later stages of infection with eventual findings of focal ring enhancing or hemorrhagic lesions. Other brain imaging modalities include proton magnetic resonance spectroscopy with MRI, which has been reported to be useful in the evaluation of infection due to zygomycosis (mucormycosis) and cryptococcosis *(2)*. A wide variety of radiologic findings can be found, although intracerebral masses and meningeal enhancement predominate in these infections (Table 5.1).

2.1. CNS Mass Lesions

Intracerebral masses are one of the more common findings in fungal brain infections. Predominantly, granulomas or solid enhancing lesions are reported. In *Aspergillus* infections, these have sometimes been referred to as "aspergillomas." Likewise, in patients with cryptococcal infections, the term "cryptococcoma" has been used. Most of these lesions are found in the basal ganglia. On T2 weighted images (T2WI), cryptococcomas can be single or multiple punctate hyperintense round lesions usually less than 3 mm in size *(3,4)*. Intraparenchymal cryptococcomas show low signal intensity on T1 weighted images (T1W1) and high intensity on T2 WI *(5,6)*. Persistence of cryptococcomas over a prolonged period of time has been documented and found to be inconsistent with active disease *(7)*. Single or multiple enhancing brain lesions have also been reported in *Histoplasma*, *Candida*, and *Paracoccidioides* infections.

Abscesses are frequently found in fungal brain infections *(8)*. These lesions can be multiple, hypodense, and may exert little mass effect. They may or may not enhance *(9)* (Fig. 5.1). Although abscesses occur most commonly in the cerebral hemispheres, they have also been visualized in the cerebellum and brainstem *(10)*. Organisms reported to cause abscess formation include *Aspergillus*, *Coccidioides*, *Cryptococcus*, and *Candida*. Candidal organisms tend to cause focal necrosis producing microabscesses *(11,12)*.

Table 5.1
Abnormalities more commonly seen in central nervous system imaging of fungal infections

Radiological finding	Fungus
Granulomas or solid enhancing lesions	*Aspergillus, Cryptococcus, Histoplasma, Candida, Paracoccidioides*
Abscesses	*Aspergillus, Blastomyces* (epidural), *Coccidioides, Cryptococcus, Candida,* dematiaceous fungi, *Pseudallescheria boydii (Scedosporium apiospermum)*
Parenchymal/leptomeningeal nodules; pseudocysts	*Cryptococcus*
Hemorrhagic/infarcted lesions	*Aspergillus*
Meningeal enhancement	*Blastomyces, Coccidioides* (chronic granulomatous), *Cryptococcus, Histoplasma, Paracoccidioides, Aspergillus*
Hydrocephalus	*Cryptococcus, Coccidioides, Paracoccidioides*

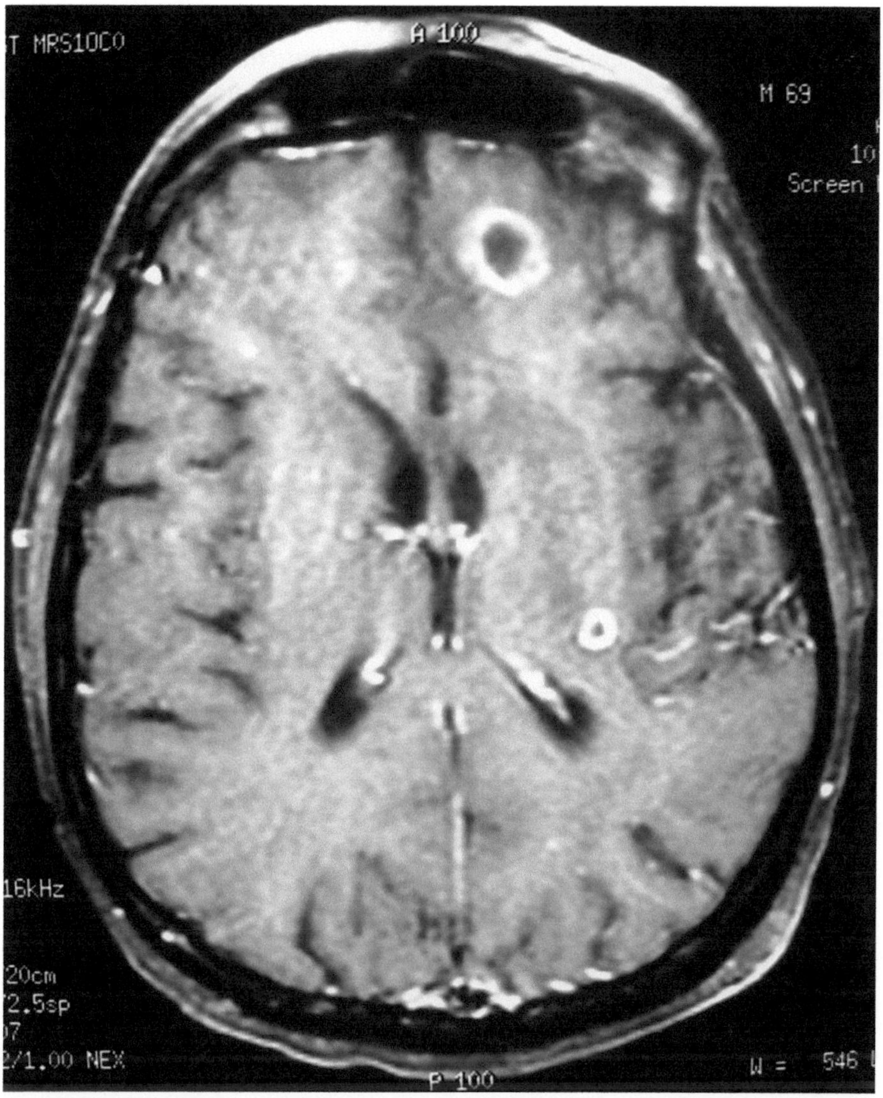

Fig. 5.1. Contrast-enhanced MRI showing multiple ring-enhancing brain abscesses in immunocompromised patient with disseminated aspergillosis. Note the lack of surrounding edema. (Courtesy of Dr. D. R. Hospenthal.).

Less commonly, the dematiaceous moulds and *Pseudallescheria boydii* have been reported to cause one or multiple brain abscesses *(13)*. CNS abscesses outside the brain parenchyma are not common, although *Blastomyces* has been reported to cause epidural abscesses *(14)*.

Other intracerebral masses associated with fungal pathogens include edematous, hemorrhagic, or infarcted lesions such as those seen in *Aspergillus* infections *(9)*. The hemorrhagic lesion, usually a consequence of an area of infarction, is an early radiologic sign owing to the angioinvasive nature of certain fungi *(8,15)*. A peripheral ring of low signal intensity relates to a dense population of hyphal elements and small areas of hemorrhage *(16)*. On cross-sectional imaging, these lesions show little or no enhancement or mass effect *(9)*. Less frequently seen intracerebral lesions include parenchymal or leptomeningeal nodules, and non-enhancing, gelatinous pseudocysts and dilated Virchow-Robin (perivascular) spaces, found mainly in cryptococcal infections *(5,17)* (Fig. 5.2).

2.2. *Meningeal Enhancement*

Diffuse enhancement of the meninges on MRI is another common radiological finding of fungal infection of the CNS, thought to be due to active inflammation (meningitis). *Histoplasma*, *Blastomyces*, *Coccidioides*, *Paracoccidioides*, *Cryptococcus*, as well as *Aspergillus* have all been observed to produce meningeal enhancement. *Coccidioides*

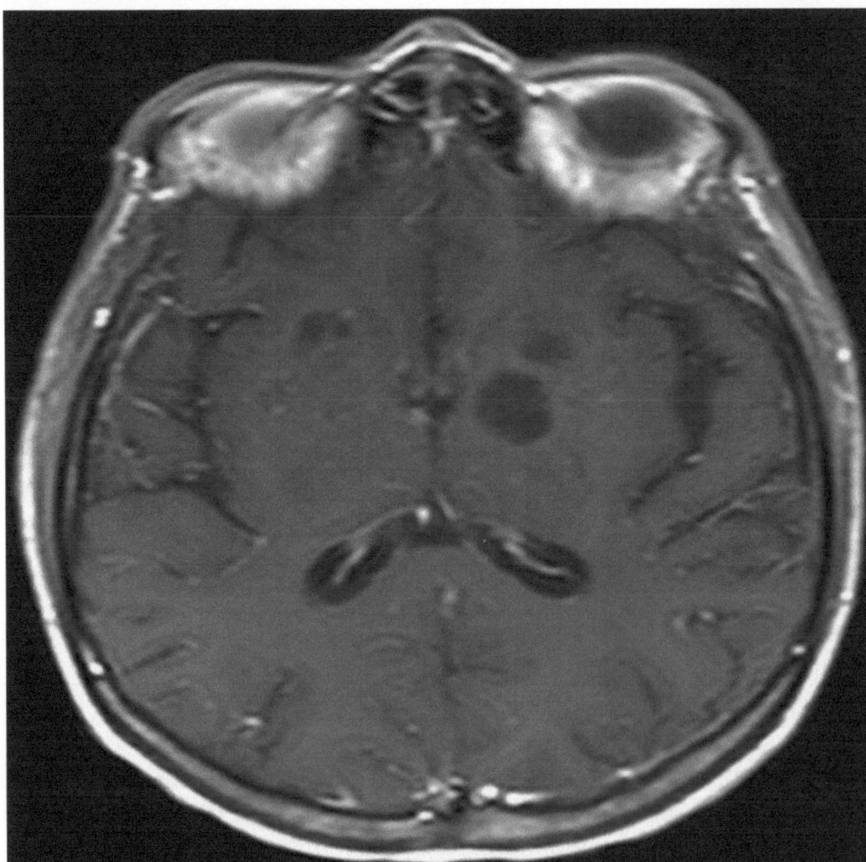

Fig. 5.2. Contrast-enhanced TI transaxial MRI image of the brain demonstrating low signal intensity lesions in the bilateral basal ganglia (left greater than right) associated with no significant enhancement, consistent with gelatinous pseudocysts of cryptococcosis. Also note mild meningeal enhancement.

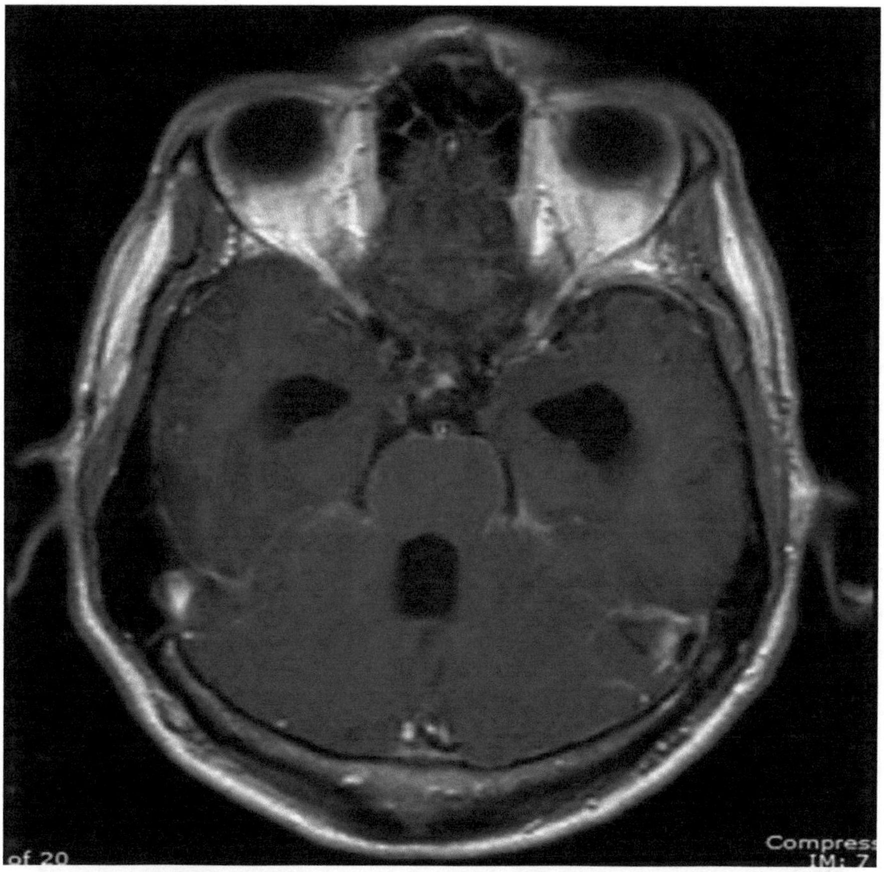

Fig. 5.3. MRI of brain revealing leptomeningeal enhancement and hydrocephalus in a patient with coccidioidomycosis.

meningitis early in its course can cause focal or nodular enhancement in the basal cisterns which represents focal organization of the fungus surrounded by inflammation *(18)*.

2.3. *Hydrocephalus*

Hydrocephalus, a consequence of meningeal involvement, is an additional finding associated with infections by *Cryptococcus*, *Coccidioides*, and *Paracoccidioides (19)* (Fig. 5.3). Although CT is helpful in identifying dilated ventricles, MRI appears better in determining the patency of the aqueduct of Sylvius. Other nonspecific CNS radiological findings include early vascular enhancement and diffuse cerebral edema.

3. RESPIRATORY TRACT IMAGING

3.1. *Sinus Imaging*

CT imaging is a useful initial test to evaluate the extent of fungal sinus disease. The CT scan defines soft tissue invasion, necrosis, early bone erosion, and cavernous sinus thrombosis *(20)*. When findings are suggestive of fungal sinusitis but the diagnosis is uncertain, MRI with or without gadolinium is the best radiological means to further evaluate the disease *(21)*. Central areas of hyperattenuation on CT correspond to hypointense signals on T1WI and signal void with T2WI MRI. Early changes in major vessels and intracranial extension are also best seen on MRI, as is possible cavernous sinus thrombosis and embolic phenomena. It is thought that fungal sinusitis also has characteristic high signal intensity on T1WI and very low signal intensity on T2WI.

The paranasal sinuses are the most frequently affected, with the maxillary and ethmoid sinuses being the most commonly involved, followed by the sphenoid sinuses. Bilateral involvement is slightly more common than unilateral involvement *(22)*. Radiologic findings include opacification of multiple paranasal sinuses, with possible demonstration of sinus cavity expansion and erosion of the involved sinus wall. Bone destruction, erosion, and osteomyelitis have been reported in both the invasive and allergic form of *Aspergillus* sinusitis, as well as in infections due to zygomycetes *(21,23)* (Fig. 5.4). A soft tissue mass or a sinus "aspergilloma" is reported as a major CT finding of the invasive granulomatous form of fungal sinusitis from *Aspergillus*. It can appear as sinus opacification associated with flocculent calcifications *(24)* (Fig. 5.5). The mass may either present as a homogenous density or have components of lower attenuation. Intraorbital and/or intracranial extension may occasionally occur. Air-fluid levels may be found though these are rare in either the invasive or noninvasive forms of fungal sinusitis *(20)*. Other findings include scattered intrasinus high attenuation areas amid mucosal thickening on unenhanced CT scans.

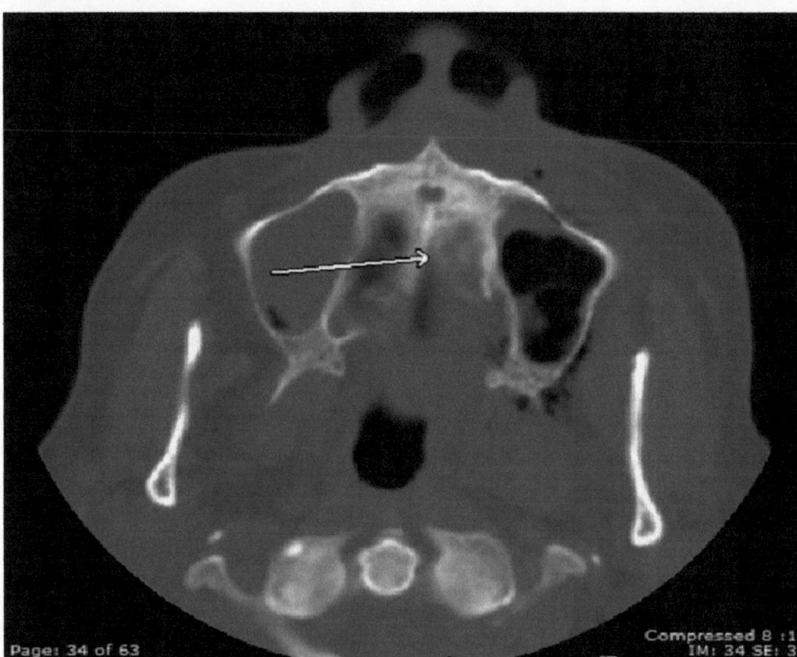

Fig. 5.4. Transaxial sinus CT of patient with zygomycosis demonstrating osteolysis of the hard palate (arrow) and left maxillary sinus mucosal thickening with surrounding soft tissue air.

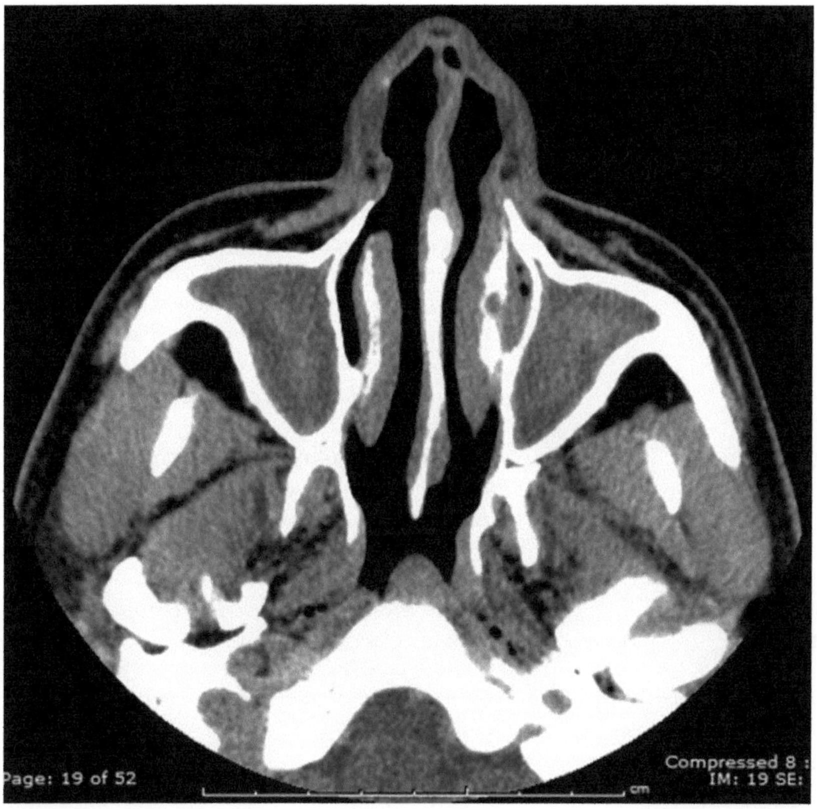

Fig. 5.5. Transaxial CT image through the sinuses demonstrating high-density opacification of the maxillary sinuses consistent with fungal sinusitis.

3.2. Pulmonary Imaging

Definitive diagnosis of a pulmonary fungal infection by radiological imaging alone is not possible as other infectious organisms, and likewise, noninfectious pulmonary syndromes, can mimic radiological findings *(25)*. The most useful tools to assess lung infections include chest roentgenography and CT *(26)*. Chest radiography in the earlier stages of fungal disease may be normal; thus CT is the superior imaging modality as it has been shown to reveal abnormalities much earlier than chest x-ray films. MRI, although reported to have been useful in the work-up for *Pneumocystis* disease, has not been recognized as a significant diagnostic tool for the majority of pulmonary fungal infections. Fungal infection of the lung presents generally with a wide variety of nonspecific radiographic patterns (Table 5.2).

3.2.1. Airspace and Interstitial Opacities

Nonspecific airspace opacities are the most frequent radiologic findings found with any pulmonary infectious process. Alveolar, "patchy," "air-space," or "mass-like" opacities have been identified in many fungal diseases, often progressing to areas of consolidation in the lung. Alveolar opacities have been noted in both endemic

Table 5.2
Abnormalities more commonly seen in pulmonary imaging of fungal infections

Radiological finding	Fungus
Alveolar infiltrates	*Aspergillus, Blastomyces, Candida, Coccidioides, Cryptococcus, Histoplasma, Pneumocystis,* zygomycetes
Interstitial infiltrates	*Aspergillus, Coccidioides, Cryptococcus, Histoplasma, Paracoccidioides, Penicillium, Pneumocystis*
Nodules	*Aspergillus*/zygomycetes (halo sign), *Candida, Coccidioides, Cryptococcus, Histoplasma, Paracoccidioides, Pneumocystis*
Masses	*Aspergillus, Blastomyces, Coccidioides, Cryptococcus,* zygomycetes
Cavitation	*Aspergillus*/Zygomycetes (air crescent sign), *Blastomyces, Coccidioides, Cryptococcus, Histoplasma, Paracoccidioides, Pneumocystis*
Abscesses	*Candida, Pseudallescheria (Scedosporium),* zygomycetes
Adenopathy	*Coccidioides, Cryptococcus, Histoplasma*
Pleural effusion	*Candida, Coccidioides, Cryptococcus, Histoplasma, Pneumocystis*

and opportunistic fungal infections. Airspace opacities have been noted as a frequent initial pattern in invasive pulmonary aspergillosis (IPA). Opacities may be unifocal or multifocal and then progress to diffuse consolidation, although segmental areas of consolidation has been noted as one of the most common CT patterns in IPA *(27,28)* (Fig. 5.6). Other disease processes resulting from *Aspergillus* infection such as bronchopneumonia, hypersensitivity pneumonitis, chronic necrotizing aspergillosis, and semi-invasive aspergillosis have also presented with alveolar opacities, often progressing to consolidation *(26,27,29)*.

Interstitial, "reticular," "reticulonodular," and "linear" opacities have also been observed in many fungal infections. Diffuse bilateral interstitial opacities in a perihilar distribution *(25,30,31)* is the most common pattern seen in *Pneumocystis* infection (Fig. 5.7). Chest CT often reveals perihilar ground glass opacity in a mosaic pattern with patchy distribution of affected lung interspersed with areas of normal lung, and noted thickening of the interlobular septa *(26)*. Interstitial opacities are also the most common pattern seen in cryptococcosis *(32)*. Ground-glass attenuation may be seen in acquired immunodeficiency syndrome (AIDS) patients with this infection. *Aspergillus* can affect the lung in a variety of ways, most of which can present in an interstitial pattern. These range from nodular opacities of invasive and semi-invasive disease, mimicking the radiologic findings of reactivation tuberculosis (TB), to coarse reticulation found in chronic hypersensitivity pneumonitis *(26,27)*. A miliary or reticulonodular pattern is commonly seen in *Blastomyces* infection. *Coccidioides* pneumonia has been noted with diffuse reticulonodular lesions, especially in the

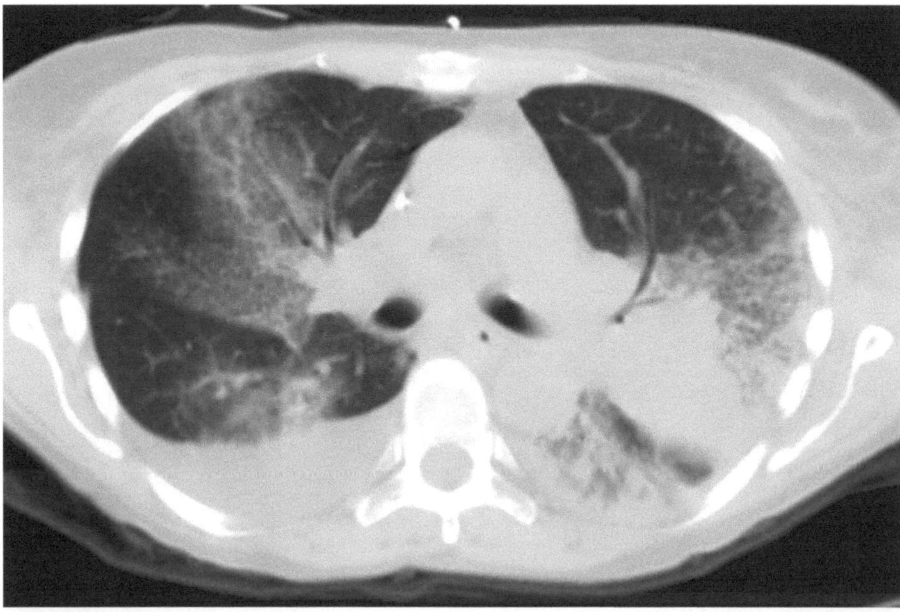

Fig. 5.6. Transaxial CT image through the chest of patient with invasive pulmonary aspergillosis demonstrating diffuse ground-glass opacity and bibasilar consolidation. (Courtesy of Dr. D. R. Hospenthal.).

setting of AIDS. Heavy exposure to *Histoplasma* can similarly present with diffuse reticulonodular opacities, such as those occurring in acute disseminated disease *(33)*. Other organisms commonly demonstrating interstitial opacities include *Penicillium marneffei* in the setting of human immunodeficiency virus (HIV) infection and paracoccidioidomycosis. In *Paracoccidioides* infection, the "reversed halo sign" of ground-glass opacity, surrounded by denser air space consolidation of crescent and ring shapes, has been reported in 10% of patients *(34)*.

Distribution and location of opacities are also nonspecific. Opacities may be confined to a lobe or they may be diffuse as seen in disseminated disease. Hematogenous candidal spread can manifest as perivascular pulmonary opacities [35]. *Pneumocystis* infection is observed with bilateral hilar opacities with a peripheral spread. For persons on prophylactic aerosolized pentamidine, the infection may present as an upper lobe infiltrative process suggestive of TB. Allergic bronchopulmonary aspergillosis often presents with fleeting or migratory upper lobe opacities *(27)*. Phantom opacities that resolve in one segment and then reappear in another lung field have also been seen in coccidioidomycosis *(35)*.

The shape of infiltrates can sometimes aid in the diagnosis. Wedge-shaped opacities, reflecting invasion of blood vessels with subsequent lung infarction, are suggestive of invasive *Aspergillus* or zygomycetes *(36)*.

Uncommon pathogens that can cause infections presenting with nonspecific pulmonary opacities include *Fusarium*, *Trichosporon*, *Malassezia furfur*, and the phaeohyphomycetes *(37)*.

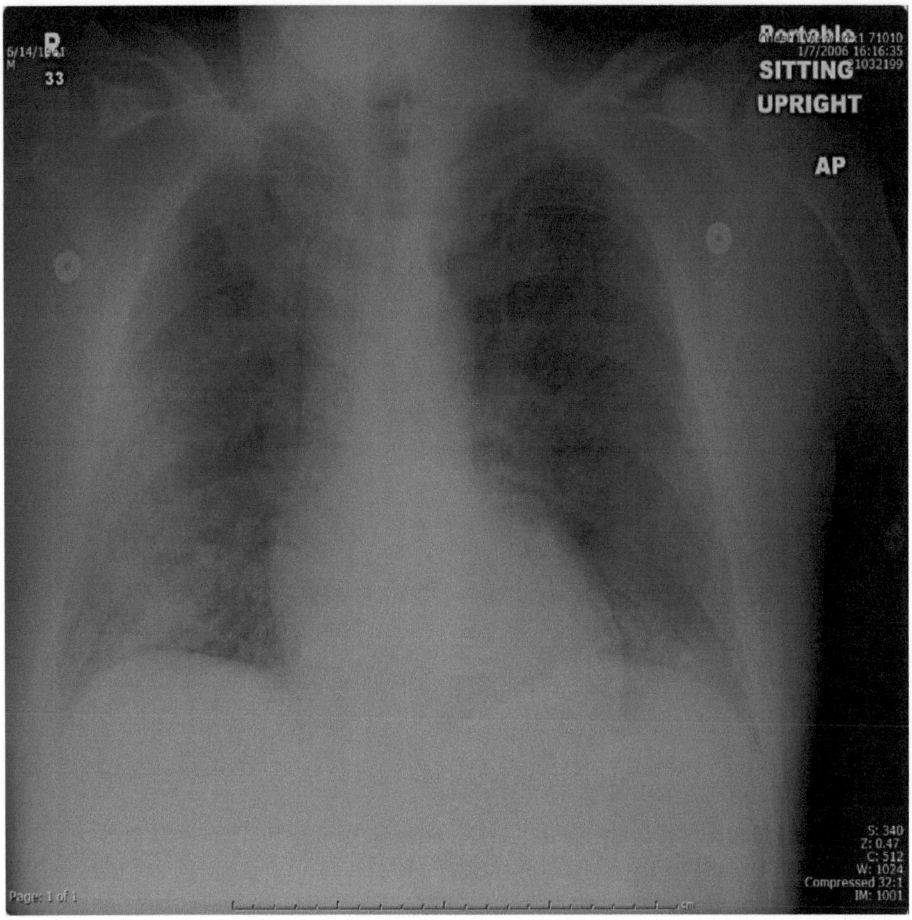

Fig. 5.7. Chest radiograph showing interstitial prominence and ground-glass opacity in a patient with *Pneumocystis* pneumonia.

3.2.2. Nodules

A well defined nodule, either single or multiple, has been reported as a frequent initial radiographic pattern of IPA *(38)*. This nodular lesion may be surrounded by a rim of hemorrhage from thrombosis of fungi within pulmonary vessels *(39)*. Days to weeks after treatment of neutropenia, patients infected with *Aspergillus* may present with ground-glass attenuation around the nodules recognized as the "halo sign" *(27,40,41)* (Fig. 5.8). The "halo sign" is highly suggestive of angioinvasive aspergillosis, but is nonspecific. It is thought that the surrounding ground-glass opacity may be related to hemorrhage from the vascular involvement. Other infectious processes including the zygomycosis, *Candida*, herpes simplex virus, and cytomegalovirus infections, as well as noninfectious processes such as Wegener's granulomatosis, Kaposi's sarcoma, and hemorrhagic metastatic malignancies, have also presented with halo signs *(42,43)*. Nodular lesions may also be observed with branching linear opacities recognized

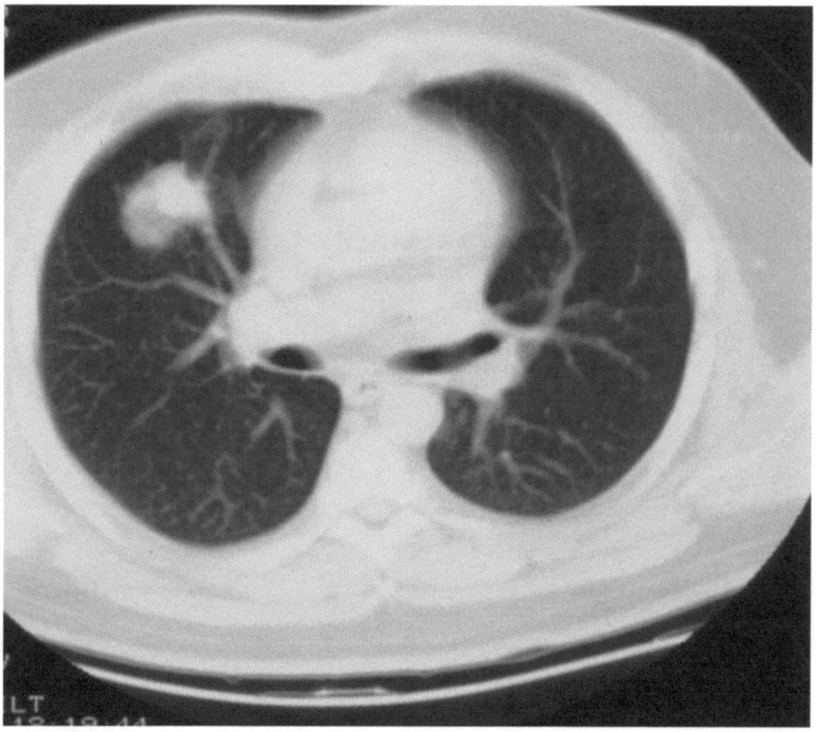

Fig. 5.8. Transaxial CT image of the chest with a right middle lobe nodule with surrounding ground glass opacity (halo sign). This is consistent with invasive aspergillosis in an immunocompromised patient.

as the "tree in bud" pattern seen in *Aspergillus* bronchiolitis *(26)*. A tree in bud pattern suggests a small airways process, a disease process that may be spread endobronchially. Similar lesions are found in endobronchial spread of mycobacterial, viral, and mycoplasma pneumonia. Nodules from zygomycetes can be indistinguishable from IPA. The most common finding in pulmonary cryptococcosis are nodules, solitary or multiple, with or without cavitation, ranging from 5 mm to 20 mm in size with smooth or irregular margins, associated with other parenchymal findings such as masses and consolidation *(44–46)*. Miliary nodules are less commonly found in AIDS patients with cryptococcosis *(47)*. Other organisms that can present with diffuse nonspecific nodular lesions include disseminated *Candida* and *Histoplasma*. Nodules can turn to "buck shot" calcifications in pulmonary histoplasmosis *(36)*. Approximately 5% of persons who develop *Coccidioides* pneumonia may develop solitary pulmonary nodules. Infections with *Pneumocystis*, *Scedosporium*, and *Paracoccidioides* have also demonstrated pulmonary nodules.

3.2.3. *Masses*

Parenchymal masses may include aspergillomas, 3 to 5 cm mobile, round or oval masses, usually solitary, and seen in the upper lobe within a preexisting cavity (Fig. 5.9). These masses may be partially surrounded by a radiolucent crescent (Monod's sign) of

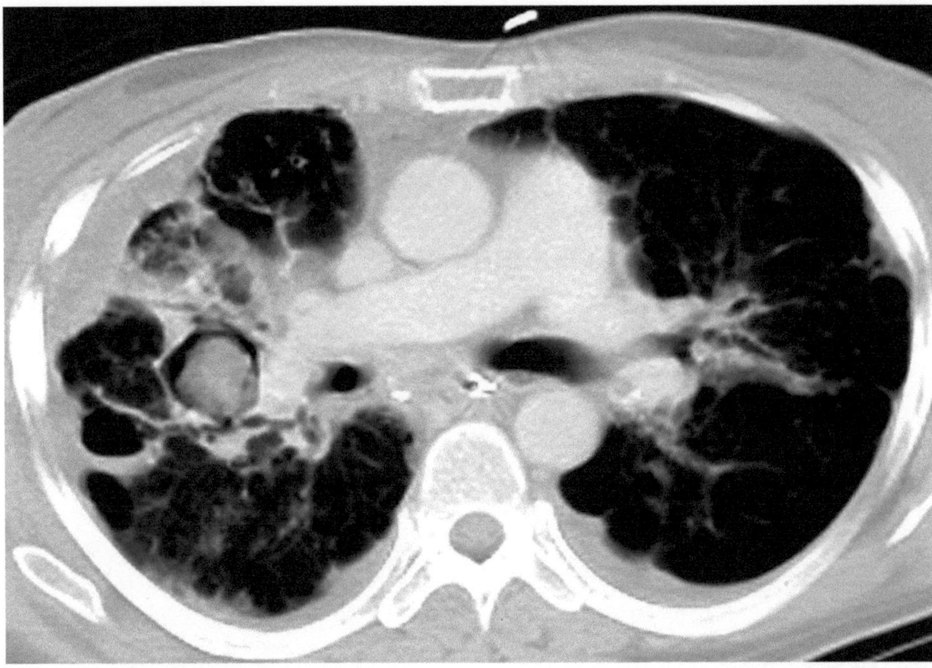

Fig. 5.9. Transaxial CT image of the chest showing bilateral upper lobe bronchiectasis, right pleural thickening, and right upper lobe ground-glass opacity and aspergilloma (soft tissue mass in preexisting cavity).

varying thickness *(27,48)*. Occasionally, coccidioidal infections may leave persistent lesions on chest x-ray exam, most commonly in the peripheral cavity *(35)*. The occasional "fungus ball" can form inside the cavity, rupture into the pleural space, and produce an air-fluid level on an upright chest x-ray study. Nonspecific mass lesions have been reported in infections with *Cryptococcus*, *Pneumocystis*, and the zygomycetes.

Nonparenchymal masses may be seen in the hilar or mediastinal areas. Chronic pulmonary blastomycosis might present with a single large perihilar mass that often warrants a thoracotomy to rule out possible carcinoma. Other findings of cryptococcosis in AIDS patients include mediastinal masses.

3.2.4. Cavitation

Virtually any nodular lesion has the potential to cavitate. Nodular lesions seen in *Aspergillus* and zygomycetes infections may progress to cavitate to what is recognized as the "air crescent sign" *(27,41,42,49)*. The air crescent sign represents cavitation of nodules caused by resorption of necrotic tissue by returning neutrophils *(39)* (Fig. 5.10). It is usually unilateral and frequently in the upper lobes *(26)*. Other nodules, single or multiple, can cavitate and then proceed to either diffuse pulmonary consolidation or abrupt development of large wedge-shaped pleural based lesions mimicking bland infarction. Thin- or thick-walled cavities as well as cavitary infiltrates can appear in subacute invasive aspergillosis and chronic progressive coccidioidomycosis, both of

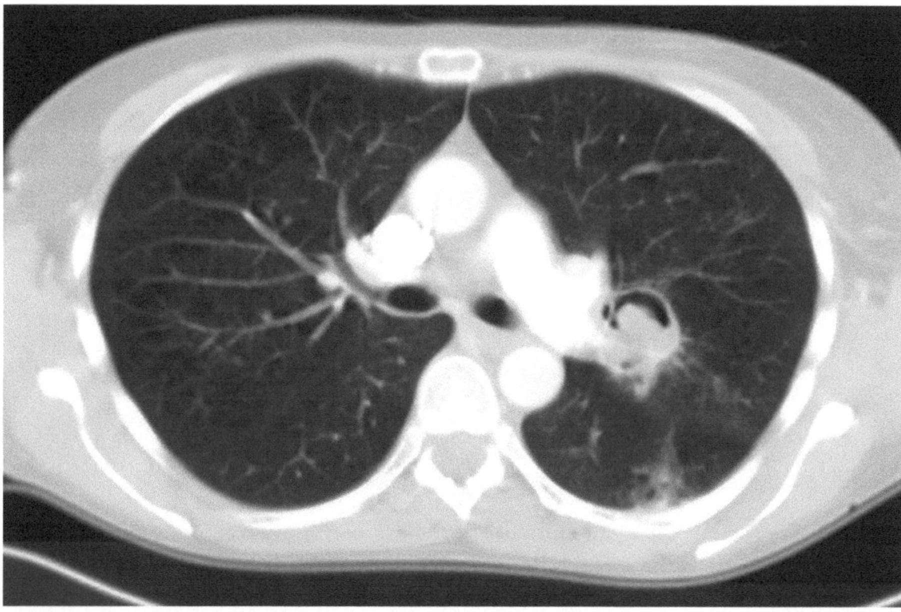

Fig. 5.10. Transaxial CT scan of the chest demonstrates a cavity in the left upper lobe with dependent soft tissue in a patient with invasive aspergillosis (air crescent sign). (Courtesy of Dr. D. R. Hospenthal.).

which can mimic TB *(36)*. Approximately 5% of persons who develop *Coccidioides* pneumonia develop thin-walled solitary cavities, typically near the pleura (Fig. 5.11). A chronic form of *Coccidioides* pneumonia presents as a slowly progressive fibrocavitary process of biapical fibronodular lesions with retraction and cavitation. In pulmonary histoplasmosis, upper lobe cavities are common, except in persons with HIV infection. Cavitary infiltrates have also been demonstrated in disseminated disease. Fibrotic apical infiltrates with cavitation have been reported in chronic pulmonary histoplasmosis which can be confused with TB infection or coinfection on chest x-ray examination *(36)*. Other fungal infections reported to cause cavitary disease include sporotrichosis and paracoccidioidomycosis; nodular areas are sometimes confluent, often in the lower lobes; cavitation occurs in one-third of cases. Cavitation from blastomycosis is unusual and not as commonly seen as in mycobacterial or *Histoplasma* infections. Cryptococcal infection may present with cavitary masses or nodules, though this is uncommonly seen in the setting of AIDS infection. In cancer patients infected with *Pneumocystis* previously given prophylactic aerosolized pentamidine, upper lobe infiltrative disease suggestive of tuberculosis may be seen, but cavitary lesions are very uncommon.

3.2.5. Adenopathy

Adenopathy has been observed commonly in histoplasmosis, coccidioidomycosis, and cryptococcosis. In acute histoplasmosis, a common finding in a low-level exposure includes enlarged hilar or mediastinal lymphadenopathy. In heavy exposure,

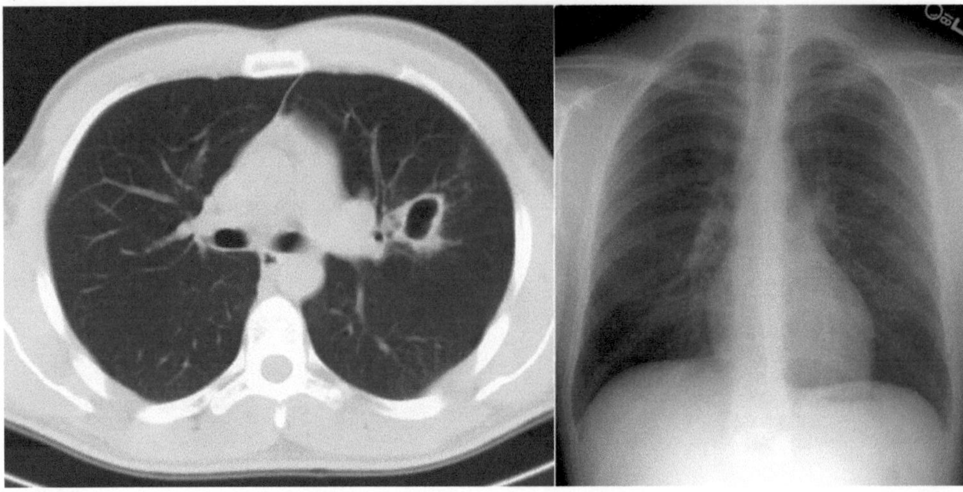

Fig. 5.11. Transaxial CT scan through the chest and chest radiograph demonstrating a thin-walled cavity in the left upper lobe in an asymptomatic patient proven to have coccidioidomycosis. (Courtesy of Dr. D. R. Hospenthal.).

the mediastinal adenopathy is usually accompanied by diffuse reticulonodular infiltrates as mentioned previously. Lymph nodes can potentially calcify. Occasionally, these lymph nodes coalesce and form granulomas which may rupture and result in chronic inflammation with subsequent fibrosis *(50)*. This process, known as fibrosing mediastinitis, can partially obstruct airways, vessels, and the esophagus. Mediastinal lymphadenopathy is uncommon in disseminated histoplasmosis, occurring at less than 10% in one series. Coccidioidomycosis is also noted to present with bilateral hilar adenopathy. Prominent hilar adenopathy is occasionally seen in cryptococcosis. Radiologic findings vary widely in *Pneumocystis* infections but lymphadenopathy is extremely rare.

3.2.6. Pleural Abnormalities

The effect of fungal infections on the pleura and pleural cavity is not as common as the other previously described radiologic findings. Pleural thickening with concomitant upper lobe consolidation potentially progressing to cavitation over weeks to months can be seen in semi-invasive pulmonary aspergillosis *(27)*. Pleural effusions have been noted in candidal pneumonia. Large parapneumonic effusions have been documented in coccidioidomycosis. Other organisms that have demonstrated pleural effusions include *Cryptococcus*, *Histoplasma*, and *Scedosporium*. Effusions are unusual in *Blastomyces* and *Pneumocystis* infections.

3.2.7. Airway Abnormalities

Tracheal or bronchial wall mucosal thickening along with airway plaques can be seen in invasive aspergillosis *(26,27)*. *Cryptococcus* infection of the larynx can present on CT soft tissue images of the neck as vocal cord irregularities and asymmetric enlargement *(51)*. Cylindric bronchiectasis in a central distribution, as well as traction bronchiectasis, have also been noted on CT images of various forms of *Aspergillus* as well as *Paracoccidioides* infections *(27,52)*.

3.2.8. Miscellaneous

Hematogenous spread of *Candida* can cause multiple abscesses in the body, including the lungs *(53)*. Zygomycosis and pseudallescheriasis have also been reported to cause pulmonary abscesses *(54,55)*. Atelectasis, which may appear as bilateral lower lobe consolidation, has been noted in various pathologic processes caused by *Aspergillus (27)*. Thin-walled cysts or pneumatoceles can form in *Pneumocystis* infections, especially in patients receiving prophylaxis with aerosolized pentamidine and trimethoprim/sulfamethoxazole (TMP/SMX) *(30)*. These upper lobe lesions increase the risk of developing pneumothoraces. End-stage honeycombing can be seen in the chronic form of hypersensitivity pneumonitis secondary to *Aspergillus (27)*. Pseudoaneurysm of the aortic arch has been noted in IPA *(56)*.

A new imaging modality has recently been used to study invasive aspergillosis. Multidetector CT (MDCT) angiography takes advantage of the angioinvasive nature of *Aspergillus* and allows direct detection of vessel occlusion up to a peripheral lesion, with high-resolution images demonstrating possibly the earliest sign of disease from *Aspergillus (57)*.

4. ABDOMINAL IMAGING

CT or MRI should be the initial imaging modality used to evaluate the abdomen for signs of fungal infection. Ultrasonography, a safer, low-cost method, may then be obtained to follow up noted disease processes. Serial ultrasounds every 3 to 4 weeks may be used to monitor response to therapy, typically observed as decreasing size and number of lesions, or may be useful in detecting evolution of new lesions *(58)*. Once the ultrasound is clear, a repeat CT or MRI is suggested. Similar to other affected organs mentioned in the preceding text, radiologic findings of abdominal fungal infections are varied to include nonspecific lesions, organomegaly, and lymphadenopathy.

4.1. *Target Lesions*

Candida is one of the main fungi to cause abdominal disease. Involvement of the liver, biliary tree, pancreas, and spleen has been documented in disseminated disease *(59)*. Target lesions seen in the spleen and liver resulting from candidal infection are most commonly detected on CT or MRI after the resolution of neutropenic episodes *(58)* (Fig. 5.12). On abdominal CT, chronic disseminated (formerly hepatosplenic) candidiasis is characterized by small, round, low-attenuation lesions scattered through the liver and spleen with occasional peripheral enhancement *(60)*. Occasionally, multiple small low attenuation lesions in the spleen and kidneys are seen without lymph node enlargement or hepatosplenomegaly *(61)*. Four dominant findings on ultrasound have been described. Most commonly, uniform hypoechoic lesions are noted and can be seen in conjunction with the other three patterns. A "wheel within a wheel" pattern can be seen representing an outer hypoechoic area of fibrosis surrounding a hyperechoic area of inflammation. A "bull's eye" measuring from 1 to 4 cm may

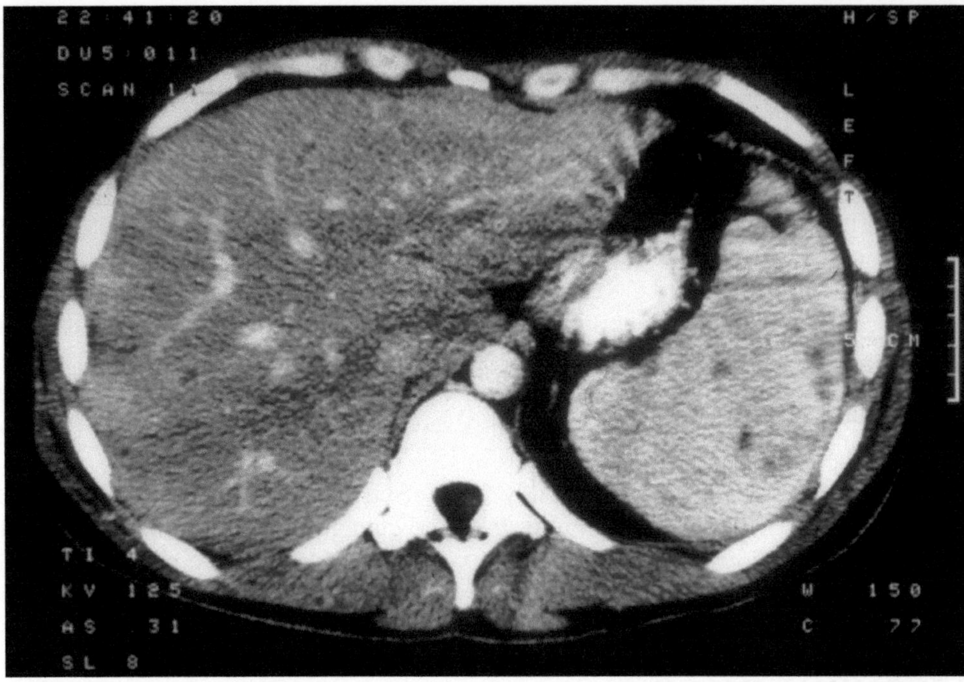

Fig. 5.12. Contrast-enhanced CT scan through the abdomen showing multiple subcentimeter low attenuation hepatic and splenic lesions in patient with chronic disseminated candidiasis. (Courtesy of Dr. D. R. Hospenthal.).

evolve from primary lesions. "Echogenic foci," usually seen late, correlate with central fibrosis, calcifications, or both *(62)*. MRI has been reported to be superior to CT in characterizing chronic disseminated candidiasis. *Coccidioides* infections have also been reported to present with splenic lesions with central areas of low attenuation on CT imaging *(61)*.

4.2. Organomegaly

Moderate to marked enlargement of the liver, spleen, and adrenals have been noted in disseminated histoplasmosis *(61,63)*. Cryptococcal infections have also been reported to produce marked splenomegaly and mild hepatomegaly *(61)*.

4.3. Lymphadenopathy

Enlarged lymph nodes with or without central or diffuse low attenuation are seen in the majority of patients with abdominal histoplasmosis *(61)*. On CT imaging, enlarged lymph nodes have also been noted in the case of cryptococcal infection.

4.4. Miscellaneous

Abdominal abscesses have been reported in deeply invasive candidiasis *(59)*. Uncommon findings in disseminated histoplasmosis include colonic wall thickening, and omental and mesenteric infiltration *(61)*. Adrenal masses, vascular occlusion, and extensive necrosis have also been noted. Multiple scattered low-attenuation foci can persist from focal scarring and granulomatous change, which may eventually result in calcifications.

5. MUSCULOSKELETAL IMAGING

Bone scans are the imaging modality of choice in assessing fungal infections of the skeletal system (Fig. 5.13). Technetium uptake is dependent on blood flow, while gallium uptake is dependent on the presence of leukocytes in the area of inflammation *(64)*. Although positive bone scans may be seen as early as 24 hours after the onset of infection, a normal scan may be the result of scanning before the onset of reactive hyperperfusion. Osteomyelitis is the most frequent radiologic finding associated with skeletal fungal infections, although radiographic appearance is nonspecific and indistinguishable among fungi or from bacterial or neoplastic disease. Bone MRI may be sensitive for picking up early lesions of osteomyelitis.

5.1. Osteomyelitis

In blastomycosis, the vertebral column is infrequently involved. The skull, ribs, and the epiphyseal ends of long bones are more commonly affected *(65)*. In the tubular

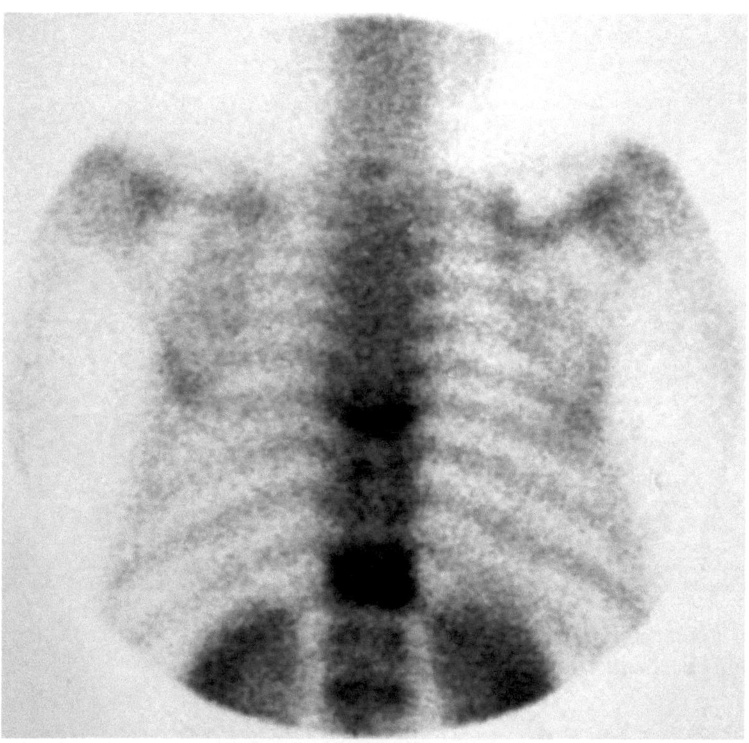

Fig. 5.13. Bone scan demonstrates increased uptake at approximately T8, T11, and T12. Although this patient had coccidioidomycosis, these findings are nonspecific and could represent another infection or inflammatory or neoplastic process..

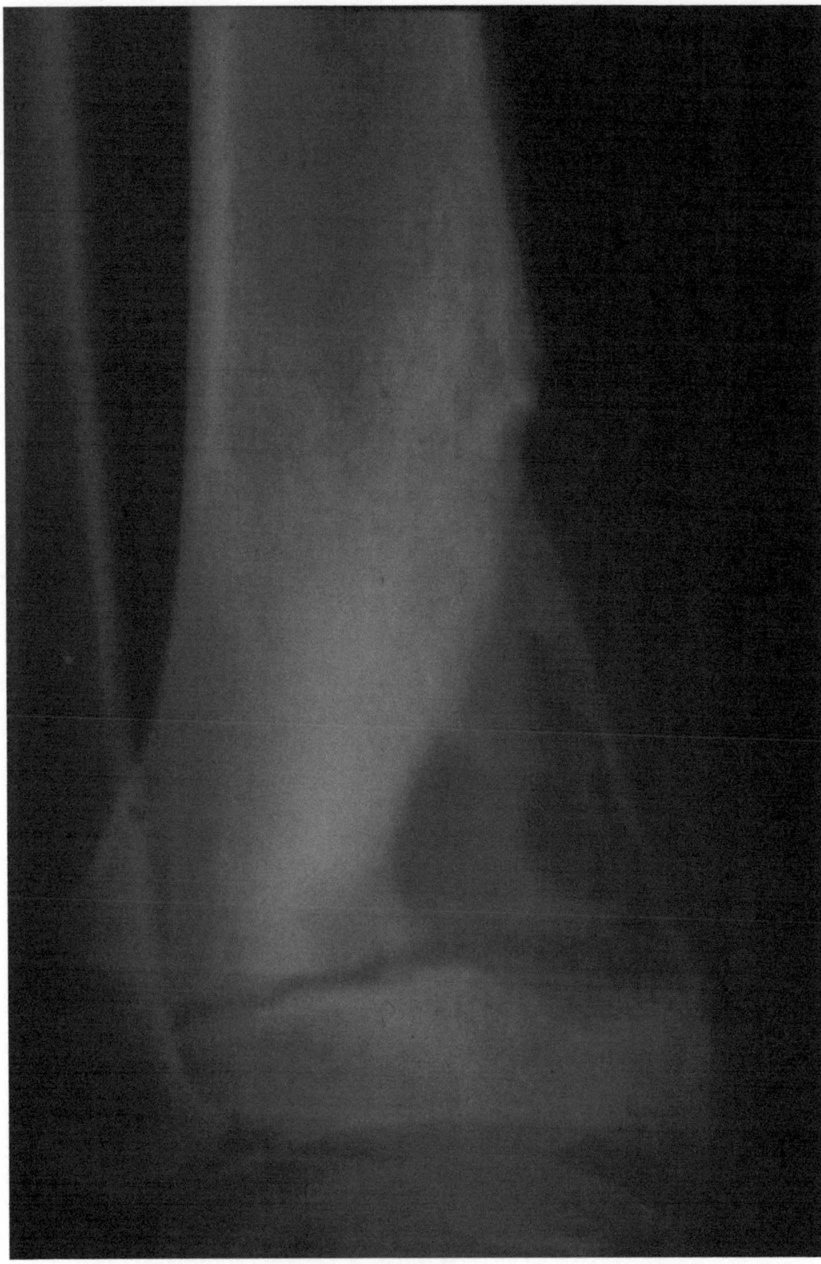

Fig. 5.14. Plain radiograph of the right ankle showing a lytic lesion in the medial aspect of the distal tibia secondary to coccidioidomycosis.

bones of the extremities, eccentric saucer-shaped erosions may be seen beneath a cutaneous abscess. Epiphyseal or metaphyseal focal or diffuse osteomyelitis has been reported as well as cystic foci or diffuse "moth-eaten" areas in the carpal or tarsal areas *(66)*. Histoplasmosis similarly affects the pelvis, skull, ribs, and small tubular bones.

Radiologically, osteoporosis, joint space narrowing, and bony erosion may be seen similar to tuberculosis. *Candida* osteomyelitis usually occurs in the setting of disseminated candidiasis, affecting primarily the axial spine of adults and the long bones of children *(66)*. Soft tissue swelling, joint space narrowing, and irregularities of subchondral bone are noted *(67)*. Coccidioidomycosis also primarily affects the vertebral column and ribs. There is a tendency to involve multiple segments of the vertebrae, sometimes with "skip lesions" *(65)*. Radiographs reveal periostitis as well as multiple well-demarcated lytic foci in the metaphyses of long tubular bones and in bony prominences. In the spine, one or more vertebral bodies may be involved, typically with paraspinal masses and contiguous rib lesions *(67)* (Fig. 5.14). Cryptococcosis presents with nonspecific radiographic features to include osteolytic lesions with discrete margins, mild or absent surrounding sclerosis, and little or no periosteal reaction. Zygomycosis generally causes osteolytic changes to the skull or face *(67)*. With Madura foot (eumycotic mycetoma), a chronic granulomatous disease of the subcutaneous tissues and bone, standard x-ray films may reveal abnormalities, though CT has been reported to be more sensitive in the earlier stages of the disease. Typically, single or multiple bony defects with extensive soft tissue and bony disruption occurring with sclerosis and periostitis are seen *(67)*. Other organisms reported to cause radiologic abnormalities of soft tissue and bone include *Scedosporium*, *Paecilomyces*, *Pseudallescheria boydii*, and *Sporothrix schenckii (13,55,67)*. Osseous and disk space destruction and a paraspinal mass resembling those of TB have been reported in aspergillosis *(67)*.

REFERENCES

1. Aribandi M, Bazan C, Rinaldi MG. Magnetic resonance imaging findings in fatal primary cerebral infection due to *Chaetomium strumarium*. Australas Radiol 2005;49:166–169.
2. Siegal JA, Cacayorinb ED, Nassif AS, et al. Cerebral mucormycosis: proton MR spectroscopy and MR imaging. Magn Reson Imaging 2000;18:915–920.
3. Miszkiel KA, Hall-Craggs MA, Miller RF, et al. The spectrum of MRI findings in CNS cryptococcosis in AIDS. Clin Radiol 1996;51:842–850.
4. Tan CT, Kuan BB. Cryptococcus meningitis, clinical–CT scan considerations. Neuroradiology 1987;29:43–46.
5. Ho TL, Lee H-J, Lee K-W, Chen W-L. Diffusion-weighted and conventional magnetic resonance imaging in cerebral cryptococcoma. Acta Radiol 2005;46:411–414.
6. Kamezawa T, Shimozuru T, Niiro M, Nagata S, Kuratsu J. MRI of a cerebral cryptococcal granuloma. Neuroradiology 2000;42:441–443.
7. Hospenthal DR, Bennett JE. Persistence of cryptococcomas on neuroimaging. Clin Infect Dis 2000;31:1303–1306.
8. DeLone DR, Goldstein RA, Petermann G, et al. Disseminated aspergillosis involving the brain: distribution and imaging characteristics. AJNR Am J Neuroradiol 1999;20: 1597–1604.
9. Okafuji T, Yabuuchi H, Nagatoshi Y, Hattanda Y, Fukuya T. CT and MR findings of brain aspergillosis. Comput Med Imaging Graph 2003;27:489–492.
10. Banuelos AF, Williams PL, Johnson RH, et al. Central nervous system abscesses due to *Coccidioides* species. Clin Infect Dis 1996;22:240–250.
11. Chaabane M, Krifa H, Ladeb MF, et al. Cerebral candidiasis: CT appearance. Pediatr Radiol 1989;19:436.

12. Lai PH, Lin SM, Pan HB, Yang CF. Disseminated miliary cerebral candidiasis. Am J Neuroradiol 1997;18:1303–1306.
13. Fleming RV, Walsh TJ, Anaissie EJ. Emerging and less common fungal pathogens. Infect Dis Clin North Am 2002;16:915–933.
14. Roos KL, Bryan JP, Maggio WW, Jane JA, Scheld WM. Intracranial blastomycosis. Medicine (Baltimore) 1979;66:224–235.
15. Yamada Y, Shrier DA, Rubio A, et al. Imaging findings in intracranial Aspergillosis. Acad Radiol 2002;9:163–171.
16. Cox J, Murtagh FR, Wilfong A, Brenner J. Cerebral aspergillosis: MR imaging and histopathologic correlation. Am J Neuroradiol 1992;13:1489–1492.
17. Cheng YC, Ling JF, Chang FC, et al. Radiological manifestations of cryptococcal infection in central nervous system. J Chin Med Assoc 2003;66:19–26.
18. Erly WK, Bellon RJ, Seeger JF, Carmody RF. MR Imaging of acute coccidioidal meningitis. Am J Neuroradiol 1999;20:509–514.
19. Gasparetto EL, Liu CB, de Carvalho Neto A, Rogacheski E. Central nervous system paracoccidioidomycosis: Imaging findings in 17 cases. J Comput Assist Tomogr 2003;27:12–17.
20. Blitzer A, Lawson W. Fungal infections of the nose and paranasal sinuses: part I. Otolaryngol Clin North Am 1993;26:1007–1035.
21. Manning SC, Merkel M, Kriesel K, Vuitch F, Marple B. Computed tomography and magnetic resonance diagnosis of allergic fungal sinusitis. Laryngoscope 1997;107: 170–176.
22. Dahniya MH, Makkar R, Grexa E, et al. Appearances of paranasal fungal sinusitis on computed tomography. Br J Radiol 1998;71:340–344.
23. Terk MR, Underwood DJ, Zee CS, Colletti PM. MR imaging in rhinocerebral and intracranial mucormycosis with CT and pathological correlation. Magn Reson Imaging 1992;10:81–87.
24. Yoon JH, Na DG, Byun HS, Koh YH, Chung SK, Dong HJ. Calcification in chronic maxillary sinusitis: comparison of CT findings with histopathologic results. Am J Neuroradiol 1999;20:571–574.
25. Boiselle PM, Tocino I, Hooley RJ, et al. Chest radiograph interpretation of *Pneumocystis carinii* pneumonia, bacterial pneumonia, and pulmonary tuberculosis in HIV-positive patients: accuracy, distinguishing features, and mimics. J Thorac Imaging 1997;12: 47–53.
26. Franquet T, Gimenez A, Hidalgo A. Imaging of opportunistic fungal infections in the immunocompromised patient. Eur J Radiol 2004;51:130–138.
27. Gotway MB, Dawn SK, Caoili EM, Reddy GP, Araoz PA, Webb WR. The radiologic spectrum of pulmonary *Aspergillus* infections. J Comput Assist Tomogr 2002;26: 159–173.
28. Kami M, Kishi Y, Hamaki T, et al. The value of the chest computed tomography halo sign in the diagnosis of invasive pulmonary aspergillosis: an autopsy-based retrospective study of 48 patients. Mycoses 2002;45:287–294.
29. Kim SY, Lee KS, Han J, et al. Semiinvasive pulmonary aspergillosis: CT and pathologic findings in six patients. AJR Am J Roentgenol 2000;174:795–798.
30. Goodman PC. *Pneumocystis carinii* pneumonia. J Thorac Imaging 1991;6:16–21.
31. Primack SL, Muller NL. High resolution computed tomography in acute diffuse lung disease in the immunocompromised patients. Radiol Clin North Am 1994;32:731–744.
32. Feigin DS. Pulmonary cryptococcosis: radiologic-pathologic correlates of its three forms. AJR Am J Roentgenol 1983;141:1263–1272.
33. Conces DJ, Stockberger SM, Tarver RD, Wheat LJ. Disseminated histoplasmosis in AIDS: findings on chest radiographs. AJR Am J Roentgenol 1993;160:15–19.

34. Gasparetto EL, Escuissato DL, Davaus T, et al. Reversed halo sign in pulmonary paracoccidioidomycosis. AJR Am J Roentgenol 2005;184:1932–1934.
35. Bayer AS. Fungal pneumonias: pulmonary coccidioidal syndromes (part I). Chest 1981;79:575–583.
36. Davies SF. An overview of pulmonary fungal infections. Clin Chest Med 1987;8:495–512.
37. Walsh TJ, Hiemenz JW, Anaissie E. Recent progress and current problems in treatment of invasive fungal infections in neutropenic patients. Infect Dis Clin North Am 1996;10: 365–400.
38. Orr DP, Myerowitz RL, Dubois PJ. Patho-radiologic correlation of invasive pulmonary aspergillosis in the immunocompromised host. Cancer 1978;41:2028–2039.
39. Tanaka N, Matsumoto T, Miura G, Emoto T, Matsunaga N. HRCT findings of chest complications in patients with leukemia. Eur Radiol 2002;12:1512–1522.
40. Kim Y, Lee KS, Jung KJ, Han J, Kim JS, Suh JS. Halo sign on high resolution CT: findings in spectrum of pulmonary diseases with pathologic correlation. J Comput Assist Tomogr 1999;23:622–626.
41. Kuhlman JE, Fishman EK, Siegelman SS. Invasive pulmonary aspergillosis in acute leukemia: characteristic findings on CT, the CT halo sign, and the role of CT in early diagnosis. Radiology 1985;157:611–614.
42. McAdams HP, Rosado de Christenson M, Strollo DC, Patz EF. Pulmonary mucormycosis: radiologic findings in 32 cases. AJR Am J Roentgenol 1997;168:1541–1548.
43. Primack SL, Hartman TE, Lee KS, Muller NL. Pulmonary nodules and the CT halo sign. Radiology 1994;190:513–515.
44. Khoury MB, Godwin JD, Ravin CE, Gallis HA, Halvorsen RA, Putman CE. Thoracic cryptococcosis: immunologic competence and radiologic appearance. AJR Am J Roentgenol 1984;141:893–896.
45. Zinck SE, Leung AN, Frost M, Berry GJ, Muller NL. Pulmonary cryptococcosis: CT and pathologic findings. J Comput Assist Tomogr 2002;26:330–334.
46. Zlupko GM, Fochler FJ, Goldschmidt ZH. Pulmonary cryptococcosis presenting with multiple pulmonary nodules. Chest 1980;77:575.
47. Cameron ML, Barlett JA, Gallis HA, Waskin HA. Manifestations of pulmonary cryptococcosis in patients with acquired immunodeficiency syndrome. Rev Infect Dis 1991;13: 64–67.
48. Irwin A. Radiology of the aspergilloma. Clin Radiol 1966;18:432–438.
49. Lee FY, Mossad SB, Adal KA. Pulmonary mucormycosis: the last 30 years. Arch Intern Med 1999;159:1301–1309.
50. Sherrick AD, Brown LR Harms GF, Myers JL. The radiographic findings of fibrosing mediastinitis. Chest 1994;106:484–489.
51. McGregor DK ,Citron D, Shahab I. Cryptococcal infection of the larynx simulating laryngeal carcinoma. South Med J 2003;96:74–77.
52. Funari M, Kavakama J, Shikanai-Yasuda MA, et al. Chronic pulmonary paracoccidioidomycosis (South American blastomycosis): high resolution CT findings in 41 patients. AJR Am J Roentgenol 1999;173:59–64.
53. Masur H, Rosen PP, Armstrong D. Pulmonary disease caused by *Candida* species. Am J Med 1977;63:914–925.
54. Rinaldi MG. Zygomycosis. Infect Dis Clin North Am 1989;3:19–41.
55. Travis LB, Roberts GD, Wilson WR. Clinical significance of *Pseudallescheria boydii*: a review of 10 years' experience. Mayo Clin Proc 1985;60:531–537.
56. Koral K, Hall TR. Mycotic pseudoaneurysm of the aortic arch: an unusual complication of invasive pulmonary aspergillosis. Clin Imaging 2000;24:279–282.

57. Sonnet S, Buitrago-Tellez CH, Tamm M, Christen S, Steinbrich W. Direct detection of angioinvasive pulmonary aspergillosis in immunosuppressed patients: preliminary results with high-resolution 16-MDCT angiography. Am J Roentgenol 2005;184:746–751.
58. Karthaus M, Huebner G, Elser C, Geissler RG, Heil G, Ganser A. Early detection of chronic disseminated *Candida* infection in leukemia patients with febrile neutropenia: value of computer-assisted serial ultrasound documentation. Ann Hematol 1998;77:41–45.
59. Ostrosky-Zeichner L, Rex JH, Bennett J, Kullberg BJ. Deeply invasive candidiasis. Infect Dis Clin North Am 2002;16:821–835.
60. Kontoyiannis DP, Luna MA, Samuels BI, Bodey GP. Hepatosplenic candidiasis: a manifestation of chronic disseminated candidiasis in infections of the liver. Infect Dis Clin North Am 2000;14:721–739.
61. Radin R. HIV infection: analysis in 259 consecutive patients with abnormal abdominal CT findings. Radiol 1995;197:712–722.
62. Pastakia B, Shawker TH, Thaler M, O'Leary T, Pizzo PA. Hepatosplenic candidiasis: wheels within wheels. Radiology 1988;166:417–421.
63. Radin DR. Disseminated histoplasmosis: abdominal CT findings in 16 patients. AJR Am J Roentgenol 1991;157:955–958.
64. Bonakdar-pour A, Gaines VD. The radiology of osteomyelitis. Orthop Clin North Am 1983;14:21–37.
65. Sapico FL, Montogmerie JZ. Vertebral osteomyelitis. Infect Dis Clin North Am 1990;4:539–550.
66. Katzenstein D. Isolated *Candida* arthritis. Report of a case and definition of a distinct clinical syndrome. Arthritis Rheum 1985;28:1421–1424.
67. Chhem RK, Wang S, Jaovisidha S, et al. Imaging of fungal, viral, and parasitic musculoskeletal and spinal diseases. Radiol Clin North Am 2001;39:357–378.

SUGGESTED READINGS

Davies SF. An overview of pulmonary fungal infections. Clin Chest Med 1987;8:495–512.

DeLone DR, Goldstein RA, Petermann G, et al. Disseminated aspergillosis involving the brain: distribution and imaging characteristics. AJNR Am J Neuroradiol 1999;20:1597–1604.

Franquet T, Gimenez A, Hidalgo A. Imaging of opportunistic fungal infections in the immunocompromised patient. Eur J Radiol 2004;51:130–138.

Gotway MB, Dawn SK, Caoili EM, Reddy GP, Araoz PA, Webb WR. The radiologic spectrum of pulmonary *Aspergillus* infections. J Comput Assist Tomogr 2002;26:159–173.

Manning SC, Merkel M, Kriesel K, Vuitch F, Marple B. Computed tomography and magnetic resonance diagnosis of allergic fungal sinusitis. Laryngoscope 1997;107:170–176.

Radin R. HIV infection: analysis in 259 consecutive patients with abnormal abdominal CT findings. Radiol 1995;197:712–722.

Som PM. Imaging of paranasal sinus fungal disease. Otolaryngol Clin North Am 1993;26: 983–994.

III

Antifungal Agents

6
Antifungal Agents

Russell E. Lewis, PharmD
and Annette W. Fothergill, MA, MBA

1. INTRODUCTION

Until the 1950s, relatively few drugs were available for the treatment of superficial or invasive mycoses. The era of antifungal chemotherapy effectively began in 1955, with the discovery of the polyene antifungals nystatin and amphotericin B, followed closely by the discovery of the first topical azole antifungal agent, chlormidazole, in 1958 (Fig. 6.1). Although amphotericin B was to remain the mainstay of therapy for serious fungal infections for more than 40 years, infusion-related side effects and dose-limiting nephrotoxicity associated with its use prompted continued the search for equally effective but less toxic alternatives. In the 1960s, a synthetic fluorinated pyrimidine analogue originally developed as an antineoplastic agent, flucytosine, was found to have potent antifungal activity against common yeasts. Unfortunately, resistance to flucytosine developed rapidly when the drug was administered as monotherapy, thus restricting its use to combination therapy with amphotericin B. The next major milestone in antifungal therapy was not realized until 1981, when the first orally bioavailable systemic azole, ketoconazole, was introduced into clinical practice. For almost a decade, it would be regarded as the drug of choice for chronic mucocutaneous candidiasis, mild to moderate blastomycosis, histoplasmosis, paracoccidioidomycosis and coccidioidomycosis, and occasionally deep-seated *Candida* and *Cryptococcus* infections in patients who could not tolerate amphotericin B *(1)*. Because ketoconazole is a highly lipophilic weak base, it has many undesirable physiochemical characteristics that increased its toxicity and limited its usefulness in critically ill patients including:

- Limited absorption of the drug at elevated gastric pH
- Lack of an intravenous formulation
- Requirement for extensive cytochrome P450 biotransformation before elimination, resulting in a high propensity for drug–drug interactions
- Dose-related gastrointestinal, hepatic, and adrenal toxicity

From: *Infectious Disease: Diagnosis and Treatment of Human Mycoses*
Edited by: D. R. Hospenthal and M. G. Rinaldi © Humana Press Inc., Totowa, NJ

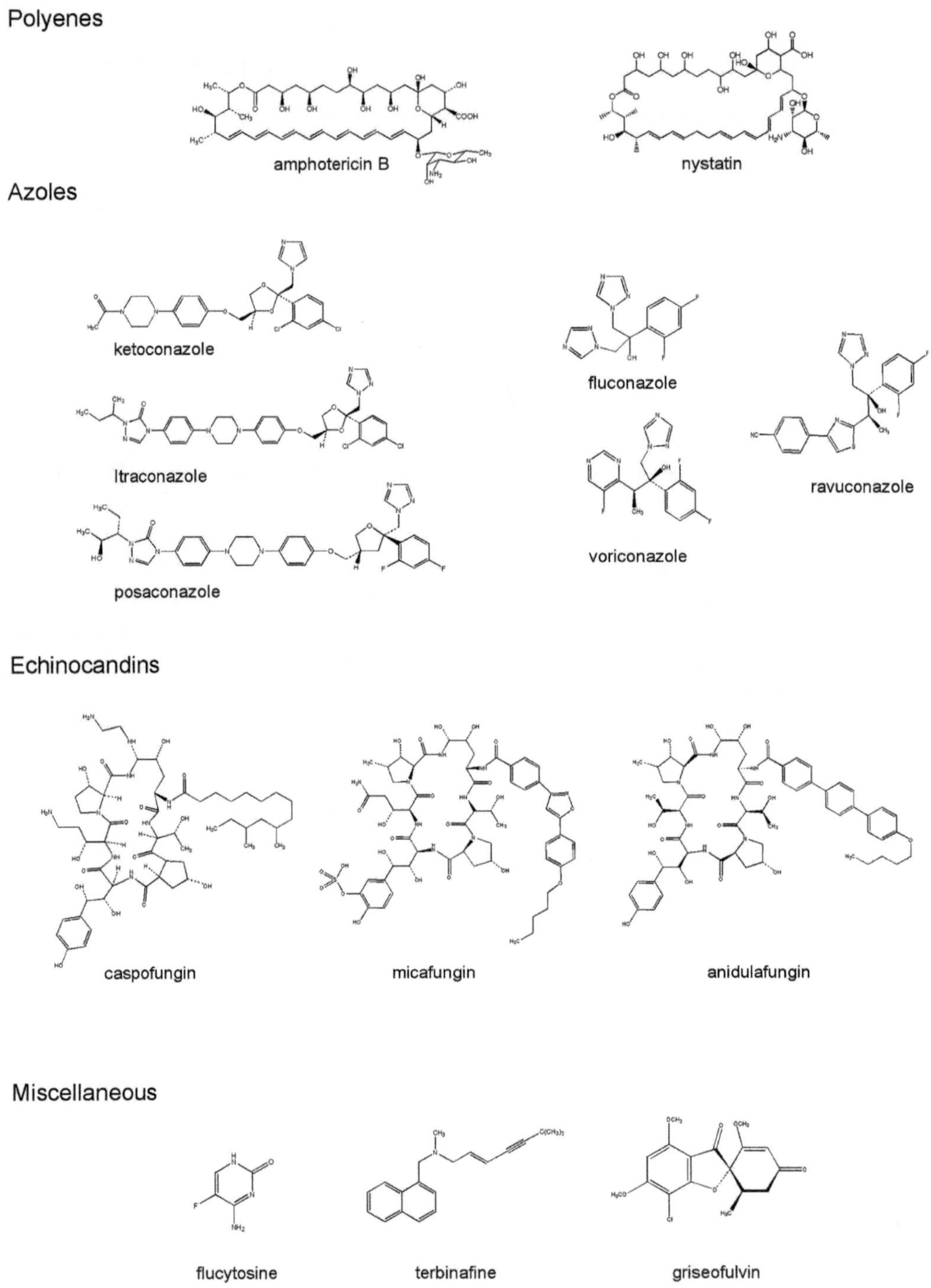

Fig. 6.1. Representative structures of systemic antifungal agents.

- Limited penetration into anatomically restricted sites such as the cerebrospinal fluid (CSF)

In an attempt to address these limitations, a new chemical group of azoles was developed (triazoles) with improved physiochemical characteristics and spectrum of activity. Fluconazole, the first triazole introduced on the market in early 1990s, could be administered intravenously or orally and had predictable pharmacokinetics, excellent oral bioavailability, and improved penetration into anatomically restricted sites such as the vitreous humor and CSF. Importantly, fluconazole was well tolerated and was associated with few serious drug interactions in critically-ill patients. As a result, during the 1990s fluconazole quickly became one of the most widely prescribed antifungal agents for superficial and life-threatening infections due to yeast *(1)*. The lack of activity against opportunistic moulds (i.e., *Aspergillus*, *Fusarium*, and the Zygomycetes) and intrinsic resistance among some non-*albicans* *Candida* species (*Candida glabrata* and *Candida krusei*), however, created a need for broader-spectrum alternatives in the treatment of severely immunocompromised patients. The development of itraconazole and the broader-spectrum triazole derivatives, voriconazole and posaconazole, has largely addressed the spectrum limitations of fluconazole among these high-risk patients. Yet, these broader spectrum triazoles still carry a potential for cross-resistance with fluconazole *(2)* and exhibit more complex pharmacokinetic profiles, and a higher propensity for drug interactions. Hence, less toxic alternatives to triazole antifungal therapy would be desirable in critically ill patients, especially patients at higher risk of pharmacokinetic drug–drug interactions.

The final milestone of antifungal drug discovery during the 20th century was the identification and development of the echinocandins, lipopeptide molecules that inhibit glucan synthesis leading to damage of the cell wall *(3)*. Because of the importance of the fungal cell wall survival and the lack of this target in mammalian cells, echinocandins were predicted to be well tolerated antifungal agents with little collateral toxicity in humans. Yet, the first echinocandin tested in humans, cilofungin, had to be abandoned before large-scale clinical trials owing to difficulties in its preparation and the toxicity of its intravenous formulation *(4)*. Subsequent semisynthetic echinocandin derivatives demonstrated improved solubility and potency and were well tolerated even at high dosages. In 2001, caspofungin became the first echinocandin approved by the US Food and Drug Administration (FDA) for the treatment of invasive fungal infections in humans. Two other echinocandin derivatives with a similar spectrum as caspofungin, anidulafungin and micafungin, subsequently progressed through Phase III clinical trials and have been approved or have pending approval for clinical use in patients with oroesophageal candidiasis or invasive candidiasis.

Although the arrival of new antifungal agents has clearly advanced the management of invasive fungal infections, drug therapy failures are still common and many patients may not tolerate particular antifungal agents because of hypersensitivity reactions, renal or hepatic toxicity, or the potential for serious drug interactions. Therefore, no single antifungal agent is appropriate for all patients for any given mycosis. Moreover, breakthrough infections with intrinsically resistant pathogens have become more common with prolonged treatment courses and improved survival of chronically immunocompromised hosts. This trend has created an urgent need for laboratory support in the treatment of invasive fungal infections including *(1)* the rapid identification of fungal pathogens to the species level, and where appropriate, *(2)* in vitro susceptibility testing of clinical isolates to guide the selection of antifungal therapy. This chapter reviews key components of antifungal pharmacology with a special emphasis on systemic antifungal agents and common resistance patterns among opportunistic mycoses in humans.

2. TARGETS OF ANTIFUNGAL THERAPY

Despite differences in the composition of the cell membrane and the presence of a cell wall, much of the cellular machinery of fungi shares remarkable homology to mammalian cells. Consequently, development of drugs that selectively target pathogenic fungi without producing collateral damage to mammalian cells is a daunting pharmacological challenge. Indeed, many of the toxicities and drug interactions observed with contemporary antifungal therapies can be attributed to "nonselective" interactions with homologous enzyme or cell membrane systems found in mammalian host cells *(5)*.

With the exception of flucytosine, currently available systemic antifungals act primarily through direct or indirect interactions with the fungal cell wall and plasma membrane, and the fungal membrane sterol ergosterol and its biosynthetic pathways (Fig. 6.2). The fungal cell envelope has several properties that make it an ideal target for antifungal therapy *(4)*:

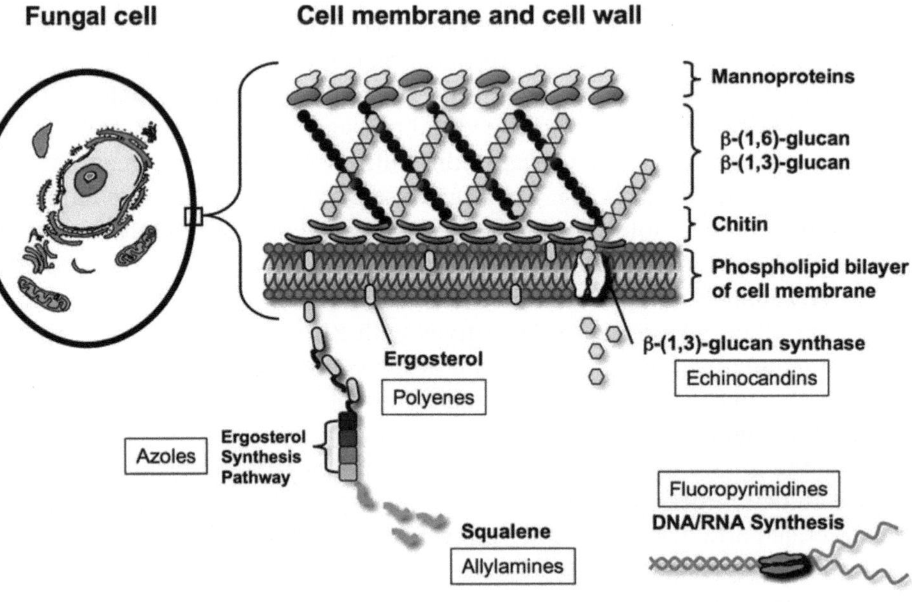

Fig. 6.2. Targets of antifungal therapy. [Figure in color on CD-ROM].

- In contrast to the cholesterol-rich cell membranes of mammalian cells, the predominant cell membrane sterol in pathogenic fungi is ergosterol. Indirect or direct targeting of ergosterol results in selective toxicity to the fungal cells.
- Mammalian cells lack a true cell wall. Drugs that target synthesis of the fungal cell wall have a low potential to cause collateral toxicity in mammalian cells.
- The cellular wall and membranes are important for ion exchange, filtration, and are a critical area for localization of enzymes involved in the metabolism and catabolism of complex nutrients *(6)*. Drugs that disrupt growth of the cell membrane and wall produce a number of pleotropic effects are selectively lethal to fungi.

2.1. Polyene Mechanisms of Action

Polyene antifungals (amphotericin B) bind to ergosterol, the principal sterol in the fungal cell membrane, disrupting the structure of the fungal cell membrane to the point of causing leakage of intracellular contents. Although this binding typically results in rapid cell death, the precise mechanism of fungicidal activity remains unknown. Structurally, the fungal sterol ergosterol exhibits a more cylindrical three-dimensional structure than the mammalian sterol cholesterol, which largely explains the greater affinity of amphotericin B binding to ergosterol (Fig. 6.3) *(4)*. However, amphotericin B also can bind to cholesterol in mammalian cell membranes; a mechanism that could account for the direct toxicity of the drug to the distal tubules of the kidney *(5)*.

2.2. Azole Mechanisms of Action

In contrast to the direct interactions of the polyene antifungals with ergosterol, azole antifungals indirectly affect the fungal cell membrane through inhibition of ergosterol biosynthesis. Azole antifungal compounds inhibit cytochrome P-450 sterol 14α-demethylase (Erg11p or CYP51p depending on nomenclature), an enzyme that catalyzes the oxidative removal of 14α-methyl group of lanosterol in the ergosterol

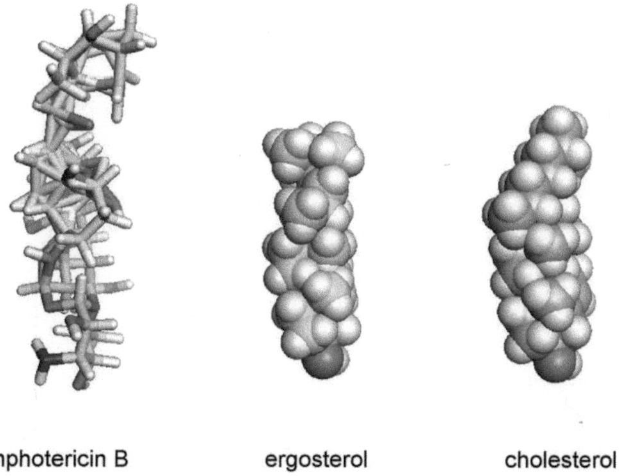

Fig. 6.3. Amphotericin B, ergosterol and cholesterol visualized in three dimensions. [Figure in color on CD-ROM].

biosynthetic pathway. Inhibition of 14α-demethylase by azoles results in an accumulation of 14α-methylated sterols in the cytoplasmic membrane, which disrupt phospholipid organization and impair membrane-bound enzyme systems such as ATPase and enzymes of the electron transport system, thus arresting fungal cell growth. CYP51p enzyme binding is accomplished through coordination of the triazole nitrogen, N3 or imidazole N4 of the azole ring with the cytochrome P-450 heme target site, while the remainder of the drug molecule binds to the apoprotein in a manner dependent on the individual structure of the azole (Fig. 6.4) *(4)*. Differences in the exact conformation of the active site between fungal species and drug structure largely define the spectrum of each agent. For molecules derived from the ketoconazole pharmacophore (e.g., itraconazole, posaconazole), extension of the side chain enhances binding of the azole to the P450 apoprotein, and expands the potency and spectrum against both yeast and filamentous fungi. For molecules derived from fluconazole (e.g., voriconazole) inclusion of an α-*O*-methyl group confers activity against *Aspergillus* and other filamentous fungi *(7)*.

One drawback of targeting fungal CYP-450 enzymes involved in ergosterol biosynthesis is the homology the fungal enzyme systems share with mammalian CYP 450 enzymes involved in drug metabolism (Fig. 6.4). Indeed, all azoles inhibit to varying degrees the mammalian CYP P450 enzymes involved in drug metabolism *(8)*. Azole therapy can predispose patients to a number of clinically significant pharmacokinetic drug–drug interactions when these antifungals are administered concurrently with drugs that are either substrates or inducers of CYP P450 enzymes in humans. Unfortunately, modifications of the azole pharmacophore designed to enhance binding to fungal CYP51p frequently enhance binding of mammalian CYP P450 enzymes. Therefore,

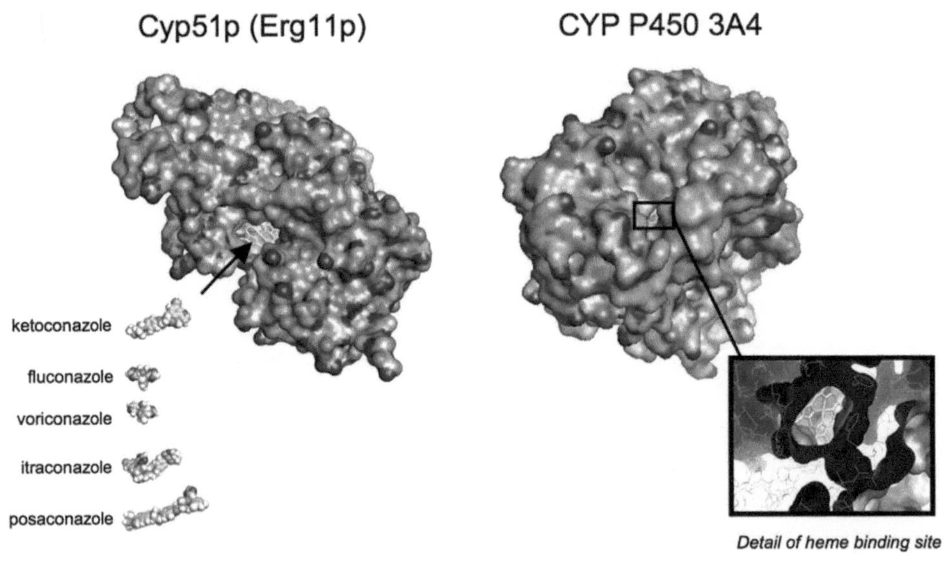

Fig. 6.4. Cyp51p and CYP P450 3A4 visualized in three dimensions highlighting the heme binding site for the imidazole (ketoconazole) and triazole rings. [Figure in color on CD-ROM].

improvement in the spectrum of azole antifungals is often accompanied by an increased potential for drug interactions.

2.3. Allylamine Mechanisms of Action

Similar to azoles, allylamines inhibit ergosterol biosynthesis before 14 α-demethylase by inhibition of the squalene monooxygenase (formally epoxidase). This enzyme is responsible for conversion of squaline to squalene epoxide, a precursor of lanosterol in the ergosterol biosynthetic pathway. After exposure to allylamines such as terbinafine, the fungal cell membrane accumulates squalene while becoming deficient in ergosterol, resulting in arrest of cell growth. Although allylamines do not appear to produce the same degree of cross-inhibition of mammalian CYP P450 enzymes as azole antifungals, strong inducers of mammalian CYP-P450 enzymes such as rifampin still increase the metabolism of squalene monooxygenase inhibitors such as terbinafine.

2.4. Echinocandin Mechanisms of Action

Of the currently available antifungal agents, only one class of agents, the echinocandins, are known to specifically target fungal cell wall synthesis. Echinocandins inhibit the synthesis of 1,3-β-D-glucan polymers, which serve as essential cross-linking structural components of the cell wall. Depletion of 1,3-β-D-glucan polymers in susceptible fungi leads to an structurally impaired cell wall, osmotic instability, and lysis in rapidly growing cells. The presumed target of the echinocandins is thought to be β-1,3-D-glucan synthase, although formal proof of this target in pathogenic fungi has been complicated by technical difficulties in studying the membrane-bound protein complex. In *Saccharomyces cerevisiae*, where the enzyme complex has been best studied, the echinocandins are known to bind to the Fks1p component of the two proteins (Fks1p and Fks2p) regulated by the GTP-binding peptide, Rho1p, that comprise the transmembrane β-1,3-D-glucan synthase complex *(9)*.

The degree of β-1,3-D-glucan polymerization in the cell wall and expression of the β-1,3-D-glucan synthase target chiefly defines the spectrum and lethality of the echinocandins in pathogenic fungi. In *Candida* species, the fungal cell wall is rich in β-1,3-D-glucans and the enzyme complex is highly expressed during rapid cell growth. Hence, echinocandins exhibit fungicidal activity against most rapidly growing *Candida* species. However, echinocandins lack clinically useful activity against *Cryptococcus neoformans* owing in part to the limited use of β-1,3-D-glucan in the cell wall of this species *(10)*. Among hyaline moulds, the cell wall of *Aspergillus* species contain the greatest degree of β-1,3- and β-1,6-D-glucan polymers. The β-1,3-D-glucan synthase complex, is expressed predominantly on the growing apical tips of the hyphae. Therefore, echinocandins kill only the growing hyphal tips of the fungus, resulting in abnormal, hyperacute branching and aberrant growth, with minimal effects on the viability of subapical components (Fig. 6.5) *(11)*. Other filamentous fungi such as *Fusarium* species and *Zygomycetes* utilize α-1,3-glucans in the cell wall matrix and chitosan polymers *(10)*. As such, echinocandins lack pronounced activity in vitro against these opportunistic fungi.

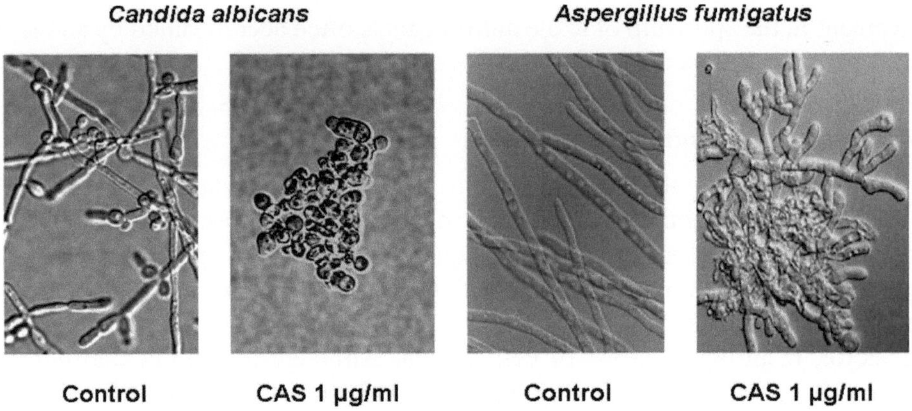

Fig. 6.5. In vitro effects of caspofungin (CAS) on fungal morphology.

2.5. *Pyrimidine Mechanisms of Action*

Flucytosine (5-fluorocytosine, 5-FC) works as an antifungal agent after conversion to 5-fluorouracil within fungal cells (Fig. 6.2). Once inside cells, 5-fluorouracil inhibits thmidylate synthase, a key enzyme in DNA synthesis, and incorporates into RNA, causing premature chain termination. The uptake and conversion of flucytosine requires the activity of two enzymes, cytosine permease and cytosine deaminase. Mammalian cells and many filamentous fungi lack or have very low activity of these enzymes, thus restricting the activity of the flucytosine to pathogenic yeast *(5)*. In humans, however, resident intestinal flora may convert flucytosine to fluorouracil, resulting in nausea, vomiting, diarrhea, and bone marrow suppression *(5)*.

3. ANTIFUNGAL RESISTANCE

Antifungal resistance is a broad concept describing the failure of a fungal infection to respond to antifungal therapy. Resistance has been traditionally classified as either primary (intrinsic, i.e., present before exposure to antifungal) or secondary (acquired, i.e., that which develops after antifungal exposure owing to stable or transient genotypic alterations) *(12,13)*. A third type of antifungal resistance could be described as "clinical resistance," which encompasses progression or relapse of infection by a pathogenic fungus that appears, by laboratory testing, to be fully susceptible to the antifungal agent used to treat the infection. Clinical resistance is most commonly a result of persistent and profound immune defects (e.g., AIDS, neutropenia, graft versus host disease and its treatment) or infected prosthetic materials (i.e., central venous catheters), which become encased in protective biofilm, thus limiting drug activity *(12,13)*. In some cases, suboptimal drug concentrations at the site of infection resulting from poor drug absorption, drug interactions, or infrequent dosing may contribute to clinical resistance.

Primary or secondary antifungal resistance can arise through a number of complex mechanisms and may be expressed over a wide phenotypic spectrum *(12)*. At one extreme, fungi may be susceptible to the effects of an antifungal agent but growth may not be completely inhibited in vitro. This so-called trailing growth may be observed for antifungals during laboratory testing (particularly azoles and flucytosine) even at high concentrations, but is generally considered a testing artifact and not indicative of true resistance. Similarly, some echinocandins may exhibit a paradoxical attenuation of activity at higher drug concentrations without clear evidence of diminished drug activity at higher dosages in animal models or patients. Heterogeneous resistance, the presence of subpopulations of fungal cells with varying degrees of resistance to an antifungal agent in a susceptible population, may indicate an increased propensity for the development of antifungal resistance. This type of resistance may not be detected unless specialized testing methods are used in the laboratory. Inducible or transiently expressed (epigenetic) antifungal resistance mechanisms have also been described in fungi, but little is known about the clinical significance of these resistance patterns in human infections *(12)*. The other extreme in the phenotypic expression of antifungal resistance is represented by isolates with stable and persistent growth even at high antifungal concentrations. It is important to note that most studies of antifungal resistance focus on isolates with a stable resistance phenotype. Molecular mechanisms of resistance have been best described in *C. albicans* isolates recovered from AIDS patients with chronic, recurring fluconazole-refractory oropharyngeal candidiasis *(13)*. The chronic nature of these mucosal infections allows the longitudinal collection of serial, matched *Candida* isolates that exhibit progressively stable, higher degrees of resistance to antifungals. By contrast, acute bloodstream candidiasis, aspergillosis, or other less common life-threatening mycoses do not typically allow for the study of serial, matched isolates, thus complicating genotypic–phenotypic correlation of resistance development.

3.1. Laboratory Detection of Resistance

Standardization of in vitro tests used to determine the activity of antifungals has been a long process. In 1982, the Clinical Laboratory and Standards Institute (CLSI, formerly NCCLS) established a subcommittee to assess the need for such testing. It was not until 1985 that the first report of this subcommittee was released. That document, NCCLS M20-CR, Antifungal Susceptibility Testing; Committee Report, was based on responses from hospitals and reference laboratories from across the nation. The committee found that approximately 20% of the laboratories that responded were in fact conducting antifungal susceptibility testing. Many methods existed, but most of the respondents utilized a broth method and were testing yeast only. Comparison testing of isolates between collaborating laboratories was unacceptably low.

Based on this study, the decision was made to develop a standardized method, the goal being to correlate not between isolate and patient outcome but rather between laboratories. Methods that existed included broth, agar, and disk diffusion. The committee decided that the standard method should be a macrobroth dilution method and that only a synthetic medium should be chosen. Several centers collaborated and a preliminary method was introduced in 1992, M27-P *(14)*. Parameters were set to include medium, inoculum preparation and size, incubation temperature and duration, and end point criteria. The procedure has been refined and is now an approved method, M27-A2 *(15)*. Subsequent publications include M38-A *(16)* and M44-A *(17)*. M38-A utilizes similar methods for mould testing while M44-A provides guidelines for disk diffusion testing of yeast. As a result of approved methods, industry now provides kits that enable routine microbiology laboratories to perform testing in-house rather than sending isolates off for reference testing. Before doing this, however, laboratories should have sufficient requests for this testing to ensure the volume of work needed to maintain accuracy and reproducibility.

Interpretive guidelines have been established only for fluconazole, itraconazole, and 5-fluorocytosine. Categories for 5-fluorocytosine include susceptible (S), intermediate (I), and resistant (R) while those for the azoles include susceptible (S), susceptible dose-dependent (SDD), and resistant (R). The susceptible dose-dependent category relates to yeast testing only and is not interchangeable with the intermediate category associated with bacterial and 5-fluorocytosine breakpoints. This category is in recognition that yeast susceptibility is dependent on achieving maximum blood levels. By maintaining blood levels with higher doses of antifungal, an isolate with an SDD endpoint may be successfully treated with a given azole *(17)*.

One important problem with any approach toward in vitro susceptibility testing is the correlation of the minimum inhibitory concentration (MIC) with patient outcome. Some assumptions can be made, however, about MIC and patient outcome. Rex and Pfaller proposed the "90–60 Rule" as a general guide for establishing clinically relevant interpretative breakpoints for resistance *(18)*. This rule states that infections caused by isolates that have MICs considered susceptible respond favorably to appropriate therapy approximately 90% of the time whereas infections caused by isolates with MICs considered resistant respond favorably in approximately 60% of cases.

3.2. Mechanisms of Resistance

Many aspects of antifungal resistance are still poorly understood, particularly with respect to the regulation and expression of resistance mechanisms after exposure to antifungal agents (secondary resistance). Nevertheless, advances in molecular biology and genome sequencing of pathogenic fungi have yielded progress in our understanding of the mechanisms most frequently leading to antifungal resistance. These mechanisms can be grouped into five general categories (Fig. 6.6):

- Decreased drug import or increased drug export (efflux pumps)
- Alteration in drug target binding site
- Changes in biosynthetic pathways (particularly sterol synthesis) that circumvent or attenuate the effects of antifungal inhibition
- Alterations in intracellular drug processing
- Upregulation of homeostatic stress-response pathways to deal with antifungal-associated damage

It is important to note that multiple resistance mechanisms are often expressed simultaneously after antifungal exposure and that a single mechanism is unlikely to result in a resistant strain. Depending on the mechanisms concurrently expressed, cross-resistance may or may not be observed between different antifungals. Whole genome expression profiles of *C. albicans* have revealed transient upregulation of several resistance mechanisms (i.e., ergosterol biosynthesis— *ERG 3*, *ERG11*; efflux pumps—*CDR1*, *CDR2*) following a single exposure to azole antifungals *(19)*. Development of resistance in

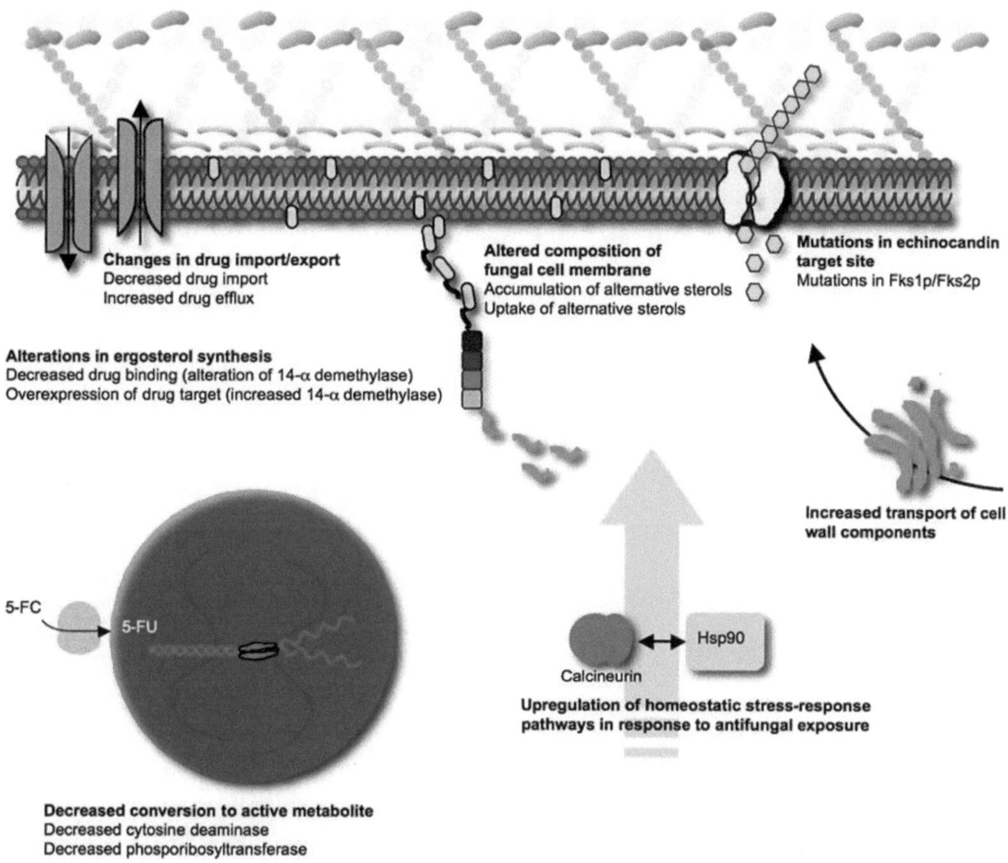

Fig. 6.6. Mechanisms of antifungal resistance. [Figure in color on CD-ROM].

longitudinally collected clinical strains in patients who fail a course of progressively higher dosages of antifungals generally demonstrates a gradual accumulation of several alternations that result in a detectable resistance *(12)*.

Changes in drug import and export are probably the most common mechanisms associated with primary and secondary antifungal resistance *(12)*. Decreased drug import is consistently associated with primary resistance to flucytosine and azole antifungals. For example, poor uptake of flucytosine due to alterations in cytosine permease or decreased availability of this enzyme largely accounts for the limited spectrum of this agent against opportunistic moulds. Similarly, differences in azole susceptibility between fluconazole and itraconazole against *C. krusei* have been reported to be more closely associated with intracellular accumulation than differences in drug binding affinity to the 14α-demethylase target *(20)*. Drug import may also be affected by the sterol composition of the plasma membrane. Several studies have demonstrated that when the ergosterol component of the membrane is altered in favor of other 14α-methyl sterols there is a concomitant permeability change in the membrane to antifungals and a decrease in membrane fluidity *(12)*.

Similar to other eukaryotic cells, fungi are known to contain two types of efflux pumps that contribute to drug resistance: ATP binding cassette (ABC) transporters and major facilitators (MF). Overexpression of the ATP-dependent ABC transporters typically confers a multidrug resistance phenotype. In contrast, MF pumps, which expel antifungal though protonmotive force (H^+ gradient across membrane), have a much narrower spectrum of substrate specificity. In *Candida albicans*, overexpression of ATP-dependent efflux pumps *CDR1* and *CDR2* confer cross-resistance to all azole antifungals *(12)*. In contrast, overexpression of MF pump *MDR1* affects only the accumulation of fluconazole and does not result in cross-resistance to itraconazole or ketoconazole. Overexpression of ATP-dependent efflux pumps is the most prevalent mechanism of efflux-mediated resistance reported in clinical isolates *(12)*. Recently, overexpression of ABC transporters was reported to confer a degree of cross-resistance between azoles and echinocandins in a laboratory strain of *C. albicans (21)*.

Besides drug efflux, the most common mechanism associated with antifungal resistance involves changes in the binding site of the drug. Several genetic alternations in *ERG11,* the gene encoding 14α-demethylase, have been attributed to decreases in azole activity, including point mutations that result in changes in the active pocket site or overexpression of *ERG11*. Similar alterations in other enzymes of the ergosterol biosynthetic pathway, particularly *ERG 3* (C-5-sterol desaturase), which is upregulated with inhibition of 14α-demethylase, have also been documented in azole-resistant clinical strains. Binding site alteration is also likely to be an important mechanism of echinocandin resistance. Point mutations in the *FKS1* gene have been reported in laboratory-derived caspofungin-resistant mutants of *C. albicans (3)*.

Changes in the target expression in the ergosterol biosynthetic pathway alter the fungal cell membrane sterol content. Substitution of alternative sterols for ergosterol, or alterations in the sterol:phospholid ratio in the cell membrane, can decrease intracellular accumulation of azoles and reduce the binding of amphotericin B to the cell membrane. Indeed, many polyene-resistant yeasts recovered from patients with clear microbiological failure on amphotericin B have dimished ergosterol concentrations in their fungal cell membranes. Several studies have even suggested that pathogenic fungi can scavenge free sterols for the cell membrane, including cholesterol, resulting in resistance to polyene and azole antifungals *(22)*.

Alterations in intracellular drug processing and/or degradation and metabolism are probably the least well studied pathways of resistance in fungi, even though these mechanisms are well characterized in other prokaryotic and eukaryotic systems. Resistance to flucytosine has been associated with alterations in cystosine deaminase, which results in decreased intracellular conversion of flucytosine to its active form.

Recent studies of antifungal resistance have begun to focus on homeostatic stress-response pathways in fungi that may be unpregulated after exposure to antifungals. Disruption of the evolutionarily conserved protein kinase C (PKC) cell wall integrity and calcineurin pathways enhances azole and echinocandin killing in fungi *(23)*. Upregulation of these pathways also diminishes the lethal effects of antifungals through upregulation of ergosterol and glucan biosynthesis, increases in chitin content in the fungal cell wall, as well as increased export of cell wall components for cell wall repair.

Recently, the molecular chaperone heat shock protein 90 (Hsp90) was reported to play a critical role in regulating resistance to antifungal agents through the calcineurin pathway *(24,25)*. Future efforts toward combating antifungal resistance are likely to exploit this important and evolutionarily conserved mechanism for maintaining and expressing resistance mechanisms to antifungals.

4. AMPHOTERICIN B

Conventional amphotericin B (Fungizone®) has long been considered to be the cornerstone of therapy for deeply invasive fungal infections. Toxicity, including infusion-related fever, chills, rigors, headache, and dose-limiting nephrotoxicity, often limits the effectiveness of this agent in severely ill patients. Consequently, three lipid-based formulations (Ambisome®, Abelcet®, Amphotec®) were developed that offer several advantages over conventional amphotericin B including *(1)* the ability to administer higher daily dosages of drug, *(2)* decreased infusion-related side effects (especially for the liposomal formulation), and *(3)* a reduced rate of nephrotoxicity (Table 6.1). Despite the improved therapeutic index of these formulations, there is still relatively few data from prospective clinical trials to suggest these formulations are more effective than conventional amphotericin B. Moreover, the higher acquisition cost of the lipid formulations has required many institutions to restrict the use of these formulations to patients with preexisting renal failure, or in patients who are at high risk for developing nephrotoxicity while receiving amphotericin B (e.g., patients on concomitant nephrotoxic therapies). Currently, there is no consensus opinion on the clinical or pharmacoeconomic threshold for using lipid amphotericin B formulations as first-line therapy for most invasive mycoses.

4.1. Spectrum and Susceptibility

Amphotericin B should be administered only to patients with progressive and possibly fatal infections. Acceptable activity can be measured in vitro against almost all fungi including *Candida*, *Cryptococcus*, *Aspergillus*, *Blastomyces*, *Histoplasma*, *Coccidioides*, *Sporothrix*, and agents of zygomycosis (mucormycosis, including *Rhizopus*, *Mucor*, and *Absidia*), as well as other less frequently recovered strains.

A few species exhibit elevated MICs when tested against amphotericin B and are known to possess innate resistance to this drug. Resistant species include both *Scedosporium apiospermum* and *S. prolificans* in addition to *Paecilomyces lilacinus*, *Aspergillus terreus,* and some *Fusarium* species. Early reports have revealed *Candida lusitaniae* resistance to amphotericin B and have shown that this species possesses the ability to develop resistance while the patient is on treatment. The first report involved a patient whose initial isolate was susceptible but whose subsequent isolates had developed amphotericin B resistance *(26)*. Later reports have shown amphotericin B resistance may exist even before exposure to amphotericin B *(27)*. The expected rate of resistance for *C. lusitaniae* is 8% to 10% of any microbiology lab stock collection.

Table 6.1
Systemic antifungal therapies

Antifungals	Trade name(s)	Usual adult dose	Mechanism of action	Toxicities	Spectrum/comments
			Polyenes		
Amphotericin B	Fungizone	0.25–1.5 mg/kg IV q24h	Bind to ergosterol and intercalates with the fungal cell membrane, resulting in increased membrane permeability to univalent and divalent cations	Acute—Fever, chills, rigor, arthralgia with infusion. Thrombophlebitis, dyspnea (rare), arrhythmias (rare)	Drug of choice for severe infections caused by endemic dimorphic fungi, most *Candida* species, and common hyalohyphomycetes (including *Aspergillus*) and zygomycosis.
				Delayed—Azotemia (26%), tubular acidosis, hypokalemia, hypomagnesemia, anemia	Nephrotoxicity is the dose-limiting side-effect, reduced with lipid amphotericin B formulations and saline pre and post hydration.
Lipid formulations of amphotericin B:					
Liposomal (L)-AMB	Ambisome,	3–10 mg/kg q24h			Infusion related reactions: Ambisome < Abelcet < Amphotec
ABLC	Abelcet,	5 mg/kg/q24h			
ABCD	Amphotec	3–4 mg/kg q24h			

Azoles					
Ketoconazole	Nizoral	200–800 mg PO q24h Divided doses recommended $\geq$ 400 mg/day	Inhibition of cytochrome P450 14α-demethylase, decreased production of ergosterol, accumulation of lanosterol leading to perturbation of fungal cell membrane, fungistatic	Gastrointestinal (20–50%) including nausea and vomiting, anorexia, rash (2%), transient increases in hepatic enzymes, severe hepatotoxicity (rare), alopecia, inhibition of adrenal steroid synthesis (especially at dosages > 600 mg/day)	Oral formulation only. Inconsistencies in oral absorption/poor gastrointestinal tolerance limits use for treatment of deep mycoses. Potent inhibitor of mammalian cytochrome P450 can lead to potentially severe drug interactions when administered concomitantly with other P450-metabolized drugs.
Itraconazole	Sporanox	200–400 mg PO q24h IV 200–400 mg q12h, then q24h Divided doses recommended $\geq$ 400 mg/day	Similar to ketoconazole, but more selective for fungal P450 demethylase	Gastrointestinal (20%) including nausea and vomiting, and diarrhea, rash (2%), taste disturbance (oral solution), transient increases in hepatic enzymes, severe hepatotoxicity (rare), alopecia, inhibition of adrenal steroid synthesis (especially at dosages > 600 mg/day). Accumulation of hydroxy-propyl--cyclodextran vehicle in patients with CrCl < 30 ml/min (intravenous formulation). Congestive heart failure (rare)	Spectrum similar to fluconazole with enhanced activity against *C. krusei* and *Aspergillus*. Not active against *Fusarium* and zygomycosis. Drug of choice for mild to moderate infections caused by endemic dimorphic fungi. Bioavailability of oral solution is improved over capsules by 30% under fed conditions and 60% in fasting conditions. Potent inhibitor of mammalian cytochrome P450 enzymes. Serum level monitoring is occasionally recommended, trough levels measured by HPLC should exceed 0.5 µg/ml

(*Continued*)

Table 6.1
(Continued)

Fluconazole	Diflucan	3–12 mg/kg PO/IV q24h Dosage adjustment required in renal impairment	Similar to ketoconazole, but more selective inhibitor of 14α demethylase	Gastrointestinal (5–10%), rash, headache, transient increases in hepatic enzymes, hepatotoxicity (rare), alopecia	Spectrum includes most *Candida* species, *Cryptococcus neoformans*, and endemic dimorphic fungi. Less active against *Candida glabrata. Candida krusei* is intrinsically resistant. Not clinically active for deep mycoses caused by invasive moulds. Higher daily dosages are recommended (e.g., 12 mg/kg per day) in critically-ill patients or in institutions where *Candida glabrata* is common
Voriconazole	Vfend	6 mg/kg IV q12h × 2 doses, then 4 mg/kg q12h 200 mg PO q12h if ≥ 40 kg, 100 mg PO q12h if < 40 kg	Similar to fluconazole, but higher affinity for fungal 14α-demethylase	Transient photopsia (reported up to 30%), rash, hallucinations (2%), transient increases in hepatic enzymes, severe hepatotoxicity (rare).Accumulation of sulfo-butyl ester cyclodextran vehicle may occur in patients with CrCl < 50 ml/min receiving intravenous formulation.	Spectrum similar to itraconazole with enhanced activity against *Aspergillus*, *Fusarium*, and *Scedosporium apiospermum* (*Pseudallescheria boydii*). Retains activity against some fluconazole-resistant *C. glabrata*. Inhibitor of mammalian cytochrome P450 enzymes.
Posaconazole	Noxafil	600–800 mg/day in divided doses	Similar to voriconazole	Gastrointestinal (5–15%), fever, headache, musculoskeletal pain (5%)	Spectrum similar to voriconazole with enhanced activity against *Fusarium*, zygomycosis, and black moulds (phaeohyphomycetes). Inhibitor of mammalian cytochrome P450 3A4

(Continued)

			Echinocandins		
Caspofungin	Cancidas	70 mg IV day 1, then 50 mg q24h	Inhibition of cell wall glucan synthesis, leading to osmotic instability of fugal cell.	Fever, chills, phlebitis/thrombophelibitis (peripheral line), rash. Drug concentrations decreased with P450 3A4 inducers. Decreases tacrolimus blood levels by ~25%	Spectrum includes most *Candida* species including fluconazole-resistant *Candida krusei* and *Candida glabrata*. Higher dosages may be required for *C. parapsilosis*. Active against *Aspergillus* species.Not active against *Cryptococcus neoformans*, Trichosporon, *Fusarium*, zygomycosis, or black moulds (phaeohyphomycetes).
Micafungin	Mycamine	50–150 mg IV q24h	Similar to caspofungin	Clearance not affected by P450 3A4 inducers	Similar to caspofungin
Anidulafungin	Eraxis	200 mg IV day 1 then 100 mg/day	Similar to caspofungin	Clearance not affected by P450 3A4 inducers	Similar to caspofungin
			Fluoropyrimidines		
Flucytosine (5-FC)	Ancobon	100 mg/kg daily PO divided q6h Dosage adjustment required in renal impairment	Drug is transported into susceptible fungi by cytosine permease, and then deaminated to active form (5-FU) by cytosine deaminase where the drug interferes with DNA/RNA synthesis	Increase in serum transaminases (7%), nausea and vomiting (5%); diarrhea, abdominal pain, rash, entercolitis (rare)Less common- leucopenia, thrombocytopenia, anemia	Narrow spectrum for deep mycoses: *Candida* and *Cryptococcus neoformans* only. Resistance is common when used as monotherapy. Typically administered in combination with amphotericin B for cryptococcal meningitis.Risk of bone marrow suppression increased with persistent flucytosine levels >100 μg/ml. Careful dosage adjustment is required in patients with renal dysfunction.

PO, Orally; IV, intraveneously; q6h, every 6 hours; q12h, every 12 hours; q24h, every 24 hours; P450, cytochrome P450.

4.2. *Pharmacokinetics*

Amphotericin B deoxycholate has negligible oral absorption and must be administered intravenously. After intravenous administration, the drug is released from its carrier and is highly bound by plasma proteins (91% to 95%) including lipoproteins, erythrocytes, and cholesterol in the plasma. Amphotericin B then redistributes from the bloodstream into tissue with an apparent volume of distribution (V_d) of 4 liters/kg *(5)*. In adults, infusion of 0.6 mg/kg of amphotericin B deoxycholate yields peak serum concentrations of approximately 1 to 3 μg/ml *(28)*. Concentrations in other body fluids outside the serum are less than 5% of concurrent serum concentrations, with poor penetration into bronchial secretions, pleura, peritoneum, synovium, and aqueous humor. Although amphotericin B poorly penetrates the CSF, fungal infections of the brain have been successfully treated with amphotericin B *(5)*.

Tissue concentrations of amphotericin B are highest in the kidney, followed by the liver, spleen, heart, skeletal, muscle, and brain. The formulation of amphotericin B into phospholipid sheets (Abelcet), cholesterol disks (Amphotec), or liposome carriers (Ambisome) alters drug distribution (particularly to the kidney) and the elimination profile of the drug *(5)* (Table 6.2).

Recent studies have suggested that amphotericin B undergoes relatively little metabolism, with a terminal elimination half-life of greater than 11 to 15 days. After 168 hours, approximately 60% of a single dose can be recovered from the feces (~40%) and urine (20%) *(29)*. Because a relatively lower fraction of the daily dosage is slowly excreted in urine and bile, dosage modification is not necessary to prevent drug accumulation in patients with renal or hepatic failure, but may be judicious in a patient with declining renal function. Because amphotericin B behaves as a colloid in aqueous solutions and is highly protein bound, hemodialysis does not remove significant amounts of the drug unless the patient is hyperlipidemic; which enhances amphotericin B binding to the dialysis membrane *(5)*.

4.3. *Adverse Effects*

The most common acute toxicity of amphotericin B formulations is infusion-related reactions, which are characterized by fever, chills, rigors, anorexia, nausea, vomiting, myalgias, arthralgias, and headache. Hypotension, flushing and dizziness are less common, but bronchospasm and true anaphylactic reactions have been reported with both the conventional and lipid formulations of amphotericin B *(5)*. Severe hypokalemia and cardiac arrhythmias have also been described in patients with central venous catheters who have received rapid infusions or excessive doses of conventional amphotericin B. Therefore, slower infusion rates (4 to 6 hours or more) and EKG monitoring should be considered in patients with underlying cardiac conduction abnormalities. Thrombophlebitis is a common local side effect with infusion, which often necessitates the placement of a central venous line for therapy more than 1 week. Slower infusion rates, rotation of infusion sites, application of hot packs, low-dose heparin, and avoidance of concentrations greater than 1 mg/ml can minimize thrombophlebitis.

Acute reactions generally subside over time and with subsequent amphotericin B infusions. In the past, a test dose of amphotericin B deoxycholate (i.e., 1 to 5 mg) was recommended before initiating therapy. This is no longer considered

Table 6.2
Comparative pharmacokinetics of the antifungal agents

	AMB	ABCD	ABLC	L-AMB	Flu	Itra[a]	Vori	Posa	Anid	Cas	Mica	5FC
Oral bioavailability (%)	<5	<5	<5	<5	95	50	96	60	<5	<5	<5	>80
Distribution												
Total C_{max} (μg/ml)		4	0.3–1	131	0.7	11	4.6	7.8	0.83	0.27	0.24	80
AUC (mg * h/L)	17	43	14	555	400	29.2	20.3	8.9	99[e]	119	158[e]	
Protein binding (%)	>95	>95	>95	>95	10	99.8	58	99	84	97.	99	4
CSF (%)	0–4				>60	<10		60	<5	<5	<5	75
Eye (%)	0–38[b,c]	0–38[b,c]	0–38[b,c]	0–38[b,c]	28–75[b,c] (10–70 μg/ml)	10[†](0.22 μg/ml)	18[b](0.81 μg/ml)	26(0.25 μg/ml)	ND	ND	ND	ND
Urine (%)[d]	3–20			4.5	90	1–10	<2	<2	<2	<2	<2	90
Metabolism	Unk	Unk	Unk	Unk	+	++	+++	++	None	Hep	Hep	None
Elimination	Urine/ bile	Unk	Unk	Unk	Renal	Hep	Renal	Feces	Feces	Urine	Feces	Renal
Half-life (h)	50	30	173	100–153	31	24	6	25	24	30	15	3–6

AMB, amphotericin B deoxycholate; ABCD, amphotericin B cholesterol dispersion; ABLC, amphotericin B lipid complex; L-AMB, liposomal amphotericin B; Flu, fluconazole; Itra, itraconazole; Vori, voriconazole; Posa, posaconazole; Anid, anidulafungin; Cas, caspofungin; Mica, micafungin; 5FC, 5-fluorocytosine or flucytosine; ND, no data available; Unk, unknown; Hep, hepatic.

[a]Data are for oral solution.

[b]Human.

[c]Animal.

[d]% of active drug or metabolites.

[e]For doses of 100 mg/day.

useful for screening patients for hypersensitivity reactions. Premedications such as low-dose hydrocortisone (1 mg/kg), diphenhydramine, meperidine (0.5 mg/kg), and nonsteroidal anti-inflammatory agents are often administered before amphotericin B infusions to blunt symptoms of acute reactions. Premedication is also recommended before infusions of the lipid amphotericin B formulations, despite the reduced rates of infusion reactions seen with these drugs. Nephrotoxicity is the most significant, delayed toxicity of amphotericin B and can be classified into glomerular or tubular mechanisms. Amphotericin B directly constricts the afferent arterioles, resulting in decreased renal blood flow and a drop in glomerular filtration (increased serum creatinine), eventually leading to azotemia. Amphotericin-induced azotemia can be reduced by ensuring patients are well hydrated before starting therapy and by sodium loading—the practice of administering intravenous normal saline (0.5 to 1 liters) before and after amphotericin B infusion to maintain renal blood flow and adequate glomerular filtration pressure. Two small nonrandomized studies have also suggested that the administration of amphotericin B deoxycholate by continuous infusion can preserve glomerular function in the short term *(30,31)*; however, this dosing approach has not been widely adopted. Azotemia with amphotericin B is generally reversible, although 5% to 10% of patients may have persistent renal impairment after discontinuation of therapy.

Amphotericin B is directly toxic to the distal tubules, resulting in impaired urinary acidification, impaired urinary concentrating ability, and wasting of potassium and magnesium. Hypokalemia is common in patients receiving either conventional or lipid formulations of the drug. Patients may require the administration of up to 15 mmol of supplemental potassium per hour *(4)*. Hypokalemia and low serum magnesium levels frequently precede decreases in glomerular filtration (increased serum creatinine), especially in patients who are adequately hydrated or receiving lipid formulations of amphotericin B. Continued tubular damage, however, eventually results in decreases in renal blood flow and glomerular filtration through tubuloglomerular feedback mechanisms that constrict the afferent arteriole. Hence, sodium loading should still be considered for patients receiving lipid amphotericin B formulations.

Patients who receive prolonged courses of amphotericin B frequently develop normochromic, normocytic anemia due to the inhibitory effects of amphotericin B on renal erythropoietin synthesis. Patients may experience decreases in hemoglobin of 15% to 35% below baseline that return to normal within several months of discontinuation of the drug. Administration of recombinant erythropoietin may be required in patients with symptomatic anemia.

5. AZOLES

The availability of azole antifungals, particularly the oral triazoles itraconazole, fluconazole, and more recently, voriconazole and posaconazole, fulfills a critical need for effective and better tolerated alternatives to amphotericin B. Miconazole was the first systemic azole approved for use in humans, but the relatively toxic intravenous formulation limited its use to severely ill patients. Similarly, ketoconazole was not effective in critically ill patients because of its lack of an intravenous formulation and erratic absorption in patients with relative achlorhydria. The triazoles have proven to be much more effective in the prevention and treatment of both primary and opportunistic mycoses. All three currently approved triazoles are available in table/capsule, oral solution, and intravenous formulations, providing clinicians with added flexibility in therapy selection. Because all azoles are potentially teratogenic, they should be avoided during pregnancy.

5.1. Spectrum and Susceptibility

The triazoles are more easily tolerated, but are primarily considered fungistatic as opposed to fungicidal (lethal) drugs. However, clear definitions of cidality are often more difficult to ascertain with antifungal agents. Although similar in mechanisms of action, each agent has a slightly different spectrum of activity.

Fluconazole is principally used for yeast infections including those caused by most *Candida* and *Cryptococcus* species. Although this drug has been used to successfully manage meningitis caused by *Coccidioides*, it is not typically a drug of choice for infections caused by other moulds.

Of primary concern is acquired resistance by yeasts. *Candida krusei* is well documented to possess intrinsic resistance to fluconazole, so much so that susceptibility testing against this isolate is not recommended. Some reports place the rate of outright *C. glabrata* resistance at about 15% of any given population of isolates *(32)*, but both *C. albicans* and *C. glabrata* are capable of developing resistance after prolonged therapy or after therapy with inappropriate dosing. Overall, by in vitro testing, about 88% of *Cryptococcus neoformans* and 95% of *C. albicans* strains appear susceptible to fluconazole.

Itraconazole possesses a wide spectrum of activity, including activity against both yeasts and moulds. It is useful in treating aspergillosis, blastomycosis, coccidioidomycosis, histoplasmosis, and candidiasis. In addition, itraconazole possess low MIC end points against the dematiaceous fungi and may be considered the drug of choice for treatment of infections caused by fungi from this group. Cross-resistance is of concern between drugs within the azole class. Comparison of resistance patterns between itraconazole and fluconazole reveal similar percentages of resistance among *Candida* species.

Voriconazole is noted to have activity against *Aspergillus*, *S. apiospermum*, and *Fusarium solani*. This is remarkable because both *S. apiospermum* and *F. solani* are notoriously resistant to other antifungal agents. In addition, voriconazole may possess lethal activity against the aspergilli as opposed to the static activity expected with the azoles. Susceptibility patterns with the yeasts are similar to those of both itraconazole and fluconazole. An important exception is the extremely low incidence of resistance seen with *C. krusei*, in contrast to near 100% resistance of this species to fluconazole and about 10% resistance to itraconazole.

Posaconazole is a very promising investigational azole with a broad spectrum of activity. Clinical trials are underway to assess activity in aspergillosis, candidiasis, fusariosis, coccidioidomycosis, and zygomycosis (mucormycosis). Results against species such as *Rhizopus* and *Mucor* show that this drug may provide alternative therapy to amphotericin B for infections caused by this group of fungi. Resistance has not been noted but some cross-resistance may occur.

5.1.1. Fluconazole

Among the triazole antifungals, fluconazole (Diflucan®) is clearly the best tolerated agent and has the most desirable pharmacological properties including high bioavailability, high water solubility, low degree of protein binding, linear pharmacokinetics, and a wide volume of distribution including the CSF, eyes, and urine *(27)*. Unlike other azoles, fluconazole is eliminated primarily unchanged through the kidneys and is less susceptible to clinically significant drug interactions through mammalian cytochrome P450 enzymes at standard dosages used to treat superficial (100 to 200 mg/day) or systemic (400 mg/day) infections.

5.1.2. Itraconazole

Itraconazole (Sporanox®) was initially introduced in the early 1990s as a capsule formulation that was effective for superficial fungal infections and mild to moderately severe endemic mycosis, but erratic absorption in the critically ill patient limited its effectiveness for opportunistic mycoses. The subsequent reformulation of this triazole into an oral and intravenous solution with hydroxy-β-propyl cyclodextran significantly improved the blood levels that could be reliably obtained in critically ill and immunocompromised patients. Itraconazole is a relatively broad-spectrum triazole with activity against many common fungal pathogens including most *Candida*, *Cryptococcus*, endemic dimorphic fungi (*Histoplasma*, *Blastomyces* , and *Coccidioides*), and *Aspergillus*. The drug is lipophilic, highly protein bound, and has a long half-life, nonlinear pharmacokinetics, and limited distribution into some body fluids, including the CSF and urine (Table 6.2). The drug is metabolized in the liver and to a lesser extent in the gut into more hydrophilic metabolites, one of which retains potent antifungal activity (hydroxyitraconazole). The most common adverse effects associated with itraconazole therapy are gastrointestinal (especially with the oral solution), rash, and transient increases in hepatic transaminases. Prolonged therapy can be associated with metabolic disturbances (suppression of adrenal steroid synthesis) and idiopathic congestive heart failure. Itraconazole is a substrate and potent inhibitor of mammalian cytochrome P450 enzymes and is therefore susceptible to a number of clinically significant drug interactions (see Section 5.2, Azole Drug Interactions).

5.1.3. Voriconazole

Voriconazole (Vfend®) is a methylated analogue of fluconazole with enhanced activity against yeast as well as important opportunistic moulds including *Aspergillus* and *Fusarium* (Table 6.1). Like fluconazole, voriconazole is well absorbed orally, has limited protein binding, and distributes widely throughout the body, including the CSF. Like itraconazole, intravenous voriconazole is formulated in a cyclodextran solution (sulfobutylether cyclodextran) and has nonlinear pharmacokinetics in adults. Voriconazole is metabolized to inactive metabolites through the liver and is an inhibitor of mammalian cytochrome P450 enzymes (Table 6.2). In addition to the common adverse effects seen with other triazole antifungals (gastrointestinal, rash, increases in hepatic enzymes), voriconazole can cause transient visual disturbances in 15% of 30% of patients that manifest as photophobia, perception of blinking or flashing lights (even with the eyes closed), and occasionally hazy or blurred vision. Symptoms tend to occur during the first week of therapy and disappear with continued therapy in most patients. Occasionally, visual disturbances are intensified by hallucinations—a separate side effect seen in 2% to 8% of patients receiving voriconazole (often with concomitant benzodiazepines and narcotic analgesic therapy). Visual disturbances are thought to be a result of temporary alterations in electrical conduction of photoreceptors in the rods and cones of the retina, which revert to normal once therapy is stopped. No permanent damage to the retina has been noted in human or animal studies of voriconazole *(33,34)*.

5.1.4. *Posaconazole*

Posaconazole (Noxafil®) is triazole analogue of itraconazole with enhanced activity against opportunistic moulds including *Aspergillus*, *Fusarium*, and (notably) the agents of zygomycosis. Posaconazole will initially be available as an oral suspension with an intravenous formulation still in development. Absorption of posaconazole suspension is dose limited at 800 mg/day and can be improved if the suspension is administered with a high-fat meal or in divided doses (twice to four times daily) (Table 6.1) *(35)*. Once absorbed, posaconazole is widely distributed into tissues throughout the body and is highly protein bound (98%). Elimination of posaconazole occurs predominantly (90%) in the feces as unchanged drug and in the urine (10%) as an inactive metabolite (Table 6.2). Despite its lack of phase I metabolism, posaconazole is a potent inhibitor of mammalian cytochrome P450 3A4 and has a similar potential for drug interactions as itraconazole when coadministered with drugs metabolized through this pathway.

5.2. *Azole Drug Interactions*

As mentioned previously, an inherent limitation of azole pharmacology is that the target of antifungal activity in pathogenic fungi, the cytochrome P450 enzyme 14-α-demethylase, shares considerable homology with mammalian cytochrome P450 enzymes involved in drug metabolism. As a result, azole antifungals can be both substrates and inhibitors of cytochrome P450 systems in humans *(8)*. Significant drug interactions with azole antifungals are summarized in Table 6.3. Many of these drug interactions are potentially severe and concomitant use should be avoided. Some azole drug interactions are less predictable and possibly dosage dependent. For example, fluconazole is a weak inhibitor of cytochrome P450 3A4 at dosages of 50 to 200 mg/day and is excreted primarily (80%) through the urine. However, as daily dosages are increased, fluconazole has a greater potential for inhibition of cytochrome P450 3A4 and a larger percentage of the drug is metabolized via the P450 system *(8)*. Cytochrome P450 3A4 inducers increase metabolism of all azoles to varying degrees regardless of their primary excretion pathways. Coadministration of rifampin, for example, can reduce fluconazole serum concentrations by approximately 50% and concentrations of itraconazole, voriconazole, and posaconazole by greater than 90% *(8)*. Azole antifungal therapy should be avoided, whenever possible, during use of high-dose conditioning chemotherapy with busulfan or cyclophosphamide owing to an increased risk of acute liver toxicity and accumulation of toxic chemotherapy metabolites *(36)*. Although azoles themselves do not appear to exert major effects on cardiac conduction, their combined use with drugs that affect potassium channels and are metabolized through CYP 450 mechanisms (e.g., cisapride, haloperidol, certain tricyclic antidepressants) has the potential to cause life-threatening arrhythmias.

Table 6.3
Drug interactions of the azole antifungals.

Drug Interaction		Outcome
Azole + Cytochrome P450 Inducers	Carbamazepine Phenobarbitol Phenytoin Isoniazid Rifabutin Rifampin Nevirapine	↓ Azole concentration
Azole + Cytochrome P450 Inhibitors	Erythromycin Azithromycin Clarithromycin	↑ Azole concentration
Azole + Cytochrome P450 Metabolites	Statins Cyclosporine Tacrolimus Sirolimus Protease inhibitors (saquinavir, ritonavir) Ca^{2+} channel blockers (diltiazem, verapamil, nifedipine, nisoldipine)	↑ Metabolite concentration

6. ECHINOCANDINS

Despite some modest differences in pharmacokinetics and potency, the echinocandins are pharmacologically similar and probably interchangeable *(3)*. All three currently approved agents, caspofungin, micafungin, and anidulafungin, are large semisynthetic lipopeptides that are available only as intravenous formulations. All have linear pharmacokinetics, are widely distributed (with the possible exception of the CSF and urine), and have prolonged elimination half-lives that permit once-daily dosing. Slight differences in the metabolism and excretion are seen between the echinocandins, which may account for some differences in the drug interaction profile of these agents.

6.1. Spectrum and Susceptibility

Caspofungin is indicated for candidiasis and for aspergillosis in patients who are refractory to other therapies. Use for infections caused by other moulds has not been as extensively studied. Activity is fungicidal against the yeasts while static against the aspergilli. End points against *Aspergillus* are determined differently than with other antifungals. End points are determined as minimum effective concentration (MEC). While growth is substantial with in vitro systems, it is evident that the growth is grossly abnormal. The MEC is considered the lowest concentration of drug that causes the abnormal growth of hyphae in this species (Fig. 6.5). End points for other moulds would be read in like manner.

The echinocandins have not been evaluated by the CLSI (NCCLS) to standardize testing parameters. Many investigators feel that they should be tested in RPMI but results in RPMI are as high as six dilutions higher than results in antibiotic medium 3 (M3). Investigational animal studies do not support the results seen with RPMI and some researchers feel that the M3 results are more representative of true MICs. Resistance has not been widely reported for this class of antifungals. However, there are a few occurrences of isolates with high MICs. *Candida parapsilosis* and *C. guilliermondii* are two species with notoriously increased MICs. Some clinical isolates of *C. albicans* and *C. glabrata* exist with elevated MICs but it is unclear if these isolates are truly resistant in vivo.

Activity of the echinocandins is similar across the class. Micafungin has low MICs in both RPMI and M3 as opposed to caspofungin and anidulafungin, both of which exhibit high MICs in RPMI but lower results in M3.

6.2. Pharmacokinetics

All three echinocandins are available as intravenous formulations only, have (mostly) linear pharmacokinetics, are widely distributed (with the possible exception of the CSF and urine), have prolonged elimination half-lives, and are metabolized by chemical degradation followed by hepatic metabolism (Table 6.2). Dosage adjustment is recommended for caspofungin in patients with severe hepatic dysfunction (Child Pugh score 7 to 9), but is not required for micafungin or anidulafungin.

6.3. Adverse Effects

All three echinocandins were well tolerated in Phase II/III clinical trials, with the most common adverse effects being phlebitis/venous irritation, headache, fever, and rash. Infusion-related reactions analogous to the "red person's syndrome" observed with vancomycin infusions have been described with all three echinocandins due to histamine release during infusions. The most common adverse effects reported with echinocandin therapy are venous irritation when infused through a peripheral vein and transient abnormalities in hepatic transaminases and bilirubin. The echinocandins are neither substrates nor inhibitors of cytochrome P450 enzymes of P-glycoprotein enzymes. For reasons not completely understood, coadministration of caspofungin with inducers of P450 3A4 (e.g., rifampin, phenytoin) results in modest (25% to 50%) decrease in the area under the curve (AUC), which can be overcome with higher dosages. P450 inducers do not appear to have as pronounced effect on the clearance of micafungin or anidulafungin. Caspofungin modestly (~20%) decreases the AUC of concomitant tacrolimus therapy. Micafungin modestly increases the AUC of nifedipine and sirolimus. No clinically significant drug interactions have been identified thus far for anidulafungin.

7. FLUOROPYRIMIDINES

Flucytosine (5-fluorocytosine, 5-FC) is the only agent among the fluoropyrimidine class of antifungal agents approved for the treatment of invasive fungal infections. In the United States it is available only in oral capsule formulation. The usefulness of flucytosine for treating invasive mycoses is hampered by its relatively narrow spectrum, high rates of acquired resistance among common pathogens (i.e., *Candida* species), and significant potential for toxic effects. For these reasons, flucytosine is not used as monotherapy and has a minimal role in the treatment of most mycoses.

7.1. *Spectrum and Susceptibility*

5-Fluorocytosine has activity against both *Candida* and *Cryptococcus* species and is not recommended for the treatment of infections caused by other fungal species. The rate of resistance against *Candida* species is expected in about 5% of isolates while for *Cryptococcus* species resistance occurs in about 2% of isolates tested.

7.2. *Pharmacokinetics*

Because flucytosine widely distributes throughout the body, including the CSF, after oral administration, it is a useful adjuvant agent for difficult to treat infections in these anatomically restricted sites. Several randomized prospective studies of cryptococcal meningitis in patients with AIDS have shown that the addition of flucytosine to amphotericin B therapy results in more rapid sterilization of the CSF, decreased early mortality, and fewer relapses after completion of "induction" antifungal therapy.

7.3. *Adverse Effects*

Flucytosine was originally developed as an antitumor chemotherapy before it was discovered to have antifungal activity against common yeasts. Not surprisingly, the most common side effects are nausea and vomiting, increases in serum transaminases, and bone marrow suppression. The risk of bone marrow suppression can be reduced if serum levels are maintained at less than 100 μg/ml. Because flucytosine is eliminated unchanged through the kidney, serum level monitoring and dosage adjustments are required in patients receiving flucytosine in combination with amphotericin B or other nephrotoxic agents.

Gastrointestinal side effects are seen in up to 6% patients receiving oral flucytosine including diarrhea, nausea, and vomiting. Reversible elevations in hepatic serum transmaninases and alkaline phosphatase have also been reported in 4% to 10% of patients receiving flucytosine. The most serious toxicity associated with flucytosine, however, is bone marrow suppression, which occurs in 6% of patients. Some evidence has accumulated in the last two decades that marrow toxicity is enhanced if serum concentrations of flucytosine exceed 100 μg/ml.

8. COMBINATION ANTIFUNGAL THERAPY

Because of their unique mechanism of action, the introduction of the echinocandins has renewed interest in the use of combination antifungal therapy for invasive mycoses. The most common reasons for consideration of combination therapy are to *(1)* broaden the spectrum of antifungal coverage of opportunistic mycoses; particularly in severely immunocompromised patients; *(2)* to enhance the activity of an antifungal regimen through (presumably) synergistic antifungal effects, especially in severely immunocompromised patients with progressive disease; and *(3)* to overcome the pharmacokinetic limitations of a single antifungal agent in the treatment of life-threatening mycoses in an anatomically restricted sites such as the CNS (e.g., combined use of flucytosine and amphotericin B for cryptococcal meningitis) *(37)*. With the possible exception of cryptococcal meningitis, there are surprisingly few data from controlled clinical trials supporting the use of combination therapy for deep mycoses. The majority of data suggesting a possible benefit for combination therapy with echinocandin-based combinations are still derived from in vitro studies and animal models. For this reason, combination antifungal therapy is not routinely recommended as a first-line strategy in the treatment of opportunistic mycoses, but may be considered as a salvage approach in patients with refractory or breakthrough infections on antifungal prophylaxis.

REFERENCES

1. Maertens JA. History of the development of azole derivatives. Clin Microbiol Infect 2004;10 (Suppl 1):1–10.
2. Pfaller MA, Diekema DJ, Messer SA, Boyken L, Hollis RJ, Jones RN. In vitro susceptibilities of rare *Candida* bloodstream isolates to ravuconazole and three comparative antifungal agents. Diagn Microbiol Infect Dis 2004;48:101–105.
3. Denning DW. Echinocandin antifungal drugs. Lancet 2003;362:1142–1151.
4. Odds FC, Brown AJ, Gow NA. Antifungal agents: mechanisms of action. Trends Microbiol 2003;11:272–279.
5. Groll AH, Piscitelli SC, Walsh TJ. Clinical pharmacology of systemic antifungal agents: a comprehensive review of agents in clinical use, current investigational compounds, and putative targets for antifungal drug development. Adv Pharmacol 1998;44:343–500.
6. Kurtz MB, Rex JH. Glucan synthase inhibitors as antifungal agents. Adv Protein Chem 2001;56:423–475.
7. Sheehan DJ, Hitchcock CA, Sibley CM. Current and emerging azole antifungal agents. Clin Microbiol Rev 1999;12:40–79.
8. Gubbins PO, McConnell SA, Penzak SR. Antifungal agents. In: Piscitelli SC, Rodvold KA, eds. Drug interactions in infectious diseases. Totowa, NJ: Humana Press, 2001:185–217.
9. Denning DW. Echinocandin antifungal drugs. Lancet 2003;362:1142–1151.
10. Hector RF. Compounds active against cell walls of medically important fungi. Clin Microbiol Rev 1993;6:1–21.
11. Kurtz MB, Heath IB, Marrinan J, Dreikorn S, Onishi J, Douglas C. Morphological effects of lipopeptides against *Aspergillus fumigatus* correlate with activities against (1,3)-beta-D-glucan synthase. Antimicrob Agents Chemother 1994;38:1480–1489.
12. White TC. Mechanisms of resistance to antifungal agents. In: Murray PR, Baron EJ, Jorgensen JH, Pfaller MA, Yolken RH, eds. Manual of clinical microbiology. 8th Ed. Washington, DC: ASM Press, 2003:1869–1879.
13. Kontoyiannis DP, Lewis RE. Antifungal drug resistance of pathogenic fungi. Lancet 2002;359:1135–1144.
14. NCCLS. Reference method for broth dilution antifungal susceptibility testing of yeasts; proposed standard. NCCLS document M27-P. Wayne, PA: National Committee for Clinical Laboratory Standards, 1992.
15. NCCLS. Reference method for broth dilution antifungal susceptibility testing of yeasts; approved standard. NCCLS document M27-A2. Wayne, PA: National Committee for Clinical Laboratory Standards, 2002.

16. NCCLS. Reference method for broth dilution antifungal susceptibility testing of conidial-forming filamentous fungi. Approved standard. NCCLS M38-A. Wayne, PA: National Committee for Clinical Laboratory Standards, 2002.
17. NCCLS. Reference Method for Antifungal Disk Diffusion Susceptibility Testing of Yeasts; Approved Guideline. NCCLS document M44-A. Wayne, PA: National Committee for Clinical Laboratory Standards, 2004.
18. Rex JH. Pfaller MA. Has antifungal susceptibility testing come of age? Clin Infect Dis 2002;35:982–989.
19. Liu TT, Lee RE, Barker KS, et al. Genome-wide expression profiling of the response to azole, polyene, echinocandin, and pyrimidine antifungal agents in *Candida albicans*. Antimicrob Agents Chemother 2005;49:2226–2236.
20. Marichal P, Gorrens J, Coene MC, Le Jeune L, Vanden Bossche H. Origin of differences in susceptibility of *Candida krusei* to azole antifungal agents. Mycoses 1995;38:111–117.
21. Schuetzer-Muehlbauer M, Willinger B, Krapf G, Enzinger S, Presterl E, Kuchler K. The *Candida albicans* Cdr2p ATP-binding cassette (ABC) transporter confers resistance to caspofungin. Mol Microbiol 2003;48:225–235.
22. Tsai HF, Bard M, Izumikawa K, et al. Candida glabrata erg1 mutant with increased sensitivity to azoles and to low oxygen tension. Antimicrob Agents Chemother 2004;48: 2483–2489.
23. Sanglard D, Ischer F, Marchetti O, Entenza J, Bille J. Calcineurin A of Candida albicans: involvement in antifungal tolerance, cell morphogenesis and virulence. Mol Microbiol 2003;48:959–976.
24. Heitman J. Cell biology. A fungal Achilles' heel. Science 2005;309:2175–2176.
25. Cowen LE, Lindquist S. Hsp90 potentiates the rapid evolution of new traits: drug resistance in diverse fungi. Science 2005;309:2185–2189.
26. Pappagianis D, Collins MS, Hector R, Remington J. Development of resistance to amphotericin B in *Candida lusitaniae* infecting a human. Antimicrob Agents Chemother 1979;16:123–126.
27. Merz WG. *Candida lusitaniae*: frequency of recovery, colonization, infection, and amphotericin B resistance. J Clin Microbiol 1984;20:1194–1195.
28. Atkinson AJ, Bennett JE. Amphotericin B pharmacokinetics in humans. Antimicrob Agents Chemother 1978;13:271–276.
29. Bekersky I, Fielding RM, Dressler DE, Lee JW, Buell DN, Walsh TJ. Pharmacokinetics, excretion, and mass balance of liposomal amphotericin B (AmBisome) and amphotericin B deoxycholate in humans. Antimicrob Agents Chemother 2002;46:828–833.
30. Imhof A, Walter RB, Schaffner A. Continuous infusion of escalated doses of amphotericin B deoxycholate: An open-label observational study. Clin Infect Dis 2003;36:943–951.
31. Eriksson U, Seifert B, Schaffner A. Comparison of effects of amphotericin B deoxycholate infused over 4 or 24 hours: randomised controlled trial. Br Med J 2001;322:579–582.
32. Pfaller MA, Messer SA, Hollis RJ, et al. Trends in species distribution and susceptibility to fluconazole among blood stream isolates of *Candida* species in the United States. Diagn Microbiol Infect Dis 1999;33:217–222.
33. Lewis RE. Pharmacotherapy of *Candida* bloodstream infections: new treatment options, new era. Expert Opin Pharmacother 2002;3:1039–1057.
34. Johnson LB, Kauffman CA. Voriconazole: a new triazole antifungal agent. Clin Infect Dis 2003;36:630–637.
35. Ezzet F, Wexler D, Courtney R, Krishna G, Lim J, Laughlin M. Oral bioavailability of posaconazole in fasted healthy subjects: comparison between three regimens and basis for clinical dosage recommendations. Clin Pharmacokinet 2005;44:211–220.

36. Marr KA, Leisenring W, Crippa F, et al. Cyclophosphamide metabolism is affected by azole antifungals. Blood 2004;103:1557–1559.
37. Kontoyiannis DP, Lewis RE. Toward more effective antifungal therapy: the prospects of combination therapy. Br J Haematol 2004;126:165–175.

SUGGESTED READINGS

Boucher HW, Groll AH, Chiou CC, Walsh TJ. Newer systemic antifungal agents: pharmacokientics, safety and efficacy. Drugs 2004:64:1997–2020.

Rex JH, Pfaller MA. Has antifungal susceptibility testing come of age? Clin Infect Dis 2002;35:982–989.

Sheehan DJ, Hitchcock CA, Sibley CM. Current and emerging azole antifungal agents. Clin Microbiol Rev 1999;12:40–79.

Gonzales GM, Fothergill AW, Sutton DA, Rinaldi MG, Lobenberg D. In vitro activities of new and established triazoles against opportunistic filamentous and dimorphic fungi. Med Mycol 2005;43:281–284.

IV

Mycoses

7
Candidiasis

Jack D. Sobel, MD

1. INTRODUCTION

Candida species are ubiquitous fungi and the most common fungal pathogens affecting humans *(1,2)*. The growing problem of mucosal and systemic candidiasis reflects the enormous increase in the pool of patients at risk and the increased opportunity for *Candida* to invade tissues normally resistant to invasion. *Candida* are true opportunistic pathogens that exploit recent technological advances to gain access to the vascular circulation and deep tissues. *Candida* in particular affects high-risk patients who are either immunocompromised or critically ill.

2. ETIOLOGIC AGENTS

Candida are yeast-like fungi that can form true hyphae and pseudohyphae. These yeasts are typically confined to human and animal reservoirs; however, they are frequently recovered from the hospital environment, including from food, countertops, air conditioning vents, floors, respirators, and medical personnel. They are also normal commensals of diseased skin and mucosal surfaces of the gastrointestinal (GI), genitourinary, and respiratory tracts.

More than 100 species of *Candida* exist, but only a few are recognized as causing disease in humans *(1)*. The medically significant *Candida* species are shown in Table 7.1. *Candida glabrata* and *Candida albicans* account for 70% to 80% of yeasts isolated from patients with invasive candidiasis. *C. glabrata* has become important because of its increasing worldwide incidence and because it is intrinsically less susceptible to azoles and amphotericin B. Two uncommon *Candida* species, *C. lusitaniae* and *C. guilliermondii*, are important because of their innate resistance to amphotericin B. *C. krusei*; although not as common as some *Candida* species, is clinically significant because of its intrinsic resistance to fluconazole and decreased susceptibility to all other antifungals, including amphotericin B (Table 7.1) *(3)*.

From: *Infectious Disease: Diagnosis and Treatment of Human Mycoses*
Edited by: D. R. Hospenthal and M. G. Rinaldi © Humana Press Inc., Totowa, NJ

Table 7.1
General patterns of susceptibility of *Candida* species

Candida species	Fluconazole	Itraconazole	Flucytosine	Amphotericin B	Voriconazole	Echinocandins[a]
C. albicans	S	S	S	S	S	S
C. tropicalis	S	S	S	S	S	S
C. parapsilosis	S	S	S	S	S	S (to I?)
C. glabrata	S-DD to R	S-DD to R	S	S-I	S to I	S
C. krusei	R	S-DD to R	I-R	S-I	S to I	S
C. lusitaniae	S	S	S	S to R	S to I	S
C. Kefyr	S	S	S	S	S	S
C. guilliermondii	S	S	S	S to R	S	S
C. dubliniensis	S	S	S	S	S	S

S, susceptible; R, resistant; S-DD, susceptible-dose dependent.

[a]Susceptibility methods for the echinocandin antifungal agents (caspofungin, micafungin, and anidulafungin) are not standardized, and interpretive criteria are not available. All three drugs show generally similar susceptibility patterns and therefore are shown as a class.

3. EPIDEMIOLOGY

Candida species are the most common cause of fungal infection, primarily affecting immunocompromised patients *(4–7)*. Oropharyngeal colonization is found in 30% to 55% of healthy young adults, and *Candida* may be detected in 40% to 65% of normal fecal flora. Clinical and autopsy studies have confirmed the marked increase in the incidence of disseminated candidiasis, reflecting a parallel increase in the frequency of candidemia. This increase is multifactorial in origin, reflecting an increased recognition as well as a growing population of patients at risk (i.e., patients undergoing complex surgical procedures and those with indwelling vascular devices). The increase in disseminated candidiasis also reflects the improved survival of patients with underlying neoplasms, collagen vascular disease, and immunosuppression. Candidiasis causes more fatalities than any other systemic mycosis. Early studies observed that in febrile neutropenic patients who die of sepsis, there was a 20% to 40% chance of finding evidence of invasive candidiasis at autopsy. Bodey described 21% of fatal infections in leukemic patients as the result of invasive fungal disease, in contrast with 13% and 6% of fatal infections in patients with lymphoma and solid tumors, respectively *(8)*. Systemic candidiasis has been described in 20% to 30% of patients undergoing bone marrow transplantation. *Candida* species are now the fourth most commonly isolated pathogens from blood cultures in hospitals *(4–7)*. A dramatic increase in the incidence of candidemia has occurred in the last four decades. Epidemiologic data indicate that at least 10% to 12% of all nosocomial infections and 8% to 15% of all nosocomial bloodstream infections are caused by *Candida*.

Candidemia and disseminated candidiasis mortality rates have not improved markedly over the past few years and remain in the 30% to 40% range, resulting in a serious economic impact *(9)*. Candidemia is associated with considerable prolongation of the length of hospital stay (70 days versus 40 days in matched patients) *(10,11)*. Although mucocutaneous fungal infections such as oral thrush and *Candida* esophagitis are common in acquired immunodeficiency syndrome (AIDS) patients, candidemia and disseminated candidiasis are not.

Within the hospital setting, areas with the highest rates of candidemia include intensive care units (ICUs), surgical units, trauma units, and neonatal ICUs. In fact, 25% to 50% of all nosocomial candidemia occurs in critical care units. Neutropenic patients, formerly the highest risk group, are no longer the most vulnerable subpopulation, likely as a result of the widespread use of fluconazole prophylaxis during neutropenia *(12)*. In some tertiary care centers, *C. albicans* is no longer the most frequent bloodstream isolate, having been replaced by C. glabrata, which has replaced *C. tropicalis* as the most prevalent non-*albicans* species, now causing 3% to 35% of all candidemias. Non-*albicans Candida* have also become an increasing problem in ICUs, attributed to the more widespread use of fluconazole in this population *(13)*.

Risk factors for *Candida* bloodstream infections include broad-spectrum antibiotic use, chemotherapy, corticosteroids, intravascular catheters, receipt of total parenteral nutrition (TPN), recent surgery, hospitalization in ICU, malignancy, neutropenia, and fungal colonization. The most important risk factor for invasive candidiasis is a prolonged stay in the ICU *(11)*.

4. PATHOGENESIS AND IMMUNOLOGY

Host defects play a significant role in the development of candidal infections *(1)*. The intact skin constitutes a highly effective, impermeable barrier to *Candida* penetration. Disruption of the skin from burns, wounds, and ulceration permits invasion by colonizing opportunistic organisms. Similarly, indwelling intravascular devices provide an efficient conduit that bypasses the skin barrier. The major defense mechanisms operating at the mucosal level to maintain colonization and prevent invasion include normal protective bacterial flora and cell-mediated immunity. The importance of the latter mechanism is highlighted by chronic mucocutaneous candidiasis, a congenital *Candida* antigen-specific deficiency manifested by chronic, intractable, and severe mucocutaneous infection. However, candidemia and disseminated candidiasis are rare in the presence of an intact humoral and phagocytic system.

An effective phagocytic system is the critical defense mechanism that prevents *Candida* deep tissue invasion, thereby limiting candidemia and preventing dissemination. Polymorphonuclear and monocytic cells are capable of ingesting and killing blastoconidia and hyphal phases of *Candida*, a process that is enhanced by serum complement and specific immunoglobulins. Severe leukocyte qualitative dysfunction (e.g., chronic granulomatous disease) is associated with disseminated, often life-threatening candidal infections. Myeloperoxidase deficiency also results in increased susceptibility to invasive infection.

Several *Candida* virulence factors contribute to their ability to cause infection, including surface molecules that permit adherence of the organism to other structures (human cells, extracellular matrix, prosthetic devices), acid proteases, phospholipase, and the ability to convert from yeast to hyphal form.

Candidal colonization is at the highest levels in patients at the extremes of age—neonates and adults older than 65 years. Numerous risk factors are associated with increased colonization. Once the colonized mucosal surface is disrupted by chemotherapy or trauma, organisms penetrate the injured areas and gain access to the bloodstream. Although the yeast phase of *Candida* is capable of penetrating intact mucosal cells, the more virulent hyphal phase is more often associated with tissue invasion. Indwelling central venous catheters appear to be a frequent route of bloodstream invasion, accounting for at least 20% of candidemias. Hyperalimentation (TPN) constitutes an independent risk factor. The risk of fungemia is increased with prolonged duration of catheterization, which also increases the risk of local phlebitis, occasionally progressing to suppurative thrombosis. Tunneled catheters (e.g., Hickman and Broviac) are less commonly the source of candidemia, but the intravascular portion may become colonized and infected as the result of candidemia originating from a second independent focus or portal of entry. Fungal invasion from colonized wounds occurs rarely, except in patients with extensive burns. Similarly, the respiratory tract, although frequently colonized, is not a common site for *Candida* invasion and rarely is a source of dissemination.

After invasion of the bloodstream, efficient phagocytic cell function rapidly clears the invading organisms, especially when the inoculum is small. More prolonged candidemia is likely in granulocytopenic patients, especially when diagnosis and treatment are delayed. This results in increased risk of hematogenous spread and metastatic seeding of multiple visceral sites, primarily the kidney, eyes, liver, skin, and central nervous system. Manifestations of metastatic infection may be apparent immediately or may be delayed several weeks or even months, long after predisposing factors (e.g., granulocytopenia) have resolved.

A third route for bloodstream invasion is persorption via the GI wall, following massive colonization with a high titer of organisms that pass directly into the bloodstream. Candidemia and disseminated candidiasis almost invariably follow serious bacterial infections, especially bacteremia.

5. CLINICAL MANIFESTATION

Candida infections can present in a wide spectrum of clinical syndromes, depending on the site of infection and the degree of immunosuppression of the host.

5.1. Cutaneous Candidiasis Syndromes

Generalized cutaneous candidiasis manifests as a diffuse eruption over the trunk, thorax, and extremities. Patients have a history of generalized pruritus with increased severity in the genitocrural folds, anal region, axillae, hands, and feet. Physical examination reveals a widespread rash that begins as individual vesicles and spreads into large confluent areas.

Intertrigo affects any site where skin surfaces are in close proximity, providing a warm, moist environment. A red pruritic rash develops, beginning with vesiculopustules, enlarging to bullae, which then rupture causing maceration and fissuring. The area involved typically has a scalloped border, with a white rim consisting of necrotic epidermis that surrounds the erythematous macerated base. Satellite lesions are frequently found. These may coalesce and extend into larger lesions. *Candida* folliculitis is predominantly found in hair follicles and rarely becomes extensive. Paronychia and onychomycosis are frequently associated with immersion of the hands in water, especially in patients with diabetes mellitus. These patients usually have a history of a painful and erythematous area around and underneath the nails and nail beds.

Chronic mucocutaneous candidiasis describes a unique group of individuals with *Candida* infections of the skin, hair, nails, and mucous membranes that tend to have a protracted and persistent course. Most infections begin in infancy or the first two decades of life; whereas onset in people older than 30 years is rare. These chronic and recurrent infections frequently result in a disfiguring form called *Candida* granuloma. Most patients survive for long periods and rarely experience disseminated fungal infections. Chronic mucocutaneous candidiasis is frequently associated with multiple endocrinopathies. Examination reveals disfiguring lesions of the face, scalp, hands, and nails occasionally associated with oral thrush and vitiligo.

5.2. Oropharyngeal Candidiasis

Oropharyngeal candidiasis (OPC) occurs in association with serious underlying conditions such as diabetes, leukemia, neoplasia, corticosteroid use, antimicrobial therapy, radiation therapy, dentures, and human immunodeficiency virus (HIV) infection. Persistent OPC in infants may be the first manifestation of childhood AIDS or chronic mucocutaneous candidiasis. Samonis et al. reported that 28% of cancer patients not receiving antifungal prophylaxis developed OPC *(14)*. In a similar immunocompromised, hospitalized population, Yeo et al. observed OPC in 57% of patients *(15)*.

Approximately 80% to 90% of patients with HIV infection will develop OPC at some stage of their disease. The presence of OPC should alert the physician to the possibility of underlying HIV infection. Untreated, 60% of HIV-infected patients develop an AIDS-related infection or Kaposi's sarcoma within 2 years of the appearance of OPC. Many HIV-positive patients experience recurrent episodes of OPC and esophageal candidiasis as HIV progresses, and multiple courses of antifungals administered may contribute to the development of antifungal resistance. Antifungal agents are less effective and take longer to achieve a clinical response in HIV-positive patients than in cancer patients. There has been a significant increase in the incidence of non-*albicans Candida* recovered from HIV-positive patients.

C. albicans remains the most common species responsible for OPC (80% to 90%). *C. albicans* adheres better in vitro to epithelial cells than non-*albicans Candida* does.

The manifestations of OPC (commonly called thrush) vary significantly, from none to a sore, painful mouth, burning tongue, and dysphagia. Frequently, patients with severe objective (examination) changes are asymptomatic. Clinical signs include a diffuse erythema with white patches (pseudomembranes) that appear as discrete lesions on the surfaces of the mucosa, throat, tongue, and gums. With some difficulty, the plaques can be wiped off, revealing a raw, erythematous, and sometimes bleeding base. OPC impairs quality of life and results in a reduction in fluid or food intake. The most serious complication of untreated OPC is extension to the esophagus. Fungemia and disseminated candidiasis are uncommon.

Chronic atrophic stomatitis or denture stomatitis is a very common form of OPC, with soreness and burning of the mouth. Characteristic signs are chronic erythema and edema of the portion of the palate that comes into contact with dentures. Denture stomatitis is found in 24% to 60% of denture wearers and is more frequent in women than in men. Notably, *C. glabrata* has been identified in 15% to 30% of all cultures, a higher prevalence than generally found in the mouth. Angular cheilitis (perlèche), also called cheilosis, is characterized by soreness, erythema, and fissuring at the corners of the mouth. Chronic hyperplastic candidiasis (*Candida* leukoplakia) produces oral white patches, or leukoplakia, which are discrete, transparent-to-whitish, raised lesions of variable sizes found on the inner surface of the cheeks and, less frequently, on the tongue. Midline glossitis (median rhomboid glossitis, acute atrophic stomatitis) refers to symmetrical lesions of the center dorsum of the tongue characterized by loss of papillae and erythema.

5.3. Esophageal Candidiasis

Candida esophagitis occurs in predisposed individuals. C. *albicans* is the most common cause. The prevalence of *Candida* esophagitis has increased because of AIDS and the increased numbers of transplant, cancer, and severely immunocompromised patients.

Esophageal candidiasis in an HIV-infected patient may be the first manifestation of AIDS. *Candida* esophagitis tends to occur later in the natural history of HIV infection and almost invariably at a much lower CD4 count. In cancer patients, factors predisposing to esophagitis include recent exposure to radiation, cytotoxic chemotherapy, antibiotic and corticosteroid therapy, and neutropenia. Clinical features include dysphagia, odynophagia, and retrosternal pain. Constitutional findings, including fever, occur only occasionally. Rarely, epigastric pain is the dominant symptom. Although esophagitis may occur as an extension of OPC, in more than two thirds of published reports, the esophagus was the only site involved; more often infection involved the distal two thirds of the esophagus. *Candida* esophagitis in AIDS patients may occur in the absence of symptoms despite extensive objective esophageal involvement. Kodsi classified *Candida* esophagitis on the basis of its endoscopic appearance *(16)*. Type I cases refer to a few white or beige plaques up to 2 mm in diameter. Type II plaques are larger and more numerous. In the milder grades, plaques may be hyperemic or edematous, but there is no ulceration. Type III plaques may be confluent, linear, nodular, and elevated, with hyperemia and frank ulceration, and type IV plaques additionally have increased friability of the mucosa and occasional narrowing of the lumen. Uncommon complications of esophagitis include perforation, aortic–esophageal fistula formation, and rarely, candidemia or bacteremia.

A reliable diagnosis can be made only by histologic evidence of tissue invasion in biopsy material. Nevertheless, antifungal therapy is frequently initiated empirically with minimal criteria in a high-risk patient. The mere presence of *Candida* within an esophageal lesion as established by brushings, smear, or culture does not provide sufficient evidence to distinguish *Candida* as a commensal from *Candida* as the responsible invasive pathogen.

Radiographic studies have been replaced by endoscopy, which not only provides a rapid and highly sensitive diagnosis, but also is the only reliable method of differentiating among the various causes of esophagitis. The characteristic endoscopic appearance is described as yellow-white plaques on an erythematous background, with varying degrees of ulceration. Differential diagnosis includes radiation esophagitis, reflux esophagitis, cytomegalovirus, or herpes simplex virus infection. In AIDS patients, it is not uncommon to identify more than one etiologic agent causing esophagitis.

5.4. Respiratory Tract Candidiasis

Laryngeal candidiasis is seen primarily in HIV-infected patients and occasionally in those with hematologic malignancies. The patient presents with a sore throat and hoarseness and the diagnosis is made by direct or indirect laryngoscopy.

Candida tracheobronchitis is a rare form of candidiasis seen in HIV-positive or severely immunocompromised subjects complaining of fever, productive cough, and shortness of breath. Physical examination reveals dyspnea and scattered rhonchi. The diagnosis generally is made during bronchoscopy.

Candida pneumonia is also a rare form of candidiasis. The most common form of infection appears to be multiple lung abscesses due to the hematogenous dissemination of *Candida*. As there may be a high degree of colonization and isolation of *Candida* from the upper respiratory tract, diagnosis requires the visualization of *Candida* invasion on histopathology. Patient history usually reveals similar risk factors for disseminated candidiasis, and patients complain of shortness of breath, cough, and fever. Sputum or endotracheal secretions positive for *Candida* usually indicate upper respiratory tract colonization and have low predictive value for pneumonia.

5.5. *Vulvovaginal Candidiasis*

In the United States, *Candida* vaginitis is the second most common vaginal infection. During the childbearing years, 75% of women experience at least one episode of vulvovaginal candidiasis (VVC), and 40% to 50% of these women experience a second episode. A small subpopulation of women experiences repeated, recurrent episodes of *Candida* vaginitis. *Candida* may be isolated from the genital tract of about 10% to 20% of asymptomatic, healthy women of childbearing age.

Candida vaginitis can be classified as complicated or uncomplicated, depending on factors such as severity and frequency of infection and the causative *Candida* species (Table 7.2). Increased rates of asymptomatic vaginal colonization with *Candida* and *Candida* vaginitis are seen in pregnancy (30% to 40%), with the use of oral contraceptives with a high estrogen content, and in uncontrolled diabetes mellitus. The hormonal dependence of the infection is illustrated by the fact that *Candida* is seldom isolated from premenarchal girls, and the prevalence of *Candida* vaginitis is lower after menopause, except in women taking hormone replacement therapy (HRT). Other factors include corticosteroid and antimicrobial therapy, the use of an intrauterine device, high frequency of coitus, and refined-sugar eating binges.

Vulvar pruritus is the most common symptom of VVC and is present in most symptomatic patients. Vaginal discharge is often minimal and occasionally absent. Although described as being typically "cottage cheese-like" in character, the discharge may vary from watery to homogeneously thick. Vaginal soreness, irritation, vulvar burning, dyspareunia, and external dysuria are common. Malodorous discharge is characteristically absent. Typically, symptoms are exacerbated during the week before menses, while the onset of menstrual flow frequently brings some relief.

Examination reveals erythema and swelling of the labia and vulva, often with discrete pustulopapular peripheral lesions. The cervix is normal. Vaginal mucosal erythema with adherent whitish discharge is typically present.

In most symptomatic patients, VVC is readily diagnosed by microscopic examination of vaginal secretions. A wet mount of saline preparation has a sensitivity of only 40% to 60%. A 10% potassium hydroxide preparation (KOH) is more sensitive in diagnosing the presence of budding yeast. Patients with *Candida* vaginitis have a normal vaginal

Table 7.2
Classification of *Candida* vaginitis

	Uncomplicated (90%)	Complicated (10%)
Severity	Mild or moderate	Severe
Frequency	Sporadic	Recurrent
Organism	*Candida albicans*	Non-*albicans* species of *Candida*
Host	Normal	Abnormal (e.g., uncontrolled diabetes mellitus)

pH (4.0 to 4.5). A pH of more than 4.5 suggests bacterial vaginosis, trichomoniasis, or mixed infection. Routine cultures are unnecessary, but in suspicious cases with negative microscopy cases vaginal culture should be performed. Although vaginal culture is the most sensitive method available for detecting *Candida*, a positive culture does not necessarily indicate that *Candida* is responsible for the vaginal symptoms.

5.6. Urinary Tract Candidiasis

Candiduria is rare in otherwise healthy people. Although epidemiologic studies have documented candiduria in approximately 10% of individuals sampled, many of these culture results reverted to negative when a clean-catch technique was used. The incidence of fungal urinary tract infections (UTIs), specifically candiduria, has dramatically increased recently, especially among patients with indwelling urinary catheters.

Platt et al. reported that 26.5% of all urinary tract infections related to indwelling catheters were caused by fungi. *Candida* are the organisms most frequently isolated from the urine samples of patients in surgical ICUs and 10% to 15% of nosocomial UTIs are caused by *Candida (17)*.

Diabetes mellitus may predispose patients to candiduria by enhancing *Candida* colonization of the vulvovestibular area (in women), by enhancing urinary fungal growth in the presence of glycosuria, by lowering host resistance to invasion by fungi as a consequence of impaired phagocytic activity, and by promoting stasis of urine in those with neurogenic bladder.

Antibiotics also increase colonization of the GI tract by *Candida*, which are normally present in approximately 30% of immunocompetent adults. In patients receiving antibiotics, colonization rates approach 100%. Candiduria is almost invariably preceded by bacteriuria. Indwelling urinary catheters serve as a portal of entry for microorganisms into the urinary drainage system. Other risk factors include the extremes of age, female sex, use of immunosuppressive agents, venous catheters, interruption of urine flow, radiation therapy, and genitourinary tuberculosis.

In a large multicenter study by Kauffman et al., *C. albicans* was found in 51.8% of 861 patients with funguria. The second most common pathogen (134 patients) was C. glabrata *(18)*. Other non-*albicans Candida* are also very common and far more prevalent than in other sites (i.e., oropharynx and vagina), possibly as a function of urine composition and pH selectivity for non-*albicans* species. In approximately 10% of patients, more than one species of *Candida* are found simultaneously.

Ascending infection is by far the most common route for infection of the bladder. It occurs more often in women because of a shorter urethra and frequent vulvovestibular colonization with *Candida* (10% to 35%). Ascending infection that originates in the bladder can infrequently lead to infection of the upper urinary tract, especially if vesicoureteral reflux or obstruction of urinary flow occurs. This may eventually result in acute pyelonephritis and, rarely, candidemia. A fungus ball consisting of yeast, hyphal elements, epithelial and inflammatory cells, and, sometimes, renal medullary tissue secondary to papillary necrosis may complicate ascending or descending infections.

Hematogenous spread is the most common route for renal infection (i.e., renal candidiasis). *Candida* have a tropism for the kidneys; one study revealed that 90%

of patients with fatal disseminated candidiasis had renal involvement at autopsy. Frequently, when renal candidiasis is suspected, blood cultures are no longer positive.

The finding of *Candida* organisms in the urine may represent contamination, colonization of the drainage device, or infection. Contamination of a urine specimen is common, especially with suboptimal urine collection from a catheterized patient or from a woman who has heavy yeast colonization of the vulvovestibular area. Given the capacity of yeast to grow in urine, small numbers of yeast cells that migrate into the collected urine sample may multiply quickly. Therefore, high colony counts could be the result of yeast contamination or colonization. Colonization usually refers to the asymptomatic adherence and settlement of yeast, usually on drainage catheters or other foreign bodies in the urinary tract (i.e., stents and nephrostomy tubes), and it may result in a high concentration of the organisms on urine culture. Simply culturing the organism does not imply clinical significance, regardless of the concentration of organisms in the urine. Accordingly, some clinicians require confirmation of *Candida* presence by a second urine sample examination before they initiate treatment or further investigation.

Infection is caused by superficial or deep tissue invasion. Kozinn showed that colony counts of greater than 10^4 colony-forming units (cfu)/ml of urine were associated with infection in patients without indwelling urinary catheters, although clinically significant renal candidiasis has been reported with colony counts of 10^3 cfu/ml of urine *(19)*. Pyuria supports the diagnosis of infection in patients with a urinary catheter but can result from mechanical injury of the bladder mucosa by the catheter or from coexistent bacteriuria. In summary, absence of pyuria and low colony counts tend to rule out *Candida* infection, but the low specificity of pyuria and counts greater than 10^3 cfu/ml require that results be interpreted in their clinical context. The number of yeast cells in urine has little value in localizing the anatomical level of infection. Rarely, a granular cast containing *Candida* hyphal elements is found in urine, allowing localization of the infection to the renal parenchyma. Declining renal function suggests urinary obstruction or renal invasion. For candiduria patients with sepsis, is it not only necessary to obtain blood cultures, but also, given the frequency with which obstruction and stasis coexist, essential to perform radiographic visualization of the upper tract. Any febrile patient for whom therapy for candiduria is considered necessary should be investigated for the anatomic source of candiduria. In contrast, patients without sepsis require no additional studies unless candiduria persists after the removal of catheters.

Candiduria is most often asymptomatic, usually in hospitalized or nursing home patients with indwelling catheters. These patients usually show none of the signs or symptoms associated with UTI. Symptomatic *Candida* cystitis is uncommon. Cystoscopy, although rarely indicated, reveals soft, pearly white, elevated patches with friable mucosa underneath and hyperemia of the bladder mucosa. Emphysematous cystitis is a rare complication of lower UTI, as is prostatic abscess.

Upper UTIs present with fever, leukocytosis, and costovertebral angle tenderness, indistinguishable from bacterial pyelonephritis and urosepsis. Ascending infection almost invariably occurs in the presence of urinary obstruction and stasis, especially in patients with diabetes or nephrolithiasis.

A major complication of upper UTI is obstruction caused by fungus balls (bezoars), which can be visualized on ultrasonography. Renal colic may occur with the passage of fungal "stones," which are actually portions of these fungus balls.

Patients with hematogenous seeding of the kidneys caused by candidemia may present with high fever, hemodynamic instability, and variable renal insufficiency. Blood culture results are positive for *Candida* in half of these patients. Retinal or skin involvement may suggest dissemination, but candiduria and a decline in renal function are often the only clues to systemic candidiasis in a febrile, high-risk patient.

5.7. Abdominal Candidiasis, Including Peritonitis

Candida infection has been increasingly recognized as a cause of abdominal sepsis and is associated with a high mortality. Peritoneal contamination with *Candida* follows either spontaneous GI perforation or surgical opening of the gut. However, after contaminating the peritoneal cavity, *Candida* organisms do not inevitably result in peritonitis and clinical infection. Risk factors for peritonitis, include recent or concomitant antimicrobial therapy, inoculum size, and acute pancreatitis. Translocation of *Candida* across the intact intestinal mucosa has been shown experimentally in animals and in a volunteer. Additional risk factors for invasive candidiasis include diabetes, malnutrition, ischemia, hyperalimentation, neoplasia, and multiple abdominal surgeries. Pancreatic transplantation, especially with enteric drainage, is associated with intraabdominal *Candida* abscess formation. *Candida* have a unique affinity for the inflamed pancreas, resulting in intrapancreatic abscesses or infecting accompanying pseudocysts. In *Candida* peritonitis, *Candida* usually remains localized to the peritoneal cavity, with the incidence of dissemination at about 25%.

The clinical significance of *Candida* isolated from the peritoneal cavity during or after surgery has been controversial. Several earlier studies concluded that a positive culture did not require antifungal therapy. Calandra et al., in a review of *Candida* isolates from the peritoneal cavity, determined that *Candida* caused intraabdominal infection in 19 of 49 (39%) patients *(20)*. In 61% of patients, *Candida* isolation occurred without signs of peritonitis. Accordingly, in each patient, clinicians should consider the clinical signs of infection and other risk factors when deciding whether to initiate antifungal therapy *(21)*.

Candida peritonitis as a complication of continuous ambulatory peritoneal dialysis (CAPD) is more common, but it infrequently results in positive blood cultures or hematogenous dissemination. In a series of CAPD patients followed for 5 years, fungal peritonitis, most commonly due to *Candida*, accounted for 7% of episodes of peritonitis. Seventeen cases of fungal peritonitis were reported, with eight associated deaths. Few risk factors have emerged except for recent hospitalization, previous episodes of peritonitis, and antibacterial therapy. Clinically, fungal peritonitis cannot be differentiated from bacterial peritonitis except by Gram stain and culture of dialysate.

Yeast in the bile is not uncommon, especially after biliary surgery, and has the same significance as asymptomatic bactibilia (i.e., colonization only); however *Candida* is an infrequent cause of cholecystitis and cholangitis. Other risk factors include diabetes, immunosuppression, abdominal malignancy, and the use of biliary stents.

Biliary infection is usually polymicrobial, and when isolated, *Candida* is a pathogen that should not be ignored.

5.8. Candida *Osteomyelitis and Arthritis*

Although previously rare, *Candida* osteomyelitis is now not uncommon, usually as the result of hematogenous dissemination, with seeding of long bones in children and the axial skeleton in adults. Sites of bone infection include the spine (vertebral and intravertebral disk), wrist, femur, humerus, and costochondral junctions.

Osteomyelitis may present weeks or months after the causal candidemic episode; therefore, at presentation, blood cultures are usually negative and radiologic findings nonspecific. A bone biopsy is usually required for diagnosis .

Occasionally, postoperative wound infections may spread to contiguous bone such as the sternum and vertebrae. Regardless of the source, manifestations resemble bacterial infection but run a more insidious course, with a significant delay in diagnosis.

Candida arthritis generally represents a complication of hematogenous candidiasis and rarely follows local trauma, surgery, or intra-articular injections. Patients with underlying joint disease (e.g., rheumatoid arthritis, prosthetic joints) are at increased risk. *Candida* arthritis can occur in any joint, is usually monoarticular (knee), but has been reported to affect multiple joints in up to 25% of cases. Infection resembles bacterial septic arthritis, but chronic infection often develops with secondary bone involvement because of the delay in diagnosis and suboptimal treatment.

5.9. Candidemia and Disseminated Candidiasis

Clinical presentation of candidemia varies from fever alone and absence of any organ-specific manifestations to a wide spectrum of manifestations, including fulminant sepsis *(22)*. Accordingly, acute candidemia is indistinguishable from bacterial sepsis and septic shock. In general, there are no specific clinical features associated with individual *Candida* species.

Candidemia may also present with manifestations of systemic and invasive metastatic candidiasis, although when these occur, blood cultures have frequently become negative. Accordingly, candidemia is a marker, although insensitive, of deep invasive candidiasis. Only 50% of patients with disseminated candidiasis will have positive blood cultures, and an antemortem diagnosis is even lower (15% to 40%). Dissemination to multiple organs may occur with candidemia, especially to the kidney, eye, brain, myocardium, liver, and spleen in leukemia patients, but infection can also involve the lungs, skin, vertebral column, and endocardium.

The possibility of asymptomatic disseminated infection drives the treatment principles of candidemia. Transient candidemia can occur from any source but most often follows intravascular catheter infection, with prompt resolution of candidemia following catheter removal. Prolonged candidemia, especially when blood cultures remain persistently positive on appropriate antifungal treatment, suggests a persistent focus or source (e.g., intravascular catheter, abscess, suppurative thrombophlebitis, endocarditis, severe neutropenia) or antifungal resistance, which albeit rare, is more common with some of the non-*albicans Candida*. When candidemia is diagnosed, a general physical examination rarely reveals clinical signs of dissemination, but a thorough examination, including a dilated funduscopic examination, is mandatory. The crude mortality rate reported in patients with candidemia ranges from 40% to 60%, with an attributable mortality of 38%, exceeding that of most bacteremias. McNeil et al. reported a 50% reduction in national mortality rates for invasive candidiasis since 1989 after a steady increase in mortality in the previous decades, reaching 0.62 death/100,000 population *(9)*. The decrease in mortality, despite increased invasive disease, may be related to increased awareness, earlier diagnosis, and increased therapeutic options, primarily fluconazole and echinocandins.

5.10. Ocular Candidiasis

Candida organisms gain access to the eye by one of two routes: direct inoculation during eye surgery or trauma, or as the result of hematogenous spread (endogenous). Once endophthalmitis occurs, therapy, especially if delayed, is often insufficient to prevent blindness. Given the recent increased incidence of nosocomial candidemia, a parallel increase in endophthalmitis has occurred. Endophthalmitis should raise the suspicion of concomitant, widely disseminated candidiasis. Estimates of the incidence of eye involvement during candidemia have been as high as 37%, but recent studies indicate a reduced rate of less than 10%. Only half of patients diagnosed with endophthalmitis have a history of recent candidemia.

Symptoms of chorioretinitis vary; may be absent in patients too ill to complain; and include visual blurring, floaters, scotomata, and blindness. Funduscopic examination reveals white, cotton ball-like lesions situated in the chorioretinal layer that may progress rapidly to extend into the posterior vitreous. Indirect ophthalmoscopy with pupillary dilation is necessary to achieve complete visualization. To be visible, the lesions require the presence of leukocytes; thus, in the presence of neutropenia, ocular lesions may be absent.

5.11. Cardiac and Endovascular Candidiasis

Candida myocarditis is the result of hematogenous dissemination with formation of microabscesses within the myocardium usually detected only on autopsy. Franklin et al. reported that 62% of 50 patients with disseminated candidiasis had myocardial involvement at autopsy *(23)*.

Candida may reach the pericardium from adjacent endocarditis or myocarditis, but pericardial involvement is most often the result of hematogenous seeding or direct inoculation during cardiac surgery. Pericarditis is purulent in nature, resembles bacterial infection, and may be complicated by constrictive pericarditis.

The advent of prosthetic cardiac valve replacement surgery and the increase in intravenous drug abuse have resulted in a dramatic increase in the incidence of *Candida* endocarditis, which previously had been rare. Fungal endocarditis is responsible for fewer than 10% of all cases of infective endocarditis.

Endocarditis following prosthetic valve surgery (PVE) remains the most common form of *Candida* endocarditis (>50%). Most episodes occur within 2 months of surgery, although endocarditis can also occur much later (>12 months). Specific risk factors for PVE include complicated surgery, antibiotics, prolonged postoperative use of catheters, and candidemia, even if transient. Non-*albicans Candida* species are increasingly responsible for prosthetic valve endocarditis, especially *C. parapsilosis*. Damaged endocardium and prosthetic material, especially suture lines, serve as foci for *Candida* adherence. Pacemaker-associated endocarditis from *Candida* has also been reported.

Clinical findings and complications in *Candida* endocarditis are similar to those seen in bacterial endocarditis, with the exceptions of increased frequency of large vegetations and large emboli to major vessels. Aortic and mitral valve involvement is the most common. The higher incidence of embolization is frequently manifested as focal and global neurologic deficits. Some studies have found a reduced incidence of cardiac failure, charging heart murmurs, and splenomegaly. Prosthetic valve endocarditis may recur several years after a putative cure with medical therapy, so long-term follow up is necessary.

Most patients with *Candida* endocarditis have positive blood cultures. Improved diagnosis is the result of greater awareness of the significance of candidemia, newer blood culture techniques, and echocardiography. Visualizing large vegetations via echocardiogram in patients with negative blood culture is strong circumstantial evidence of *Candida* endocarditis. Mycologic examination including culture and histopathology should be performed on all surgically removed emboli.

Candida endocarditis mortality remains high. Before cardiac surgery was available, mortality exceeded 90%. With combined treatment using surgery and aggressive antifungal therapy, mortality rates of approximately 45% are now typical.

Phlebitis due to *Candida* is common and often associated with subcutaneous catheters. Delay in treatment often results in extensive vascular thrombosis and suppuration. Prolonged candidemia, despite adequate antifungal treatment, is not uncommon. Venous thrombi, even after removal of responsible catheters, impair drug penetration and contain persistent microabscesses, with resultant prolonged candidemia. Surgical excision of thrombi is often required in addition to prolonged antifungal therapy. Complications include superior vena cava obstruction, tricuspid valve endocarditis, right-sided mural endocarditis, and pulmonary vein thrombosis.

5.12. Chronic Systemic Candidiasis

Hepatosplenic candidiasis (HSC) is a chronic form of disseminated candidiasis that develops as a complication of invasive candidiasis during granulocytopenia. Many now prefer the term chronic systemic candidiasis because other organs (eyes, skin, soft tissue) may also be involved. In the last 2 decades, reports of HSC have increased, probably as a result of improved diagnostic imaging and increased rates of candidemia. Candidemia, although frequently secondary to intravascular catheter infection, generally follows *Candida* colonization of the gut, together with disruption of the GI mucosa, organism reach the submucosal blood vessels that drain into the portal venous system and into the liver, where focal lesions are established. Thus, many patients with chronic systemic candidiasis have no history of documented candidemia. As patients recover from neutropenia, the lesions that were established during the neutropenic phase become more prominent, especially in the liver, spleen, and kidneys.

Clinically, most patients have a history of a hematologic malignancy, cytotoxic chemotherapy, or recent recovery from neutropenia, during which time they were febrile and received antibacterial therapy. On recovery from neutropenia, symptoms of antibiotic-resistant fever and abdominal pain begin and worsen as the neutrophils infiltrate foci of *Candida* in the liver and spleen. Serum alkaline phosphatase increases, paralleling the increase in leukocytes, although hepatic transaminases are not commonly elevated.

6. DIAGNOSIS

In superficial candidiasis, wet mount smears use scrapings or smears from skin, nails, oral or vaginal mucosa examined under the microscope to identify hyphae, pseudohyphae, or budding yeast cells. Potassium hydroxide smear, gram stain, or methylene blue stain may help directly demonstrate fungal cells. For diagnosis of invasive candidiasis, laboratory studies are nonspecific and lack sensitivity. Clinicians are required to act definitively based on a high index of suspicion. In the past, many patients with life-threatening candidiasis died without receiving antifungal therapy. For therapy to be effective, clinicians must act early, often empirically in patients who are febrile and at risk.

In candidemia and disseminated candidiasis, blood cultures are helpful, but they are positive in only 40% to 60% of cases of disseminated disease. Urinalysis may be helpful and may be indicative of colonization or renal candidiasis. Non-culture, antigen-based diagnostic assays are not available in the United States. Occasionally, blood cultures obtained via central catheters may indicate contamination. Nevertheless, febrile patients with a single positive blood culture for *Candida* should always initially be considered to have a proven infection. Given the low sensitivity of blood cultures, as well as the lack of an adequate test for the diagnosis of invasive candidiasis, detection of hematogenous dissemination remains poor.

Cultures of nonsterile sites, although not useful in establishing a diagnosis, may demonstrate high degrees of candidal colonization. This may be useful in deciding whether to initiate antifungal therapy in patients with fever unresponsive to broad-spectrum antimicrobials. Positive blood cultures and cultures from sterile sites, on the other hand, are indicative of definite infection using recently established international definitions of the European Organization for Research and Treatment of Cancer/Mycoses Study Group (EORTC/MSG). Lesions of HSC may be detected by imaging techniques such as computed tomography (CT) scan, ultrasonography, and magnetic resonance imaging (see Fig. 5.12, Chapter 5). The characteristic "bull's-eye" lesions seen on ultrasound and/or CT are not detectable until neutrophil recovery. However, the lesions are not specific for HSC. As they resolve during therapy, they may either disappear completely or calcify. Ultrasonography appears to be less sensitive but possibly more specific than CT scanning in demonstrating these lesions. Diagnosis may be confirmed by histopathologic examination and culture of hepatic tissue obtained by either percutaneous biopsy or laparoscopy. The appearance of hyphae in a granulomatous lesion is itself not specific for *Candida* and may be caused by other fungi such as *Trichosporon, Fusarium,* and *Aspergillus*. In addition, metastatic tumors may simulate the appearance of HSC. Diagnosis of *Candida* endophthalmitis is usually made on the basis of clinical context and characteristic funduscopic picture. Aspiration of the anterior chamber is justified, but often culture-negative; vitrectomy is often helpful. Polymerase chain reaction (PCR) studies on the aspirate may prove the presence of *Candida*.

Species identification of *Candida* is critically important because of the increase in non-*albicans Candida* infections. CHROMagar *Candida* media allows for the presumptive identification of several *Candida* species by using enzymatic reactions in specialized media that produce differing colony colors. Several biochemical assays, usually based on fermentation reactions, can be used to identify the different *Candida* species with more accuracy. Assays that evaluate the assimilation of a number of carbon substrates and generate profiles are used in the identification of different fungal species.

Recently, a new sensitive commercial test for diagnosis of fungal infection has been introduced. The Fungitell™ assay measures the amount of β-D-glucan released from the fungal cell wall. Sensitivity for *Candida* infections of greater than 80% has been reported. The test often provides a positive test days before clinical signs and symptoms appear, allowing earlier initiation of therapy *(24)*.

The CLSI (formerly NCCLS) microbroth dilution methodology has standardized antifungal susceptibility testing for *Candida* species. Although not used as a standard of care, it may be helpful in guiding difficult therapeutic decisions. Most of these difficult decisions involve antifungal therapy of refractory oral or esophageal candidiasis in patients with AIDS or of patients with persistent candidemia, including infective endocarditis.

7. TREATMENT

Treatment of *Candida* infections varies considerably and is based on the anatomic location of the infection, the patient's underlying disease and immune status, the patient's risk factors for infection as well as the species of *Candida* responsible for infection, and, in some cases, the susceptibility of the strain to antifungal drugs (Tables 7.1, 7.3, 7.4, and 7.5). In 2004, the Infectious Diseases Society of America published updated practice guidelines for the treatment of candidiasis *(26)*.

Azoles have become the mainstay of therapy, including many topical and systemic agents. Polyenes include amphotericin B, lipid-based amphotericin B formulations, and

Table 7.3
In vitro susceptibility of *Candida* species to azoles antifungal agents[a]

Candida species	Fluconazole (MIC_{50})	Voriconazole (MIC_{50})	Itraconazole (MIC_{50})	Posaconazole (MIC_{50})
C. albicans	1	0.06	0.5	0.13
C. tropicalis	1	2	1	1
C. glabrata	16	0.5	0.25	1
C. parapsilosis	1	0.06	0.13	0.13
C. krusei	64	1	0.5	0.5
C. lusitaniae	2	0.06	0.25	0.13

MIC50, median minimum inhibitory concentration (μg/ml).
[a]Based on 2047 blood culture isolates collected from January 1997 through December 2000. Susceptibilities were calculated on the basis of NCCLS methodology. Pfaller et al.*(25)*.

Table 7.4
In vitro susceptibility of *Candida* species to other antifungal agents[a]

Candida species	Amphotericin B[b] (MIC_{50})	Flucytosine[b] (MIC_{50})	Caspofungin[c] (MIC_{50})	Anidulafungin[c] (MIC_{50})	Micafungin[c] (MIC_{50})
C. albicans	0.5	< 0.25	0.5	0.03	0.03
C. tropicalis	0.25	< 0.25	1	0.06	0.06
C. glabrata	0.5	< 0.25	2	0.06	0.06
C. parapsilosis	0.25	< 0.25	2	2	2
C. krusei	0.25	16	2	0.25	0.13
C. lusitaniae	≥1	< 0.25	1	1	0.25

MIC_{50}, median minimum inhibitory concentration (μg/ml).
[a]Susceptibilities were calculated on the basis of NCCLS methodology.
[b]Pfaller et al.*(5)*.
[c]Ostrosky-Zeichner L et al.*(3)*.

Table 7.5
Interpretive breakpoints for *Candida* species

Drug	Minimum inhibitory concentration (MIC, *μg/ml)* S	S-DD or I	R
Fluconazole	≤8	S-DD, 16–32	>32
Itraconazole	≤0.125	S-DD, 0.25–0.5	>0.5
Flucytosine	≤4	I, 8–16	>16
Voriconazole	≤1	S-DD, 2	>4

S, susceptible; R, resistant; S-DD, susceptible-dose dependent; I, intermediate.

topical nystatin. The echinocandin class of antifungals has excellent fungicidal activity against *Candida* species.

7.1. Cutaneous Candidiasis

Most localized, cutaneous candidiasis infections can be treated with topical antifungal agents, such as clotrimazole, econazole, ciclopirox, miconazole, ketoconazole, and nystatin. If the infection is a paronychium, the most important aspect of the therapy is drainage of the abscess, followed by oral antifungal therapy with either fluconazole or itraconazole. In cases of extensive cutaneous infections, infections in immunocompromised patients, folliculitis, or onychomycosis, systemic antifungal therapy is recommended. For *Candida* onychomycosis, oral itraconazole appears to be the most efficacious of azoles. Two treatment regimens are available: a single daily dose of itraconazole taken for 3 to 6 months or a pulsed-dose regimen that requires a slightly higher dose daily for 7 days, followed by 3 weeks off therapy. The cycle is

Table 7.6
Oropharyngeal and esophageal candidiasis treatment options

Drug/formulation	Dose	Comments
Nystatin		
Pastilles or lozenge	200,000 U qid[a]	Unpleasant taste; may cause nausea and gastrointestinal disturbances
Suspension	500,000 U by swish and swallow qid	
Vaginal tablet	100,000 U dissolve 1 tablet tid	Vaginal tablets in combination with unsweetened mints or chewing gum better tolerated; not recommended for esophagitis
Clotrimazole Troches	Dissolve in mouth 5 times each day	More palatable than nystatin but contains dextrose, which may promote dental caries; not recommended for esophagitis
Fluconazole Oral suspension or Tablet	100 mg/day; loading dose of 200 mg for severe disease	Superior to nystatin, clotrimazole, ketoconazole. High doses (up to 800 mg/day) can be used in difficult cases. Success has been obtained even in cases with in vitro resistance
Itraconazole		
Solution	200 mg (20 ml) by swish and swallow daily	Solution has been tested only among HIV patients, but is much better absorbed and has shown efficacy equivalent to that of fluconazole
Capsule	200 mg/day (with food) × 14–28 days	Limited bioavailability; absorption improved if taken with fatty meal; efficacy of capsules is thought equal to that of ketoconazole
Ketoconazole Tablet	200–400 mg/day	Limited bioavailability; requires acidic environment for best absorption; liver toxicity; less efficacious than fluconazole and itraconazole and less frequently used
Amphotericin B		
Suspension	1 ml (1 mg/ml) swish and swallow qid	Agent considered second-line option; reserved for severe cases and documented failures to azoles; parenteral dosing necessary for esophagitis
Lozenge	100 mg qid	
Tablet	10 mg qid	
Parenteral	0.4–0.6 mg/kg per day IV	

U, units; qid, four times daily; tid, three times daily; IV, intravenously.
[a]All given for 7–14 days for oropharyngeal candidiasis and up to 21 days for esophageal candidiasis orally, unless otherwise stated.

repeated every month for 3 to 6 months. Also effective and well-tolerated is terbinafine 250 mg daily for 6 weeks.

7.2. Gastrointestinal Candidiasis

Oropharyngeal candidiasis may be treated with topical antifungal agents (nystatin, clotrimazole, amphotericin B oral suspension) or with systemic oral azoles (fluconazole, itraconazole) (Table 7.6).

Candida esophagitis requires systemic therapy, usually with fluconazole or itraconazole for at least 14 to 21 days. Parenteral therapy with fluconazole may be required initially if the patient is unable to take oral medications. Daily suppressive antifungal therapy with fluconazole 100 to 200 mg/day is effective in preventing recurrent episodes, but it should be used only if the recurrences become frequent or are associated with malnutrition from poor oral intake and wasting syndrome. In patients with advanced AIDS and severe immunodeficiency, recurrent candidal esophagitis due to azole-resistant *C. albicans* or *C. glabrata* can be treated effectively with voriconazole or caspofungin *(27,28)*.

Table 7.7
Azole therapy for vaginal candidiasis

Drug	Formulation	Dosage
Butoconazole	2% cream	5 g × 3 d (single dose)
	2% vaginal suppository	1 suppository (5g) once daily × 7–14 d
Clotrimazole	1% cream	5 g × 7–14 days
	10% cream	5 g single application
	100-mg vaginal tablet	1 tablet × 7 days
	100-mg vaginal tablet	2 tablets × 3 days
	500-mg vaginal tablet	1 tablet once
Econazole	150-mg vaginal tablet	1 tablet × 3 days
Fenticonazole	2% cream	5 g × 7 days
Miconazole	2% cream	5 g ×7 days
	100-mg vaginal suppository	1 suppository × 7 days
	200-mg vaginal suppository	1 suppository × 3 days
	1200-mg vaginal suppository	1 suppository once
Tioconazole	2% cream	5 g × 3 days
	6.5% cream	5 g single dose
Terconazole	0.4% cream	5 g × 7 days
	0.8% cream	5 g × 3 days
	80-mg vaginal suppository	80 mg × 3 days
Fluconazole	Oral tablet	150 mg single dose
Ketoconazole	200-mg tablet	400 mg × 5 days
Itraconazole	100-mg tablet	200 mg × 3 days

7.3. Genital Tract Candidiasis

Vulvovaginal candidiasis can be managed with either topical antifungal agents or single-dose oral fluconazole in uncomplicated infections (Table 7.7). Single-dose (150 mg) oral fluconazole is the preferred method of treatment and typically preferred by women. This therapy has been shown to have clinical and microbiologic efficacy as good as that of topical antifungal agents.

A small percentage of women (<5%) suffer from chronic recurrent VVC infections, which often require chronic or prophylactic oral azole therapy for control. In women who suffer from recurrent attacks, the recommended regimen is fluconazole at a dose of 150 mg every third day for three doses, followed by weekly fluconazole at a dose of 150 mg for 6 months. This regimen prevents recurrent infections in more than 90% of women, although symptomatic recurrence is common after cessation of maintenance suppressive prophylaxis *(29)*.

7.4. Urinary Tract Candidiasis (Candiduria)

Asymptomatic candiduria in urinary catheterized patients is extremely common and most commonly reflects yeast colonization of the catheter and lower urinary tract and hence no antifungal therapy is not indicated. Symptomatic candiduria reflects deep tissue or parenchymal invasion and results in organ specific as well as constitutional symptoms (e.g., fever, frequency, dysuria [lower urinary tract] or fever, renal angle pain, nausea, vomiting, and even sepsis [pyelonephritis]). While amphotericin B IV has been the mainstay of indicated therapy, accompanying drug nephrotoxicity limits its use. Fluconazole, 400 mg daily, achieves high urinary concentrations and has emerged as the drug of first choice with small dose adjustments required for coexistent renal insufficiency. None of the other azoles, including voriconazole, are excreted in urine. Similarly, the echinocandins achieve minimal subtherapeutic urine concentrations. A useful agent for eradicating non-*albicans* candidemia, especially *C. glabrata*, is oral flucytosine in the absence of renal failure. Deep tissue invasion of kidneys or bladder can be treated by all the systemically active antifungals.

7.5. Candidemia and Acute Disseminated Candidiasis

Candidemia requires treatment in all patients (Tables 7.8 and 7.9) and is related to the presence of an intravascular catheter in up to 80% of non-neutropenic patients. Removal of intravascular catheters shortens the duration of candidemia and has been associated with reduced mortality. Although some patients have been cured by catheter removal alone, even transient episodes of candidemia can be associated with hematogenous spread and subsequent diagnosis of endophthalmitis or osteomyelitis. Thus, all episodes of candidemia mandate antifungal therapy. A dilated retinal examination is important in all candidemic patients.

Although amphotericin B has been the standard approach, two prospective randomized trials and two retrospective reviews compared amphotericin B with fluconazole *(2)*. The studies demonstrated that amphotericin B at 0.5 to 0.6 mg/kg per day and fluconazole at 400 mg/day are equivalent as effective therapy of candidemia in non-neutropenic patients. In all studies, most isolates were *C. albicans*. The strength

Table 7.8
First-line therapy for candidemia and invasive candidiasis

Polyenes
Amphotericin B deoxycholate 0.5–0.7 mg/kg IV daily
Liposomal amphotericin B 3–5 mg/kg IV daily
Lipid complex amphotericin B 3–5 mg/kg IV daily
Azoles
Fluconazole 400–800 mg IV daily
Itraconazole 200 mg IV q12h × 4 doses, followed by 200 mg IV daily
Voriconazole 6 mg/kg IV q12h × 2 doses, followed by 3 mg/kg IV q12h
Posaconazole PO (not yet approved)
Echinocandins
Caspofungin 70 mg IV × 1 dose, followed by 50 mg IV daily
Micafungin 100 mg IV daily[a]
Anidulafungin 200 mg IV × 1 dose, followed by 100 mg IV daily

IV, intravenously; PO, by mouth; q12h, every 12 hours.
[a]Suggested, but not finalized dose.

of the study data is equally convincing for non-*albicans Candida* species. Certain non-*albicans Candida*, especially *C. glabrata,* have higher fluconazole minimum inhibitory concentrations, so higher antifungal doses may be required for optimal outcome *(3)*. Caspofungin was also approved for candidemia and invasive candidiasis, based on data from one study that showed caspofungin to be as good as, if not superior to, amphotericin B in patients with candidemia *(30)*. The broad-spectrum anti-*Candida* activity of echinocandins together with rapid fungicidal action makes the echinocandin class highly suitable for therapy, especially given their safety profile and ease of use in renal failure and liver disease: In a recent study, anidulafungin was found to be non-inferior to fluconazole in candidemic patients *(31)*. Voriconazole has been shown to be equivalent to a strategy of amphotericin B therapy followed by fluconazole *(32)*.

Table 7.9
Management of candidemia and disseminated candidiasis

For *C. albicans, C. parapsilosis, C. tropicalis, C. lusitaniae, C. dubliniensis*
Fluconazole 800 mg IV × 1 dose, followed by 400 mg
Caspofungin 70 mg IV × 1 dose, followed by 50 mg IV daily
For *C. glabrata* (select therapy on the basis of MICs)
Caspofungin (as above)
Voriconazole 6 mg/kg IV q12h × 2 doses, followed by 3 mg/kg IV q12h
Amphotericin B 0.7–1.0 mg/kg IV daily
Fluconazole 800 mg IV daily
For *C. krusei*
Caspofungin (as above)
Voriconazole (as above)

IV, intravenously; PO, by mouth; q12h, every 12 hours.

Accordingly, a number of potent antifungal agents can be empirically selected in the initial therapy candidemia.

Many clinicians treat *C. glabrata* fungemia with intravenous (IV) fluconazole 800 mg/d (12 mg/kg) in adults with normal renal function *(26,33)*. The results of only one noncomparative study suggest that 800 mg/day may produce a better response rate than 400 mg/day for *C. albicans* fungemia. Choosing between the initial polyene, triazole or echinocandin, is somewhat arbitrary; however, in unstable, critically ill patients with little margin for error, or in patients previously exposed to fluconazole, initiating treatment with amphotericin B or an echinocandin is recommended *(33)*. Moreover, a study by the Mycoses Study Group suggests a possible advantage in initiating treatment with a combination of fluconazole and amphotericin B. Combinations of either fluconazole or amphotericin B with flucytosine at 100 to 150 mg/kg per day may be useful in some patients, but the precise role of this combination is unclear. The required duration of antifungal therapy is undetermined, but therapy is usually continued for about 2 weeks after the last positive blood culture *(26)*. With this approach, the rate of subsequent recurrent infection at a hematogenously seeded site is about 1%.

Although the gut has been implicated as a potential source of candidemia only in non-neutropenic patients, it appears likely that the GI tract is the most common source of candidemia in neutropenic patients. In these patients, removal of intravenous catheters may still be important. One notable exception is *C. parapsilosis* fungemia, which is highly associated with intravascular catheters in cancer patients. Recovery of marrow function is critical, and no therapeutic approach is consistently successful in the face of persistent leukopenia. In this setting, most available experience is with the use of amphotericin B at 0.6 to 1.0 mg/kg per day, given until recovery of marrow function. The optimal dose of amphotericin B is not certain, but non-*albicans Candida* require higher doses (0.8 to 1.0 mg/kg per day) of amphotericin B. This appears to be especially true of *C. krusei* and *C. glabrata.* Use of flucytosine in neutropenic patients is generally limited because of its potential for marrow suppression and the lack of a readily available intravenous formulation.

Patients may develop candidemia while receiving antifungal therapy, including prophylactic antifungals. Such breakthrough candidemia may be the result of an infected unremoved intravascular catheter. In cancer patients, breakthrough candidemia has been associated with a higher mortality and has occurred more often during an ICU stay, during prolonged neutropenia, and with the use of corticosteroids. In this setting, immunosuppression should be reduced and factors that might alter antifungal drug delivery or clearance excluded. Intravenous catheters should be changed and the possibility of drug resistance considered, especially since non-*albicans Candida* are frequently responsible. Antifungal drug susceptibility tests should be performed and therapy should be changed to an antifungal of a different class.

Central tunneled catheters in febrile neutropenic patients do not require mandatory removal because alternate vascular access sites are less available, removal is more difficult, and, most importantly, such catheters are less likely to be the source of candidemia, although they may become infected secondarily to bloodstream infection.

Occasionally, these valuable access sites can be salvaged using the controversial antibiotic lock method using amphotericin B, but results are unpredictable.

7.6. Chronic Disseminated Candidiasis

Therapy of chronic disseminated candidiasis or HSC traditionally consists of prolonged therapy with amphotericin B alone, but this approach has not been uniformly successful. Amphotericin B 0.5 to 1.0 g, followed by a prolonged course of fluconazole 200 to 400 mg/day for 2 to 14 months, is associated with cure rates of greater than 90%. Use of fluconazole is sometimes successful when therapy with amphotericin B is not. Lipid-based amphotericin B has also been used successfully. If the lesions have stabilized and the patient is clinically improved, antineoplastic therapies (including those that induce neutropenia) may be restarted, while antifungal therapy is continued. The duration of antifungal therapy is determined by imaging studies of the liver and spleen.

8. PREVENTION

8.1. Prophylaxis of Candidiasis in Transplant Patients

Invasive candidal infections are a concern in these high-risk groups. Institutions with recipients of solid organ and bone marrow transplants usually consider prophylaxis with fluconazole for the prevention of candidiasis in selected patients only *(34)*. Fluconazole is generally started 1 day before neutropenia, and although controversial, some investigators support its use for 75 to 100 days after bone marrow transplantation. In liver transplants, short-term fluconazole prophylaxis is indicated in selected high-risk patients.

8.2. Prophylaxis of Superficial Candidiasis in HIV-Positive Patients

There is little support for primary or secondary prevention of OPC, esophageal candidiasis, or vaginal candidiasis in HIV-positive patients. Concern about potential development of resistance or colonization by resistant species or strains of *Candida* exists. Prophylaxis may be indicated in a select group of patients with recurrent episodes of symptomatic candidiasis only.

*8.3. Empirical Anti-*Candida *Treatment*

Empirical use of antifungal agents in febrile patients in ICUs is widely used without data to support its use. Given the existent difficulties in diagnosing invasive candidiasis, it appears reasonable to recommend empirical antifungal therapy in selected febrile, high-risk patients with persistent antibiotic resistant fever. Although caspofungin with its broad spectrum may be preferable, less expensive, empirical fluconazole is recommended. The use of empirical antifungals in low-risk patients is not justified *(35)*.

REFERENCES

1. Calderone RA. *Candida* and candidiasis. Washington, DC: ASM Press, 2001.
2. Edwards JE. *Candida* species. In: Mandell GL, Bennett JE, Dolin R, eds. Mandell, Douglas, and Bennett's principles and practice of infectious diseases. 6th ed. Philadelphia: Elsevier Churchill Livingstone, 2005;2938–2957.

3. Ostrosky-Zeichner L, Rex JH, Pappas PG, et al. Antifungal susceptibility survey of 2,000 bloodstream *Candida* isolates in the United States. Antimicrob Agents Chemother 2003;47:3149–3154.
4. Jarvis WR. Epidemiology of nosocomial fungal infections, with emphasis on *Candida* species. Clin Infect Dis 1995;20:1526–1530.
5. Morgan J. Global trends in candidemia: review of reports from 1995–2005. Curr Infect Dis Rep 2005;7:429–439.
6. Pfaller MA, Jones RN, Messer SA, Edmond MB, Wenzel RP. National surveillance of nosocomial bloodstream infection due to *Candida* albicans: frequency of occurrence and antifungal susceptibility in the SCOPE Program. Diagn Microbiol Infect Dis 1998;31: 327–332.
7. Pappas PG, Rex JH, Lee J, et al. A prospective observational study of candidemia: epidemiology, therapy, and influences on mortality in hospitalized adult and pediatric patients. Clin Infect Dis 2003;37:634–643.
8. Bodey GP, Anaissie EJ, Edwards JE. Definition of *Candida* infections. In: Bodey GP, ed. Candidiasis: pathogenesis, diagnosis, and treatment. New York: Raven Press Ltd, 1993:407–409.
9. McNeil MM, Nash SL, Hajjeh RA, et al. Trends in mortality due to invasive mycotic diseases in the United States, 1980–1997. Clin Infect Dis 2001;33:641–647.
10. Gudlaugsson O, Gillespie S, Lee K, et al. Attributable mortality of nosocomial candidemia, revisited. Clin Infect Dis 2003;37:1172–1177.
11. Pittet D, Tarara D, Wenzel RP. Nosocomial bloodstream infection in critically ill patients. Excess length of stay, extra costs, and attributable mortality. JAMA 1994;271:1598–1601.
12. Marr KA, Seidel K, White TC, Bowden RA. Candidemia in allogeneic blood and marrow transplant recipients: evolution of risk factors after the adoption of prophylactic fluconazole. J Infect Dis 2000;181:309–316.
13. Abi-Said D, Anaissie E, Uzun O, Raad I, Pinzcowski H, Vartivarian S. The epidemiology of hematogenous candidiasis caused by different *Candida* species. Clin Infect Dis 1997;24:1122–1128.
14. Samonis G, Anaissie EJ, Rosenbaum B, Bodey GP. A model of sustained gastrointestinal colonization by *Candida albicans* in healthy adult mice. Infect Immun 1990;58:1514–1517.
15. Yeo E, Alvarado T, Fainstein V, Bodey GP. Prophylaxis of oropharyngeal candidiasis with clotrimazole. J Clin Oncol 1985;3:1668–1671.
16. Kodsi BE, Wickremesinghe C, Kozinn PJ, Iswara K, Goldberg PK. Candida esophagitis: a prospective study of 27 cases. Gastroenterology 1976;71:715–719.
17. Platt R, Polk BF, Murdock B, Rosner B. Risk factors for nosocomial urinary tract infection. Am J Epidemiol 1986;24:977–985.
18. Kauffman CA, Vazquez JA, Sobel JD, et al. Prospective multicenter surveillance study of funguria in hospitalized patients. The National Institute for Allergy and Infectious Diseases (NIAID) Mycoses Study Group. Clin Infect Dis 2000;30:14–18.
19. Kozinn PJ, Taschdjian CL, Goldberg PK, Wise GJ, Toni EF, Seelig MS. Advances in the diagnosis of renal candidiasis. J Urol 1978;19:184–187.
20. Calandra T, Bille J, Schneider R, Mosimann F, Francioli P. Clinical significance of *Candida* isolated from peritoneum in surgical patients. Lancet 1989;2:1437–1440.
21. Eggimann P, Garbino J, Pittet D. Management of *Candida* species infections in critically ill patients. Lancet Infect Dis 2003;:772–785.
22. Pappas PG, Rex JH, Lee J, et al. A prospective observational study of candidemia: epidemiology, therapy, and influences on mortality in hospitalized adult and pediatric patients. Clin Infect Dis 2003;3:634–643.

23. Franklin WG, Simon AB, Sodeman TM. *Candida* myocarditis without valvulitis. Am J Cardiol 1976;38:924–928.
24. Odabasi Z, Mattiuzzi G, Estey E, et al. Beta-D-glucan as a diagnostic adjunct for invasive fungal infections: validation, cutoff development, and performance in patients with acute myelogenous leukemia and myelodysplastic syndrome. Clin Infect Dis 2004;39:199–205.
25. Pfaller MA, Diekema DJ, Jones RN, Messer SA, Hollis RJ, SENTRY Participants Group. Trends in antifungal susceptibility of *Candida* spp. isolated from pediatric and adult patients with bloodstream infections: SENTRY Antimicrobial Surveillance Program, 1997 to 2000. J Clin Microbiol 2002;40:852–856.
26. Pappas PG, Rex JH, Sobel JD, et al. Guidelines for treatment of candidiasis. Clin Infect Dis 2004;38:161–189.
27. Ally R, Schurmann D, Kreisel W, et al. A randomized, double-blind, double-dummy, multicenter trial of voriconazole and fluconazole in the treatment of esophageal candidiasis in immunocompromised patients. Clin Infect Dis 2001;33:1447–1454.
28. Villanueva A, Gotuzzo E, Arathoon EG, et al. A randomized double-blind study of caspofungin versus fluconazole for the treatment of esophageal candidiasis. Am J Med 2002;113:294–299.
29. Sobel JD, Wiesenfeld HC, Martens M, et al. Maintenance fluconazole therapy for recurrent vulvovaginal candidiasis. N Engl J Med 2004;351:876–883.
30. Mora-Duarte J, Betts R, Rotstein C, et al. Comparison of caspofungin and amphotericin B for invasive candidiasis. N Engl J Med 2002;347:2020–2029.
31. Reboli A, Robstein C, Pappas P, Schrantz J, Krause D, Walsh T. Anidulafungin versus fluconazole for treatment of candidemia and invasive candidiasis. 45th Interscience Conference of Antimicrobial Agents and Chemotherapy, Washington DC, 2005, Dec 16–19, Abstract M-718, p 418.
32. Kullberg BJ, Sobel JD, Ruhnke M, et al. Voriconazole versus a regimen of amphotericin B followed by fluconazole for candidemia in non-neutropenic patients: a randomized non-inferiority trial. Lancet 2005;366:1435–1442.
33. Spellberg BJ, Filler SG, Edwards Jr JE. Current treatment strategies for disseminated candidiasis. Clin Infect Dis 2006;42:244–251.
34. Goodman JL, Winston DJ, Greenfield RA, et al. A controlled trial of fluconazole to prevent fungal infections in patients undergoing bone marrow transplantation. N Engl J Med 1992;326:845–851.
35. Golan Y, Wolf MP, Pauker SG, Wong JB, Hadley S. Empirical anti-*Candida* therapy among selected patients in the intensive care unit: a cost-effectiveness analysis. Ann Intern Med 2005;143:857–869.

SUGGESTED READINGS

Calderone RA. *Candida* and candidiasis. Washington, DC: ASM Press, 2001.

Edwards JE. *Candida* species. In: Mandell GL, Bennett JE, Dolin R, eds. Mandell, Douglas, and Bennett's principles and practice of infectious diseases. 6th ed. Philadelphia: Elsevier Churchill Livingstone, 2005:2938–2957.

Pappas PG, Rex JH, Lee J, et al. A prospective observational study of candidemia: epidemiology, therapy, and influences on mortality in hospitalized adult and pediatric patients. Clin Infect Dis 2003;3:634–643.

Pappas PG, Rex JH, Sobel JD, et al. Guidelines for treatment of candidiasis. Clin Infect Dis 2004;38:161–189.

Spellberg BJ, Filler SG, Edwards Jr JE. Current treatment strategies for disseminated candidiasis. Clin Infect Dis 2006;42:244–251.

8
Infection Due to Non-Candidal Yeasts

Jose A. Vazquez, MD

1. INTRODUCTION

Yeasts exist throughout nature in association with soil, plants, mammals, fish, and insects, and as a result, humans are constantly exposed to many yeast genera through varying routes. Depending on the interaction between host defense mechanisms and fungal virulence factors, the association between yeast and humans can be either transient or persistent, and can associated with either local infection or systemic disease. Most yeast organisms are of low virulence and generally require significant alterations or reductions in host defenses before tissue invasion. Recently, however, because of the increased population of immunocompromised patients, the frequency of invasive infections due to yeast as well as the number of organisms causing disease continue to grow *(1,2)* (Table 8.1).

2. *TRICHOSPORON*

Trichosporon asahii was first described in 1865 by Beigel, who identified it as the causative agent of hair infections *(3)*. Infections due to *Trichosporon* may be classified as superficial or deep. Disseminated infections are increasingly recognized in the compromised host over the past decade and are frequently fatal *(1,2)*. One of the first reported cases of disseminated disease was described in a 39-year-old woman with lung cancer who subsequently developed a brain abscess *(4)*.

2.1. *Etiologic Agents*

The genus *Trichosporon* was first reported by Behrend *(5)*. Gueho and colleagues have suggested that the species known as *T. asahii* may include several different *Trichosporon* species with epidemiological and pathogenic differences *(6)*. Kemker et al., using isoenzyme delineation and polymerase chain reaction (PCR) DNA fingerprinting suspect that strains that produce superficial infections are distinctly different from those strains that produce invasive infection *(7)*. There are currently seven species of *Trichosporon*. These include *T. asahii* (formerly, *T. beigelii*), the most frequently recovered species from invasive infections, and *T. mucoides* and *T. inkin,* also known

From: *Infectious Disease: Diagnosis and Treatment of Human Mycoses*
Edited by: D. R. Hospenthal and M. G. Rinaldi © Humana Press Inc., Totowa, NJ

Table 8.1
Yeasts other than *Candida* and *Cryptococcus* that occasionally cause human infection

Trichosporon
T. asahii (T. beigelii)
T. inkin
T. Mucoides
Saccharomyces
S. cerevisiae
S. boulardii
Rhodotorula
R. mucilaginosa (rubra)
R. glutinis
Malassezia
M. furfur
M. pachydermatis
Blastoschizomyces capitatus
(Geotrichum capitatum, Trichosporon capitatum)
Sporobolomyces
S. Salmonicolor
S. holsaticus

to cause systemic infections *(1,2,8)*. *T. asteroides* and *T. cutaneum* generally produce superficial skin infections, while *T. ovoides* generally causes white piedra of the scalp and *T. inkin,* white piedra of the pubic hair. *Trichosporon capitatum* is now known as *Blastoschizomyces capitatus (5,6)*.

Trichosporon species are characterized by true hyphae, pseudohyphae, arthroconidia, and blastoconidia *(5)* (Fig. 8.1). *T. asahii* grows readily on Sabouraud dextrose agar, producing smooth, shiny gray to cream colored yeast-like colonies with cerebriform radiating furrows that become dry and membranous with age. All *Trichosporon* species are easily identified via commercially available carbohydrate assimilation assays.

2.2. *Epidemiology*

T. asahii is generally found in the soil, but may also be recovered from air, rivers and lakes, sewage, and bird droppings *(1,2)*. It rarely colonizes the inanimate environment, but can colonize the mucosal surfaces of the oropharynx, the lower gastrointestinal tract, and the skin of humans *(9)*.

More than 100 documented cases of disseminated infection due to Trichosporon species have been reported, most due to *T. asahii (1,2,5)*. The major risk factors associated with infection include hematologic malignancies (acute leukemia, chronic leukemia, multiple myeloma), solid tumors, and neutropenia *(1,2)*. In non-neoplastic, non-neutropenic cases, the major risk factors include corticosteroids, prosthetic valve replacement, solid organ transplantation, chronic active hepatitis, and occasionally intravenous drug use (Table 8.2). The most common portal of entry appears to be the

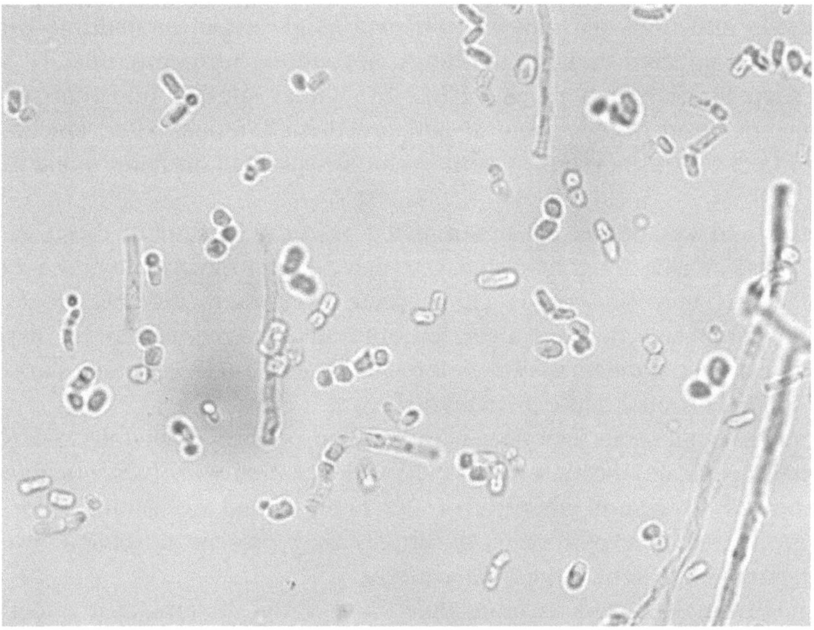

Fig. 8.1. *Trichosporon* species produce yeast-like colonies in culture and are unique in their production of hyphae, pseudohyphae, arthroconidia, and blastoconidia (budding) both in culture and in disease. (Courtesy of D. R. Hospenthal.) [Figure in color on CD-ROM].

either the respiratory or gastrointestinal tracts. Infrequently, central venous catheters and other vascular devices have also been implicated *(10,11)*.

2.3. Clinical Manifestations

Trichosporonosis is classified into superficial infections (white piedra [hair shaft infection], onychomycosis, and otomycosis) and invasive infections.

Table 8.2
Risk factors associated with *Trichosporon* infection

Hematologic malignancy
Solid organ transplantation (kidney, heart, liver)
Neutropenia
Broad-spectrum antibiotics
Corticosteroids
Use of intravenous lipids
Bone marrow transplant
Chronic active hepatitis
IVDU
Central venous catheters
CAPD
Burns

Deep tissue infections may involve either a single organ or multiple organs. The most commonly infected tissue is the lungs, accounting for approximately 33% of all localized deep tissue infections *(1,2,10,12,13)*. Other sites of infection may include the peritoneum, heart valves (natural and prosthetic), retina, liver, spleen, kidneys, gallbladder, and central nervous system (brain abscess and chronic fungal meningitis) *(1,2,10,12,13)*.

The signs and symptoms of disseminated infection resemble those of systemic candidiasis and include fungemia with associated organ infection. Moreover, disseminated infections may present as either acute or chronic disease. Acute disseminated trichosporonosis often has a sudden onset and progresses rapidly, especially in neutropenic patients. Patients may develop skin lesions (~33%), pulmonary infiltrates (~30% to 60%), or renal and ocular involvement.

The metastatic cutaneous lesions generally begin as an erythematous rash with raised papules on the trunk and the extremities. The rash eventually evolves into macronodular lesion, followed by central necrosis of the nodules and occasionally formation of hemorrhagic bullae. The pulmonary infiltrates may present as lobar consolidations, bronchopneumonia, or reticulonodular patterns.

Renal involvement occurs in more than 75% of the disseminated infection cases. Renal disease may manifest as proteinuria, hematuria, red blood cell casts, with either acute renal failure or acute glomerulonephritis *(10)*. Urine cultures are frequently positive for *Trichosporon* and suggest disseminated disease, especially in immunocompromised patients.

Chorioretinitis is not uncommon in disseminated infection and may be a cause of visual alterations due to retinal vein occlusion or retinal detachment *(10)*. For unexplained reasons, *Trichosporon* has been found to have tropism for the choroid and retina. However, unlike candidal endophthalmitis, Trichosporon infects uveal tissues including the iris, but spares the vitreous *(14)*.

During disseminated infection, any tissue in the body may become infected. The organs most frequently include the liver, spleen, gastrointestinal tract, lymph nodes, myocardium, bone marrow, pleura, brain, adrenal gland, and thyroid gland *(1,2,10,11)*.

In chronic disseminated infection subtle manifestations may be present for several weeks and frequently include persistent fever of unknown etiology *(1,2,10)*. The infection is similar to the entity known as chronic disseminated (hepatosplenic) candidiasis. It is generally a chronic infection of the liver, spleen, and other tissues after recovery from neutropenia. Laboratory studies frequently reveal an elevated alkaline phosphatase. Computed tomography (CT) scan or magnetic resonance imaging (MRI) frequently reveals hepatic or splenic lesions compatible with abscesses. A tissue biopsy is needed to confirm the diagnosis.

2.4. Diagnosis

The diagnosis is made with a biopsy of the skin or involved organs. Blood cultures may occasionally be useful in deep tissue infection, but are positive only late in the course of infection. *Trichosporon* grows readily in conventional blood culture and on standard fungal media including Sabouraud dextrose agar *(5)*. The presence of *Trichosporon* in the urine of a high-risk patient should increase the suspicion of disseminated infection.

Although there are no standardized serologic assays, the serum latex agglutination test for *C. neoformans* may be positive. A potential usefulness of this assay has been postulated based on the report of positive serum latex agglutination test for *C. neoformans* in several patients with disseminated *Trichosporon* infection *(15,16)*.

2.5. Treatment

Disseminated trichosporonosis has a mortality rate of approximately 60% to 70% *(1,2)*. In most cases, however, the underlying disease contributes greatly to the overall mortality. First-line, optimal antifungal therapy has not been established. The initial step in the management of disseminated *Trichosporon* infection should be to decrease or reverse immunosuppression.

In vitro susceptibility studies of *Trichosporon* species are limited (Table 8.3). In vitro susceptibility assays of *T. asahii,* reveal fluconazole MIC_{90} (minimal inhibitory concentration for 90% of isolates) of 4.0 μg/ml, itraconazole MIC_{90} of 0.25 μg/ml, and an amphotericin B MIC_{90} of 4.0 μg/ml. In general, most strains have relatively high MICs for polyenes, flucytosine, and echinocandins, with relatively low MICs for the azoles. Among the newer triazoles, voriconazole and posaconazole have demonstrated excellent in vitro activity *(17)*. In vitro and animal models suggest that azoles and not polyenes are more effective in the eradication of *Trichosporon* species *(1,2,13,14)*. Suggested therapy for the treatment of disseminated disease includes the use of either voriconazole 3 mg/kg IV or 200 mg orally twice daily, fluconazole 400 to 800 mg/day, or itraconazole 400 to 600 mg/day (Table 8.4). A potential option in patients failing azole therapy may also include a combination of an azole with an echinocandin. Serena et al. demonstrated in vitro synergy and improved outcomes in an animal model of trichosporonosis with either the combination of amphotericin B–micafungin or fluconazole–micafungin *(18)*. However, because of the high MICs to polyenes and echinocandins, these antifungals should not be used alone or as first-line therapy. In a patient with disseminated infection and poor response to therapy, in vitro susceptibility testing of recovered isolates may be a helpful adjunct.

3. SACCHAROMYCES

Saccharomyces is an ascomycetous yeast found throughout nature. *Saccharomyces* is commonly known as "brewer's yeast" or "baker's yeast." It is best known for its commercial use in beer and wine production, in health food supplements, and more recently, its use in DNA recombinant technology. Occasionally, these yeasts have been reported to cause severe infection in immunocompromised hosts *(5)*. Species include *S. cerevisiae, S. boulardii* (a subtype of *S. cerevisiae*), *S. fragilis,* and *S. carlsbergensis. Saccharomyces* may occasionally be part of the normal flora of the gastrointestinal and genitourinary tracts *(1,2,19)*. Recently, *S. cerevisiae* has been found to cause mucosal and disseminated infection in humans, primarily in immunocompromised hosts *(19–22)*.

Table 8.3
In vitro antifungal activity against emerging yeast infections

	Minimum inhibitory concentration (MIC; μg/ml) range[a]								
Organism	Flu	Itra	Vori	Posa	Mica	Cas	Anid	AMB	5FC
Trichosporon	1–16	0.06– 0.25	0.03–>16	0.06–>16	16–654	4–>16	16–>16	1–8	16–>512
Saccharomyces	0.5–64	0.03–4	0.016–2	0.12–1.0	NA	0.25–1	0.25–1	0.032–4	< 0.125–1
Rhodotorula	0.5–>64	0.25–>16	0.25–>8	0.25–>8.0	>64	8–>64	>64	0.12–1.0	0.6–0.25
Malassezia	1.0–16	0.03–0.25	0.03–0.125	0.03–32	NA	NA	NA	0.3–2.5	>100
Blastoschizomyces	1–32	0.03–0.50	0.03–0.50	0.12–0.25	NA	NA	1–4	0.6–0.25	0.12–16
Sporobolomyces	1.25–>64	1.0–2.0	0.25–4.0	NA	>64	NA	NA	0.14–1.0	NA

Flu, fluconazole; Itra, itraconazole; Vori, voriconazole; Posa, posaconazole; Mica, micafungin; Cas, caspofungin; Anid, anidulafungin; AMB, amphotericin B; 5FC, flucytosine; NA, data not available.
[a]Clinical Laboratory Standards Institute (CLSI) testing criteria and breakpoints have not been established for any of these fungi.

Table 8.4
Suggested antifungal agents for use in treatment of emerging yeast infections

Yeast	Antifungal therapy[a]
Trichosporon	Fluconazole 400 mg/day
	Voriconazole 200 mg bid
	Itraconazole 400–600 mg /day
Saccharomyces	Amphotericin B
	5-Flucytosine
	Azoles (ketoconazole, clotrimazole, miconazole)
Rhodotorula	Amphotericin B + 5-flucytosine
Malassezia	Fluconazole 400 mg/day
	Voriconazole 200 mg bid
	Amphotericin B 0.7 mg/kg/day
Blastoschizomyces	Amphotericin B 1–1.5 mg/kg/day
Sporobolomyces	Amphotericin B
	Azoles (ketoconazole, itraconazole, fluconazole)

[a]No antifungal agents have specific FDA approval for therapy of any of these infections. No randomized clinical trials have been performed. Selections are based on in vitro data, limited animal studies, and/or individual case reports.

3.1. *Etiologic Agents*

Cells are oval to spherical and exist as either haploids or diploids. When present, ascospores, one to four in number, are in either tetrahedral or linear arrangement and stain gram negative; vegetative cells stain gram positive. Colonies are smooth, moist, and either white or cream-colored. *Saccharomyces* are generally nonpathogenic because of innate low virulence *(23–25)*. Investigators evaluating more than 3300 yeast cultures obtained from cancer patients found only 19 isolates of *S. cerevisiae*. Recent studies by Clemons et al. using an animal model have been able to show that some strains of *S. cerevisiae*, when introduced into CD-1 mice, can proliferate and resist clearance in vivo, supporting the role of *S. cerevisiae* as a cause of clinical infection in humans *(25)*.

3.2. *Epidemiology*

Isolation of *Saccharomyces* species from human surfaces is rarely of any clinical significance. It has been recovered from the bloodstream, lungs, peritoneal cavity, esophagus, urinary tract and vagina *(19,23,26)*. Genotyping studies evaluating the relatedness between clinical strains and commercial strains of *S. cerevisiae* have demonstrated that commercial products may occasionally be a contributing factor in human colonization and infection *(27)*. Nyirjesy et al. reported that four women suffering from recurrent *S. cerevisiae* vaginitis had also experienced exposure to bread dough that contained identical strains *S. cerevisiae (22)*.

The risk factors associated with *Saccharomyces* infections are similar to the risk factors associated with candidemia and systemic candidiasis, including central venous catheters, neutropenia, use of antimicrobials, gastrointestinal tract surgery, and occasionally HIV *(21,28–30)*. The portal of entry for invasive disease is most likely the oropharynx or gastrointestinal tract *(29)*.

3.3. Clinical Manifestations

Manifestations are generally nonspecific and indistinguishable from those associated with candidemia and invasive candidiasis. In addition, *Saccharomyces* has been associated with bloodstream infections, endocarditis, peritonitis, disseminated disease and vaginitis *(1,2,19,22,26,28–32)*

Fungemia is the most common form of infection, occurring in approximately 70% of reported cases. As in invasive candidiasis, it is seen primarily in the immunocompromised host and tends to be associated with use of intravascular catheters, chemotherapy, and/or antimicrobials *(20,21,29)*. Manifestations are similar to those of systemic candidiasis and candidemia. Overall, fever unresponsive to broad spectrum antimicrobials is the most frequent manifestation. Unlike patients with infections due to *Candida* species, most patients with *Saccharomyces* infections survive.

In addition, it is not uncommon for other organ systems to become infected, including the respiratory tract, with several documented episodes of pneumonia and empyema. Diagnosis is generally established by histopathology, because *Saccharomyces* can colonize the respiratory tract without producing invasive disease *(20,29,33)*. *Saccharomyces* has also been reported to produce peritonitis, cholecystitis, and endocarditis *(20,29)*. All cases of endocarditis were associated with prosthetic valves and intravenous heroin use. Further, two out of the three patients were cured with antifungal therapy, while only one patient had their valve replaced. There have also been several documented cases of urinary tract infections due to S. cerevisiae *(26,29)*. All patients had urologic abnormalities that were underlying or associated with fungemia *(29)*.

Mucosal infections due to *S. cerevisiae* have also been reported. Sobel et al. reported on 17 women with difficult to manage vaginitis due to *S. cerevisiae (19,22)*. In fact, the women with symptomatic vaginitis had manifestations indistinguishable from those caused by *C. albicans*. All patients had a history of chronic vaginitis unresponsive to conventional antifungals and all but two had systemic or local predisposing factors.

3.4. Diagnosis

Because of the fact that *Saccharomyces* species have a tendency to be nonpathogenic, the decision to attribute a causal role to *S. cerevisiae* is difficult. Diagnostic difficulty occurs when the organism is recovered from body sites that may be colonized by *Saccharomyces,* especially in the absence of symptoms of infection. Unless the organism is found in the bloodstream, it is frequently necessary to determine whether these yeasts are causing true infection versus colonization. This is generally done via a histopathologic examination. *S. cerevisiae* readily grows from blood culture bottles and on Sabouraud dextrose media.

3.5. Treatment

It is often difficult to assess the role of antifungal therapy in patients with infection due to *Saccharomyces*. There are several reports that document resolution of fungemia and infection just by removing the intravascular catheter without providing antifungal therapy *(28,29)*. Most experts advocate removing the focus of infection, whether it is an indwelling or tunneled intravenous catheter and the concurrent use of antifungal agents *(29)*. In vitro susceptibility studies reveal that *S. cerevisiae*, when compared to *C. albicans* isolates, are less susceptible to most antifungals, including azoles *(2,20)* (Table 8.3). Although clinical trials have not be conducted and in vitro susceptibility assays are not standardized, *Saccharomyces* species appear to be susceptible to most antifungals including amphotericin B, 5-flucytosine, ketoconazole, clotrimazole, miconazole, and terconazole *(1,2,20,34)* (Table 8.4).

4. *RHODOTORULA*

Yeasts of the genus *Rhodotorula* are found worldwide from a variety of sources and is generally considered a contaminant when identified. Infections are occasionally seen primarily in immunocompromised hosts.

4.1. *Etiologic Agents*

Yeasts of the genus *Rhodotorula* are imperfect basidiomycetous yeasts belonging to the family Cryptococcaceae. Currently, eight species in the genus *Rhodotorula* are recognized *(2,34,35)*. *Rhodotorula mucilaginosa* (formerly *R. rubra*) is the species most frequently associated with human infections. The other species include *R. glutinis, R. pilimanae, R. pallida, R. aurantiaca,* and *R. minuta.* Most *Rhodotorula* species produce red-to-orange colonies due to the presence of carotenoid pigments *(5,36)*. The yeast is mucoid, encapsulated, and readily grows on many types of culture media.

4.2. *Epidemiology*

Rhodotorula can be isolated from a variety of sources including seawater, plants, air, food, fruit juices, and occasionally from humans *(1,2,5,36)*. It is not unusual to recover it as an airborne laboratory contaminant. *Rhodotorula* can also be recovered from shower curtains, bathtub-wall junctions, and toothbrushes. In humans, *Rhodotorula* can be been recovered from skin, nails, respiratory tract, urinary tract, gastrointestinal tract, and bloodstream *(1,2,37–41)*.

R. mucilaginosa and *R. glutinis* account for approximately 0.5% of yeast isolated from the oral cavity and more than 12% of yeast isolates recovered from stool and rectal swabs *(42)*. The recovery of *Rhodotorula* from nonsterile human sources such as mucosal sites has been of questionable clinical significance. Although a number of invasive infections have been documented, risk factors include underlying immunosuppression (malignancy, neutropenia, corticosteroids, collagen vascular disease, and uncontrolled diabetes mellitus), use of broad-spectrum antimicrobials, and central venous catheters.

4.3. *Clinical Manifestations*

Manifestations are generally nonspecific, and may vary from subtle and mild, to severe, including septic shock. *Rhodotorula* have been incriminated in a wide spectrum of infections including bloodstream infections, endocarditis, peritonitis, meningitis, and disseminated disease *(34,38,41,43–46)* (Table 8.5)

Table 8.5
Clinical manifestations of *Rhodotorula* infections

Fungemia
Endocarditis
Meningitis
Peritonitis
Disseminated disease

Fungemia is the most common form of infection and is generally due to intravascular catheter infection *(1,2,34,38,41,45)*. Fever of unknown etiology that is unresponsive to broad spectrum antimicrobials is the most frequent manifestation associated with fungemia.

Meningitis has also been described in patients with acute leukemia, HIV infection, and postoperatively *(47,48)*. The organisms are generally recovered from the cerebrospinal fluid on culture, and frequently seen on an India ink stain. In addition, several case of *R. rubra* peritonitis have been described in patients undergoing continuous ambulatory peritoneal dialysis. In these patients, environmental cultures revealed a possible common source outbreak. In all patients, the symptoms were subtle and intermittent at first, consisting of abdominal pain, anorexia, nausea, and occasional diarrhea *(2,34)*.

4.4. Diagnosis

In the most proven infections, *Rhodotorula* is recovered from a sterile site of infection. In these cases, the decision to attribute a causal role to *Rhodotorula* is relatively simple, and the patient should be treated appropriately for an invasive fungal infection. The more difficult decision is when the organism is recovered from nonsterile body sites that may normally harbor *Rhodotorula* species, especially in the absence of signs or symptoms of infection. In this setting, it is essential to establish the presence of infection and not just colonization.

4.5. Treatment

As with many of the uncommon yeast isolates, it is difficult to assess the role of antifungal therapy in patients infected with *Rhodotorula*. Optimal management of patients with indwelling catheters and infection due to *Rhodotorula* has not been well defined. Several case reports document the clearance of fungemia and the resolution of infection by removing the intravascular catheter without providing antifungal therapy *(38,45)*. Several other documented case reports, however, have suggested that antifungal treatment alone may suffice without having to remove the central venous catheter. Because infections due to *Rhodotorula* have been severe and life threatening, it is probably best to manage these infections aggressively with catheter removal and antifungal therapy.

In vitro susceptibility studies reveal that *Rhodotorula* are susceptible to amphotericin B and flucytosine, but less susceptible to azoles and resistant to echinocandins *(34, 49)* (Table 8.3). Although clinical trials have not been conducted, it appears that amphotericin B with or without flucytosine is the best recommendation for antifungal therapy at this time *(1,2)*. In view of the intrinsic resistance of *Rhodotorula* to the azoles and echinocandins, these agents should not be used as monotherapy unless in vitro susceptibility activity has been assessed.

5. *MALASSEZIA*

Malassezia furfur is a yeast commonly found on human skin. It has been well documented to cause superficial skin infections such as pityriasis (tinea) versicolor and folliculitis. In addition, in immunocompromised host it may occasionally cause invasive infection.

5.1. *Etiologic Agents*

The genus Malassezia consists of several species; the two most frequently isolated species include *M. furfur* and *M. pachydermatis (1,2,5)*. The other less commonly isolated species include *M. sympodialis, M. slooffiae, M. globosa, M. obtuse,* and *M. restricta. M. furfur* is the dominant species recovered in humans as a fungal pathogen. *M. furfur* is a dimorphic, lipophilic yeast that is unable to synthesize medium or long-chain fatty acids and thus has a strict in vitro requirement for exogenous fatty acids of the C_{12} and C_{14} series *(50)*. Although it exists primarily in the yeast form, it may also form filamentous structures on the skin when the organism is associated with superficial infections *(51)*. Because of its nutritional requirements, *M. furfur* is difficult to recover from clinical specimens unless its presence is suspected and special preparations are made by the microbiology laboratory. The second most common species is *M. pachydermatis,* which is generally associated with infections in dogs producing otitis externa *(50)*. Occasionally, however, it has been implicated in human infections *(51,52)*. Both *Malassezia* species, when grown under favorable conditions produce clusters of oval to round, thick-walled yeast cells, with unipolar buds that form repeatedly from the same pole of the parent cell. This gives rise to the characteristic "collarette" at the bud site. Media such as Sabouraud dextrose agar, chocolate agar, and trypticase soy agar with 5% sheep blood all require the addition of supplements such as olive oil to permit the growth of this organism *(53)*. *M. pachydermatis,* however, does not require exogenous lipids for growth, can be recovered on conventional fungal media, and its colonies tend to be dry and white to creamy in color.

5.2. *Epidemiology*

Malassezia is frequently found on normal individuals colonizing the skin. Distribution of this colonization tends to correlate with the more oily areas, most likely because of the organisms' requirement of exogenous fatty acids found in those areas. Thus, it is found primarily on the scalp, shoulders, chest, and back *(53)*. The highest colonization rates are found in teenagers (>90%).

The isolation of *M. furfur* from newborns is reported to be less than 10% in non-intensive care settings. However, it has been reported to be greater than 80% in neonatal intensive care units (ICUs) *(51,53)*. Risk factors associated with increased colonization rates in neonates include prematurity, duration of hospitalization in the ICU, use of occlusive dressings, and prolonged antimicrobial use *(51)*. Although the epidemiology

Table 8.6
Risk factors associated with *Malassezia* infections

Prematurity
Longer duration of hospitalization
Use of occlusive dressings
Administration of antibiotics
Use of central venous catheters
Use of intravenous lipids

of disseminated infection in adults has not been well studied, there appear to be several risk factors that are frequently associated with deep-seated infections (Table 8.6). These include prematurity, central venous catheters, total parenteral nutrition, parenteral lipid preparations, and immunocompromised state *(54–57)*. Molecular epidemiologic studies using DNA fingerprinting have concluded that within the neonatal ICUs there is longitudinal persistence of both *M. furfur* and *M. pachydermatis* strains *(58)*.

5.3. Clinical Manifestations

Malassezia generally produces superficial skin infections, such as pityriasis (tinea) versicolor or folliculitis. From time to time, *Malassezia* may produce a deep-seated or hematogenous infections *(54–57)*. The first reported case of systemic infection was described in 1981 in a premature neonate who developed fungemia and vasculitis while on lipid therapy *(57)*. Since then, numerous reports describing disseminated infection have been published *(51,55)*. The manifestations of disseminated infection vary from subclinical and mild symptomatology, such as fever, to sepsis with associated multi-organ dysfunction *(51,55)*. The majority of the *Malassezia* infections are diagnosed in premature infants. Occasionally, they may be seen in adults. The most commonly reported manifestations of systemic infection include fever unresponsive to broad-spectrum antimicrobials, bradycardia, respiratory distress, hepatosplenomegaly, and lethargy.

5.4. Diagnosis

Laboratory findings include leukocytosis and thrombocytopenia. Chest x-ray examination frequently reveals bilateral pulmonary infiltrates (>50%) *(1,2,54)*. Occasionally, the diagnosis of disseminated infection can be made by a Gram stain of the buffy coat of blood. The budding yeast cells may be observed using different stains such as Giemsa, periodic acid Schiff (PAS), Gomori's methenamine silver (GMS), or Calcofluor white. Blood cultures are usually negative unless the infection is initially suspected and the laboratory uses a lipid-enriched media. The recovery of the organisms is enhanced by using the lysis centrifugation blood culture technique *(59)*. Palmitic acid (3%) supplementation may also improve the recovery of *Malassezia (59)*.

5.5. Treatment

Management of *M. furfur* fungemia and disseminated infection are controversial. Most authorities recommend prompt removal of the central venous catheter and discontinuation of intravenous lipids *(54,55)*. In most cases without a deep-seated infection, removal of the central venous catheter and discontinuation of lipids is all that is needed to clear the infection. This treatment modality accomplishes two objectives: it eradicates the nidus of infection, and removes the nutritional requirements of the organism. If fungemia persists or there is evidence of deep-seated infection, it is prudent to initiate antifungal therapy. Fortunately, *Malassezia* species are susceptible to azoles and polyenes *(1,2,34)* (Table 8.3). In vitro susceptibility assays of *M. furfur* strains demonstrate that most of the isolates are susceptible to amphotericin B, ketoconazole (MIC range $\leq$0.05 to 0.4 μg/ml), miconazole (MIC range 0.4$\geq$50 μg/ml), and fluconazole. Most of the isolates are intrinsically resistant to flucytosine (MIC_{90}>100 μg/ml) *(1,2,34)*. Although randomized clinical trials have not been conducted, in most situations, either fluconazole 400 mg/day or amphotericin B 0.7 mg/kg per day is sufficient to eradicate the infection (Table 8.4). Based on excellent in vitro activity, itraconazole and voriconazole are also alternate choices.

6. OTHER YEASTS

In addition to the yeasts discussed thus far, fewer reports have been published of infection due to other yeasts. These include *Blastoschizomyces, Sporobolomyces, Pichia* (formerly *Hansenula*), and *Exophiala.*

6.1. Blastoschizomyces

Blastoschizomyces capitatus (formerly *Geotrichum capitatum* or *Trichosporon capitatum*) infections, although less common than those due to *T. asahii*, have been well described in the literature *(60)*. *B. capitatus* is found in wood and poultry, but has also been recovered from sputum and normal intact skin *(5)*. Geographically, it appears to be the opposite of *T. asahii*, with *B. capitatus* infections found primarily in Europe and *T. asahii* found in North America *(61)*. In most cases, the major risk factors include neutropenia and underlying hematologic malignancies. Although the portal of entry is unknown, it is suspected to be the either the respiratory tract, gastrointestinal tract, or central venous catheters *(35,61)*.

Infection may involve a single organ or multiple organs and may be associated with fungemia. The clinical spectrum of disseminated infection is similar to that of systemic candidiasis and includes fungemia with or without organ infection *(1,2,61)*. By and large, the manifestations begin with fever of unknown etiology and unresponsive to antimicrobials. Diagnosis can be made with blood cultures or on biopsy of the skin or affected organs. Blood cultures have been reported to be positive in more than 80% of cases *(61)*. *B. capitatus* easily grows in blood culture bottles and on fungal specific media *(5)*. Although skin lesions are commonly seen, fungal stains and cultures from biopsied skin lesions are frequently negative *(5,61)*.

Mortality rates between 60% and 80% are generally described *(61)*. However, underlying disease, persistent neutropenia and concurrent infections are significant contributing factors to this overall mortality rate. Optimal therapy has not yet been established. Until recently, however, most patients have received amphotericin B *(2)*. As with all fungal infections, the initial step is to decrease or reverse the immunocompromised state. In vitro susceptibility studies demonstrate that the organism is susceptible to amphotericin B (MIC_{90} 0.12 μg/ml), and less susceptible to azoles such as fluconazole and ketoconazole (0.04 to 32μg/ml), but appears to be susceptible to itraconazole and voriconazole. Most isolates are resistant to flucytosine *(5)* (Table 8.3). The current recommendation is to use amphotericin B at a dose of 1 to 1.5 mg/kg per day *(1,2)*. However, since the newer azoles, voriconazole and posaconazole, have demonstrated good in vitro activity they may also be suitable alternatives *(62)*.

6.2. Sporobolomyces

Sporobolomyces are yeast-like organisms that belong to the family Sporobolomycetaceae. These yeast are found throughout the world in soil, bark, and decaying organic material. They have occasionally been associated with infections in humans. There are seven known species of *Sporobolomyces*, but only three have been documented to cause disease—*S. salmonicolor*, *S. holsaticus*, and *S. roseus*. To date, there have been only six documented cases of *Sporobolomyces* infections: a nasal polyp, one case of dermatitis, one case of infected skin blisters, one case of mycetoma, and two cases of disseminated infection in patients with acquired immunodeficiency syndrome (AIDS; lymph node and bone marrow) *(2,63)*. In vitro susceptibility studies show that *S. salmonicolor* is susceptible to amphotericin B and the imidazoles *(1,2,5)* (Table 8.3). Despite the fact that these organisms are saprophytic, the case reports indicate their potential ability to produce invasive infection in humans, especially in a compromised host.

REFERENCES

1. Hospenthal DR. Uncommon fungi. In: Mandell GL, Bennett JE, Dolin R, eds. Mandell, Douglas, and Bennett's principles and practice of infectious diseases. 6th ed. Philadelphia: Elsevier Churchill Livingstone, 2005;3068–3079.
2. Vazquez JA. *Rhodotorula, Malassezia, Trichosporon,* and other yeast-like fungi. In: Dismukes WE, Pappas PG, Sobel JD, eds. Clinical mycology. New York: Oxford University Press, 2003:206–217.
3. Beigel H. The human hair: its growth and structure (1865), as cited by Langenon M. In Darier S, et al: Nouvelle Praqt Dermatol (Paris, Masson, Cie) 1936;2:377.
4. Watson KC, Kallichurum S. Brain abscess due to *Trichosporon cutaneum.* J Med Microbiol 1970;3:191–193.
5. Kwon-Chung KJ, Bennett JE. Infections due to *Trichosporon* and other miscellaneous yeast-like fungi. In: Medical mycology. Philadelphia: Lea & Febiger, 1992:768–794.
6. Gueho E, de Hoog GS, Smith MT, Meyer SA. DNA relatedness, taxonomy, and medical significance of *Geotrichum capitatum.* J Clin Microbiol 1997;25:1191–1194.
7. Kemeker BJ, Lehman PF, Lee JW, Walsh TJ. Distinction of deep vs. superficial clinical and non-clinical environmental isolates of *Trichosporon beigelii* by isoenzymes and restriction fragment length polymorphisms of rDNA generated by the polymerase chain reaction. J Clin Microbiol 1991;29:1677–1683.
8. Behrend G. *Ubertrichomycosis nodosa.* Berlin Lin Wochenschr 1890;27:464.
9. Haupt HM, Merz WG, Beschorner WE, Vaughan WP, Saral R. Colonization and infection with *Trichosporon* species in the immunosuppressed host. J Infect Dis 1983;147:199–203.
10. Walsh TJ. Trichosporonosis. Infect Dis Clin North Am 1989;3:43–52.
11. Ebright JR, Fairfax MR, Vazquez JA. *Trichosporon asahii*, a non-*Candida* yeast that caused fatal septic shock in a patient without cancer or neutropenia. Clin Infect Dis 2001;33:28–30.
12. Keay S, Denning D, Stevens DA. Endocarditis due to *Trichosporon beigelii*: in vitro susceptibility of isolates and review. Rev Infect Dis 1991;13:383–386.

13. Sheikh HA, Mahgoub S, Badi K. Postoperative endophthalmitis due to *Trichosporon cutaneum*. Brit J Ophthalmol 1986;58:591–594.
14. Walsh TJ, Lee JW, Melcher GP, et al. Experimental *Trichosporon* infection in persistently granulocytopenia rabbits: Implications for pathogenesis, diagnosis, and treatment of an emerging opportunistic mycosis. J Infect Dis 1992;166:121–133.
15. Seeliger HPR, Schroter R. A serologic study on the antigenic relationships of the form genus *Trichosporon*. Sabouraudia 1963;2:248–263.
16. Campbell CK, Payne AL, Teall AJ, Brownell A, Mackenzie DW. Cryptococcal latex antigen test positive in a patient with *Trichosporon beigelii*. Lancet 1985;2:43–44.
17. Paphitou NI, Ostrosky-Zeichner L, Paetznick VL, Rodriguez JR, Rex JH. In vitro antifungal susceptibilities of *Trichosporon* species. J Clin Microbiol 2003; 46:1144–1146.
18. Serena C. Pastor FJ, Gilgado F, Mayayo E, Guarro J.. Efficacy of micafungin in combination with other drugs in a murine model of disseminated *Trichosporonosis*. Antimicrob Agents Chemother 2005;49:497–502.
19. Sobel JD, Vazquez J, Lynch M, Meriwether C, Zervos MJ.. Vaginitis due to *Saccharomyces cerevisiae*: epidemiology, clinical aspects, and therapy. Clin Infect Dis 1993;16:93–99.
20. Enache-Angoulvant A, Hennequin C. Invasive *Saccharomyces* Infection: a comprehensive review. Clin Infect Dis 2005;41:1559–1568.
21. Nielsen H, Stenderup J, Bruun B. Fungemia with Saccharomycetaceae. Report of four cases and review of the literature. Scand J Infect Dis 1990;22:581–584.
22. Nyirjesy P, Vazquez JA, Ufberg DD, Sobel JD, Boikov DA, Buckley HR. *Saccharomyces cerevisiae* vaginitis: transmission from yeast used in baking. Obstet Gynecol 1995;86: 326–329.
23. Morrison VA, Haake RJ, Weisdorf DJ. The spectrum of non-*Candida* fungal infections following bone marrow transplantation. Medicine 1993;72:78–89.
24. Holzschu DL, Chandler FW, Ajello L, Ahearn DG. Evaluation of industrial yeast for pathogenicity. Sabouradia 1979;17:71–78.
25. Clemons KV, McCusker JH, Davis RW, Stevens DA. Comparative pathogenesis of clinical and non-clinical isolates of *Saccharomyces cerevisiae*. J Infect Dis 1994;169:859–867.
26. Eng RH, Drehmel R, Smith SM, Goldstein EJ. *Saccharomyces cerevisiae* infections in man. Sabouraudia 1984;22:403–407.
27. McCullough MJ, Clemons KV, Farina C, McCusker JH, Stevens DA. Epidemiological investigation of vaginal *Saccharomyces cerevisiae* isolates by a genotypic method. J Clin Microbiol 1998;36:557–562.
28. Cimolai N, Gill MJ, Church D. *Saccharomyces cerevisiae* fungemia: case report and review of the literature. Diagn Microbiol Infect Dis 1987;8:113–117.
29. Aucott JN, Fayen J, Grossnicklas H, Morrissey A, Lederman MM, Salata RA. Invasive infection with *Saccharomyces cerevisiae*: report of three cases and review. Rev Infect Dis 1990;12:406–411.
30. Sethi N, Mandell W. *Saccharomyces* fungemia in a patient with AIDS. NY State J Med 1988;88:278–279.
31. Rubinstein E, Noriega ER, Simberkoff MS, Holzman R, Rahal Jr JJ. Fungal endocarditis: analysis of 24 cases and review of the literature. Medicine 1975;54:331–344.
32. Canafax DM, Mann HJ, Dougherty SH. Postoperative peritonitis due to *Saccharomyces cervisiae* treated with ketoconazole. Drug Intell Clin Pharm 1982;16:698–699.
33. Chertow GM, Marcantonio ER, Wells RG. *Saccharomyces cerevisiae* empyema in a patient with esophagopleural fistula complicating variceal sclerotherapy. Chest 1991;99: 1518–1519.
34. Hazen KC. New and emerging yeast pathogens. Clin Microbiol Rev 1995;8:462–478.

35. Fell JW, Tallman AS, Ahearn DG. Genus *Rhodotorula* Harrison. In: Kreger-van Rij NJW, ed. The yeasts: a taxonomic study. 3rd ed. Amsterdam: Elsevier Science Publishers, 1984:893–905.
36. Rippon JW. Medical mycology. The pathogenic fungi and pathogenic actinomycetes. 3rd ed. Philadelphia: W.B. Saunders, 1988:610–611.
37. Mackenzie DWH. Yeasts from human sources. Sabouraudia 1961;1:8–14.
38. Kiehn TE, Gorey E, Brown AE, Edwards FF, Armstrong D. Sepsis due to *Rhodotorula* related to use of indwelling central venous catheters. Clin Infect Dis 1992;14:841–846.
39. Ahearn DG, Jannach JR, Roth FJ. Speciation and densities of yeasts in human urine specimens. Sabouraudia 1966;5:110–119.
40. Saez H. Etude ecologique sur les *Rhodotorula* des homotherms. Rev Med Vet 1979;130:903–908.
41. Anaissie E, Bodey GP, Kantarjian H, et al. New spectrum of fungal infections in patients with cancer. Rev Infect Dis 1989;11:369–378.
42. Rose HD, Kurup VP. Colonization of hospitalized patients with yeast-like organisms. Sabouraudia 1977;15:251–256.
43. Leeber DA, Scher I. *Rhodotorula* fungemia presenting as "endotoxic" shock. Arch Intern Med 1969;123:78–81.
44. Rusthoven JJ, Feld R, Tuffnell PG. Systemic infection by *Rhodotorula* spp. in the immunocompromised host. J Infect 1984;8:241–246.
45. Braun DK, Kauffman CA. *Rhodotorula* fungemia: a life-threatening complication of indwelling central venous catheters. Mycoses 1992;35:305–308.
46. Louria DB, Greenberg SM, Molander DW. Fungemia caused by certain nonpathogenic strains of the family *Cryptococcaceae*. N Engl J Med 1960;263:1281–1284.
47. Pore RS, Chen J. Meningitis caused by *Rhodotorula*. Sabouraudia 1976;14:331–335.
48. Gyaurgieva OH, Bogomolova TS, Gorshkova GI. Meningitis caused by *Rhodotorula rubra* in an HIV-infected patient. J Med Vet Mycol 1996;34:357–359.
49. Diekema DJ, Petroelje B, Messer SA, Hollis RJ, Pfaller MA. Activities of available and investigational agents against *Rhodotorula* species. J Clin Microbiol 2005;43:476–478.
50. Nazzaro-Porro MN, Passi S, Caprilli F, Nazzaro P, Morphogo G. Growth requirements and lipid metabolism of *Pityrosporum orbiculare*. J Invest Dermatol 1976;66:178–182.
51. Marcon MJ, Powell DA. Human infections due to *Malassezia* spp. Clin Microbiol Rev 1992;5:101–119.
52. Gueho E, Simmons RB, Pruitt WR, Meyer SA, Ahearn DG. Association of *Malassezia pachydermatis* with systemic infections of humans. J Clin Microbiol 1987;25:1789–1790.
53. Ingham E, Cunningham AC. *Malassezia furfur*. J Med Vet Mycol 1993;31:265–288.
54. Marcon MJ, Powell DA. Epidemiology, diagnosis and management of *M. furfur* systemic infection. Diagn Microbiol Infect Dis 1987;10:161–175.
55. Klotz SA. *Malassezia furfur*. Infect Dis Clin Am 1989;3:53–63.
56. Barber GR, Brown AE, Kiehn TE, Edwards FF, Armstrong D. Catheter-related *Malassezia furfur* fungemia in immunocompromised patients. Am J Med 1993;95:365–370.
57. Weiss SJ, Schoch PE, Cunha BA. *Malassezia furfur* fungemia associated with central venous catheter lipid emulsion infusion. Heart Lung 1991;20:87–90.
58. van Belkum A, Boekhout T, Bosboom R. Monitoring spread of *Malassezia* infections in a neonatal intensive care unit by PCR-medicated genetic typing. J Clin Microbiol 1994;32:2528–2532.
59. Nelson SC, Yau YC, Richardson SE, Matlow AG. Improved detection of *Malassezia* species in lipid-supplemented peds plus blood culture bottles. J Clin Microbiol 1995;33:1005–1007.

60. Gemeinhardt H. Lungenpathogenitat von *Trichosporon capitatum* beim menschen. Zentrablatt fur Bakteriolgie (Series A) 1965;196:121–133.
61. Martino P, Venditti M, Micozzi A, et al. *Blastoschizomyces capitatus*: an emerging cause of invasive fungal disease in leukemia patients. Rev Infect Dis 1990;12:570–582.
62. Espinel-Ingroff A. Comparison of in vitro activities of the new triazole SCH56592 and the echinocandins MK-0991 (L-743,872) and LY303366 against opportunistic filamentous and dimorphic fungi and yeast. J Clin Microbiol 1998;36:2950–2956.
63. Morris JT, Beckius M, McAllister CK. *Sporobolomyces* infection in an AIDS patient. J Infect Dis 1991;164:623–624.

SUGGESTED READINGS

Diekema DJ, Petroelje B, Messer SA, Hollis RJ, Pfaller MA. Activities of available and investigational agents against *Rhodotorula* species. J Clin Microbiol 2005;43:476–478.

Enache-Angoulvant A, Hennequin C. Invasive *Saccharomyces* infection: a comprehensive review. Clin Infect Dis 2005;41:1559–1568.

Espinel-Ingroff A. Comparison of in vitro activities of the new triazole SCH56592 and the echinocandins MK-0991 (L-743,872) and LY303366 against opportunistic filamentous and dimorphic fungi and yeast. J Clin Microbiol 1998;36:2950–2956.

Hospenthal DR. Uncommon fungi. In: Mandell GL, Bennett JE, Dolin R, eds. Mandell, Douglas, and Bennett's principles and practice of infectious diseases. 6th ed. Philadelphia: Elsevier Churchill Livingstone, 2005:3068–3079.

Marcon MJ, Powell DA. Human infections due to *Malassezia* spp. Clin Microbiol Rev 1992;5:101–119.

Martino P, Venditti M, Micozzi A, et al. *Blastoschizomyces capitatus*: an emerging cause of invasive fungal disease in leukemia patients. Rev Infect Dis 1990;12:570–582.

Vazquez JA. *Rhodotorula, Malassezia, Trichosporon,* and other yeast-like fungi. In: Dismukes WE, Pappas PG, Sobel JD, eds. Clinical mycology. New York: Oxford University Press, 2003:206–217.

9
Aspergillosis

Helen W. Boucher, MD and Thomas F. Patterson, MD

1. INTRODUCTION

Aspergillosis is caused by *Aspergillus*, a hyaline responsible not only for invasive aspergillosis, but also for a variety of noninvasive or semi-invasive conditions. These syndromes range from colonization to allergic responses to *Aspergillus* including allergic bronchopulmonary aspergillosis (ABPA) to semi-invasive or invasive infections, spanning a spectrum from chronic necrotizing pneumonia to invasive pulmonary aspergillosis.

The genus *Aspergillus* was first recognized in 1729 by Micheli, in Florence, who noted the resemblance between the sporulating head of an *Aspergillus* species and an aspergillum used to sprinkle holy water (Fig. 9.1). In 1856, Virchow published the first complete microscopic descriptions of the organism *(1)*.

The frequency and severity of invasive fungal infections in immunocompromised patients have increased steadily over the past 2 decades with the growing population of patients undergoing transplantation and the persistent challenges in preventing, diagnosing and treating these infections *(2)*. Mortality due to documented invasive aspergillosis approaches 80% to 100% in high-risk patients, including those with underlying hematologic malignancy or bone marrow or solid organ transplantation, and may be related to several factors, including diagnostic and therapeutic inadequacies *(3–5)*. Apart from organ transplant recipients, individuals with acquired immunodeficiency syndrome (AIDS), and patients hospitalized with severe illnesses, major increases in invasive fungal infections have been observed in patients with hematologic malignancies who receive induction or consolidation chemotherapy and those who undergo hematopoietic stem cell transplantation (HSCT) *(5)*.

Successful therapy depends not only an early diagnosis—which is often difficult to establish—but even more importantly, on reversal of underlying host immune defects, such as neutropenia or high-dose immunosuppressive therapy *(2)*. Non-culture-based tests and radiological approaches can be used to establish an early diagnosis of infection and may result in improved outcomes of infection *(2,6,7)*. Even when therapy is begun

From: *Infectious Disease: Diagnosis and Treatment of Human Mycoses*
Edited by: D. R. Hospenthal and M. G. Rinaldi © Humana Press Inc., Totowa, NJ

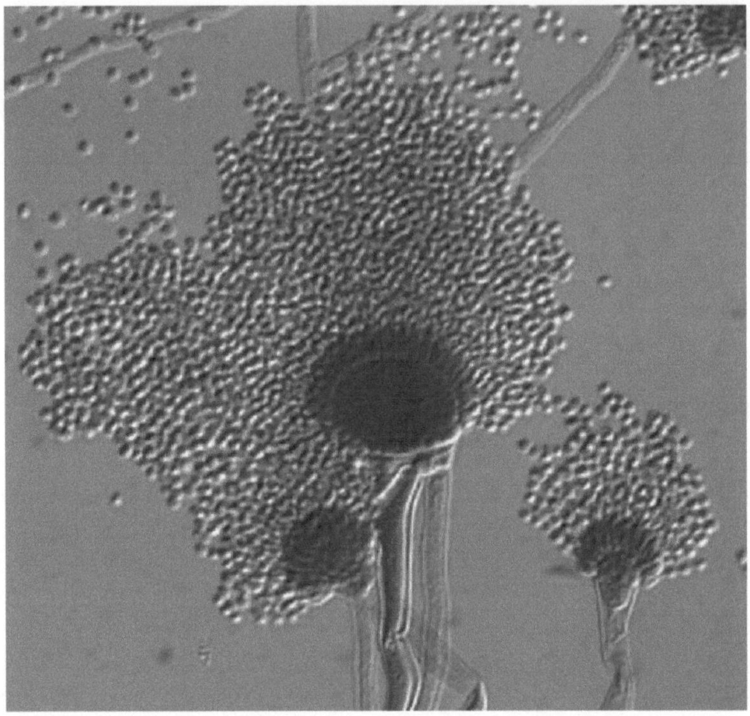

Fig. 9.1. Microscopic morphology of *Aspergillus fumigatus* showing a single role of phialides (uniseriate) bearing smooth conidia in a columnar fashion. (Courtesy of www.doctorfungus.org). [Figure in color on CD-ROM].

promptly, efficacy of many treatment regimens, including amphotericin B deoxycholate, is poor, particularly in patients with disseminated or central nervous system disease *(2,3,5)*. New diagnostic approaches have been introduced and new antifungal agents have been developed for this disease including the newer azoles, lipid formulations of amphotericin B, and a new drug class—the echinocandins *(8)*.

2. ETIOLOGIC AGENTS

Aspergillus fumigatus is one of the most ubiquitous of the airborne saprophytic fungi *(9)*. *A. fumigatus* has emerged worldwide as a frequent cause of nosocomial infection and may be regarded as the most important airborne pathogenic fungus *(10)*. As *Aspergillus* species can be readily found in the environment, invasive aspergillosis is widely believed to occur as a consequence of exogenous acquisition of the conidia (spores) of the species *(10)*. The most common route of transmission of *Aspergillus* infection is the airborne route. *Aspergillus* conidia are resilient and may survive for long periods in fomites (any substance that can absorb, retain, and transport infectious species, e.g., woolen clothes or bedding) *(11)*. *Aspergillus* infection occurs less frequently through damaged mucocutaneous surfaces (e.g., following surgery or through contaminated dressings). However, the sources of *Aspergillus* may be broader than have traditionally been thought, as waterborne transmission of *Aspergillus* conidia through contaminated aerosols has been suggested *(12)*.

Table 9.1
Characteristics of common *Aspergillus* species

Aspergillus species	Mycological characteristics	Clinical significance	Mycoses
A. flavus	Olive to lime green colonies	Second most common species, produces aflatoxin, may be less susceptible to polyenes	Sinusitis, cutaneous infection, pulmonary and disseminated disease
A. fumigatus	Smoky, blue- or gray green, small, smooth conidia (2–2.5 µm)	Most common species causing invasive infection	Invasive pulmonary aspergillosis, disseminated infection, CNS, others
A. niger	Typically black colonies, radiate conidial head, large rough conidia	Common cause of otomycosis, produces oxalate crystals which may be seen in host	Otomycosis, cutaneous, endophthalmitis, aspergilloma, invasive pulmonary or disseminated disease less common
A. terreus	Beige to buff colonies, globose accessory conidia along hyphae	Increasing frequency, associated with soil, usually resistant to polyenes	Pulmonary, disseminated, cutaneous, keratitis, CNS
A. lentulus	Poorly sporulating variant of *A. fumigatus*	May be multidrug resistant, recently described variant, may be underdiagnosed	Invasive pulmonary, disseminated, other sites

The most common species causing invasive aspergillosis include *Aspergillus fumigatus,* by far the most common, *A. flavus, A. terreus*, and, less commonly for invasive infection, *A. niger (5)* (Table 9.1). Recent studies have shown emergence of less common species, including *A. terreus* (which is frequently resistant to polyenes) and other unusual less pathogenic species as the etiologic agents of invasive infection *(13)*.

3. EPIDEMIOLOGY

The incidence of invasive aspergillosis has increased substantially during the last few decades because of the use of more intensive cytotoxic anticancer chemotherapy and the introduction of novel immunosuppressive therapies for organ transplant recipients, both of which have prolonged the period of risk for many individuals. The increasing number of patients undergoing solid organ, bone marrow, and hematopoietic stem cell transplantation, and the implementation of aggressive surgical interventions has also contributed to the increased incidence *(10)*. The changes in epidemiology of invasive aspergillosis may also be the result of growing awareness of aspergillosis among clinicians, the introduction of noninvasive diagnostic tools, and improved microbiological laboratory techniques.

Invasive fungal infections are an important cause of morbidity and mortality among patients with severely compromised immune systems. Although there have been significant advances in the management of immunosuppressed patients, invasive aspergillosis remains an important life-threatening complication, and is the leading cause of infection-related mortality in many immunocompromised individuals.

Immunosuppression and breakdown of anatomical barriers, such as the skin, are the major risk factors for fungal infections *(7)*. Individuals at risk for invasive aspergillosis include those with severely comprised immune systems as a result of anticancer chemotherapy, solid organ or bone marrow transplantation, AIDS, or use of high-dose corticosteroids. Patients with hematological disorders, such as prolonged and severe neutropenia, those undergoing transplantations, and those treated with corticosteroids and newer immunosuppressive therapies such as the tumor necrosis factor-α antagonists (e.g., inflixamab) are considered to be at highest risk for invasive aspergillosis *(7,14)*.

4. PATHOGENESIS AND IMMUNITY

Invasive aspergillosis most frequently originates via inhalation of *Aspergillus* conidia into the lungs, although other routes of exposure such as inhalation of water aerosols contaminated with *Aspergillus* conidia have been suggested *(12)*.

In the absence of effective pulmonary host defenses, the inhaled small resting conidia enlarge and germinate, then transform into hyphae with subsequent vascular invasion and eventual disseminated infection. The incubation period for conidial germination in pulmonary tissue is variable, ranging from 2 days to months *(15)*. Hydrocortisone significantly increases the growth rates of *Aspergillus*; likely one of the reasons corticosteroids pose a risk factor for invasive disease *(16)*.

Although infection in apparently normal hosts can occur, invasive aspergillosis is extremely uncommon in immunocompetent hosts *(5)*. Normal pulmonary defense mechanisms usually contain the organism in a host with intact pulmonary defenses. The first line of defense against *Aspergillus* is ciliary clearance of the organism from the airways and limited access to the alveoli due to conidia size. This feature is one reason for the increased pathogenicity of *A. fumigatus* as compared with other species of *Aspergillus (16)*. Once conidia reach the alveoli, pulmonary macrophages are generally capable of ingesting and killing *Aspergillus* conidia *(17)*. When macrophages fail to kill the conidia (e.g., high fungal inoculum, decreased number or function of macrophages), conidia germinate and begin to form hyphae. Polymorphonuclear leukocytes are recruited via complement activation and production of neutrophil chemotactic factors and extracellularly kill both swollen conidia and hyphae *(18)*. Antibodies against *Aspergillus* are common due to the ubiquitous nature of the organism, although they are not protective nor are they useful in the diagnosis of infection in high-risk patients due to the lack of consistent seroconversion after exposure or infection *(19)*.

Corticosteroids play a major role in increasing susceptibility to *Aspergillus* by decreasing oxidative killing of the organism by pulmonary macrophages and by increasing the linear growth rate by as much as 30% to 40% and cell synthesis by greater than 150% *(16)*.

Many *Aspergillus* species produce toxins including aflatoxins, ochratoxin A, fumagillin, and gliotoxin. Gliotoxin works in several ways to help evade host defenses:

- Inhibition of phagocyte NADPH oxidase activation (key in host defense versus filamentous fungi)
- Inhibition of macrophage ingestion of *Aspergillus*
- Suppression of functional T cell responses *(9,20)*

In tissues, invasive aspergillosis causes extensive destruction across tissue planes via vascular invasion with resulting infarction and necrosis of distal tissues.

5. CLINICAL MANIFESTATIONS

The clinical syndromes associated with aspergillosis are diverse, ranging from allergic responses to the organism including allergic bronchopulmonary aspergillosis (ABPA), asymptomatic colonization, superficial infection, and acute or subacute and chronic invasive disease. The clinical presentation generally corresponds to the underlying immune defects and risk factors associated with each patient group, with greater immune suppression correlating with increased risk for invasive disease. Although this chapter focuses on invasive aspergillosis, a brief description of other presentations follows. The reader is encouraged to reference other sources for more in-depth discussion of those conditions *(1)*.

5.1. Allergic Bronchopulmonary Aspergillosis

Allergic bronchopulmonary aspergillosis (ABPA) is a chronic allergic response to *Aspergillus* characterized by transient pulmonary infiltrates due to atelectasis. The incidence of ABPA is estimated to range from 1% to 2% in patients with persistent asthma and in approximately 7% (with a range from 2% to 15%) of patients with cystic fibrosis *(21)*. Specific criteria are used to establish the diagnosis of ABPA as no single finding except for central bronchiectasis in a patient with asthma is diagnostic for the condition *(21–23)*. ABPA typically progresses through a series of remissions and exacerbations but can eventually lead to pulmonary fibrosis, which is associated with a poor long-term prognosis *(23)*. Management of ABPA is directed at reducing acute asthmatic symptoms and avoiding end-stage fibrosis. Corticosteroid therapy is commonly used for treating exacerbations, although few randomized trials have been conducted for their use *(24)*. The role for antifungal therapy was evaluated with a randomized double-blind, placebo-controlled trial that showed itraconazole at 200 mg/day for 16 weeks significantly reduced daily corticosteroid use, reduced levels of immunoglobulin E (IgE), and improved exercise tolerance and pulmonary function *(22,25)*.

5.2. Aspergilloma

A pulmonary fungus ball due to *Aspergillus* or "aspergilloma" is a solid mass of hyphae growing in a previously existing pulmonary cavity, typically in patients with chronic lung disease such as bullous emphysema, sarcoidosis, tuberculosis, histoplasmosis, congenital cyst, bacterial lung abscess or, very rarely, in a pulmonary bleb from *Pneumocystis* pneumonia in AIDS *(26,27)*. On chest radiograph, a pulmonary aspergilloma appears as a solid round mass in a cavity (see Fig. 5–9, Chapter 5). In many patients the fungus ball due to *Aspergillus* remains asymptomatic, but in a significant number, hemoptysis occurs and can be fatal *(28)*. Surgical resection is considered the definitive therapy but the dense pleural adhesions adjacent the fungus ball and the poor pulmonary reserve of most patients makes surgery hazardous. Contamination of the pleural space with *Aspergillus* and the common complication of bronchopleural fistula in the postoperative period can lead to chronic *Aspergillus* empyema. Dense adhesions make pleural drainage difficult, often requiring pleural stripping or an Eloesser procedure, further compromising lung function *(28)*.

Aspergillus can also be associated with fungal balls of the sinuses without tissue invasion *(27)*. The maxillary sinus is the most common site for a sinus aspergilloma to occur *(27)*. Clinical presentation is similar to that for any chronic sinusitis. Management is usually directed at surgical removal and a generous maxillary antrostomy for sinus drainage, along with confirmation that invasive disease has not occurred.

5.3. *Other Superficial or Colonizing Syndromes*

Other superficial or colonizing syndromes of aspergillosis include otomycosis, a condition of superficial colonization typically due to *A. niger (29)*; onychomycosis which, although rare, can become chronic and respond poorly to antifungal agents *(30)*; and keratitis, particularly following trauma or corneal surgery *(31)*.

5.4. *Chronic Pulmonary Aspergillosis*

Denning and colleagues have described three distinct syndromes of chronic pulmonary aspergillosis to better characterize patients who develop chronic pulmonary disease related to *Aspergillus (32)*. These conditions include chronic cavitary pulmonary aspergillosis, which is characterized by the formation and expansion of multiple cavities, which may contain fungus balls, chronic fibrosing aspergillosis, which as its name suggests involves extensive fibrosis, and chronic necrotizing aspergillosis or subacute aspergillosis, in which slowly progressive infection occurs usually in a single thin-walled cavity. In all of these conditions, the diagnosis is suggested by radiological and clinical features and the role for therapy remains speculative, although it appears that long-term antifungal therapy may be beneficial in a subset of patients, perhaps even with the extended spectrum triazole antifungals *(32,33)*.

5.5. *Invasive Pulmonary Aspergillosis*

Invasive pulmonary aspergillosis is the most common form of invasive aspergillosis in immunocompromised patients and occurs after approximately 2 weeks of neutropenia *(34)* or during the course of graft versus host disease, now the most common risk factor in hematopoietic stem cell transplant recipients *(35)*. Symptoms include fever (may be absent in the presence of high-dose corticosteroid therapy), dry cough, shortness of breath, pleuritic chest pain, hemoptysis as well as pulmonary infiltrates all of which lag behind disease progression. In lung transplant patients and those with AIDS, *Aspergillus* tracheobronchitis can present with cough, wheezing, and shortness of breath and chest radiographs show normal lungs with or without atelectasis *(36)*.

5.6. Disseminated Aspergillosis

A variety of signs and symptoms are seen with disseminated invasive aspergillosis according to the organs involved. Involved organs include the kidneys, liver, spleen, and central nervous system (signs and symptoms of stroke or meningitis) most frequently, followed by the heart, bone, skin, and other organs *(1)*. Aspergillosis of the skin can occur either as a manifestation of disseminated disease or by direct extension from a local inoculation, for example, from an intravenous catheter *(37)*.

5.7. Sinusitis

Aspergillosis of the sinuses presents in a clinically like rhinocerebral zygomycosis, but is more common in neutropenic patients than in those with diabetic ketoacidosis, and inflammatory signs may thus be less frequent. Fever, nasal congestion, and facial pain can progress to visual changes, proptosis, and chemosis if the infection spreads to the orbit. Posterior extension to the brain can lead to cranial nerve palsies, other focal neurologic deficits, as well as a depressed level of consciousness *(38)*.

5.8. Endocarditis

Aspergillus endocarditis is the second most common form of fungal endocarditis after that caused by *Candida* species and occurs in prosthetic valve recipients and in native cardiac valves in intravenous drug users and patients with indwelling central venous catheters *(39)*. Clinically, these patients present with fever and embolic complications. Blood cultures are rarely positive even with extensive disease *(40)*.

6. DIAGNOSIS

Current diagnostic modalities are limited and the clinician must rely on the combination of knowledge of risk factors, a high index of suspicion, clinical judgment, and the finding of fungi in tissue specimens and/or cultures from the presumed site of infection. The diagnosis of proven invasive aspergillosis requires both tissue biopsy demonstrating invasion with hyphae and culture positive for *Aspergillus* species *(41)*. *Aspergillus* produce hyaline, 3 to 6 μm wide septate hyphae that typically branch at acute angles *(42)* (Fig. 9.2). In tissue these features can often distinguish *Aspergillus* from agents of zygomycosis, but they cannot distinguish *Aspergillus* from a large number of other opportunistic moulds, including *Fusarium* and *Scedosporium* (*Pseudallescheria*). Thus, culture is needed to confirm the diagnosis *(42)*. Unfortunately, invasive, or even less invasive, procedures such as bronchoscopy are often contraindicated in immunosuppressed patients, many of whom have low platelets as a result of chemotherapy and other complications. In this setting, positive culture can support the diagnosis of invasive aspergillosis.

Plain chest radiography is of limited utility in invasive aspergillosis, as it has low sensitivity and specificity in this disease6. In contrast, chest computed tomography (CT) scans have proven useful in early diagnosis of invasive pulmonary aspergillosis, as the "halo sign" of low attenuation surrounding a pulmonary nodule has been used successfully as a marker for early initiation of therapy in high-risk patients with neutropenia or who have undergone hematopoietic stem cell transplantation *(43–45)* (see Fig. 5.8, Chapter 5). Of note, these radiographic findings are also consistent with

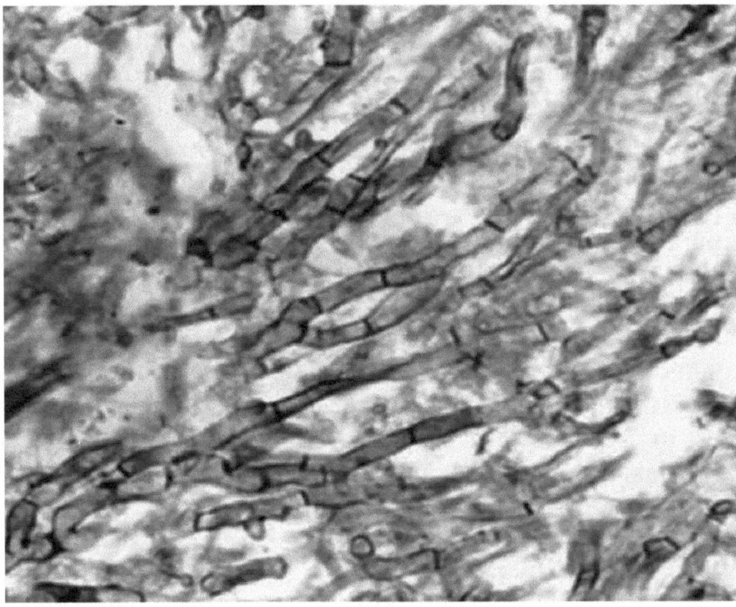

Fig. 9.2. Periodic acid-Schiff (PAS) stained tissue section of lung showing dichotomously branched, septate hyphae of *Aspergillus fumigatus*. (Courtesy of www.doctorfungus.org). [Figure in color on CD-ROM].

other infections such as *Nocardia* species, and may increase over the first week of therapy even when the patient is improving; follow-up scans should be ordered and interpreted cautiously with full attention to the clinical progress of the patient *(43)*.

Non-culture diagnostic tests have also been used to diagnose aspergillosis and in attempts to preempt difficult to treat proven disease. A sandwich enzyme immunoassay (EIA) that utilizes a monoclonal antibody to *Aspergillus* galactomannan (Platelia *Aspergillus*, Sonofi Diagnostics Pasteur, Marnes-la-Coquette, France; BioRad, Redmond, WA) is currently US Food and Drug Administration (FDA)-approved and available and is being used with varying success around the world *(46,47)*. Questions remain regarding the value of routine surveillance testing, frequency of testing, role of false positives, importance of prior antifungal therapy, and correlation of serum galactomannan results with clinical outcome.

Several reports demonstrate the potential for using polymerase chain reaction (PCR) as an early diagnostic marker, which appears more sensitive than other methods including galactomannan *(48,49)*. These assays may be associated with false-positive results due to the ubiquitous nature of *Aspergillus* conidia, are not standardized, and remain investigational at the present time *(50)*.

Other non-culture-based methods for the diagnosis of invasive aspergillosis include detection of the nonspecific fungal marker 1,3-β-D-glucan using a variation of the *Limulus* amebocyte assay. This assay (Fungitell™, Associates of Cape Cod, Falmouth, MA) has been approved for diagnostic purposes by the FDA and is a colorimetric assay that can indirectly determine the concentration of 1,3-β-D-glucan in serum samples *(51)*. The test appears promising as an indicator of infection due to many

Table 9.2
Diagnosis of invasive aspergillosis

Diagnostic method	Comment
Respiratory culture	Not frequently positive early in course of infection; positive result in high risk patient (bone marrow transplant, neutropenia) highly correlates with infection; may indicate colonization in other populations (chronic pulmonary diseases, lung transplant)
Galactomannan	*Aspergillus* Platelia system (Bio-Rad, Redmond, WA) with variable sensitivity - low (~40%) with single samples or prior antifungal therapy or prophylaxis; better yield with reduced threshold for positivity, serial samples, testing on BAL samples. False positives with pipercillin–tazobactam, dietary, neonates
1,3-β-D-glucan	Nonspecific detection of cell wall glucan. Commercially available Fungitell™ assay (Associates of Cape Cod, Falmouth, MA), limited validation and availability.
PCR	Remains investigational due to lack of standardized reagents and methods, both false positives and negatives may occur, some recent studies have suggested less sensitive than other assays
Computed tomography	In high-risk patient, "halo" sign and/or pulmonary nodules without other documented cause may be a frequent and early sign of invasive pulmonary aspergillosis

BAL, bronchoalveolar lavage.

fungi, including *Aspergillus* and *Candida* but not *Cryptococcus* or Zygomycetes (which contain little or no β-D-glucan). One study suggested the utility of the assay in early diagnosis of invasive fungal infection in a leukemic population, but validation remains limited *(52)*.

Diagnosis of invasive aspergillosis is summarized in Table 9.2.

7. TREATMENT

The goals of treatment of patients with invasive aspergillosis are to control infection and to reverse any correctable immunosuppression. Patients at high risk of developing invasive aspergillosis should be treated based on clinical or radiological criteria alone if microbiological or histological diagnosis would significantly delay treatment *(2)*.

Treatment of *Aspergillus* infection is challenging due to difficulty in diagnosis, the presence of advanced disease in many by the time of diagnosis and the presence of severe, often irreversible, immunosuppression. Mortality rates are high in patients with invasive aspergillosis and the efficacy of currently available treatments is limited by spectrum of activity and serious toxicity. Treatment failure with currently available antifungal medication in patients with invasive aspergillosis has been reported to be at least 50% *(3,4)*. New antifungal therapies with activity against *Aspergillus* have been developed, including lipid formulations of amphotericin B, the broad-spectrum triazoles (voriconazole, posaconazole, and ravuconazole), and the echinocandins (caspofungin, micafungin, and anidulafungin), all of which offer new options for therapy of this disease *(53,54)* (Table 9.3).

7.1. Amphotericin B

Amphotericin B deoxycholate has been the "gold standard" therapy in patients with invasive aspergillosis for more than 40 years *(2)*. A number of recent studies have consistently documented the limited efficacy and substantial toxicity with

Table 9.3
Antifungal agents for treating invasive aspergillosis

Agent	Typical dose/route of administration	Comments
		Polyene
Amphotericin B deoxycholate	1.0–1.5 mg/kg IV daily	Prior "gold standard"; associated with significant toxicity and limited efficacy in severely immunosuppressed patients; attempts to reduce toxicity by 24-hour infusions with limited efficacy data and concerns regarding concentration dependent killing *(80)*
Liposomal amphotericin B	3–6 mg/kg IV daily	Well tolerated; limited nephrotoxicity or infusion related reactions; anecdotal reports of efficacy with higher doses (7.5 mg/kg per day or more), but limited clinical data *(59)*; indicated for salvage therapy and empirical use *(54)*
Amphotericin B lipid complex	5 mg/kg IV daily	Indicated for salvage therapy or intolerance to standard agents, generally well tolerated *(81)*
Amphotericin B colloidal dispersion	3–6 mg/kg IV daily	Less nephrotoxic than amphotericin B deoxycholate, but associated with more infusion related and pulmonary toxicity than other lipid formulations *(63)*
		Azole
Itraconazole	200 mg IV q12h × 4 doses, then 200 mg IV daily or 200 mg PO bid (oral suspension)	Erratic bioavailability, improved with oral solution; drug interactions including chemotherapeutic agents; limited data with intravenous formulation *(2)*
Voriconazole	6 mg/kg IV q12 h × 2 doses, then 4 mg/kg IV q12 h; 200 mg PO bid (step down after 2 weeks IV)	Better efficacy and improved survival compared with amphotericin B deoxycholate; current recommended primary therapy for invasive aspergillosis; drug interactions common, hepatic toxicity (10–15%) may be dose limiting; visual effects common (~30%) but not usually dose limited and no long-term toxicity reported *(82)*

Voriconazole	6 mg/kg IV q12 h × 2 doses, then 4 mg/kg IV q12 h; 200 mg PO bid (step down after 2 weeks IV)	Better efficacy and improved survival compared with amphotericin B deoxycholate; current recommended primary therapy for invasive aspergillosis; drug interactions common, hepatic toxicity (10–15%) may be dose limiting; visual effects common (~30%) but not usually dose limited and no long-term toxicity reported *(82)*
Posaconazole	200 mg PO qid loading, 400 PO bid maintenance; oral solution only	Recent European approval for salvage therapy; studies in prophylaxis; P450 drug interactions; limited metabolism with favorable tolerance in clinical studies *(83)*
Ravuconazole	Investigational	In vitro activity but limited clinical development at present *(54)*
		Echinocandin
Caspofungin	70 mg × 1 dose, then 50 mg IV daily	Indicated for salvage therapy of aspergillosis, experimental and clinical data for use in combination therapy; well tolerated *(69)*
Micafungin	Investigational for aspergillosis (IV)	Used in doses of 100 mg/day in salvage studies; 50 mg/day for prophylaxis; well tolerated *(72)*
Anidulafungin	Investigational for aspergillosis (IV)	In vitro activity; studied at doses of 100 mg/day in other fungi; well tolerated *(84)*

IV, intravenous; PO, orally; bid, twice daily; qid, four times daily.

amphotericin B deoxycholate in high-risk patients *(44,55,56)*. The overall response rates of amphotericin B deoxycholate are less than 25%, with responses of only 10% to 15% in more severely immunosuppressed patients *(5,44)*. Wingard and colleagues recently documented increased morbidity and mortality associated with conventional amphotericin B (amphotericin B deoxycholate) in patients receiving bone marrow transplantation and those receiving concomitant nephrotoxic agents *(56)*. Similar finding were documented by Bates and colleagues, who found that renal toxicity occurred in approximately 30% of patients receiving conventional amphotericin B and that this toxicity was associated with a sixfold increase in mortality as well as a dramatic increase in hospital costs *(55)*. These unacceptably high mortality rates and significant toxicities have highlighted the need for new therapeutic approaches in this disease, so that for most patients with invasive aspergillosis, primary therapy with amphotericin B can no longer be recommended *(57)*.

The lipid formulations of amphotericin B were developed to decrease toxicity and allow the administration of higher doses of drug *(58,59)*. To date, few comparative studies of the efficacy of lipid formulations of amphotericin B in treating invasive aspergillosis have been conducted, although studies of these drugs as salvage therapy led to the approval of three lipid formulations *(60)*. Clinical experience has nevertheless been favorable, which is consistent with preclinical studies in animal models *(61)*. One small study by Leenders and colleagues compared liposomal amphotericin B at 5 mg/kg per day to standard amphotericin B at 1.0 mg/kg day for proven or suspected invasive mycoses *(62)*. Overall outcomes of both groups in this small study were similar, but analysis of patients with proven invasive aspergillosis favored the lipid preparation of amphotericin B. A recent study evaluated amphotericin B colloidal dispersion for primary therapy for invasive aspergillosis *(63)*. In this study of severely immunosuppressed patients with invasive aspergillosis, success rates with the lipid formulation were not better than those for conventional amphotericin B, although toxicity was minimally decreased. These results suggest that although lipid formulations of amphotericin B are dramatically more expensive than standard amphotericin B, hidden costs of standard amphotericin B in terms of morbidity and mortality as well as resource utilization may justify the use of lipid formulation of amphotericin B in certain high-risk patients *(55)*.

7.2. Azoles

Voriconazole is a potent, broad-spectrum, triazole that has cidal activity against many *Aspergillus* species, including *A. terreus*; is approved for therapy of invasive aspergillosis; and has become the recommended primary therapy for most patients with invasive aspergillosis *(53,64)*. This recommendation is based on data from a randomized trial that compared voriconazole to conventional amphotericin B for the primary treatment of invasive aspergillosis, with each agent followed by other licensed antifungal therapy if needed for intolerance or progression of disease, in severely immunocompromised patients with invasive aspergillosis *(44)*. In this trial, voriconazole was superior to amphotericin B, with successful outcomes in 52% of patients as compared to only 31% in those receiving amphotericin B. In addition, voriconazole demonstrated a survival advantage to amphotericin B, with an absolute 13% difference in mortality between treatment groups.

In clinical trials, voriconazole has been adequately tolerated and the drug exhibits a favorable pharmacokinetic profile. There are a number of issues to consider, including important drug interactions, especially those with immunosuppressive agents such as cyclosporine, tacrolimus, and sirolimus, the latter of which is contraindicated for use with voriconazole, and intolerance to the drug. The most common adverse event has been a transient and reversible visual disturbance described as an altered perception of light which has been reported in approximately 30% of treated patients, but has not been associated with pathologic changes *(44)*. Other less frequently reported adverse events include liver function test abnormalities in 10% to 15%, and skin rash in 6% (sometimes associated with sun exposure).

Among the other azole antifungal agents, itraconazole is approved for use as salvage therapy of aspergillosis. Its utility has been limited because until recently it has been available only in an oral formulation that is poorly absorbed; drug interactions further complicate use of this agent. An intravenous formulation of itraconazole has only recently been approved for up to 2 weeks of clinical use *(65)*. For these reasons, itraconazole is more frequently used in less immunosuppressed patients who are able to take oral therapy and for use as sequential oral therapy *(5)*. Other second-generation triazoles, including posaconazole and ravuconazole, were developed with an expanded spectrum of activity to include *Aspergillus (64,66)*. Posaconazole is available in only an oral formulation, has demonstrated in vitro and in vivo activity against *Aspergillus*, and has shown clinical activity in an open-label trial which led to its 2005 approval in the EU for salvage therapy of invasive aspergillosis *(67)*. Ravuconazole has been evaluated in early phase clinical trails and has also shown activity in animal models of invasive aspergillosis *(68)*.

7.3. Echinocandins

Echinocandins are natural cyclic hexapeptide antifungal compounds that noncompetitively inhibit 1,3-β-D-glucan synthase, an enzyme complex that is unique to a number of fungi, which forms glucan polymers in the fungal cell wall *(54)*. These agents are active against *Candida* species and *Pneumocystis*. Specific modifications to the *N*-acyl aliphatic or aryl side chains expand the antifungal spectrum to include *Aspergillus (54)*. These agents are all poorly bioavailable and produced in intravenous formulation only.

Caspofungin is approved for treating patients refractory to or intolerant of standard therapies for invasive aspergillosis based on an open-label trial that demonstrated therapeutic efficacy in 22 of 54 (41%) patients studied *(69)*. Caspofungin has been very well tolerated in clinical trials; in the aspergillosis study, only approximately 5% of patients discontinued therapy. Drug interactions with cyclosporine may occur, but have not been a significant issue *(69,70)*. In March 2005, micafungin was approved for the treatment of esophageal candidiasis and prevention of *Candida* infections. In the one prophylaxis study used to support this approval, micafungin may have reduced the number of *Aspergillus* infections as compared to standard prophylaxis with fluconazole *(71)*. Micafungin also demonstrated efficacy when used as salvage therapy *(72)*. Anidulafungin is another echinocandin with activity against *Aspergillus* spp. that appears to have a favorable toxicity profile similar to the other echinocandins. It was approved by the FDA in February 2006 for candidemia and other *Candida* infections (including abdominal abscess, peritonitis, and esophagitis). Notably, these agents are neither classically fungicidal nor fungistatic for *Aspergillus,* but exert their effect on the growing hyphal tips where the glucan synthase target is located *(73)*. For this reason, they have not frequently been used for primary therapy and have been more frequently used as salvage therapy or more recently in combination regimens *(74,75)*.

7.4. Other Therapies and Therapeutic Approaches

Outcomes for patients with invasive aspergillosis remain poor despite the advent of newer antifungal agents. This, together with the availability of several antifungal drugs and drug classes against *Aspergillus*, has increased interest in combination antifungal therapy for this infection *(76,77)*. Marr and colleagues reported on a historical control study of caspofungin and voriconazole compared with voriconazole alone in patients who failed amphotericin formulations in 2004. In this study, the use of combination salvage therapy was associated with an improved 3-month survival rate and the authors conclude that further studies of this strategy are warranted *(75)*. Adjuvant therapies including surgical resection or use of granulocyte transfusions and growth factors in invasive aspergillosis can augment antifungal therapy, although their utility has not been established in randomized trials. Surgical resection of isolated pulmonary nodules prior to additional immunosuppressive therapies has been shown to improve outcome of infection *(6,78)*. Recent studies suggest that the majority of patients will have bilateral infection when the diagnosis is first made, limiting the utility of this approach. Surgical resection may also be indicated in patients with severe hemoptysis or lesions near the hilar vessels or pericardium. The guidelines for treating invasive aspergillosis published by the Infectious Diseases Society of America were produced before the introduction of the newest available agents; a revised document is currently in press *(2)*. Unfortunately, few randomized, controlled trials exist to be used to formulate specific guidelines for therapy. A prompt diagnosis and aggressive initial therapy are both critical in improving the outcome of this infection *(79)*. Radiography and use of galactomannan EIA may facilitate an early detection of aspergillosis in high risk patients, for whom outcomes are especially poor *(45)*. Most patients should receive primary therapy with voriconazole, which has been shown to be superior to amphotericin B, the other agent approved for primary therapy of this infection *(44)*. However, in patients who are intolerant of voriconazole, have a contraindication to the drug, or have progressive infection, alternative agents include lipid formulations of amphotericin B, the echinocandins, or another triazole *(58,61,69)*. Primary use of combination therapy is not recommended at the present time because of lack of prospective clinical trial data, but the addition of another agent in a salvage setting may be considered, owing to the poor outcomes of a single agent in progressive infection *(75)*. Sequential therapy with oral azoles after initial intravenous therapy may be a useful option *(5)*. Although the optimal duration of antifungal therapy is not known, improvement in underlying host defenses is crucial to successful therapy. While substantial advances have recently been made in the management of invasive aspergillosis, newer approaches to therapy including the potential of combination therapy and newer diagnostic tools are needed to improve the outcome of this disease.

REFERENCES

1. Patterson TF. *Aspergillus* species. In: Mandell GL, Bennett JE, Dolin R, eds. Mandell, Douglas, and Bennett's principles and practice of infectious diseases. 6th ed. Philadelphia: Elsevier Churchill Livingstone, 2005:2958–2973.
2. Walsh TJ, Anaissie EJ, Denning DW, et al. Treatment of aspergillosis: clinical practice guidelines of the Infectious Diseases Society of America (IDSA). Clin Infect Dis (In press).
3. Lin SJ, Schranz J, Teutsch SM. Aspergillosis case-fatality rate: systematic review of the literature. Clin Infect Dis 2001;32:358–366.
4. McNeil MM, Nash SL, Hajjeh RA, et al. Trends in mortality due to invasive mycotic diseases in the United States, 1980–1997. Clin Infect Dis 2001;33:641–647.
5. Patterson TF, Kirkpatrick WR, White M, et al. Invasive aspergillosis. Disease spectrum, treatment practices, and outcomes. I3 Aspergillus Study Group. Medicine (Baltimore) 2000;79:250–260.
6. Caillot D, Casasnovas O, Bernard A, et al. Improved management of invasive pulmonary aspergillosis in neutropenic patients using early thoracic computed tomographic scan and surgery. J Clin Oncol 1997;15:139–147.
7. Maertens J, Vrebos M, Boogaerts M. Assessing risk factors for systemic fungal infections. Eur J Cancer Care (Engl) 2001;10:56–62.
8. Patterson TF. Advances and challenges in management of invasive mycoses. Lancet 2005;366:1013–1025.
9. Latge JP. *Aspergillus fumigatus* and aspergillosis. Clin Microbiol Rev 1999;12:310–350.

10. Hajjeh RA, Warnock DW. Counterpoint: invasive aspergillosis and the environment rethinking our approach to prevention. Clin Infect Dis 2001;33:1549–1552.
11. Woodcock AA, Steel N, Moore CB, Howard SJ, Custovic A, Denning DW. Fungal contamination of bedding. Allergy 2006;61:140–142.
12. Anaissie EJ, Stratton SL, Dignani MC, et al. Pathogenic moulds (including *Aspergillus* species) in hospital water distribution systems: a 3-year prospective study and clinical implications for patients with hematologic malignancies. Blood 2003;101:2542–2546.
13. Iwen PC, Rupp ME, Langnas AN, Reed EC, Hinrichs SH. Invasive pulmonary aspergillosis due to *Aspergillus terreus*: 12-year experience and review of the literature. Clin Infect Dis 1998;26:1092–1097.
14. Warris A, Bjorneklett A, Gaustad P. Invasive pulmonary aspergillosis associated with infliximab therapy. N Engl J Med 2001;344:1099–1100.
15. Walsh TJ, Petraitis V, Petraitiene R, et al. Experimental pulmonary aspergillosis due to *Aspergillus terreus*: pathogenesis and treatment of an emerging fungal pathogen resistant to amphotericin B. J Infect Dis 2003;188:305–319.
16. Brummer E, Kamberi M, Stevens DA. Regulation by granulocyte-macrophage colony-stimulating factor and/or steroids given in vivo of proinflammatory cytokine and chemokine production by bronchoalveolar macrophages in response to *Aspergillus* conidia. J Infect Dis 2003;187:705–709.
17. Kan VL, Bennett JE. Lectin-like attachment sites on murine pulmonary alveolar macrophages bind *Aspergillus fumigatus* conidia. J Infect Dis 1988;158:407–414.
18. Levitz SM, Selsted ME, Ganz T, Lehrer RI, Diamond RD. In vitro killing of spores and hyphae of *Aspergillus fumigatus* and *Rhizopus oryzae* by rabbit neutrophil cationic peptides and bronchoalveolar macrophages. J Infect Dis 1986;154:483–489.
19. Washburn RG, Gallin JI, Bennett JE. Oxidative killing of *Aspergillus fumigatus* proceeds by parallel myeloperoxidase-dependent and -independent pathways. Infect Immun 1987;55:2088–2092.
20. Stanzani M, Orciuolo E, Lewis R, et al. *Aspergillus fumigatus* suppresses the human cellular immune response via gliotoxin-mediated apoptosis of monocytes. Blood 2005;105:2258–2265.
21. Greenberger PA. Allergic bronchopulmonary aspergillosis. J Allergy Clin Immunol 2002;110:685–692.
22. Stevens DA, Moss RB, Kurup VP, et al. Allergic bronchopulmonary aspergillosis in cystic fibrosis–state of the art: Cystic Fibrosis Foundation Consensus Conference. Clin Infect Dis 2003;37 (Suppl 3):S225–S264.
23. Patterson R, Greenberger PA, Radin RC, Roberts M. Allergic bronchopulmonary aspergillosis: staging as an aid to management. Ann Intern Med 1982;96:286–291.
24. Wark PA, Gibson PG, Wilson AJ. Azoles for allergic bronchopulmonary aspergillosis associated with asthma. Cochrane Database Syst Rev 2004:CD001108.
25. Stevens DA, Schwartz HJ, Lee JY, et al. A randomized trial of itraconazole in allergic bronchopulmonary aspergillosis. N Engl J Med 2000;342:756–762.
26. Gillespie MB, O'Malley BW. An algorithmic approach to the diagnosis and management of invasive fungal rhinosinusitis in the immunocompromised patient. Otolaryngol Clin North Am 2000;33:323–334.
27. Ferguson BJ. Fungus balls of the paranasal sinuses. Otolaryngol Clin North Am 2000;33:389–398.
28. Kauffman CA. Quandary about treatment of aspergillomas persists. Lancet 1996;347:1640.
29. Kaur R, Mittal N, Kakkar M, Aggarwal AK, Mathur MD. Otomycosis: a clinicomycologic study. Ear Nose Throat J 2000;79:606–609.

30. Torres-Rodriguez JM, Madrenys-Brunet N, Siddat M, Lopez-Jodra O, Jimenez T. *Aspergillus versicolor* as cause of onychomycosis: report of 12 cases and susceptibility testing to antifungal drugs. J Eur Acad Dermatol Venereol 1998;11:25–31.
31. Kuo IC, Margolis TP, Cevallos V, Hwang DG. *Aspergillus fumigatus* keratitis after laser in situ keratomileusis. Cornea 2001;20:342–344.
32. Denning DW, Riniotis K, Dobrashian R, Sambatakou H. Chronic cavitary and fibrosing pulmonary and pleural aspergillosis: case series, proposed nomenclature change, and review. Clin Infect Dis 2003;37 (Suppl 3):S265–S280.
33. Jain LR, Denning DW. The efficacy and tolerability of voriconazole in the treatment of chronic cavitary pulmonary aspergillosis. J Infect 2006;52:e133–e137.
34. Gerson SL, Talbot GH, Hurwitz S, Strom BL, Lusk EJ, Cassileth PA. Prolonged granulocytopenia: the major risk factor for invasive pulmonary aspergillosis in patients with acute leukemia. Ann Intern Med 1984;100:345–351.
35. Marr KA, Carter RA, Crippa F, Wald A, Corey L. Epidemiology and outcome of mould infections in hematopoietic stem cell transplant recipients. Clin Infect Dis 2002;34:909–917.
36. Miller WT, Sais GJ, Frank I, Gefter WB, Aronchick JM, Miller WT. Pulmonary aspergillosis in patients with AIDS. Clinical and radiographic correlations. Chest 1994;105:37–44.
37. Allo MD, Miller J, Townsend T, Tan C. Primary cutaneous aspergillosis associated with Hickman intravenous catheters. N Engl J Med 1987;317:1105–1108.
38. Mylonakis E, Rich J, Skolnik PR, De Orchis DF, Flanigan T. Invasive *Aspergillus* sinusitis in patients with human immunodeficiency virus infection. Report of 2 cases and review. Medicine (Baltimore) 1997;76:249–255.
39. Ellis ME, Al-Abdely H, Sandridge A, Greer W, Ventura W. Fungal endocarditis: evidence in the world literature, 1965–1995. Clin Infect Dis 2001;32:50–62.
40. Denning DW, Stevens DA. Antifungal and surgical treatment of invasive aspergillosis: review of 2,121 published cases. Rev Infect Dis 1990;12:1147–1201.
41. Ascioglu S, Rex JH, de Pauw B, et al. Defining opportunistic invasive fungal infections in immunocompromised patients with cancer and hematopoietic stem cell transplants: an international consensus. Clin Infect Dis 2002;34:7–14.
42. Sutton DA, Fothergill AW, Rinaldi MG. Guide to Clinically Significant Fungi. Baltimore, MD: Lippincott Williams & Wilkins, 1998.
43. Caillot D, Couaillier JF, Bernard A, et al. Increasing volume and changing characteristics of invasive pulmonary aspergillosis on sequential thoracic computed tomography scans in patients with neutropenia. J Clin Oncol 2001;19:253–259.
44. Herbrecht R, Denning DW, Patterson TF, et al. Voriconazole versus amphotericin B for primary therapy of invasive aspergillosis. N Engl J Med 2002;347:408–415.
45. Herbrecht R. Improving the outcome of invasive aspergillosis: new diagnostic tools and new therapeutic strategies. Ann Hematol 2002;81 (Suppl 2):S52–S53.
46. Maertens J, Theunissen K, Verbeken E, et al. Prospective clinical evaluation of lower cut-offs for galactomannan detection in adult neutropenic cancer patients and haematological stem cell transplant recipients. Br J Haematol 2004;126:852–860.
47. Maertens J, Theunissen K, Verhoef G, et al. Galactomannan and computed tomography-based preemptive antifungal therapy in neutropenic patients at high risk for invasive fungal infection: a prospective feasibility study. Clin Infect Dis 2005;41:1242–1250.
48. Loeffler J, Hebart H, Cox P, Flues N, Schumacher U, Einsele H. Nucleic acid sequence-based amplification of *Aspergillus* RNA in blood samples. J Clin Microbiol 2001;39:1626–1629.

49. White PL, Linton CJ, Perry MD, Johnson EM, Barnes RA. The evolution and evaluation of a whole blood polymerase chain reaction assay for the detection of invasive aspergillosis in hematology patients in a routine clinical setting. Clin Infect Dis 2006;42: 479–486.
50. Donnelly JP. Polymerase chain reaction for diagnosing invasive aspergillosis: getting closer but still a ways to go. Clin Infect Dis 2006;42:487–489.
51. Odabasi Z, Mattiuzzi G, Estey E, et al. Beta-D-glucan as a diagnostic adjunct for invasive fungal infections: validation, cutoff development, and performance in patients with acute myelogenous leukemia and myelodysplastic syndrome. Clin Infect Dis 2004;39: 199–205.
52. Ostrosky-Zeichner L, Alexander BD, Kett DH, et al. Multicenter clinical evaluation of the (1–>3) beta-D-glucan assay as an aid to diagnosis of fungal infections in humans. Clin Infect Dis 2005;41:654–659.
53. Steinbach WJ, Stevens DA. Review of newer antifungal and immunomodulatory strategies for invasive aspergillosis. Clin Infect Dis 2003;37 (Suppl 3):S157–S187.
54. Boucher HW, Groll AH, Chiou CC, Walsh TJ. Newer systemic antifungal agents: pharmacokinetics, safety and efficacy. Drugs 2004;64:1997–2020.
55. Bates DW, Su L, Yu DT, et al. Mortality and costs of acute renal failure associated with amphotericin B therapy. Clin Infect Dis 2001;32:686–693.
56. Wingard JR, Kubilis P, Lee L, et al. Clinical significance of nephrotoxicity in patients treated with amphotericin B for suspected or proven aspergillosis. Clin Infect Dis 1999;29:1402–1407.
57. Ostrosky-Zeichner L, Marr KA, Rex JH, Cohen SH. Amphotericin B: time for a new "gold standard." Clin Infect Dis 2003;37:415–425.
58. Walsh TJ, Hiemenz JW, Seibel NL, et al. Amphotericin B lipid complex for invasive fungal infections: analysis of safety and efficacy in 556 cases. Clin Infect Dis 1998;26: 1383–1396.
59. Walsh TJ, Goodman JL, Pappas P, et al. Safety, tolerance, and pharmacokinetics of high-dose liposomal amphotericin B (AmBisome) in patients infected with *Aspergillus* species and other filamentous fungi: maximum tolerated dose study. Antimicrob Agents Chemother 2001;45:3487–3496.
60. Rex JH, Walsh TJ, Nettleman M, et al. Need for alternative trial designs and evaluation strategies for therapeutic studies of invasive mycoses. Clin Infect Dis 2001;33:95–106.
61. Barrett JP, Vardulaki KA, Conlon C, et al. A systematic review of the antifungal effectiveness and tolerability of amphotericin B formulations. Clin Ther 2003;25:1295–1320.
62. Leenders AC, Daenen S, Jansen RL, et al. Liposomal amphotericin B compared with amphotericin B deoxycholate in the treatment of documented and suspected neutropenia-associated invasive fungal infections. Br J Haematol 1998;103:205–212.
63. Bowden R, Chandrasekar P, White MH, et al. A double-blind, randomized, controlled trial of amphotericin B colloidal dispersion versus amphotericin B for treatment of invasive aspergillosis in immunocompromised patients. Clin Infect Dis 2002;35:359–366.
64. Espinel-Ingroff A, Boyle K, Sheehan DJ. In vitro antifungal activities of voriconazole and reference agents as determined by NCCLS methods: review of the literature. Mycopathologia 2001;150:101–115.
65. Caillot D. Intravenous itraconazole followed by oral itraconazole for the treatment of amphotericin-B-refractory invasive pulmonary aspergillosis. Acta Haematol 2003;109:111–118.
66. Sheehan DJ, Hitchcock CA, Sibley CM. Current and emerging azole antifungal agents. Clin Microbiol Rev 1999;12:40–79.

67. Raad I, Chapman S, Bradsher R. Posaconazole (POS) salvage therapy for invasive fungal infections (IFI) (abstract M-699), 44th Interscience Conference on Antimicrobial Agents and Chemotherapy, Washington, DC, 2004.
68. Kirkpatrick WR, Perea S, Coco BJ, Patterson TF. Efficacy of ravuconazole (BMS-207147) in a guinea pig model of disseminated aspergillosis. J Antimicrob Chemother 2002;49:353–357.
69. Maertens J, Raad I, Petrikkos G, et al. Efficacy and safety of caspofungin for treatment of invasive aspergillosis in patients refractory to or intolerant of conventional antifungal therapy. Clin Infect Dis 2004;39:1563–1571.
70. Marr KA, Hachem R, Papanicolaou G, et al. Retrospective study of the hepatic safety profile of patients concomitantly treated with caspofungin and cyclosporin A. Transpl Infect Dis 2004;6:110–116.
71. van Burik JA, Ratanatharathorn V, Stepan DE, et al. Micafungin versus fluconazole for prophylaxis against invasive fungal infections during neutropenia in patients undergoing hematopoietic stem cell transplantation. Clin Infect Dis 2004;39:1407–1416.
72. Denning DW, Marr KA, Lau WM, et al. Micafungin (FK463), alone or in combination with other systemic antifungal agents, for the treatment of acute invasive aspergillosis. J Infect 2006;53:337–349.
73. Bowman JC, Hicks PS, Kurtz MB, et al. The antifungal echinocandin caspofungin acetate kills growing cells of *Aspergillus fumigatus* in vitro. Antimicrob Agents Chemother 2002;46:3001–3012.
74. Kirkpatrick WR, Perea S, Coco BJ, Patterson TF. Efficacy of caspofungin alone and in combination with voriconazole in a Guinea pig model of invasive aspergillosis. Antimicrob Agents Chemother 2002;46:2564–2568.
75. Marr KA, Boeckh M, Carter RA, Kim HW, Corey L. Combination antifungal therapy for invasive aspergillosis. Clin Infect Dis 2004;39:797–802.
76. Kontoyiannis DP, Hachem R, Lewis RE, et al. Efficacy and toxicity of caspofungin in combination with liposomal amphotericin B as primary or salvage treatment of invasive aspergillosis in patients with hematologic malignancies. Cancer 2003;98:292–299.
77. Aliff TB, Maslak PG, Jurcic JG, et al. Refractory Aspergillus pneumonia in patients with acute leukemia: successful therapy with combination caspofungin and liposomal amphotericin. Cancer 2003;97:1025–1032.
78. Yeghen T, Kibbler CC, Prentice HG, et al. Management of invasive pulmonary aspergillosis in hematology patients: a review of 87 consecutive cases at a single institution. Clin Infect Dis 2000;31:859–868.
79. Patterson TF, Boucher HW, Herbrecht R, et al. Strategy of following voriconazole versus amphotericin B therapy with other licensed antifungal therapy for primary treatment of invasive aspergillosis: impact of other therapies on outcome. Clin Infect Dis 2005;41:1448–1452.
80. Imhof A, Walter RB, Schaffner A. Continuous infusion of escalated doses of amphotericin B deoxycholate: an open-label observational study. Clin Infect Dis 2003;36:943–951.
81. Wingard JR, White MH, Anaissie E, Raffalli J, Goodman J, Arrieta A. A randomized, double-blind comparative trial evaluating the safety of liposomal amphotericin B versus amphotericin B lipid complex in the empirical treatment of febrile neutropenia. L Amph/ABLC Collaborative Study Group. Clin Infect Dis 2000;31:1155–1163.
82. Keating GM. Posaconazole. Drugs 2005;65:1553–1567.
83. Murdoch D, Plosker GL. Anidulafungin. Drugs 2004;64:2249–2258.
84. Johnson LB, Kauffman CA. Voriconazole: a new triazole antifungal agent. Clin Infect Dis 2003;36:630–637.

SUGGESTED READINGS

Boucher HW, Groll AH, Chiou CC, Walsh TJ. Newer systemic antifungal agents: pharmacokinetics, safety and efficacy. Drugs 2004;64:1997–2020.

Caillot D, Casasnovas O, Bernard A, et al. Improved management of invasive pulmonary aspergillosis in neutropenic patients using early thoracic computed tomographic scan and surgery. J Clin Oncol 1997;15:139–147.

Herbrecht R, Denning DW, Patterson TF, et al. Voriconazole versus amphotericin B for primary therapy of invasive aspergillosis. N Engl J Med 2002;347:408–415.

Keating GM. Posaconazole. Drugs 2005;65:1553–1567.

Patterson TF. *Aspergillus* species. In: Mandell GL, Bennett JE, Dolin R, eds. Mandell, Douglas, and Bennett's principles and practice of infectious diseases. Philadelphia: Elsevier Churchill Livingstone, 2005;2958–2973.

Patterson TF. Advances and challenges in management of invasive mycoses. Lancet 2005; 366:1013–1025.

Patterson TF, Kirkpatrick WR, White M, et al. Invasive aspergillosis. Disease spectrum, treatment practices, and outcomes. Medicine (Baltimore) 2000;79:250–260.

Maertens J, Theunissen K, Verhoef G, et al. Galactomannan and computed tomography-based preemptive antifungal therapy in neutropenic patients at high risk for invasive fungal infection: a prospective feasibility study. Clin Infect Dis 2005;41:1242–1250.

Marr KA, Boeckh M, Carter RA, Kim HW, Corey L. Combination antifungal therapy for invasive aspergillosis. Clin Infect Dis 2004;39:797–802.

Walsh TJ, Anaissie EJ, Denning DW, et al. Treatment of aspergillosis: clinical practice guidelines of the Infectious Diseases Society of America (IDSA). Clin Infect Dis (In press).

Walsh TJ, Petraitis V, Petraitiene R, et al. Experimental pulmonary aspergillosis due to *Aspergillus terreus*: pathogenesis and treatment of an emerging fungal pathogen resistant to amphotericin B. J Infect Dis 2003;188:305–319.

10
Hyalohyphomycosis—Infection Due to Hyaline Moulds

Rhonda V. Fleming, MD and Elias J. Anaissie, MD

1. INTRODUCTION

Hyalohyphomycosis is the term used to designate infections caused by fungi noted to have hyaline (colorless) septate hyphae microscopically in clinical samples, similar to the use of phaeohyphomycosis for those infections caused by pigmented fungi (Chapter 11). This distinction is clinically useful when hyphal elements are seen on tissue examination but fail to grow. Hyalohyphomycosis typically includes infections caused by species of *Fusarium*, *Scedosporium*, *Acremonium*, *Paecilomyces*, *Scopulariopsis*, *Beauveria*, and *Penicillium*. Although *Aspergillus* produces similar hyaline septate hyphae microscopically, and is thus considered a member of this grouping of fungi, infection caused by this genus (aspergillosis) is generally discussed as a separate disease (Chapter 9). These agents may cause superficial or localized infection in immunocompetent hosts (usually as a result of direct inoculation of the fungus after trauma) and invasive or disseminated infections in immunocompromised hosts. In the latter setting, the clinical infection may be indistinguishable from that of invasive aspergillosis. A remarkable feature of some of these hyaline moulds is their ability to cause fungemia and to disseminate hematogenously, causing numerous embolic skin lesions. These infections may be clinically suspected on the basis of a constellation of clinical and laboratory findings. Definitive diagnosis requires isolation of the organism because histopathological examination reveals branching hyaline septate hyphae regardless of the pathogen, similar to the findings with *Aspergillus*. An accurate diagnosis at the species level is important because of the variable susceptibility to antifungal agents. An important component of therapy of localized infection is surgery and removal of infected prosthetic devices. Outcome is usually favorable in immunocompetent hosts, while usually very poor in the setting of persistent profound immunosuppression. We herein describe the most relevant characteristics of these organisms and the clinical spectrum and diagnosis and treatment of infections caused by these agents.

From: *Infectious Disease: Diagnosis and Treatment of Human Mycoses*
Edited by: D. R. Hospenthal and M. G. Rinaldi © Humana Press Inc., Totowa, NJ

2. *FUSARIUM*

2.1. Introduction

Fusarium species recently emerged as a cause of disseminated infections in neutropenic patients and in patients undergoing allogeneic hematopoietic stem cell transplantation (HSCT). *Fusarium* represents the second most common fungal pathogen, after *Aspergillus*, as the cause of life-threatening infection in recipients of hematopoietic transplant *(1)*. *Fusarium* causes a broad spectrum of infections in humans, including superficial and local infections in immunocompetent hosts, while disseminated infection is seen almost exclusively in immunosuppressed patients.

2.2. Etiologic Agents

Four species are most commonly involved in human infections: *F. solani* (the most common), *F. oxysporum*, *F. moniliforme*, and *F. proliferatum (2)*. *Fusarium* species are septate filamentous fungi that produce conidiophores, phialides, macroconidia, and microconidia. *Fusarium* species grow easily and rapidly in almost all fungal media. On potato dextrose agar (PDA), the colonies have a velvety or cottony surface, and are white, yellow, pink, purple salmon or gray on the surface, with a pale, red, violet, brown or sometimes blue reverse. The characteristic sickle- or banana-shaped multiseptate macroconidia with a foot cell at the base are used in identifying the genus and species of *Fusarium* (Fig. 10.1). Molecular methods may also be used for rapid identification of *Fusarium* to the species level. In tissue, the hyphae are similar to those of *Aspergillus* species, with hyaline and septate filaments that typically dichotomize in acute and right angles. In the absence of microbial growth, distinguishing fusariosis from aspergillosis and other hyalohyphomycoses is difficult, and requires the use of in situ hybridization in paraffin-embedded tissue specimens *(3)*. *Fusarium* species are toxigenic, and may cause mycotoxicosis in animals and humans *(2)*.

2.3. Epidemiology

Fusarium is ubiquitous in soil and water, taking part in water biofilms and is a human and plant pathogen *(4)*. *Fusarium* species are causative agents of superficial and localized infections in immunocompetent hosts, most commonly onychomycosis and cutaneous and subcutaneous infections including mycetoma and keratitis, the latter in contact lens wearers *(5)*. A recent large outbreak of *Fusarium* keratitis was reported in contact lens wearers in the United States and was linked to contaminated contact lens rinse solutions *(6)*. Other risk factors for keratitis are trauma and use of topical corticosteroids and antibiotics. *Fusarium* endophthalmitis may arise from keratitis or by direct inoculation after cataract surgery or trauma *(7)*. Fusariosis may also result from skin breakdown, such as burns and wounds, or the presence of foreign bodies, such as peritonitis in patients receiving continuous ambulatory peritoneal dialysis (CAPD), and catheter-associated fungemia, and thrombophlebitis *(8–10)*. Other infections include sinusitis, pneumonia, cutaneous and subcutaneous infections, septic arthritis, and osteomyelitis *(11–15)*.

Immunosuppressed patients may develop locally invasive and disseminated fusariosis *(16)*. Risk factors include prolonged neutropenia such as following chemotherapy

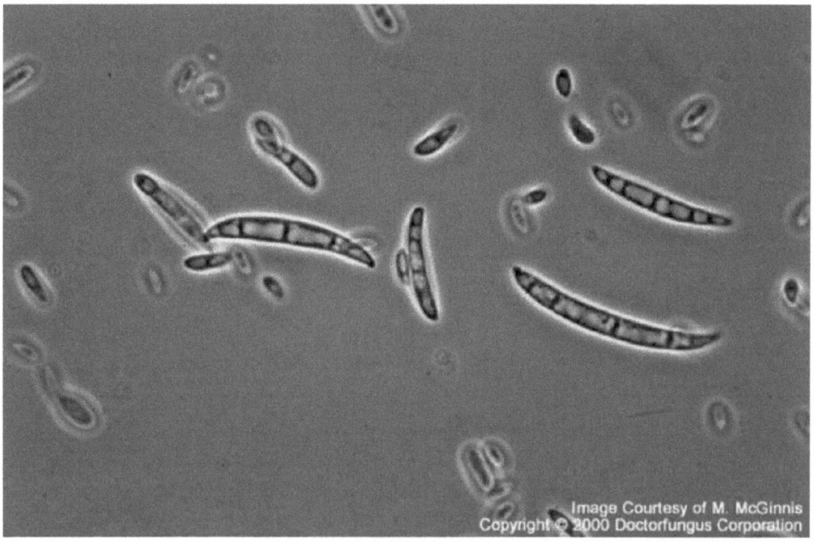

Fig. 10.1. *Fusarium oxysporum* macroconidia. Characteristic fusiform to sickle-shaped, multiseptate, mostly with an attenuated apical cell and a foot-shaped basal cell. (Courtesy of www.doctorfungus.org.) [Figure in color on CD-ROM].

for acute leukemia and T-cell immunodeficiency which occurs most commonly after HSCT *(16–18)*. In HSCT infection may develop early during neutropenia or months after neutrophil recovery, following treatment of chronic extensive graft versus host disease (GvHD). Localized infections may also develop among solid organ transplant recipients (SOT), usually as a late infection *(19)*.

Portals of entry are the respiratory tract and skin, the latter playing a significant role in patients with tissue breakdown such as onychomycosis. Hospital water systems are a potential reservoir for *Fusarium*; transmission may occur from inhalation of conidia aerosolized in the shower or from direct contact of contaminated water with sites of skin breakdown *(20–22)*.

2.4. Pathogenesis and Immunology

Similar to *Aspergillus*, this organism is highly angioinvasive and leads to tissue infarction. In contrast to *Aspergillus* however, *Fusarium* is frequently isolated from the bloodstream, likely as a result of intravascular adventitious sporulation *(23)*. Phagocytes appear to be the predominant line of defense against fusarial infections *(16–18)*.

2.5. Clinical Manifestations

Infection with *Fusarium* in immunocompetent hosts may be superficial or locally invasive, involving the skin, eyes, sinuses, lungs, and joints and bones. In immunosuppressed patients, the infection may be locally invasive, usually pneumonia and/or sinusitis, or more commonly disseminated *(16–18)*. The clinical picture resembles that of invasive aspergillosis. Unlike aspergillosis, however, fungemia and skin lesions are common (up to 40% of patients with disseminated disease). Skin lesions may represent the primary site of infection (onychomycosis) or secondary to disseminated infection *(16–18)*. Metastatic skin lesions evolve from subcutaneous painful lesions, to erythematous induration followed by ecthyma gangrenosum-like with necrotic center, which may be surrounded by a rim of erythema *(16–18)*.

2.6. Diagnosis

Two characteristics suggest the diagnosis of disseminated fusariosis in the severely immunocompromised host: metastatic skin lesions and positive blood cultures for mould *(16–18)*. Definitive diagnosis relies on cultures (tissue and/or blood) and histopathology which shows a pattern common to all hyalohyphomycosis (invasion by acute-branching, septate hyaline hyphae). The use of polymerase chain reaction (PCR) techniques and/or in situ hybridization may be required to reach the correct diagnosis in tissues *(3,24)*. The 1,3-β-D-glucan test is usually positive in invasive fusarial infections, but it cannot distinguish *Fusarium* from other fungal infections (*Candida*, *Aspergillus*, *Trichosporon* and others) that are also detected by the assay *(25)*.

2.7. Treatment

Localized infections, particularly in immunocompetent hosts, usually respond well to treatment consisting of topical therapy for fungal keratitis or excision of involved tissue (sinuses, eye, soft tissue, bone). Removal of an infected intravascular catheter may be needed in the rare cases of catheter-related fungemia.

The outcome of disseminated fusariosis in severely immunosuppressed patients remains poor despite aggressive antifungal therapy, with very high mortality rates *(16–18)*. Predictors of poor outcome are persistent neutropenia and recent therapy with corticosteroids for chronic GvHD *(17)*. Treatment options are limited by the lack of reliable and consistent activity of antifungal agents against *Fusarium* species. *F. moniliforme* is the most susceptible species, typically inhibited by amphotericin B and the newer triazoles voriconazole and posaconazole; *F. verticilloides* is commonly resistant to both antifungal classes. *F. solani* and *F. oxysporum* have an intermediate susceptibility to amphotericin B, but are resistant to the triazoles *(26)*. Hence, rapid species identification is needed and antifungal susceptibility testing should be considered because of this variable in vitro susceptibility among *Fusarium* species (Table 10.1). The echinocandins do not appear to be active against *Fusarium*.

3. *SCEDOSPORIUM*

3.1. Introduction

Two *Scedosporium* species, *S. apiospermum* (sexual state name, *Pseudallescheria boydii*) and *S. prolificans* (formerly *S. inflatum*) cause human disease *(27,28)*. A spectrum of disease, ranging from respiratory tract colonization (cystic fibrosis or SOT) to superficial and deep infections, in both immunocompetent and immunosuppressed hosts, has been reported. Rarely, disseminated infection with high mortality is seen in the setting of severe immunosuppression. *S. prolificans* belongs to the group of fungi that cause phaeohyphomycosis (dematiaceous fungi), but are briefly discussed because of its relationship to *S. apiospermum* .

Table 10.1
Overall susceptibility of hyaline fungi to available antifungals[a]

Genus/species	AmB	Itraconazole	Voriconazole	Posaconazole	Anidulafungin	Caspofungin	Ref.
Fusarium spp.	++	+	++[b]	++	0	0	*(50,51)*
F. oxysporum	++	+	++++	++	ND	ND	*(50,52)*
F. solani	+	+	+	+	ND	ND	
Scedosporium spp.							
S. prolificans	0	0	0	0	0	ND	*(51)*
S. apiospermum	0	++	++++	+++	0	0	*(51,52)*
Paecilomyces spp.	++	+++	+++	+++	++	+++	*(50,51)*
Acremonium spp.	++	0	++	ND	0	ND	*(51)*

++++, drug of choice; +++, alternative choice; ++, some strains are susceptible (< 50%); +, rarely susceptible (< 10%); 0, always resistant; ND, no data available.

[a]Susceptibility based on MIC_{50}.

[b]In the United States, the only agent indicated for invasive fusariosis.

3.2. Etiologic Agents

Scedosporium species are identified by their characteristic macroscopic (wooly to cottony, dark gray to dark brown) and microscopic (characteristic conidia, conidiophores, and hyphae) appearance. *S. prolificans* is distinguished from *S. apiospermum* by the production of terminal annelloconidia with inflated bases (cylindrical in *S. apiospermum*) and growth inhibition by cycloheximide or actidione. In tissue sections, *Scedosporium* appear as septate hyaline hyphae that cannot be reliably distinguished from *Aspergillus* or *Fusarium* unless conidia are present.

3.3. Epidemiology

Scedosporium have been isolated from soil, potting mix, compost, and animal manure and stagnant or polluted water. Infections occur worldwide, though a large number of reports come from Northern Spain *(27)*. Patients at risk for invasive and/or disseminated infection include those with human immunodeficiency virus (HIV) infection, acute leukemia and recipients of allogeneic HSCT or SOT *(29,30)*.

Infection is thought to be secondary to direct inoculation (such as after trauma) or inhalation of airborne conidia. In normal hosts, *S. apiospermum* causes infection after penetrating trauma, including keratitis, endophthalmitis, cutaneous and subcutaneous infections, bursitis, arthritis, and osteomyelitis. After near drowning accidents, sinusitis, pneumonia, meningoencephalitis, and brain abscesses may develop. Allergic bronchopulmonary disease due to *S. apiospermum* may also occur. Like *S. apiospermum, S. prolificans* causes localized infections (usually of bone or soft tissue) in immunocompetent patients after trauma, and deeply invasive infections in immunocompromised hosts, sometimes as a nosocomial outbreak *(27,29,30)*.

3.4. Clinical Manifestations

Mycetoma is the most common *S. apiospermum* infection in normal hosts (see Chapter 21), usually occurring after penetrating injury and presenting as lower extremity swelling with draining sinuses. Other infections include non-mycetoma cutaneous and subcutaneous infections, keratitis, and endophthalmitis *(29)*. Invasive *S. apiospermum* infection is usually seen in immunocompromised patients, most commonly as pneumonia. Disseminated infection is mainly associated with *S. prolificans*, and is characterized by refractory fever, pulmonary infiltrates (diffuse or nodular), central nervous system involvement (present in one third of patients), fungemia, renal failure and erythematous, and nodular skin lesions with central necrosis.

3.5. Diagnosis

The diagnosis relies on the combination of clinical signs and symptoms and recovery of *Scedosporium* from blood and/or infected tissue, with or without demonstration of colorless septate hyphae.

3.6. Treatment

Localized infections, particularly in immunocompetent hosts, usually respond well to surgical débridement. *Scedosporium apiospermum* is resistant to fluconazole and flucytosine, but susceptible to the newer azoles voriconazole, posaconazole, and ravuconazole (Table 10.1). Voriconazole is approved for use in *S. apiospermum* infections *(31,32)*. Caspofungin appears to be more active than itraconazole or amphotericin B. Variable strain-to-strain susceptibility to amphotericin B can be seen *(33)*. Surgical resection remains the only definite therapy for *S. prolificans* infections, as this organism is resistant to all available antifungal agents in vitro. In vitro synergism between terbinafine and either voriconazole or itraconazole has been reported *(34)*.

4. *PAECILOMYCES*

4.1. *Introduction*

Paecilomyces species are frequent airborne contaminants in clinical microbiology laboratories but have been increasingly reported as cause of human infection.

4.2. *Etiologic Agents*

Two *Paecilomyces* species, *P. lilacinus* (most common) and *P. varioti*, account for most human infections; although recent reports have described infection secondary to *P. marquandii* and *P. javanicus*. *Paecilomyces* grow rapidly on various agar media including blood, chocolate, Sabouraud dextrose (SDA), and PDA. *P. varioti* is thermophilic and grows well at temperatures as high as 50°C. The color of the colony and certain microscopic features help differentiate *Paecilomyces* species from each other. The colonies are flat and velvety. The color is initially white and becomes yellow-green, yellow-brown, pink or violet according to species.

4.3. *Epidemiology*

Paecilomyces are found worldwide in soil, food products, and water and causes infection in both immunocompetent and immunosuppressed patients. A strong association of *Paecilomyces* with prosthetic implants may be due to their inherent resistance to most sterilizing techniques. Prosthetic implant-related infections include keratitis in contact lens wearers and after corneal implants (rarely endophthalmitis), and in recipients of CAPD, cardiac valves, and ventriculoperitoneal shunts. Other infections involve the nails, skin, and subcutaneous tissues, bones and joints, sinuses and lungs, while disseminated infections only occur in immunosuppressed patients *(35)*.

4.4. *Clinical Manifestations*

The most common infections due to *Paecilomyces* involve the eye and eye structures (keratitis and endophthalmitis), followed by the nails (onychomycosis) and skin and soft tissues. Skin infections are characterized by erythematous macules, nodules, pustules, vesicular lesions, or necrotic crusts *(35)*. Sporotrichosis-like skin infection has also been described. Other reported infections in the competent host include peritonitis in CAPD, prosthetic-valve endocarditis, catheter-related fungemia, and arthritis/osteomyelitis. In immunocompromised patients, pneumonia and disseminated disease are most commonly observed.

4.5. *Diagnosis*

Paecilomyces infections are diagnosed with routine tissue culture. These organisms are easily cultured on SDA and on histopathology, hyaline septate hyphae can be seen with periodic acid-Schiff (PAS) staining. *Paecilomyces* may exist in various forms in tissue (conidia and phialides) and can therefore be misdiagnosed as candidiasis.

4.6. Treatment

Treatment of invasive *Paecilomyces* infections relies on surgical debridement and removal of infected prosthetic materials. Because of different susceptibilities to antifungal agents, *Paecilomyces* should be identified to the species level (Table 10.1). *P. varioti* is susceptible to amphotericin B, flucytosine, itraconazole, voriconazole, and posaconazole, whereas *P. lilacinus* is susceptible only to the latter two triazoles *(36)*.

5. ACREMONIUM

5.1. Introduction

Acremonium species are filamentous fungi of low pathogenicity commonly isolated from the environment (soil, insects, sewage, plants, and water) *(37)*.

5.2. Etiologic Agents

Seven species of *Acremonium* have been reported to cause human infection with more than 80% of infections caused by *A. strictum* (the most common), *A. falciforme*, *A. recifei*, and *A. kiliense*. *Acremonium* species grow on SDA, forming white, salmon, or yellowish-green colonies that are usually velvety or cottony with slightly raised centers. This genus is distinguished by formation of narrow hyphae bearing solitary, unbranched needle-shaped phialides. As in other hyaline moulds, septate colorless hyphae are found in tissue.

5.3. Epidemiology

Most infections occur in immunocompetent hosts and include mycetoma following trauma, keratitis in contact lenses wearers, and endophthalmitis *(37–39)*. Fungal colonization of humidifier water in a ventilator system was thought to be the source of infections in an outbreak of endophthalmitis. Invasive disease is almost exclusively seen in immunocompromised patients.

5.4. Clinical Manifestations

Mycetoma is the most common infection due to *Acremonium* and presents in a manner similar to that of mycetoma caused by *S. apiospermum*. Keratitis and endophthalmitis constitute the second most common infections. Colonization of soft contact lenses may proceed to corneal invasion. Other reported infections include onychomycosis, peritonitis, dialysis fistulae infection, pneumonia, empyema, septic arthritis, osteomyelitis, meningitis (following spinal anesthesia in an otherwise healthy individual), cerebritis in an intravenous drug abuser, and prosthetic valve endocarditis. Disseminated infection occurs exclusively in immunosuppressed hosts and has been characterized by endocarditis, meningitis, and bloodstream infection. In vivo sporulation can occur, facilitating dissemination and perhaps explaining the high rate of metastatic skin lesions and positive blood cultures with *Acremonium*.

5.5. Diagnosis

Acremonium species grow slowly on SDA. Hence, cultures must be kept at least 2 weeks. Blood cultures may isolate *Acremonium* in cases of disseminated disease. Like other hyaline moulds, septate colorless hyphae are found in histopathologic examination that stain with PAS *(39)*. *Acremonium* may be difficult to identify in tissue because of morphologic similarities with other moulds, such as *Fusarium*.

5.6. Treatment

Acremonium species have a variable susceptibility to antifungal agents *(37)* (Table 10.1). In vitro activity of amphotericin B and itraconazole against *Acremonium* is variable, while resistance to fluconazole and 5-fluorocytosine is uniform. The newer azoles, voriconazole and posaconazole, appear promising.

6. *PENICILLIUM MARNEFFEI*

6.1. Introduction

Most *Penicillium* species are frequent laboratories contaminants, but P. *marneffei* has emerged as a significant pathogen, and can cause disseminated infection in HIV-infected patients residing or traveling to Southeast Asia where the disease is endemic *(40)*.

6.2. Etiologic Agents

Penicillium marneffei is a facultative intracellular pathogen and the only known thermally dimorphic fungus of the genus *Penicillium*. At room temperature, *P. marneffei* exhibits the characteristic morphology of the genus; in contrast, it grows as a yeast when found in infected tissue or at 37°C.

6.3. Epidemiology

Infection due to *Penicillium marneffei* constitutes the third most common opportunistic infection in HIV-infected patients in certain parts of Southeast Asia and is endemic in the Guangxi province of China, Hong Kong, and Taiwan *(41)*. The incidence of penicilliosis has increased significantly, paralleling the incidence of HIV infection. Although penicilliosis is most commonly seen in adults infected with HIV, the disease has also been detected in children and adults without immunodeficiency. The mode of transmission is thought to be due to ingestion or inhalation of the fungus. Soil exposure, especially during rainy season, has been suggested to be a critical factor.

6.4. Clinical Manifestations

Penicilliosis *marneffei* can clinically resemble tuberculosis, molluscum contagiosum, cryptococcosis, and histoplasmosis. The most common clinical manifestation in penicilliosis includes low-grade fever, anemia, weight loss, cough, lymphadenopathy, and hepatosplenomegaly *(42–44)*. Skin lesions are present in up 70% of the cases and are characterized by a central necrotic umbilication resembling molluscum contagiosum. Palatal and pharyngeal lesions can also be present. Bloodstream infection is present in approximately 50% of cases. Pulmonary involvement has been described as being diffuse or focal with either a reticulonodular or alveolar pattern. The mean number of $CD4^+$ T lymphocytes at presentation is 64 cells/μl*(41)*.

6.5. Diagnosis

Diagnosis of *P. marneffei* infections is usually made by identification of the organism from smear, culture, or histopathologic sections. Rapid diagnosis of suspected infection could be obtained by direct examination of bone marrow aspirate, lymph node, or skin biopsy. Microscopic examination of Wright-stained smears reveal yeasts forms both within phagocytes and extracellularly. The intracellular forms resemble those seen with *Histoplasma capsulatum* infection. The demonstration of characteristic central septation and elongated "sausage-shaped" forms by methenamine silver stain, clearly distinguish *P. marneffei* from *H. capsulatum* (see Fig. 3.7, Chapter 3).

6.6. Treatment

Penicillium marneffei is usually susceptible to both amphotericin B and the azole antifungals. Amphotericin B is effective in the majority of the cases, whereas the azoles are preferred for mild to moderate infections. In a nonrandomized trial of 74 HIV-infected patients with disseminated penicilliosis *(45)*, high response rate (97%) was demonstrated with a regimen of amphotericin B (0.6 mg/k per day) for 2 weeks, followed by itraconazole (400 mg/day) for 10 weeks. Relapse is common 6 months after discontinuation of therapy, as high as 50% in patients who do not receive maintenance antifungal therapy. Long-term suppressive therapy with itraconazole has been recommended in patients with HIV infection and penicilliosis *(46)*. Recent noncontrolled trials, however, demonstrated safe discontinuation of secondary prophylaxis for penicilliosis in HIV-infected patients who were responding to highly active antiretroviral therapy (HAART) *(42,47)*.

7. OTHER AGENTS OF HYALOHYPHOMYCOSIS

Scopulariopsis species are common soil saprophytes and have been isolated worldwide (see Fig. 2.12, Chapter 2). Five species have been associated with human infections: *S. brevicaulis*, *S. brumptii*, *S. acremonium*, *S. fusca*, and *S. koningii*. Disease in immunocompetent hosts include onychomycosis (most common), keratitis, and rarely, posttraumatic endophthalmitis or subcutaneous infection. Rare cases of endocarditis associated with valvuloplasty or prosthetic valves have been described. Invasive and disseminated infections, particularly with *S. brevicaulis*, may occur in immunosuppressed patients, manifesting as pneumonia or disseminated infection with skin lesions and fungemia. Patients at risk include those with acute leukemia and HSCT *(48)*. Prognosis is related to immune reconstitution and the ability to perform surgical débridement on localized infections.

Beauveria are ubiquitous fungi commonly found in soil. Because of their pathogenicity to many insect species, the organisms are incorporated into pesticides worldwide. Rarely, *Beauveria* may cause infections in humans, including keratitis and subcutaneous mycosis. Disseminated infections have occurred in patients with leukemia and HSCT *(49)*. The organism appears to be susceptible to itraconazole and amphotericin B.

REFERENCES

1. Marr KA, Carter RA, Crippa F, Wald A, Corey L. Epidemiology and outcome of mould infections in hematopoietic stem cell transplant recipients. Clin Infect Dis 2002;34: 909–917.
2. Nelson PE, Dignani MC, Anaissie EJ. Taxonomy, biology, and clinical aspects of *Fusarium* species. Clin Microbiol Rev 1994;7:479–504.
3. Hayden RT, Isotalo PA, Parrett T, et al. In situ hybridization for the differentiation of *Aspergillus*, *Fusarium*, and *Pseudallescheria* species in tissue section. Diagn Mol Pathol 2003;12:21–26.
4. Elvers KT, Leeming K, Moore CP, Lappin-Scott HM. Bacterial-fungal biofilms in flowing water photo-processing tanks. J Appl Microbiol 1998;84:607–618.
5. Doczi I, Gyetvai T, Kredics L, Nagy E. Involvement of *Fusarium* spp. in fungal keratitis. Clin Microbiol Infect 2004;10:773–776.
6. *Fusarium* keratitis–multiple states, 2006. MMWR Morb Mortal Wkly Rep 2006;55: 400–401.
7. Gabriele P, Hutchins RK. *Fusarium* endophthalmitis in an intravenous drug abuser. Am J Ophthalmol 1996;122:119–121.
8. Flynn JT, Meislich D, Kaiser BA, Polinsky MS, Baluarte HJ. *Fusarium* peritonitis in a child on peritoneal dialysis: case report and review of the literature. Perit Dial Int 1996;16:52–57.
9. Velasco E, Martins CA, Nucci M. Successful treatment of catheter-related fusarial infection in immunocompromised children. Eur J Clin Microbiol Infect Dis 1995;14:697–699.
10. Murray CK, Beckius ML, McAllister K. *Fusarium proliferatum* superficial suppurative thrombophlebitis. Mil Med 2003;168:426–427.
11. Kurien M, Anandi V, Raman R, Brahmadathan KN. Maxillary sinus fusariosis in immunocompetent hosts. J Laryngol Otol 1992;106:733–736.
12. Madhavan M, Ratnakar C, Veliath AJ, Kanungo R, Smile SR, Bhat S. Primary disseminated fusarial infection. Postgrad Med J 1992;68:143–144.
13. Nucci M, Anaissie E. Cutaneous infection by *Fusarium* species in healthy and immunocompromised hosts: implications for diagnosis and management. Clin Infect Dis 2002;35: 909–920.
14. Jakle C, Leek JC, Olson DA, Robbins DL. Septic arthritis due to *Fusarium solani*. J Rheumatol 1983;10:151–153.
15. Sierra-Hoffman M, Paltiyevich-Gibson S, Carpenter JL, Hurley DL. *Fusarium* osteomyelitis: case report and review of the literature. Scand J Infect Dis 2005;37:237–240.
16. Boutati EI, Anaissie EJ. *Fusarium*, a significant emerging pathogen in patients with hematologic malignancy: ten years' experience at a cancer center and implications for management. Blood 1997;90:999–1008.
17. Nucci M, Marr KA, Queiroz-Telles F, et al. *Fusarium* infection in hematopoietic stem cell transplant recipients. Clin Infect Dis 2004;38:1237–1242.
18. Nucci M, Anaissie EJ, Queiroz-Telles F, et al. Outcome predictors of 84 patients with hematologic malignancies and *Fusarium* infection. Cancer 2003;98:315–319.
19. Sampathkumar P, Paya CV. *Fusarium* infection after solid-organ transplantation. Clin Infect Dis 2001;32:1237–1240.
20. Anaissie EJ, Kuchar RT, Rex JH, et al. Fusariosis associated with pathogenic *Fusarium* species colonization of a hospital water system: a new paradigm for the epidemiology of opportunistic mould infections. Clin Infect Dis 2001;33:1871–1878.
21. Anaissie EJ, Stratton SL, Dignani MC, et al. Cleaning patient shower facilities: a novel approach to reducing patient exposure to aerosolized *Aspergillus* species and other opportunistic moulds. Clin Infect Dis 2002;35:E86–E88.

22. Girmenia C, Arcese W, Micozzi A, Martino P, Bianco P, Morace G. Onychomycosis as a possible origin of disseminated *Fusarium solani* infection in a patient with severe aplastic anemia. Clin Infect Dis 1992;14:1167.
23. Schell WA. New aspects of emerging fungal pathogens. A multifaceted challenge. Clin Lab Med 1995;15:365–387.
24. Hue FX, Huerre M, Rouffault MA, de Bievre C. Specific detection of *Fusarium* species in blood and tissues by a PCR technique. J Clin Microbiol 1999;37:2434–2438.
25. Ostrosky-Zeichner L, Alexander BD, Kett DH, et al. Multicenter clinical evaluation of the (1–>3) beta-D-glucan assay as an aid to diagnosis of fungal infections in humans. Clin Infect Dis 2005;41:654–659.
26. Cuenca-Estrella M, Gomez-Lopez A, Mellado E, Garcia-Effron G, Monzon A, Rodriguez-Tudela JL. In vitro activity of ravuconazole against 923 clinical isolates of nondermatophyte filamentous fungi. Antimicrob Agents Chemother 2005;49:5136–5138.
27. Idigoras P, Perez-Trallero E, Pineiro L, et al. Disseminated infection and colonization by *Scedosporium prolificans*: a review of 18 cases, 1990–1999. Clin Infect Dis 2001;32: E158–E165.
28. Rainer J, De Hoog GS. Molecular taxonomy and ecology of *Pseudallescheria*, *Petriella* and *Scedosporium prolificans* (Microascaceae) containing opportunistic agents on humans. Mycol Res 2006;110:151–160.
29. Castiglioni B, Sutton DA, Rinaldi MG, Fung J, Kusne S. *Pseudallescheria boydii* (anamorph *Scedosporium apiospermum*). Infection in solid organ transplant recipients in a tertiary medical center and review of the literature. Medicine (Baltimore) 2002;81:333–348.
30. Montero A, Cohen JE, Fernandez MA, Mazzolini G, Gomez CR, Perugini J. Cerebral pseudallescheriasis due to *Pseudallescheria boydii* as the first manifestation of AIDS. Clin Infect Dis 1998;26:1476–1477.
31. Carrillo AJ, Guarro J. In vitro activities of four novel triazoles against *Scedosporium* spp. Antimicrob Agents Chemother 2001;45:2151–2153.
32. Radford SA, Johnson EM, Warnock DW. In vitro studies of activity of voriconazole (UK-109,496), a new triazole antifungal agent, against emerging and less-common mould pathogens. Antimicrob Agents Chemother 1997;41:841–843.
33. Walsh TJ, Peter J, McGough DA, Fothergill AW, Rinaldi MG, Pizzo PA. Activities of amphotericin B and antifungal azoles alone and in combination against *Pseudallescheria boydii*. Antimicrob Agents Chemother 1995;39:1361–1364.
34. Gosbell IB, Toumasatos V, Yong J, Kuo RS, Ellis DH, Perrie RC. Cure of orthopaedic infection with *Scedosporium prolificans*, using voriconazole plus terbinafine, without the need for radical surgery. Mycoses 2003;46:233–236.
35. Fleming RV, Walsh TJ, Anaissie EJ. Emerging and less common fungal pathogens. Infect Dis Clin North Am 2002;16:915–933.
36. Espinel-Ingroff A. Comparison of In vitro activities of the new triazole SCH56592 and the echinocandins MK-0991 (L-743,872) and LY303366 against opportunistic filamentous and dimorphic fungi and yeasts. J Clin Microbiol 1998;36:2950–2956.
37. Guarro J, Gams W, Pujol I, Gene J. *Acremonium* species: new emerging fungal opportunists – in vitro antifungal susceptibilities and review. Clin Infect Dis 1997;25:1222–1229.
38. Fincher RM, Fisher JF, Lovell RD, Newman CL, Espinel-Ingroff A, Shadomy HJ. Infection due to the fungus *Acremonium* (*Cephalosporium*). Medicine (Baltimore) 1991;70:398–409.
39. Liu K, Howell DN, Perfect JR, Schell WA. Morphologic criteria for the preliminary identification of *Fusarium*, *Paecilomyces*, and *Acremonium* species by histopathology. Am J Clin Pathol 1998;109:45–54.
40. Supparatpinyo K, Khamwan C, Baosoung V, Nelson KE, Sirisanthana T. Disseminated *Penicillium marneffei* infection in southeast Asia. Lancet 1994;344:110–113.

41. Sirisanthana T, Supparatpinyo K. Epidemiology and management of penicilliosis in human immunodeficiency virus-infected patients. Int J Infect Dis 1998;3:48–53.
42. Sun HY, Chen MY, Hsiao CF, Hsieh SM, Hung CC, Chang SC. Endemic fungal infections caused by *Cryptococcus neoformans* and *Penicillium marneffei* in patients infected with human immunodeficiency virus and treated with highly active anti-retroviral therapy. Clin Microbiol Infect 2006;12:381–388.
43. Supparatpinyo K, Chiewchanvit S, Hirunsri P, Uthammachai C, Nelson KE, Sirisanthana T. *Penicillium marneffei* infection in patients infected with human immunodeficiency virus. Clin Infect Dis 1992;14:871–874.
44. Duong TA. Infection due to *Penicillium marneffei*, an emerging pathogen: review of 155 reported cases. Clin Infect Dis 1996;23:125–130.
45. Sirisanthana T, Supparatpinyo K, Perriens J, Nelson KE. Amphotericin B and itraconazole for treatment of disseminated *Penicillium marneffei* infection in human immunodeficiency virus-infected patients. Clin Infect Dis 1998;26:1107–1110.
46. Supparatpinyo K, Perriens J, Nelson KE, Sirisanthana T. A controlled trial of itraconazole to prevent relapse of *Penicillium marneffei* infection in patients infected with the human immunodeficiency virus. N Engl J Med 1998;339:1739–1743.
47. Hung CC, Chen MY, Hsieh SM, Sheng WH, Hsiao CF, Chang SC. Discontinuation of secondary prophylaxis for penicilliosis marneffei in AIDS patients responding to highly active antiretroviral therapy. AIDS 2002;16:672–673.
48. Cuenca-Estrella M, Gomez-Lopez A, Mellado E, Buitrago MJ, Monzon A, Rodriguez-Tudela JL. *Scopulariopsis brevicaulis*, a fungal pathogen resistant to broad-spectrum antifungal agents. Antimicrob Agents Chemother 2003;47:2339–2341.
49. Tucker DL, Beresford CH, Sigler L, Rogers K. Disseminated *Beauveria bassiana* infection in a patient with acute lymphoblastic leukemia. J Clin Microbiol 2004;42:5412–5414.
50. Diekema DJ, Messer SA, Hollis RJ, Jones RN, Pfaller MA. Activities of caspofungin, itraconazole, posaconazole, ravuconazole, voriconazole, and amphotericin B against 448 recent clinical isolates of filamentous fungi. J Clin Microbiol 2003;41:3623–3626.
51. Pfaller MA, Diekema DJ. Rare and emerging opportunistic fungal pathogens: concern for resistance beyond *Candida albicans* and *Aspergillus fumigatus*. J Clin Microbiol 2004;42:4419–4431.
52. Sabatelli F, Patel R, Mann PA, et al. In vitro activities of posaconazole, fluconazole, itraconazole, voriconazole, and amphotericin B against a large collection of clinically important moulds and yeasts. Antimicrob Agents Chemother 2006;50:2009–2015.

SUGGESTED READINGS

Dignani MC, Anaissie E. Human fusariosis. Clin Microbiol Infect 2004;10(Suppl 1):67–75.
Fincher RM, Fisher JF, Lovell RD, Newman CL, Espinel-Ingroff A, Shadomy HJ. Infection due to the fungus *Acremonium* (*Cephalosporium*). Medicine (Baltimore) 1991;70:398–409.
Fleming RV, Walsh TJ, Anaissie EJ. Emerging and less common fungal pathogens. Infect Dis Clin North Am 2002;16:915–933.
Husain S, Alexander BD, Munoz P, et al. Opportunistic mycelial fungal infections in organ transplant recipients: emerging importance of non-*Aspergillus* mycelial fungi. Clin Infect Dis 2003;37:221–229.
Panackal AA, Marr KA. *Scedosporium/Pseudallescheria* infections. Semin Respir Crit Care Med 2004;25:171–181.
Schinabeck MK, Ghannoum MA. Human hyalohyphomycoses: a review of human infections due to *Acremonium* spp., *Paecilomyces* spp., *Penicillium* spp., and *Scopulariopsis* spp. J Chemother 2003;15 (Suppl 2):5–15.

11
Phaeohyphomycosis—Infection Due to Dark (Dematiaceous) Moulds

Sanjay G. Revankar, MD

1. INTRODUCTION

Dematiaceous, or darkly pigmented, fungi are a large heterogeneous group of organisms that have been associated with a wide variety of clinical syndromes. These are uncommon causes of human disease, but can be responsible for life-threatening infections in both immunocompromised and immunocompetent individuals. In recent years, these fungi have been increasingly recognized as important pathogens, and the spectrum of diseases they are associated with has also broadened.

These fungi may cause hypersenstivity disorders and superficial infections, but typically the term phaeohyphomycosis is limited to deeper infections. Two other more classically described clinical syndromes caused by the dark-walled fungi, typically distinguished by characteristic histologic findings, are chromoblastomycosis and mycetoma. Chromoblastomycosis and mycetoma are caused by a small group of fungi that are associated with characteristic structures in tissue and are usually seen in tropical areas *(1)*. These are discussed in the chapter on subcutaneous mycoses (Chapter 21). Phaeohyphomycosis is a term introduced by Ajello et al. in 1974 that literally means "infection caused by dark walled fungi" *(2)*. It is a catch-all term generally reserved for the remainder of clinical syndromes caused by dematiaceous fungi that range from superficial infections and allergic disease to brain abscess and widely disseminated disease *(3)*. These fungi are alternately called phaeoid, dematiaceous, dark, or black moulds. While typically phaeohyphomycosis is a term limited to infections caused by the dark moulds, there are dark yeasts that rarely cause infection, and these are also included under this grouping by many experts.

2. ETIOLOGIC AGENTS

More than 100 species and 60 genera of dematiaceous fungi have been implicated in human disease *(4)*. The common characteristic among these fungi is the presence of melanin in their cell walls, which imparts the dark color to their conidia or spores and

From: *Infectious Disease: Diagnosis and Treatment of Human Mycoses*
Edited by: D. R. Hospenthal and M. G. Rinaldi © Humana Press Inc., Totowa, NJ

Table 11.1
Clinical spectrum and treatment of phaeohyphomycosis

Clinical syndrome	Commonly associated fungi	Therapy
Allergic fungal sinusitis/Allergic bronchopulmonary mycosis (disease)	*Curvularia*, *Bipolaris*	Corticosteroids ± itraconazole or voriconazole
Onychomycosis	*Onychocola*, *Alternaria*	Itraconazole or terbinafine
Keratitis	*Curvularia*, *Bipolaris*, *Exserohilum*, *Lasiodiplodia*	Topical natamycin ± itraconazole or voriconazole
Subcutaneous infection	*Exophiala*, *Alternaria*, *Phialophora*	Surgery ± itraconazole or voriconazole
Pneumonia	*Ochroconis*, *Exophiala*, *Chaetomium*	Itraconazole or voriconazole, (amphotericin B if severe)
Brain abscess	*Cladophialophora* (*C. bantiana*), *Ramichloridium* (*R. mackenzei*), *Ochroconis*	See text
Disseminated disease	*Scedosporium* (*S. prolificans*), *Bipolaris*, *Wangiella*	See text

hyphae. Their colonies are typically brown to black in color as well. As the number of patients immunocompromised from diseases and medical therapy increases, additional species are being reported as causes of human disease, expanding an already long list of potential pathogens. Common genera associated with specific clinical syndromes are listed in Table 11.1.

Guidelines are available regarding the handling of potentially infectious fungi in the laboratory setting. It is suggested that work with cultures of certain well-known pathogenic fungi, such as *Coccidioides immitis* and *Histoplasma capsulatum*, be conducted in a Biosafety Level 3 facility, which requires a separate negative pressure room. Recently, certain agents of phaeohyphomycosis, in particular *Cladophialophora bantiana*, have been included in the list of fungi that should be kept under Biosafety Level 2 containment *(5)*. This seems reasonable given their propensity, albeit rarely, for causing life-threatening infection in normal individuals.

3. EPIDEMIOLOGY

These fungi are typically soil organisms and generally distributed worldwide *(6)*. However, there are species that do appear to be geographically restricted, such as *Ramichloridium mackenzei*, which has only been seen in patients from the Middle East *(7)*. Exposure is thought to be from inhalation or minor trauma, which may not even be noticed by the patient. Surveys of outdoor air for fungal spores routinely observe dematiaceous fungi *(8)*. This suggests that most if not all individuals are exposed to them, though they remain uncommon causes of disease. These fungi may also be found to be contaminants in cultures, making the determination of clinical significance problematic. A high degree of clinical suspicion as well as correlation with appropriate clinical findings and histopathology is required when interpreting culture results.

4. PATHOGENESIS AND IMMUNOLOGY

Little is known regarding the pathogenic mechanisms by which these fungi cause disease. One of the likely virulence factors is the presence of melanin in the cell wall, which is common to all dematiaceous fungi. It may confer a protective advantage by scavenging free radicals that are produced by phagocytic cells in their oxidative burst that normally kill most organisms *(9)*. In addition, melanin may bind to hydrolytic enzymes, thereby preventing their action on the plasma membrane *(9)*. In the yeasts *C. neoformans* and *W. dermatitidis*, disruption of melanin production leads to markedly reduced virulence in animal models *(10,11)*. Melanin has also been associated with decreased susceptibility of fungi to certain antifungals, possibly by binding these drugs *(12,13)*. It is interesting to note that almost all allergic disease and eosinophilia is caused by two genera, *Bipolaris* and *Curvularia* , though the virulence factors responsible for eliciting allergic reactions are unclear at present *(14)*.

5. CLINICAL MANIFESTATIONS

5.1. *Allergic Disease*

Relatively few species have been associated with allergic disease. *Alternaria alternata* is thought to be involved in some cases of asthma *(15)*. Whether dematiaceous fungi may be responsible for symptoms of allergic rhinitis is unclear, as it is difficult to quantitate exposure and to distinguish them from other causes *(16)*.

Bipolaris and *Curvularia* are responsible for most cases of allergic fungal sinusitis (AFS) and allergic bronchopulmonary mycosis (ABPM). Patients with AFS usually present with chronic sinus symptoms that are not responsive to antibiotics. Previously, *Aspergillus* was thought to be the most common fungus responsible for allergic sinusitis, but it is now appreciated that disease due to dematiaceous fungi actually comprises the majority of cases *(17)*. Criteria have been suggested for this disease, and include *(1)* nasal polyps; *(2)* presence of allergic mucin, containing Charcot-Leyden crystals and eosinophils; *(3)* hyphal elements in the mucosa without evidence of tissue invasion; *(4)* positive skin test to fungal allergens; and *(5)* on computed tomography (CT) scans, characteristic areas of central hyperattenuation within the sinus cavity *(18)*. Diagnosis generally depends on demonstration of allergic mucin, with or without actual culture of the organism.

Allergic bronchopulmonary mycosis (ABPM) (or disease [ABPD]) is similar in presentation to allergic bronchopulmonary aspergillosis (ABPA), which is typically seen in patients with asthma or cystic fibrosis *(19)*. Criteria for the diagnosis of ABPA in patients with asthma include *(1)* asthma, *(2)* positive skin test for fungal allergens, *(3)* elevated IgE levels, *(4)* *Aspergillus*-specific IgE, and *(5)* proximal bronchiectasis *(19)*. Similar criteria for ABPM are not established, but finding allergic mucin (Charcot-Leyden crystals and eosinophils) without tissue invasion, as in AFS, makes this diagnosis highly likely *(20)*.

5.2. Focal Infection

5.2.1. Superficial Infection

Superficial infections are the most common form of disease associated with phaeohyphomycosis. These include black piedra, tinea nigra, and onychomycosis.

Black piedra is a nodular disease of the scalp hair, typically seen in tropical climates, predominantly in South America. Caused by *Piedraia hortae*, this is chiefly a disease of only cosmetic impact to the sufferer.

Tinea nigra is primarily seen in tropical areas, and involves only the stratum corneum of the skin. Patients are generally asymptomatic, presenting with brownish-black macular lesions, almost exclusively on the palms and soles. *Hortaea werneckii* is the most commonly isolated species, though *Stenella araguata* has also been cultured from lesions *(21)*. Tinea nigra may be confused with a variety of other diseases, including dysplastic nevi, melanoma, syphilis, or Addison's disease. Diagnosis is made by scrapings of lesions and culture. As it is a very superficial infection, simple scraping or abrasion can be curative, though topical treatments such as keratolytics or imidazole creams are also highly effective *(21)*.

Dematiaceous fungi are rare causes of onychomycosis. Clinical features may include a history of trauma, involvement of only one or two toenails, and lack of response to standard systemic therapy *(22)*. *Onychocola* and *Alternaria* have been reported, with the former being highly resistant to therapy.

5.2.2. Keratitis

Fungal keratitis is an important ophthalmologic problem, particularly in tropical areas of the world. In one large series, 40% of all infectious keratitis was caused by fungi, almost exclusively moulds *(23)*. The most common fungi are *Fusarium* and *Aspergillus*, followed by dematiaceous fungi (up to 8% to 17% of cases) *(24)*. Approximately half the cases are associated with trauma; prior eye surgery, diabetes, and use of contact lens use have also been noted as important risk factors *(24)*. In a study from the United States of 43 cases of *Curvularia* keratitis, almost all were associated with trauma *(25)*. Plants were the most common source, though several cases involving metal injuries were seen as well.

5.2.3. Subcutaneous Infection

There are numerous case reports of subcutaneous infection due to a wide variety of species *(26,27)*. Minor trauma is the usual inciting factor, though it may be unrecognized by the patient. Lesions typically occur on exposed areas of the body and often appear cystic or papular. Immunocompromised patients are at increased risk of subsequent dissemination. Occasionally, these infections may involve joints or bone.

5.2.4. Pneumonia

Nonallergic pulmonary disease is usually seen in immunocompromised patients, and may be due to a wide variety of species, in contrast to allergic disease *(14,28–31)*. Clinical manifestations include pneumonia, asymptomatic solitary pulmonary nodules, and endobronchial lesions which may cause hemoptysis.

5.2.5. Brain Abscess

This is a rare but frequently fatal manifestation of phaeohyphomycosis *(32)*. Interestingly, more than half of reported cases have occurred in patients with no risk factors or known immunodeficiency. Lesions are usually solitary. Symptoms may include headache, neurologic deficits, and seizures, though the classic triad seen in bacterial brain abscess (fever, headache, and focal neurologic deficit) was not usually present. The most commonly isolated organism is *Cladophialophora bantiana*, particularly in immunocompetent patients. The pathogenesis may be hematogenous spread from an initial, presumably subclinical pulmonary focus. It remains unclear why these fungi preferentially cause CNS disease.

5.3. Disseminated Infection

This is the most uncommon manifestation of infection seen with dematiaceous fungi. Most patients are immunocompromised, though occasional patients without known immunodeficiency or risk factors have developed disseminated disease as well *(33)*. In contrast to most invasive mould infections, blood cultures are often positive. The most commonly isolated fungus, *S. prolificans*, may also be associated with septic shock. Peripheral eosinophilia, seen in 11% of these cases, was generally associated with *Bipolaris* or *Curvularia*.

6. DIAGNOSIS

In contrast to other common mycoses that cause human disease, there are no serologic or antigen tests available to detect these fungi in blood or tissue. The diagnosis of phaeohyphomycosis currently rests on pathologic examination of clinical specimens and careful gross and microscopic examination of cultures (Fig. 11.1). Hospital laboratories can generally identify the most common genera associated with human disease

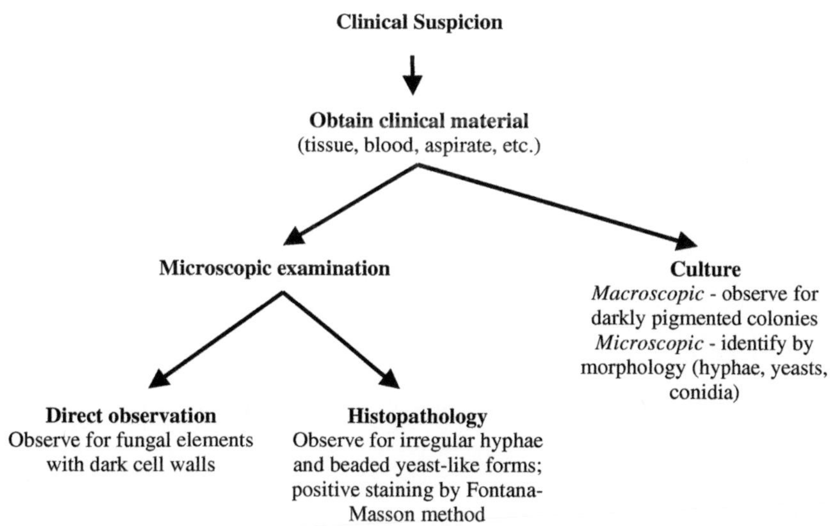

Fig. 11.1. Diagnostic approach to phaeohyphomycosis.

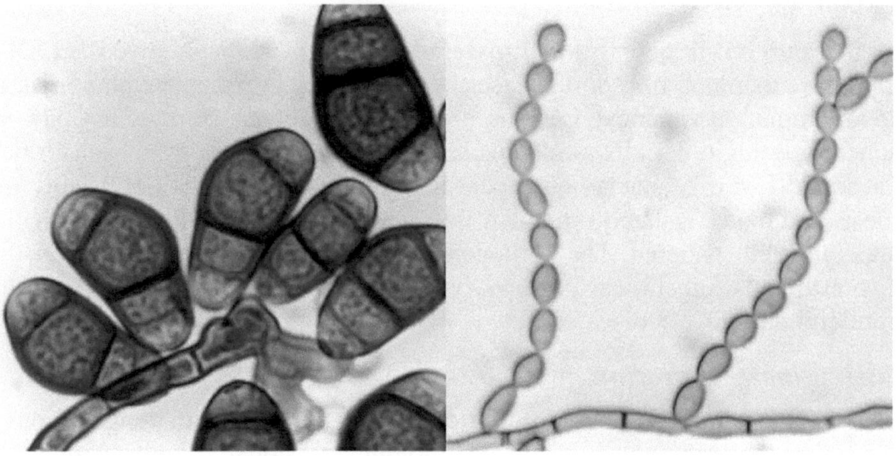

Fig. 11.2. Commonly seen fungi causing phaeohyphomycosis. **Left:** *Curvularia lunata.* **Right:** *Cladophialophora bantiana.* [Figure in color on CD-ROM].

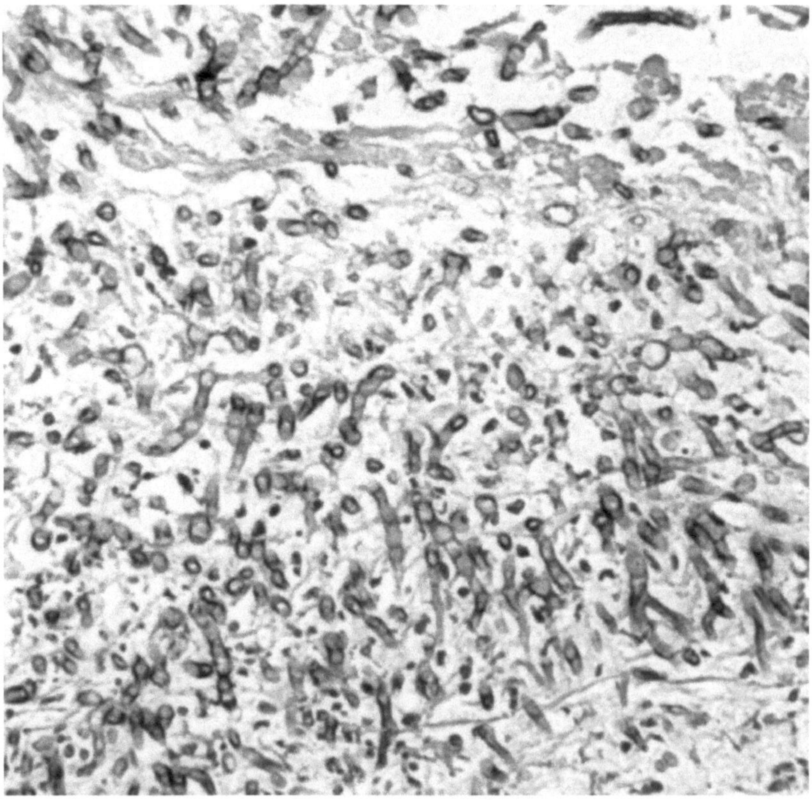

Fig. 11.3. Fontana-Masson stain of *Bipolaris* infection in the lung, demonstrating irregular hyphae and beaded yeast-like forms. [Figure in color on CD-ROM].

(Fig. 11.2) (see also Fig. 2.13, Chapter 2), though referral to a reference laboratory is often needed to identify unusual species. As many of these are rarely seen in practice, a high degree of clinical suspicion is required when interpreting culture results.

In tissue, these fungi will stain strongly with the Fontana-Masson stain, which is specific for melanin (Fig. 11.3) *(3)*. This can be helpful in distinguishing these fungi from other species, particularly *Aspergillus*. In addition, hyphae typically appear more fragmented in tissue than seen with *Aspergillus*, with irregular septate hyphae and beaded, yeast-like forms *(3)*.

7. TREATMENT

Therapy is not standardized for any of these clinical syndromes, and randomized trials are unlikely given the sporadic nature of cases. Itraconazole and voriconazole demonstrate the most consistent in vitro activity against this group of fungi, though far more clinical experience has accumulated with itraconazole *(34)*. Amphotericin B may be used for severe infections in unstable patients; high doses of lipid formulations may have a role in the treatment of refractory cases or in patients intolerant of standard amphotericin B. However, some species of dematiaceous fungi are resistant to this agent. Once the infection is under control, longer term therapy with a broad-spectrum oral azole is often reasonable until a complete response is achieved, which may require several weeks to months.

Other agents have limited roles in treating these fungi. Ketoconazole is not well tolerated, and fluconazole has poor activity against these fungi in general. Terbinafine and flucytosine have occasionally been used for subcutaneous infections in patients refractory to other therapy. Echinocandins do not appear to be very useful as single agents. Combination therapy is a potentially useful therapeutic strategy for refractory infections, particularly brain abscess and disseminated disease, though it has not been well studied. Suggested therapies for specific infections are summarized in Table 11.1.

7.1. Allergic Disease

Steroids are the mainstay of treatment for allergic disease caused by these fungi, especially in asthma, though other modalities may have a role in specific clinical situations. For example, therapy for AFS consists of systemic corticosteroids and surgery to remove the mucin, which is often tenacious. Antifungal therapy, usually in the form of itraconazole, may play a role in reducing the requirement for corticosteroids, but this is not routinely recommended *(35)*. Other azoles have only rarely been used in the treatment of this disease.

Allergic bronchopulmonary mycosis (ABPM) can be treated with systemic corticosteroids as in ABPA; prednisone at a dose of 0.5 mg/kg per day for 2 weeks, followed by a slow taper over 2 to 3 months or longer *(19)*. Itraconazole has been used as a steroid sparing agent in APBA, but its efficacy is not clear, and routine use of itraconazole is not generally recommended *(19)*.

7.2. Focal Infection

7.2.1. Superficial Infection

Itraconazole and terbinafine are the most commonly used systemic agents for onychomycosis, and may be combined with topical therapy for refractory cases *(36)*. There is no published experience with voriconazole.

7.2.2. Keratitis

For keratitis, topical 5% natamycin is used almost exclusively, with only a few severe cases requiring adjunctive therapy, usually with an azole *(23,37)*. Itraconazole has the best in vitro activity. The majority of isolates are resistant to flucytosine. Surgery, including penetrating keratoplasty, is often needed. Enucleation is occasionally required due to poor clinical response. Many patients do not recover complete visual acuity despite aggressive therapy.

7.2.3. Subcutaneous Infection

Subcutaneous lesions will often respond to surgical excision alone *(38)*. Oral systemic therapy with a broad-spectrum azole antifungal agent in conjunction with surgery is frequently employed and has been used successfully, particularly in immunocompromised patients *(39,40)*.

7.2.4. Pneumonia

Therapy consists of systemic antifungal agents, usually amphotericin B or itraconazole initially, followed by itraconazole for a more prolonged period *(14)*. Mortality rates are high in immunocompromised patients. Experience with voriconazole is currently only anecdotal *(41)*.

7.2.5. Brain Abscess

Therapy published in the literature has varied greatly depending on the case report, and there is no standard treatment. A retrospective analysis of 101 reported cases suggested that the combination of amphotericin B (high-dose lipid formulation), flucytosine, and itraconazole may be associated with improved survival, though it was not frequently used *(32)*. Voriconazole may also prove useful. High doses of azoles have been suggested as an option, though there are no studies confirming this approach. Complete excision of brain abscesses may lead to better outcomes than aspiration or partial excision. Overall mortality is greater than 70%.

7.3. Disseminated Infection

A recent literature review suggested the mortality rate is greater than 70%, despite aggressive antifungal therapy *(33)*. There were no antifungal regimens associated with improved survival in disseminated infection. High-dose lipid amphotericin B may be reasonable for initial therapy, given its fungicidal activity for many fungi. Addition of a broad-spectrum azole or echinocandin could be considered in individuals failing therapy. Infection with *S. prolificans* has been associated with a nearly 100% mortality in the absence of recovery from neutropenia, as it is generally resistant to all available antifungal agents. Recent reports have suggested that the combination of itraconazole or voriconazole with terbinafine may be synergistic against this species, though the clinical relevance of this finding is unclear *(42,43)*.

REFERENCES

1. McGinnis MR. Chromoblastomycosis and phaeohyphomycosis: new concepts, diagnosis, and mycology. J Am Acad Dermatol 1983;8:1–16.
2. Ajello L, Georg LK, Steigbigel RT, Wang CJ. A case of phaeohyphomycosis caused by a new species of *Phialophora*. Mycologia 1974;66:490–498.
3. Rinaldi MG. Phaeohyphomycosis. Dermatol Clin 1996;14:147–153.
4. Matsumoto T, Ajello L, Matsuda T, Szaniszlo PJ, Walsh TJ. Developments in hyalohyphomycosis and phaeohyphomycosis. J Med Vet Mycol 1994;32(Suppl 1):329–349.
5. Biosafety in microbiological and biomedical laboratories. 4th ed. Washington, DC: US Government Printing Office, 1999:123–124.
6. De Hoog GS. Significance of fungal evolution for the understanding of their pathogenicity, illustrated with agents of phaeohyphomycosis. Mycoses 1997;40(Suppl 2):5–8.
7. Sutton DA, Slifkin M, Yakulis R, Rinaldi MG. US case report of cerebral phaeohyphomycosis caused by *Ramichloridium obovoideum (R. mackenziei)*: criteria for identification, therapy, and review of other known dematiaceous neurotropic taxa. J Clin Microbiol 1998;36:708–715.
8. Shelton BG, Kirkland KH, Flanders WD, Morris GK. Profiles of airborne fungi in buildings and outdoor environments in the United States. Appl Environ Microbiol 2002;68:1743–1753.
9. Jacobson ES. Pathogenic roles for fungal melanins. Clin Microbiol Rev 2000;13:708–717.
10. Dixon DM, Polak A, Szaniszlo PJ. Pathogenicity and virulence of wild-type and melanin-deficient *Wangiella dermatitidis*. J Med Vet Mycol 1987;25:97–106.
11. Kwon-Chung KJ, Polacheck I, Popkin TJ. Melanin-lacking mutants of *Cryptococcus neoformans* and their virulence for mice. J Bacteriol 1982;150:1414–1421.
12. van Duin D, Casadevall A, Nosanchuk JD. Melanization of *Cryptococcus neoformans* and *Histoplasma capsulatum* reduces their susceptibilities to amphotericin B and caspofungin. Antimicrob Agents Chemother 2002;46:3394–3400.
13. Ikeda R, Sugita T, Jacobson ES, Shinoda T. Effects of melanin upon susceptibility of *Cryptococcus* to antifungals. Microbiol Immunol 2003;47:271–277.
14. Revankar SG. Dematiaceous fungi. Semin Respir Crit Care Med 2004;25:183–190.
15. Bush RK, Prochnau JJ. *Alternaria*-induced asthma. J Allergy Clin Immunol 2004;113: 227–234.
16. Bush RK, Portnoy JM, Saxon A, Terr AI, Wood RA. The medical effects of mould exposure. J Allergy Clin Immunol 2006;117:326–333.
17. Ferguson BJ. Definitions of fungal rhinosinusitis. Otolaryngol Clin North Am 2000;33: 227–235.
18. Houser SM, Corey JP. Allergic fungal rhinosinusitis: pathophysiology, epidemiology, and diagnosis. Otolaryngol Clin North Am 2000;33:399–409.
19. Greenberger PA. Allergic bronchopulmonary aspergillosis. J Allergy Clin Immunol 2002;110:685–692.
20. Hamilton BG, Humphreys CW, Conner WC, Hospenthal DR. Allergic bronchopulmonary disease secondary to *Bipolaris spicifera*: Case report. J Bronchol 2006;13:77–79.
21. Perez C, Colella MT, Olaizola C, de Capriles CH, Magaldi S, Mata-Essayag S. Tinea nigra: report of twelve cases in Venezuela. Mycopathologia 2005;160:235–238.
22. Gupta AK, Ryder JE, Baran R, Summerbell RC. Non-dermatophyte onychomycosis. Dermatol Clin 2003;21:257–268.
23. Gopinathan U, Garg P, Fernandes M, Sharma S, Athmanathan S, Rao GN. The epidemiological features and laboratory results of fungal keratitis: a 10-year review at a referral eye care center in South India. Cornea 2002;21:555–559.
24. Srinivasan M. Fungal keratitis. Curr Opin Ophthalmol 2004;15:321–327.

25. Wilhelmus KR, Jones DB. *Curvularia* keratitis. Trans Am Ophthalmol Soc 2001;99:111–130.
26. Sutton DA, Rinaldi MG, Kielhofner M. First US report of subcutaneous phaeohyphomycosis caused by *Veronaea botryosa* in a heart transplant recipient and review of the literature. J Clin Microbiol 2004;42:2843–2846.
27. Chuan MT, Wu MC. Subcutaneous phaeohyphomycosis caused by *Exophiala jeanselmei*: successful treatment with itraconazole. Int J Dermatol 1995;34:563–566.
28. Odell JA, Alvarez S, Cvitkovich DG, Cortese DA, McComb BL. Multiple lung abscesses due to *Ochroconis gallopavum*, a dematiaceous fungus, in a nonimmunocompromised wood pulp worker. Chest 2000;118:1503–1505.
29. Yeghen T, Fenelon L, Campbell CK, et al. *Chaetomium* pneumonia in patient with acute myeloid leukaemia. J Clin Pathol 1996;49:184–186.
30. Mazur JE, Judson MA. A case report of a *Dactylaria* fungal infection in a lung transplant patient. Chest 2001;119:651–653.
31. Manian FA, Brischetto MJ. Pulmonary infection due to *Exophiala jeanselmei*: successful treatment with ketoconazole. Clin Infect Dis 1993;16:445–446.
32. Revankar SG, Sutton DA, Rinaldi MG. Primary central nervous system phaeohyphomycosis: a review of 101 cases. Clin Infect Dis 2004;38:206–216.
33. Revankar SG, Patterson JE, Sutton DA, Pullen R, Rinaldi MG. Disseminated phaeohyphomycosis: review of an emerging mycosis. Clin Infect Dis 2002;34:467–476.
34. Sharkey PK, Graybill JR, Rinaldi MG, et al. Itraconazole treatment of phaeohyphomycosis. J Am Acad Dermatol 1990;23:577–586.
35. Kuhn FA, Javer AR. Allergic fungal rhinosinusitis: perioperative management, prevention of recurrence, and role of corticosteroid and antifungal agents. Otolaryngol Clin North Am 2000;33:419–433.
36. Tosti A, Piraccini BM, Lorenzi S, Iorizzo M. Treatment of nondermatophyte mould and *Candida* onychomycosis. Dermatol Clin 2003;21:491–497.
37. Thomas PA. Fungal infections of the cornea. Eye 2003;17:852–862.
38. Summerbell RC, Krajden S, Levine R, Fuksa M. Subcutaneous phaeohyphomycosis caused by *Lasiodiplodia theobromae* and successfully treated surgically. Med Mycol 2004;42: 543–547.
39. Kimura M, Goto A, Furuta T, Satou T, Hashimoto S, Nishimura K. Multifocal subcutaneous phaeohyphomycosis caused by *Phialophora verrucosa*. Arch Pathol Lab Med 2003;127: 91–93.
40. Clancy CJ, Wingard JR, Hong NM. Subcutaneous phaeohyphomycosis in transplant recipients: review of the literature and demonstration of in vitro synergy between antifungal agents. Med Mycol 2000;38:169–175.
41. Diemert D, Kunimoto D, Sand C, Rennie R. Sputum isolation of *Wangiella dermatitidis* in patients with cystic fibrosis. Scand J Infect Dis 2001;33:777–779.
42. Meletiadis J, Mouton JW, Meis JF, Verweij PE. Combination chemotherapy for the treatment of invasive infections by *Scedosporium prolificans*. Clin Microbiol Infect 2000;6:336–337.
43. Howden BP, Slavin MA, Schwarer AP, Mijch AM. Successful control of disseminated *Scedosporium prolificans* infection with a combination of voriconazole and terbinafine. Eur J Clin Microbiol Infect Dis 2003;22:111–113.

SUGGESTED READINGS

Clancy CJ, Wingard JR, Hong NM. Subcutaneous phaeohyphomycosis in transplant recipients: review of the literature and demonstration of in vitro synergy between antifungal agents. Med Mycol 2000;38:169–175.

Jacobson ES. Pathogenic roles for fungal melanins. Clin Microbiol Rev 2000;13:708–717.
Kuhn FA, Javer AR. Allergic fungal rhinosinusitis: perioperative management, prevention of recurrence, and role of steroids and antifungal agents. Otolaryngol Clin North Am 2000;33:419–433.
Revankar SG, Patterson JE, Sutton DA, Pullen R, Rinaldi MG. Disseminated phaeohyphomycosis: review of an emerging mycosis. Clin Infect Dis 2002;34:467–476.
Revankar SG, Sutton DA, Rinaldi MG. Primary central nervous system phaeohyphomycosis: a review of 101 cases. Clin Infect Dis 2004;38:206–216.
Sharkey PK, Graybill JR, Rinaldi MG, et al. Itraconazole treatment of phaeohyphomycosis. J Am Acad Dermatol 1990;23:577–586.
Srinivasan M. Fungal keratitis. Curr Opin Ophthalmol 2004;15:321–327.

12
Zygomycosis (Mucormycosis)

**Charalampos Antachopoulos, MD,
Juan C. Gea-Banacloche, MD, and Thomas J. Walsh, MD**

1. INTRODUCTION

The class Zygomycetes includes a variety of filamentous fungi that may cause life-threatening human disease and, over the past decade, have emerged as an increasingly important cause of morbidity and mortality among immunocompromised patients *(1,2)*. The first case of zygomycosis in humans was reported in 1885 by Platauf as Mycosis Mucorina. In many of the cases reported thereafter the infection was identified as "mucormycosis" or *Mucor* infection based solely on histological findings of wide, rarely septate hyphae, without culture confirmation. The use of the term "mucormycosis" was further promoted by the original classification of most of the pathogenic zygomycetes species as members of the genus *Mucor*. Many of these species were later reassigned into different genera or families *(3)*. Consequently the term "zygomycosis" should be preferred, instead of "mucormycosis," for infections caused by any of the zygomycetes species. Some authors still employ the term "mucormycosis," however, for infections caused by members of the order Mucorales *(3,4)*. Those who prefer the use of "mucormycosis" stress that the opportunistic disease due to those fungi in the order Mucorales differs substantially from disease caused by the other pathogenic zygomycetes order, Entomophthorales.

2. ETIOLOGIC AGENTS

The medically important Zygomycetes encompass two orders of filamentous fungi with distinct morphologic, epidemiologic, and pathogenic characteristics, the Mucorales and the Entomophthorales *(3,5–8)* (Table 12.1). The majority of cases of zygomycosis in humans are caused by members of the order Mucorales. Organisms of the genus *Rhizopus* are by far the most common clinical isolates, with *R. oryzae* being the most frequently recovered species. Members of the genus *Mucor* are second to *Rhizopus* in order of frequency, while *Cunninghamella, Apophysomyces, Absidia, Saksenaea, Rhizomucor* and other genera each represent a significantly smaller percentage of clinical isolates *(1,3,4)*.

From: *Infectious Disease: Diagnosis and Treatment of Human Mycoses*
Edited by: D. R. Hospenthal and M. G. Rinaldi © Humana Press Inc., Totowa, NJ

Table 12.1
Taxonomic classification of the Zygomycetes

Class	Order	Family	Genus	Species causing human disease
Zygomycetes	Mucorales	Mucoraceae	*Absidia*	*A. corymbifera*
			Apophysomyces	*A. elegans*
			Mucor	*M. circinelloides, M. ramosissimus, M. racemosus, M. hiemalis, M. rouxianus*
			Rhizomucor	*R. pusillus*
			Rhizopus	*R. oryzae (R. arrhizus), R. microsporus* var. *rhizopodiformis*
		Cunninghamellaceae	*Cunninghamella*	*C. bertholletiae*
		Mortierellaceae	*Mortierella*	(animal pathogens)
		Saksenaceae	*Saksenaea*	*S. vasiformis*
		Syncephalastraceae	*Syncephalastrum*	*S. racemosum*
		Thamnidaceae	*Cokeromyces*	*C. recurvatus*
	Entomophthorales[a]	Ancylistaceae	*Conidiobolus**	*C. coronatus, C. incongruus*
		Basidiobolaceae	*Basidiobolus**	*B. ranarum*

[a]It has been recently suggested that the order Entomophthorales should be divided into two phylogenetically distinct groups: the genus *Basidiobolus* should be classified in a new order, the Basidiobolales, while *Conidiobolus* appears to be closely related to the Mucorales and should form a distinct group *(5,8)*.

The class of Zygomycetes is characterized in culture by broad, nonseptate or sparsely septated hyphae and by the presence of sporangiophores supporting sporangia, which contain sporangiospores (see Fig. 2.7, Chapter 2). During sexual reproduction in culture zygospores may be produced. The Zygomycetes are characterized in tissue by the formation of wide, ribbonlike, hyaline, aseptate or sparsely septated hyphae with wide-angle (approximately 90°) branching. The substantial differences among these and other structures allow mycology laboratories to diagnose organisms by genus and species *(3)*.

3. EPIDEMIOLOGY

The Zygomycetes are ubiquitous in soil and can be isolated from decaying organic matter including hay, decaying vegetation, and a variety of food items. Human infection is usually acquired through inhalation of sporangiospores from environmental sources. Acquisition via the cutaneous or percutaneous route is also common, either through traumatic disruption of skin barriers or with the use of catheters and injections. Less commonly, infection through the gastrointestinal route may occur *(1,3,6)*.

Zygomycosis is approximately 10- to 50- fold less common than invasive *Candida* or *Aspergillus* infections, with a prevalence of 1 to 5 cases per 10,000 autopsies and an estimated incidence of 1.7 cases per million per year in the United States *(4,9)*. A clear male predisposition has been observed, as demonstrated by an approximate 2:1 male to female ratio among cases *(1)*. Unlike other filamentous fungi, targeting mainly immunocompromised patients, the Zygomycetes cause disease in a wider and more heterogeneous population. While the Mucorales mainly affect patients with underlying immunosuppression or other medical conditions, the Entomophthorales largely afflict immunocompetent hosts in tropical and subtropical areas of developing countries. Lately, however, infections caused by the Entomophthorales in immunocompromised hosts have occasionally been documented *(6,7,10)*.

The most common underlying condition for development of zygomycosis is diabetes, both type I and type II. A significant proportion of these patients will present with concomitant ketoacidosis, while in others zygomycosis may even present as the diabetes-defining illness. Other significant underlying conditions include the presence of hematological malignancy, solid organ or bone marrow transplantation, deferoxamine therapy, and injection drug use *(1,6)*. During the 1980s and 1990s, the percentage of patients with hematological malignancy, solid organ or bone marrow transplantation, and injection drug use among all cases of zygomycosis increased significantly *(1,11,12)*. In the aforementioned groups of hematological patients and transplant recipients, factors associated with this infection have been reported to include prolonged neutropenia, corticosteroid use, and graft versus host disease (GvHD) *(6,12)*. Less commonly, the Zygomycetes may cause invasive disease in the presence of renal failure, diarrhea, and malnutrition in low birth weight infants and in HIV patients. Occasionally zygomycosis has developed in patients with persistent metabolic acidosis secondary to causes other than diabetes *(1,6)*.

A significant proportion of zygomycosis cases have as well been observed in persons with no primary underlying disease at the time of infection. In many of these cases there was a history of penetrating trauma, surgery, or burn before the development of infection *(1,6)*.

4. PATHOGENESIS AND IMMUNOLOGY

The epidemiologic profile of zygomycosis cases (patients with diabetes, hematological malignancies or on deferoxamine therapy, transplant recipients) may in part be explained by our current understanding of the pathogenesis of these infections.

As with other filamentous fungi, an effective immune response following inoculation of sporangiospores requires the presence of adequate phagocytic activity of the host effector cells, including tissue macrophages and neutrophils. The macrophages ingest the sporangiospores to inhibit germination, while the neutrophils are involved in hyphal damage *(13)*. Consequently, the host immune response against the Zygomycetes may be compromised if the phagocytic cells are insufficient in number as in the case of chemotherapy-induced neutropenia, or dysfunctional, as in the case of corticosteroid treatment or diabetes mellitus *(3,13)*.

Experimental evidence also suggests an important role of iron in the pathogenesis of infections caused by *Rhizopus* species, whose growth is promoted in the presence of increased iron uptake. Deferoxamine, an iron chelator, has siderophore activity for these fungi, allowing significant increase in iron uptake. Further, the availability of serum iron is increased in the presence of acidic pH, suggesting an additional mechanism for the development of zygomycosis in patients with diabetic ketoacidosis *(4,13)*.

An almost universal feature in infections caused by the Mucorales is the presence of extensive angioinvasion associated with thrombosis and ischemic necrosis *(3)*. This is likely an important mechanism by which these organisms survive antifungal therapy because adequate blood supply is necessary for the delivery of antifungal agents. Recent data also have demonstrated the ability of *R. oryzae* sporangiospores or hyphae to adhere to subenthodelial matrix proteins and human endothelial cells *(4,14)*. Pregerminated sporangiospores of *R. oryzae* were able to damage endothelial cells in vitro, following adherence to and phagocytocis by these cells. *R. oryzae* viability was not required for endothelial cell damage, suggesting that in the setting of established infection even fungicidal therapy may not prevent subsequent tissue injury *(14)*.

5. CLINICAL MANIFESTATIONS

The clinical presentations of zygomycosis in humans largely depend on the causative agent (Mucorales versus Entomophthorales) and the patient's condition (intact immune response versus immunosuppresion or other underlying conditions). Thus, while the Mucorales cause rapidly progressive disease characterized by angioinvasion, thrombosis, tissue necrosis, and dissemination in susceptible hosts, infections caused by the Entomophthorales usually lack these features, inducing a chronic inflammatory response and following an indolent course in immunocompetent patients *(3,6,7)*. Consequently the patterns of human disease are described separately for these two orders of Zygomycetes, with more emphasis given to infections caused by the Mucorales, because organisms of this order are most likely to be encountered in developed countries.

The clinical manifestations of human infection caused by the Mucorales can be classified as sinus disease, localized or extended to the orbit and/or brain, pulmonary, cutaneous, gastrointestinal, disseminated and miscellaneous infection. Some of these manifestations may occur with increased frequency in patients with certain underlying conditions (Table 12.2) *(1,6)*. However, this is not always the case and zygomycosis in these patient groups may still present with any of the above patterns.

5.1. *Sinus Infection*

Sinus disease may be confined to the paranasal sinuses or may infiltrate the orbit (sino-orbital) and/or the brain parenchyma (rhinocerebral). This form represents approximately two-thirds of all cases of zygomycosis in diabetic patients *(1)*. The infection originates in the paranasal sinuses after inhalation of sporangiospores. Initial symptoms may suggest sinusitis and include sinus pain, discharge, soft tissue swelling, and perinasal cellulitis/paresthesia. Fever is variable and may be absent in up to half of cases *(4,15,16)*. The tissues involved become red, violaceous, and finally black, as vascular thrombosis leads to tissue necrosis. A blood-tinged nasal discharge may be present. Extension of the infection to the mouth may produce painful necrotic ulcerations in the hard palate. Extension into the periorbital area and ultimately the orbit

Table 12.2
Predominant site of Mucorales infection according to the patient's underlying condition

Underlying condition	Type of infection, by site
Diabetes	Sinus
Malignancy	Pulmonary
Solid organ transplantation	Pulmonary
Bone marrow transplantation	Pulmonary
Deferoxamine therapy	Pulmonary, sinus, disseminated[a]
Injection drug use	Cerebral
No underlying condition	Cutaneous

Data from ref. 1.
[a]No clear predominance among the three sites.

may be manifested by periorbital edema, lacrimation, chemosis, and proptosis. Subsequent ocular or optic nerve involvement may be suggested by pain, diplopia, blurring or loss of vision. Alteration of mental status and cranial nerve palsies may signify invasion of the central nervous system. Occasionally thrombosis of the cavernous sinus or the internal carotid artery may follow, with resultant neurological deficits, while dissemination of the infection also may occur *(4,6,16,17)*.

5.2. *Pulmonary Infection*

Pulmonary disease is most commonly observed in patients with hematological malignancies, solid organ or bone marrow transplant recipients, and in those receiving deferoxamine treatment *(1)*. Not infrequently it may occur with concomitant sinus disease (sinopulmonary infection) *(18)*. Lung involvement may be manifested as infiltrates, consolidation, and solitary nodular or cavitary lesions (Fig. 12.1) *(19,20)*. Fungal invasion of the pulmonary vessels may result in thrombosis and subsequent infarcts in the lung parenchyma (Fig. 12.2). Angioinvasion may also lead to intraparenchymal bleeding or even hemoptysis, which can be fatal if major vessels, such as the pulmonary artery, are involved. Extension of the infection to the chest wall, pericardium, myocardium, mediastinum, and diaphragm has been described *(4,6,19)*. A predilection for the upper lobes has been reported; however, any part of the lung may be involved, and bilateral disease is not uncommon *(19)*. Presenting signs and symptoms are nonspecific and include fever, cough, chest pain, dyspnea, hemoptysis, tachypnea, crackles, decreased breath sounds, and wheezing *(4,19,20)*.

5.3. *Cutaneous Infection*

Cutaneous zygomycosis is often observed in individuals with no underlying condition as a result of infection of a preexisting lesion, such as skin trauma or burn. Alternatively, it may occur in the context of disseminated disease or extensive local infection in immunocompromised hosts *(1,3,21,22)*. In the case of primary cutaneous inoculation, the lesion appears acutely inflamed with redness, swelling, induration, and frequent progression to necrosis. Extensive local invasion may occur involving the

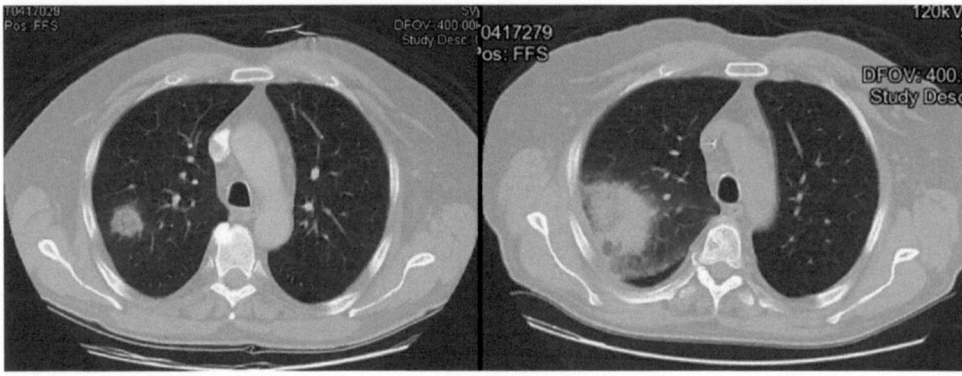

Fig. 12.1. Thoracic CT scan of profoundly neutropenic patient with pulmonary zygomycosis demonstrates rapid evolution of pulmonary nodule to involve the pleural surface and to manifest a halo sign at the interface with radiologically normal lung. The two scans are separated by 5 days. [Figure in color on CD-ROM].

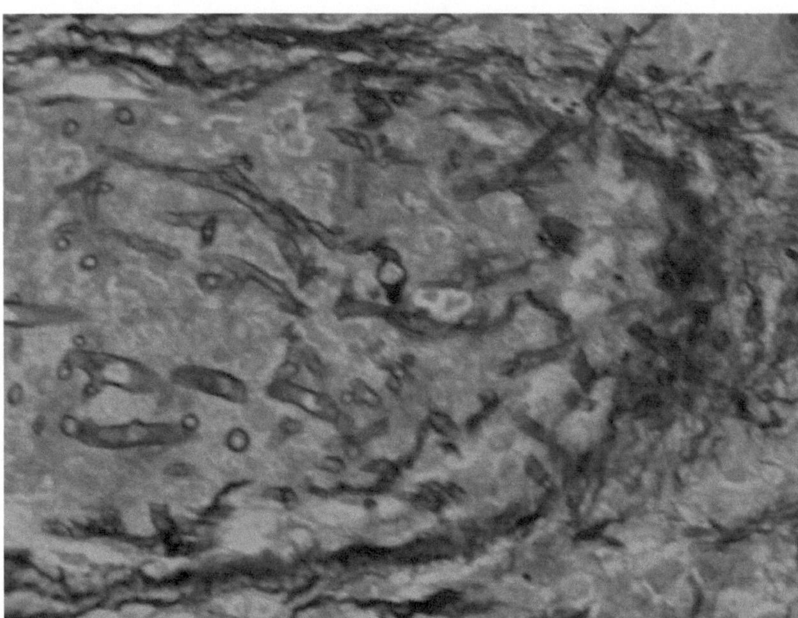

Fig. 12.2. Histopathology of pulmonary zygomycosis. Characteristic broad nonseptated ribbonlike hyphae with nondichotomous branching invading a pulmonary blood vessel. The specimen was obtained from the lung lesion seen on CT scan in Figure 12.1. GMS. [Figure in color on CD-ROM].

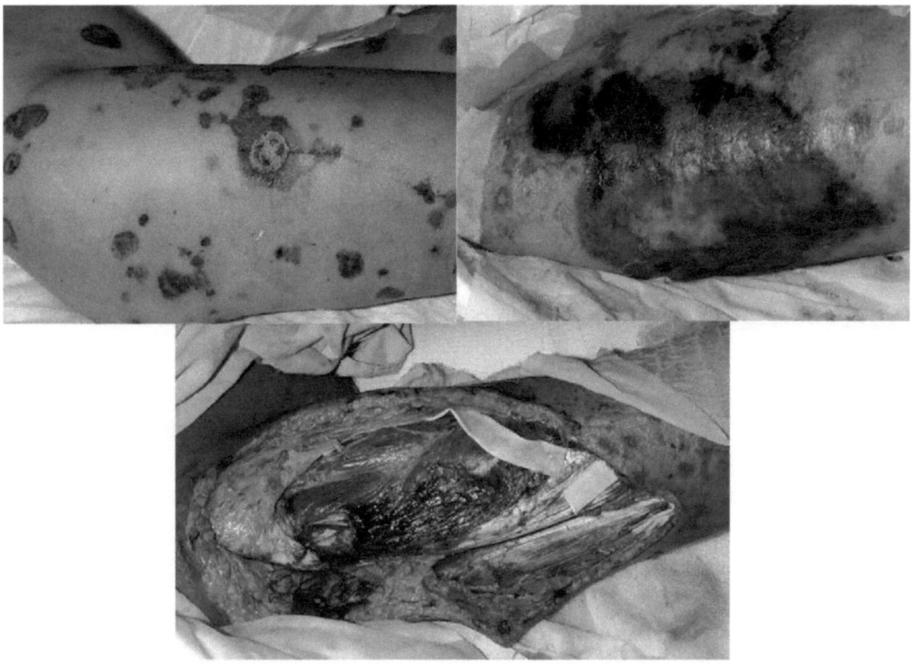

Fig. 12.3. Development of zygomycosis in the skin and subcutaneous tissues of the right lower extremity in a patient with cutaneous T-cell lymphoma. The top left panel depicts the lesions of cutaneous T-cell lymphoma, which were possibly infected by direct inoculation. The top right panel reveals the extensive necrosis and destruction of soft tissue caused by the rapidly invading zygomycete. The bottom panel demonstrates the soft tissues following extensive surgical debridement. [Figure in color on CD-ROM].

adjacent subcutaneous fat, muscle, bone tissues, and fascial layers (Fig. 12.3). When cutaneous disease is the result of disseminated infection, it usually presents as nodular subcutaneous lesions that may ulcerate *(3,6,22)*.

5.4. Gastrointestinal Infection

Gastrointestinal disease is rare, occurring mainly in malnourished patients and premature neonates, in whom it can present as necrotizing enterocolitis *(1,23)*. After ingestion of the sporangiospores, fungal invasion of the mucosa, submucosa, and vascular structures of the gastrointestinal tract may occur, often resulting in necrotic ulcers, rupture of the intestinal wall, and peritonitis. Symptoms are nonspecific, including fever, abdominal pain, distention, vomiting, and gastrointestinal hemorrhage *(3,4,23)*.

5.5. Disseminated Infection

Disseminated infection refers to involvement of at least two noncontiguous sites and is commonly observed in patients receiving deferoxamine therapy *(1)*. Dissemination occurs through the hematogenous route and may originate from any of the above sites of primary infection, although it seems to be more frequently associated with lung disease. The most common site of dissemination is the brain, but other organs may also be involved *(4,25)*.

5.6. Other Infection

Isolated cerebral zygomycosis is usually observed in injection drug users *(1)*. Endocarditis is a potential complication of cardiac surgery. Isolated peritonitis is often associated with peritoneal dialysis. Renal infection and external otitis also have been reported *(4,6)*.

5.7. Infection Due to the Entomophthorales

In contrast to the Mucorales infections, human disease caused by the Entomophthorales usually follows an indolent course, as previously mentioned. A chronic subcutaneous disease, characterized by slowly enlarging subcutaneous nodules that eventually ulcerate, is typically caused by *B. ranarum*. *C. coronatus* infections commonly present as chronic sinusitis that usually does not extend to the central nervous system *(3,7)*. Less commonly, involvement of other body sites or even aggressive disseminated infection by members of the order Entomophthorales has been reported for immunocompromised and immunocompetent patients *(3,7,10,23)*.

6. DIAGNOSIS

As infections caused by the Zygomycetes, and particularly the Mucorales, in humans may be rapidly fatal, timely diagnosis is crucial to avoid treatment delay. While confirmation of the diagnosis and species identification of the causative organism should be pursued, treatment should be initiated as soon as the diagnosis is suspected, owing to the severity of these infections.

Currently, the diagnosis of zygomycosis relies on a constellation of the following: high index of suspicion, assessment of presenting signs and symptoms, imaging studies, cultures of clinical specimens, and histopathology (Fig. 12.4).

6.1. Clinical Assessment

The high index of suspicion should be based on the knowledge of the underlying conditions that predispose to zygomycosis and the usual presentation of the infection in each of these conditions (Table 12.2). Nevertheless, less common manifestations of the disease should not be excluded. A common scenario is the development of zygomycosis in oncological patients or transplant recipients who are receiving antifungal therapy for prophylaxis or treatment of other opportunistic fungal infections, such as invasive aspergillosis. If the antifungal agents that are being administered to the patient are not active against the Zygomycetes (including, fluconazole, voriconazole, and the echinocandins), then clinical deterioration or appearance of new signs and symptoms in these patients should alert the clinician to the possibility of zygomycosis *(18)*.

Most of the signs and symptoms that are associated with the clinical manifestations of zygomycosis are nonspecific. However, their diagnostic significance may increase if they are interpreted in relation to the patient's underlying condition. For example, the development of sinusitis in a leukemic or diabetic patient should raise the suspicion of zygomycosis. Other findings have probably greater specificity for this infection,

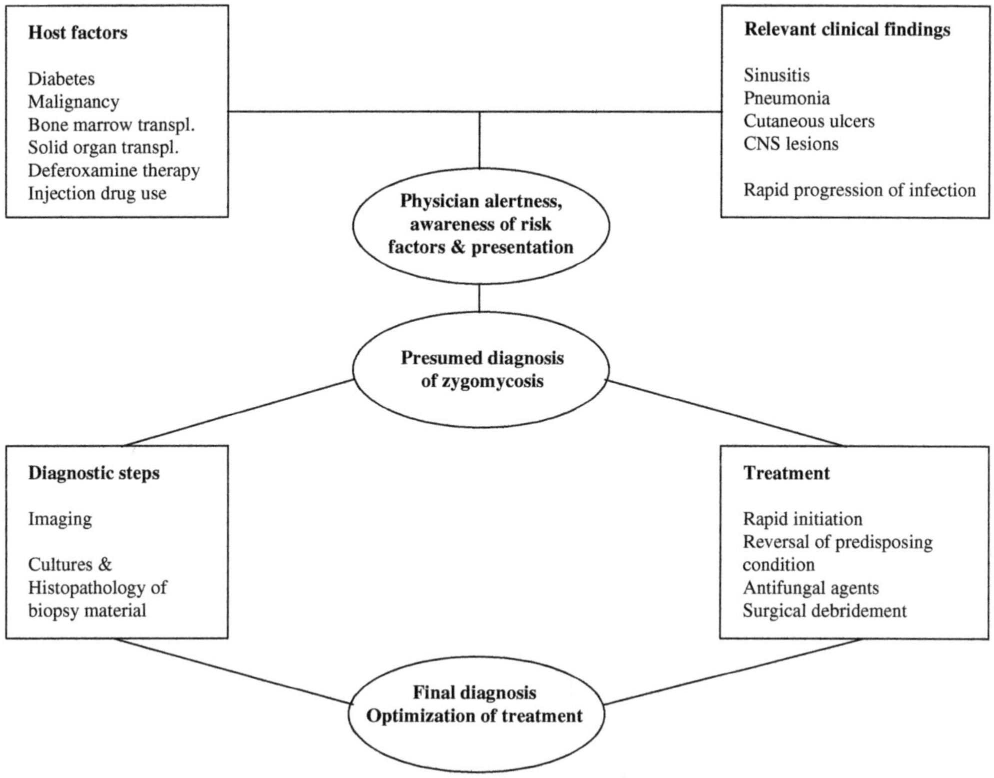

Fig. 12.4. Diagnosis and management of zygomycosis.

such as the presence of blood-tinged nasal discharge or necrotic eschars in the hard palate. In addition, the presence of hemoptysis in a susceptible host is consistent with angioinvasion and should raise the possibility of zygomycosis *(19)*. An alarming sign should also be the rapid spread of the infection. Finally, even after the diagnosis has been made, careful periodic clinical assessment should be performed in order to detect progression of the disease. For example, in a patient with pulmonary zygomycosis, palpation of the skin for subcutaneous nodules and neurological evaluation for changes in mental status and focal neurological signs should be performed repeatedly to detect dissemination to the skin and brain, respectively.

6.2. Diagnostic Imaging

Imaging studies are helpful in assessing the burden of the disease, involvement of adjacent tissues, and response to treatment. They are also helpful in guiding more invasive procedures to obtain biopsy specimens for histopathology and culture *(26)*. Although imaging findings may be suggestive of zygomycosis in the appropriate clinical setting, they are not sufficiently specific to establish the diagnosis. In sinus disease, computerized tomography (CT) detects subtle mucosal thickening or bony erosions of the sinuses, but it is less sensitive than magnetic resonance imaging (MRI) for the detection of extension of the infection to the soft tissues of the orbit *(15,27)*.

In the case of pulmonary disease, high-resolution CT is more sensitive than chest radiograph for early diagnosis of the infection and can more accurately determine the extent of pulmonary involvement. Radiographic features may be consistent with infliltrate, cavity, or consolidation (Fig. 12.1). The air crescent and halo signs, which are recognized radiologic features of invasive aspergillosis, have been reported as well for zygomycosis *(19,20,28)*. In patients with pulmonary zygomycosis the presence of an air crescent sign seems to be associated with increased risk for massive hemoptysis *(19)*. Another suggestive finding could be expansion of a mass or consolidation across tissue planes, in particular toward the great vessels in the mediastinum *(4,29)*. In the case of cutaneous disease, MRI is superior to CT scan for assessment of extension of the infection to the adjacent soft or bone tissues.

6.3. Culture

Recovery of Zygomycetes from cultures of clinical specimens would allow not only establishment of diagnosis, but also identification of the causative organism to the species level. Although the Zygomycetes may contaminate laboratory material, their isolation from clinical specimens of susceptible hosts should not be disregarded as contamination. Despite the ability of these organisms to invade tissues, they are rarely isolated from cultures of blood, urine, cerebrospinal fluid, feces, sputum, paranasal sinuses secretions, bronchoalveolar lavage, or swabs from infected areas *(3,15,19)*. The recovery of Zygomycetes from biopsy material may be compromised if processing of the specimens involves tissue grinding, a procedure that kills the nonseptate hyphae of these fungi. The recovery rate is enhanced, however, if thin slices of minimally manipulated tissue are placed onto the culture medium. Consequently, for proper handling of the specimens, the laboratory should be notified of the possibility of zygomycosis. In any case, negative cultures do not rule out the infection *(3,6)*.

6.4. Endoscopic Findings and Histopathology

Given the above limitations of cultures or imaging studies, diagnosis of zygomycosis is almost always based on histopathologic examination of appropriately collected samples. The latter should be pursued in the presence of strong suspicion for zygomycosis if the cultures or imaging studies are negative or nonspecific. Depending on the presentation of the disease, the samples may be collected by fiberoptic bronchoscopy, radiographically guided transthoracic needle aspiration, open lung biopsy, nasal endoscopy, paranasal sinus biopsy or débridement, and biopsies of skin or other infected tissues *(4,6,19,26)*. In the case of lung disease, endobronchial findings include stenosis or airway obstruction, erythematous mucosa, fungating or polypoid mass, and, less often, granulation tissue or mucosal ulceration *(19)*. In sinus disease, nasal endoscopy may show black necrotic crusts on the nasal septum and turbinates; in the early phases the mucosa may still look pink and viable *(4)*. We refer to these necrotic ulcers along the nasal mucosa or turbinates as "sentinel eschars," as they may represent an early phase of infection or may be more amenable to biopsy than a deep maxillary sinus infection.

Because the hyphae of Zygomycetes in tissue specimens may stain poorly with hematoxylin and eosin (H&E), a second more fungus-specific tissue stain should also be used, such as Gomori methenamine silver (GMS) or periodic acid Schiff (PAS) *(3)*. As previously mentioned, the hallmark of zygomycosis is the demonstration of wide, ribbonlike, aseptate (nonseptate or rarely septate) hyphae with wide-angle branching in biopsy specimens (Fig. 12.2) (see also Fig. 3.11, Chapter 3). For Mucorales infections, the hyphae are seen to invade the adjacent blood vessels. Mycotic emboli may thrombose small vessels in which they are lodged. Extensive tissue necrosis or hemorrhage may be observed *(3)*. Although histopathology is sensitive and reliable for diagnosing zygomycosis, obtaining biopsy material from hematological patients may not always be feasible owing to concomitant thrombocytopenia. Finally, because fixing and staining of the biopsy specimens takes time, a promising method for accelerating diagnosis by use of frozen sections in tissue specimens has been proposed recently *(30)*.

6.5. *Other Non-Culture Diagnosis*

Unfortunately, no reliable molecular or antigen detection methods are available to date for primary diagnosis of zygomycosis. A number of molecular techniques are currently used by research laboratories for species identification of zygomycetes isolates, epidemiologic studies, or determination of taxonomic assignments *(3,18)*.

7. TREATMENT

There are four cornerstones of successful management of zygomycosis: *(1)* rapid initiation of therapy, *(2)* reversal of the patient's underlying predisposing condition, *(3)* administration of appropriate antifungal agents, and *(4)* surgical débridement of infected tissues (Fig. 12.4) *(4,6)*. If not treated or if diagnosed with delay, infections caused by the Mucorales in humans are typically fatal *(1,11,12)*. Even if timely diagnosis is made, treatment is challenging due to a number of reasons such as the underlying condition of the patient, the rapid progression of the disease, and the high degree of angioinvasion and thrombosis that compromises the delivery of antifungal agents active against the causative organisms. As mentioned previously, in the presence of certain conditions such as diabetes, immunosuppression, and others (Table 12.2), treatment for zygomycosis should be initiated as soon as a strong suspicion for this infection is raised, without awaiting formal confirmation of the diagnosis, which may take time. Meanwhile of course, all the required actions to establish the diagnosis should be undertaken, as previously described (Fig. 12.4).

Reversal of the underlying condition can be fairly quickly achieved in certain circumstances, such as diabetic ketoacidosis, which should be promptly corrected, or deferoxamine therapy, which should be discontinued. However, timely reversal of the disease- or treatment-related immunosuppression in patients with hematological malignancies or transplant recipients is challenging. In these patients, temporary discontinuation of corticosteroid treatment or myelotoxic chemotherapy should be strongly considered until the infection is brought under control. However, even with these measures, spontaneous restoration of phagocytic activity or recovery from neutropenia are likely to occur after several days, during which time the infection may progress. In vitro and in vivo studies, as well as case reports, have suggested that the administration of cytokines, such as granulocyte colony-stimulating factor (G-CSF), granulocyte-macrophage colony-stimulating factor (GM-CSF), and interferon-γ, may accelerate immune recovery *(31,32)*. In support of these general recommendations for cytokine augmentation of host defense are recent in vitro studies demonstrating enhancement of neutrophil activity against *R. oryzae* and other species of Zygomycetes in the presence of interferon-γ and GM-CSF *(33)*. An alternative approach has been the administration of granulocyte transfusions in neutropenic patients with invasive fungal infections *(31,32)*. These immunomodulatory interventions may be considered on an individual patient basis as adjunctive therapy for zygomycosis in immunocompromised hosts. Nonetheless, as a caveat, there is a lack of adequately powered clinical trials to evaluate their clinical efficacy and potential complications *(6,31,32)*.

7.1. Amphotericin B

Amphotericin B is the drug of choice for the treatment of zygomycosis. This polyene agent exerts good in vitro and in vivo activity against the Zygomycetes. However, apparent in vitro resistance, with elevated minimal inhibitory concentrations (MICs) of amphotericin B, may be observed among clinical isolates and is relatively common among *Cunninghamella* species *(34–36)*. The efficacy of amphotericin B in the treatment of zygomycosis was demonstrated in a recent review of 929 cases, where survival was 61% for patients treated with amphotericin B deoxycholate versus 3% for those who received no treatment *(1)*. The lipid formulations of amphotericin B (mainly amphotericin B lipid complex and the liposomal formulation) also have been used in the treatment of zygomycosis. These formulations are associated with significantly less toxicity than amphotericin B deoxycholate and demonstrate at least equivalent clinical efficacy *(1,37,38)*. However, no randomized controlled trials have been conducted to compare the efficacy of deoxycholate versus lipid formulations of amphotericin B in the treatment of zygomycosis.

When treatment with amphotericin B is initiated for documented zygomycosis, full doses should be given from the onset, foregoing the past practice of dose escalation. The optimal dosage of amphotericin B formulations for the treatment of zygomycosis has not been systematically evaluated in clinical studies. A study of the safety, tolerance, and plasma pharmacokinetics of liposomal amphotericin B in patients with invasive fungal infections found no demonstrable dose-limiting nephrotoxicity or infusion-related toxicity over a dose range of 7.5 to 15 mg/kg per day *(39)*. Plasma concentrations of liposomal amphotericin B achieved an upper limit at 10 mg/kg per day and were not increased by further dosage increases. Nevertheless, the efficacy of higher dosages of liposomal amphotericin B compared to the US Food and Drug Administration (FDA)-approved dosage of 3 to 5 mg/kg per day for aspergillosis has not been investigated through clinical trials in zygomycosis. In the absence of such studies, an increase of dosage of liposomal amphotericin B to 7.5 or 10 mg/kg per day could be considered on an individual basis for patients with zygomycosis progressing through liposomal amphotericin B at 5 mg/kg per day *(39)*. Amphotericin B lipid complex has been used in a dosage of 5 mg/kg per day in salvage treatment of zygomycosis with complete or partial responses in 17 (71%) of 24 cases *(38)*.

7.2. Azoles

Of the azole agents, fluconazole and voriconazole have little or no activity against the Zygomycetes *(40)*. Itraconazole is active in vitro against some of these organisms, but has demonstrated poor efficacy in animal models *(41,42)*. The investigational azole posaconazole is active in vitro and in vivo against many of the Zygomycetes *(34,35,40–42)*. Results from two recent case series as well as a number of case reports on the use of posaconazole in patients with zygomycosis refractory to or intolerant of conventional antifungal treatment provide encouraging data regarding posaconazole as an alternative salvage therapy for zygomycosis *(43–48)*. The use of this azole, however, as monotherapy or in combination with amphotericin B, for the treatment of zygomycosis awaits further evaluation in a randomized clinical trial versus deoxycholate amphotericin B or a lipid formulation of amphotericin B.

7.3. Surgery

Appropriate and early surgical débridement is a critical intervention for the successful management of zygomycosis for a number of reasons: the infection progresses rapidly, vascular thrombosis compromises the delivery of antifungal agents to the site of infection, and there is massive tissue necrosis. Several retrospective studies have demonstrated that the survival of patients treated with antifungal therapy combined with surgical débridement was significantly higher than that of patients treated with antifungal therapy alone *(1,4,6,19)*. Surgical treatment should aim in removing all necrotic tissues and should be considered for any of the clinical presentations of zygomycosis (sinus disease, pulmonary or cutaneous). It should be performed early in the course of treatment and repeated if necessary. It may include excision of the infected sinuses, débridement of retroorbital space, or even enucleation in the case of sinus/sinoorbital disease, and wedge resection, lobectomy, or pneumonectomy in the case of pulmonary disease *(15,16,19,22,29)*. If the patient survives the infection, plastic surgery is likely to be needed to correct disfiguring resulting from débridement *(4)*.

7.4. Hyperbaric Oxygen

Besides the aforementioned important aspects of management of zygomycosis, hyperbaric oxygen is a therapeutic modality that has been occasionally used as adjunctive treatment. Hyperbaric oxygen has a theoretical potential for being beneficial in the treatment of zygomycosis because it is known to inhibit fungal growth at high pressures, correct tissue hypoxia and lactic acidosis, promote healing, and enhance phagocytosis *(49,50)*. In a number of case reports and small case series of zygomycosis, administration of hyperbaric oxygen was associated with a favorable outcome *(49)*. Currently, however, the absence of randomized controlled clinical trials on the efficacy of hyperbaric oxygen in this setting does not allow firm recommendations regarding its use as adjunctive treatment of zygomycosis.

7.5. Prognosis

The prognosis of zygomycosis largely depends on the patient's underlying condition, the clinical presentation of the infection, the time of initiation of therapy, and the type of treatment provided. Mortality may range from less than 10% for localized sinus disease to approximately 100% for disseminated infection, with an overall percentage of 47% for zygomycosis cases reported in the 1990s *(1,4)*.

8. PREVENTION

Prevention may be feasible for a proportion of cases through adequate control of diabetes and judicious use of deferoxamine and corticosteroids. For severely immunocompromised hosts, measures to reduce the risk of exposure to airborne sporangiospores should be undertaken, including Hepafiltration of air supply, positive room air pressures, exclusion of plants from the wards, and wearing of masks when leaving the room. Owing to the relatively low incidence of zygomycosis, the cost-effectiveness of prophylactic treatment is questionable; the development of a preemptive therapy approach, however, based on validated early indicators of the disease and risk assumption, should be a target for research in the near future. In the meantime, physicians caring for susceptible patients should maintain a high level of suspicion and be alert to the early signs and symptoms of zygomycosis in order to achieve early diagnosis and timely initiation of treatment.

REFERENCES

1. Roden MM, Zaoutis TE, Buchanan WL, et al. Epidemiology and outcome of zygomycosis: a review of 929 reported cases. Clin Infect Dis 2005;41:634–653.
2. Kauffman CA. Zygomycosis: reemergence of an old pathogen. Clin Infect Dis 2004;39:588–590.
3. Ribes JA, Vanover-Sams CL, Baker DJ. Zygomycetes in human disease. Clin Microbiol Rev 2000;13:236–301.
4. Spellberg B, Edwards J, Jr., Ibrahim A. Novel perspectives on mucormycosis: pathophysiology, presentation, and management. Clin Microbiol Rev 2005;18:556–569.
5. Jensen AB, Dromph KM. The causal agents of "entomophthoramycosis" belong to two different orders: a suggestion for modification of the clinical nomenclature. Clin Microbiol Infect 2005;11:249–250.
6. Gonzalez CE, Rinaldi MG, Sugar AM. Zygomycosis. Infect Dis Clin North Am 2002;16:895–914.
7. Prabhu RM, Patel R. Mucormycosis and entomophthoramycosis: a review of the clinical manifestations, diagnosis and treatment. Clin Microbiol Infect 2004;10(Suppl 1):31–47.
8. Jensen AB, Gargas A, Eilenberg J, Rosendahl S. Relationships of the insect-pathogenic order Entomophthorales (Zygomycota, Fungi) based on phylogenetic analyses of nuclear small subunit ribosomal DNA sequences (SSU rDNA). Fungal Genet Biol 1998;24: 325–334.
9. Rees JR, Pinner RW, Hajjeh RA, Brandt ME, Reingold AL. The epidemiological features of invasive mycotic infections in the San Francisco Bay area, 1992–1993: results of population-based laboratory active surveillance. Clin Infect Dis 1998;27:1138–1147.
10. Walsh TJ, Renshaw G, Andrews J, et al. Invasive zygomycosis due to Conidiobolus incongruus. Clin Infect Dis 1994;19:423–430.
11. Kontoyiannis DP, Wessel VC, Bodey GP, Rolston KV. Zygomycosis in the 1990s in a tertiary-care cancer center. Clin Infect Dis 2000;30:851–856.
12. Marr KA, Carter RA, Crippa F, Wald A, Corey L. Epidemiology and outcome of mould infections in hematopoietic stem cell transplant recipients. Clin Infect Dis 2002;34:909–917.

13. Shoham S, Levitz SM. The immune response to fungal infections. Br J Haematol 2005;129:569–582.
14. Ibrahim AS, Spellberg B, Avanessian V, Fu Y, Edwards Jr JE. Rhizopus oryzae adheres to, is phagocytosed by, and damages endothelial cells in vitro. Infect Immun 2005;73:778–783.
15. Dhiwakar M, Thakar A, Bahadur S. Improving outcomes in rhinocerebral mucormycosis—early diagnostic pointers and prognostic factors. J Laryngol Otol 2003;117:861–865.
16. Talmi YP, Goldschmied-Reouven A, Bakon M, et al. Rhino-orbital and rhino-orbito-cerebral mucormycosis. Otolaryngol Head Neck Surg 2002;127:22–31.
17. Thajeb P, Thajeb T, Dai D. Fatal strokes in patients with rhino-orbito-cerebral mucormycosis and associated vasculopathy. Scand J Infect Dis 2004;36:643–648.
18. Kontoyiannis DP, Lionakis MS, Lewis RE, et al. Zygomycosis in a tertiary-care cancer center in the era of Aspergillus-active antifungal therapy: a case-control observational study of 27 recent cases. J Infect Dis 2005;191:1350–1360.
19. Lee FY, Mossad SB, Adal KA. Pulmonary mucormycosis: the last 30 years. Arch Intern Med 1999;159:1301–1309.
20. McAdams HP, Rosado de Christenson M, Strollo DC, Patz EF, Jr. Pulmonary mucormycosis: radiologic findings in 32 cases. AJR Am J Roentgenol 1997;168:1541–1548.
21. Hay RJ. Mucormycosis: an infectious complication of traumatic injury. Lancet 2005;365:830–831.
22. Losee JE, Selber J, Vega S, Hall C, Scott G, Serletti JM. Primary cutaneous mucormycosis: guide to surgical management. Ann Plast Surg 2002;49:385–390.
23. Lyon GM, Smilack JD, Komatsu KK, et al. Gastrointestinal basidiobolomycosis in Arizona: clinical and epidemiological characteristics and review of the literature. Clin Infect Dis 2001;32:1448–1455.
24. Woodward A, McTigue C, Hogg G, Watkins A, Tan H. Mucormycosis of the neonatal gut: a "new" disease or a variant of necrotizing enterocolitis? J Pediatr Surg 1992;27:737–740.
25. Cuvelier I, Vogelaers D, Peleman R, et al. Two cases of disseminated mucormycosis in patients with hematological malignancies and literature review. Eur J Clin Microbiol Infect Dis 1998;17:859–863.
26. Maschmeyer G. Pneumonia in febrile neutropenic patients: radiologic diagnosis. Curr Opin Oncol 2001;13:229–235.
27. Fatterpekar G, Mukherji S, Arbealez A, Maheshwari S, Castillo M. Fungal diseases of the paranasal sinuses. Semin Ultrasound CT MR 1999;20:391–401.
28. Jamadar DA, Kazerooni EA, Daly BD, White CS, Gross BH. Pulmonary zygomycosis: CT appearance. J Comput Assist Tomogr 1995;19:733–738.
29. Reid VJ, Solnik DL, Daskalakis T, Sheka KP. Management of bronchovascular mucormycosis in a diabetic: a surgical success. Ann Thorac Surg 2004;78:1449–1451.
30. Hofman V, Castillo L, Betis F, Guevara N, Gari-Toussaint M, Hofman P. Usefulness of frozen section in rhinocerebral mucormycosis diagnosis and management. Pathology 2003;35:212–216.
31. Antachopoulos C, Roilides E. Cytokines and fungal infections. Br J Haematol 2005;129:583–596.
32. Pappas PG. Immunotherapy for invasive fungal infections: from bench to bedside. Drug Resist Updat 2004;7:3–10.
33. Gil-Lamaignere C, Simitsopoulou M, Roilides E, Maloukou A, Winn RM, Walsh TJ. Interferon-gamma and granulocyte-macrophage colony-stimulating factor augment the activity of polymorphonuclear leukocytes against medically important zygomycetes. J Infect Dis 2005;191:1180–1187.
34. Dannaoui E, Meletiadis J, Mouton JW, Meis JF, Verweij PE. In vitro susceptibilities of zygomycetes to conventional and new antifungals. J Antimicrob Chemother 2003;51:45–52.

35. Sun QN, Fothergill AW, McCarthy DI, Rinaldi MG, Graybill JR. In vitro activities of posaconazole, itraconazole, voriconazole, amphotericin B, and fluconazole against 37 clinical isolates of zygomycetes. Antimicrob Agents Chemother 2002;46:1581–1582.
36. Singh J, Rimek D, Kappe R. In vitro susceptibility of 15 strains of zygomycetes to nine antifungal agents as determined by the NCCLS M38-A microdilution method. Mycoses 2005;48:246–250.
37. Gleissner B, Schilling A, Anagnostopolous I, Siehl I, Thiel E. Improved outcome of zygomycosis in patients with hematological diseases? Leuk Lymphoma 2004;45: 1351–1360.
38. Walsh TJ, Hiemenz JW, Seibel NL, et al. Amphotericin B lipid complex for invasive fungal infections: analysis of safety and efficacy in 556 cases. Clin Infect Dis 1998;26:1383–1396.
39. Walsh TJ, Goodman JL, Pappas P, et al. Safety, tolerance, and pharmacokinetics of high-dose liposomal amphotericin B (AmBisome) in patients infected with *Aspergillus* species and other filamentous fungi: maximum tolerated dose study. Antimicrob Agents Chemother 2001;45:3487–3496.
40. Boucher HW, Groll AH, Chiou CC, Walsh TJ. Newer systemic antifungal agents: pharmacokinetics, safety and efficacy. Drugs 2004;64:1997–2020.
41. Dannaoui E, Meis JF, Loebenberg D, Verweij PE. Activity of posaconazole in treatment of experimental disseminated zygomycosis. Antimicrob Agents Chemother 2003;47: 3647–3650.
42. Sun QN, Najvar LK, Bocanegra R, Loebenberg D, Graybill JR. In vivo activity of posaconazole against *Mucor* spp. in an immunosuppressed-mouse model. Antimicrob Agents Chemother 2002;46:2310–2312.
43. Greenberg RN, Scott LJ, Vaughn HH, Ribes JA. Zygomycosis (mucormycosis): emerging clinical importance and new treatments. Curr Opin Infect Dis 2004;17:517–525.
44. Greenberg RN, Mullane K, van Burik JA, et al. Posaconazole as salvage therapy for zygomycosis. Antimicrob Agents Chemother 2006;50:126–133.
45. van Burik JA, Hare RS, Solomon HF, Corrado ML, Kontoyiannis DP. Posaconazole is effective as salvage therapy in zygomycosis: a retrospective summary of 91 cases. Clin Infect Dis 2006;42:e61–65.
46. Tobon AM, Arango M, Fernandez D, Restrepo A. Mucormycosis (zygomycosis) in a heart-kidney transplant recipient: recovery after posaconazole therapy. Clin Infect Dis 2003;36:1488–1491.
47. Garbino J, Uckay I, Amini K, Puppo M, Richter M, Lew D. *Absidia* posttraumatic infection: successful treatment with posaconazole. J Infect 2005;51:e135–e138.
48. Dupont B. Pulmonary mucormycosis (zygomycosis) in a lung transplant recipient: recovery after posaconazole therapy. Transplantation 2005;80:544–545.
49. John BV, Chamilos G, Kontoyiannis DP. Hyperbaric oxygen as an adjunctive treatment for zygomycosis. Clin Microbiol Infect 2005;11:515–517.
50. Gill AL, Bell CN. Hyperbaric oxygen: its uses, mechanisms of action and outcomes. QJM 2004;97:385–395.

SUGGESTED READINGS

Gonzalez CE, Rinaldi MG, Sugar AM. Zygomycosis. Infect Dis Clin North Am 2002;16: 895–914.

Greenberg RN, Scott LJ, Vaughn HH, Ribes JA. Zygomycosis (mucormycosis): emerging clinical importance and new treatments. Curr Opin Infect Dis 2004;17:517–525.

Lee FY, Mossad SB, Adal KA. Pulmonary mucormycosis: the last 30 years. Arch Intern Med 1999;159:1301–1309.

Prabhu RM, Patel R. Mucormycosis and entomophthoramycosis: a review of the clinical manifestations, diagnosis and treatment. Clin Microbiol Infect 2004;10 (Suppl 1):31–47.
Ribes JA, Vanover-Sams CL, Baker DJ. Zygomycetes in human disease. Clin Microbiol Rev 2000;13:236–301.
Roden MM, Zaoutis TE, Buchanan WL, et al. Epidemiology and outcome of zygomycosis: a review of 929 reported cases. Clin Infect Dis 2005;41:634–653.
Spellberg B, Edwards Jr J, Ibrahim A. Novel perspectives on mucormycosis: pathophysiology, presentation, and management. Clin Microbiol Rev 2005;18:556–569.

13
Pneumocystosis

Francis Gigliotti, MD and Terry W. Wright, PhD

1. INTRODUCTION

Pneumocystis is the classic opportunistic pathogen in that it does not produce any recognizable disease in an immunologically intact host, yet infection of the at-risk immunocompromised host results in a pneumonitis that is universally fatal if untreated. The organism was first identified in the early 1900s but was not appreciated to be a significant human pathogen until after World War II, when outbreaks of *Pneumocystis* pneumonia (PCP) occurred in orphanages in Europe. These young infants who developed what was termed "interstitial plasma cell pneumonitis" were suspected to be immunosuppressed secondary to severe malnutrition. Two subsequent events firmly established *Pneumocystis* as a major opportunistic pathogen; the development of successful cancer chemotherapy in the late 1950s and 1960s and the start of the acquired immunodeficiency syndrome (AIDS) epidemic in the early 1980s. In fact it was the recognition of a cluster of this "rare" pneumonia, PCP, in gay men over a short period of time that led to the recognition that a new syndrome (AIDS) and infection (human immunodeficiency virus [HIV]) had emerged *(1,2)*.

At present the population of patients at risk to develop PCP is growing steadily as we develop new modalities of therapy and potent immunosuppressive drugs to treat malignancies, organ failure, and autoimmune and inflammatory diseases. For example, in solid organ transplant recipients, as survival improves so does the recognition that these patients are at risk of developing PCP if not on specific prophylaxis. Most recently, the addition of antitumor necrosis factor (TNF) therapy to the management of patients with Crohn's disease has resulted in the occurrence of PCP in this population that had previously not been considered to be at risk for the development of PCP.

2. ETIOLOGIC AGENT

All strains of *Pneumocystis* are extracellular organisms found in the lungs of mammals. The taxonomic placement of these organisms has not been unequivocally established, largely owing to the inability to adequately culture the organism. However, nucleic acid homologies indicate it is most closely related to the fungi, despite its

From: *Infectious Disease: Diagnosis and Treatment of Human Mycoses*
Edited by: D. R. Hospenthal and M. G. Rinaldi © Humana Press Inc., Totowa, NJ

morphologic features and susceptibility to drugs that are similar to those of protozoa. Both phenotypic and genotypic analysis demonstrates that each mammalian species is infected by a unique strain of *Pneumocystis (3–5)*. A biological correlate for these differences is evidenced by animal experiments that have shown organisms are not transmissible from one mammalian species to another *(6)*. This restricted host range is the one biologic characteristic of *Pneumocystis* that might achieve the level of uniqueness sufficient to define species of *Pneumocystis*.

Two forms of *Pneumocystis* are found in the alveolar spaces, thick-walled cysts (Fig. 13.1) that are 5 to 8 μm in diameter and may contain up to eight pleomorphic intracystic sporozoites, and trophozoites, which are 2 to 5 μm diameter cells with a more typical cell membrane, thought to be derived from excysted sporozoites. The terminology sporozoites and trophozoites are based on the morphological similarities to protozoa, because there are not exact correlates for these forms of the organism among the fungi. Sporozoites are also called intracystic bodies and trophozoites are referred to as trophic forms.

As noted in the preceding text, the host-species specificity of *Pneumocystis* has led some to propose the division of *P. carinii* into multiple unique species, with the nomenclature *P. jirovecii* being used to refer to human *P. carinii (7)*. The proposal for a change in nomenclature is controversial because it also calls for species distinction

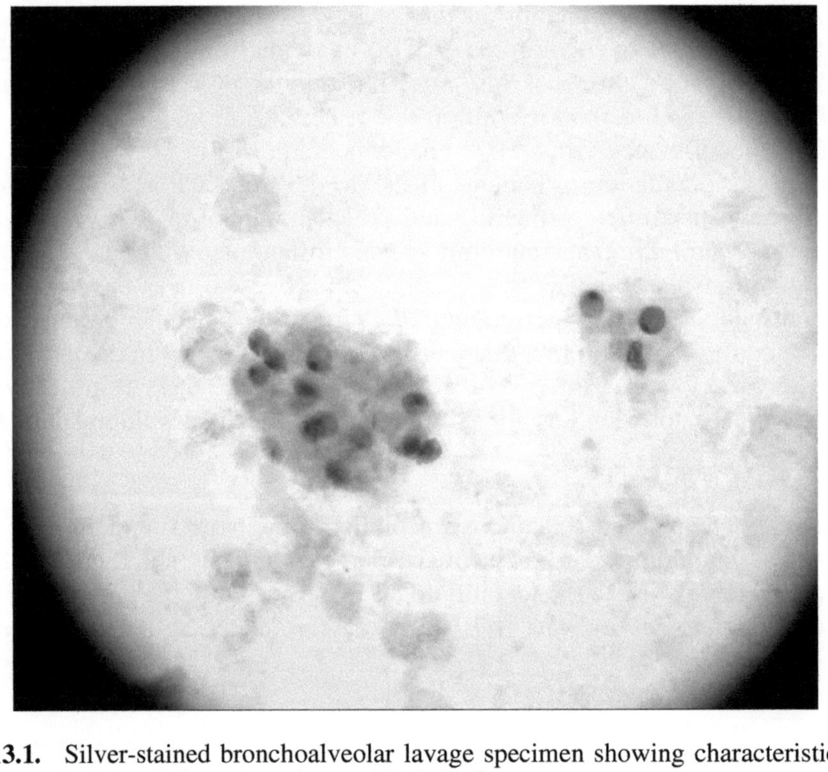

Fig. 13.1. Silver-stained bronchoalveolar lavage specimen showing characteristic clusters of *Pneumocystis* cysts. [Figure in color on CD-ROM].

based on variation in gene sequences not known to result in a unique phenotype. Opposing opinions have also been published calling for the nomenclature *P. carinii* to be retained for all *P. carinii* or at least for *P. carinii* infecting humans *(8)*. Until consensus is achieved, *P. carinii* can also be clearly defined using "special form" nomenclature (e.g., *P. carinii* f. sp. hominus for human *P. carinii*) or simply by identifying the mammalian source (e.g., mouse *P. carinii* to describe *P. carinii* isolated from mice).

3. EPIDEMIOLOGY

PCP occurs only in patients who are significantly immunosuppressed, typically with abnormalities in $CD4^+$ T lymphocytes or B cells. Serologic studies have demonstrated that a high proportion of the population has evidence of infection and that seroconversion typically occurs during childhood. A recent prospective longitudinal study demonstrated that seroconversion began in the first few months of life and by 20 months of age 85% of the infants in the study had seroconverted *(9)*.

Aside from the serologic data, *Pneumocystis* was not known to actually infect the immunologically normal host. However, animal studies have proved that *Pneumocystis* produces a typical pattern of infection, transmission, and resolution in the normal host *(10)*. The other important biological feature of *Pneumocystis* infection is that the strain (or species) of *Pneumocystis* from any given mammalian host is transmissible only to members of the same host species. Cross-species transmission has never been convincingly demonstrated. Because of the finding of early seroconversion followed by disease later in life, PCP was postulated to be the result of reactivation of latent infection. However, no evidence for latency has ever been demonstrated, and mouse and rat models of PCP have shown that latency does not develop after infection. Considering all of these features it would seem most likely that PCP is the result of new infection rather than reactivation of a latent infection. Person-to-person transmission is likely, based on the cumulative experience in animal models, but difficult to prove.

Without prophylaxis, PCP develops in approximately 70% of adults and 40% of infants and children with AIDS, and 10% of patients with organ transplants. It is often the sentinel event identifying infants with severe congenital immunodeficiencies such as severe combined immunodeficiency syndrome. PCP also is a frequent occurrence in patients being treated for malignancies, occurring with an overall frequency of 10% to 15%. The actual incidence for any given malignancy depends on the treatment regimen and is positively correlated with number of chemotherapeutic agents and intensity of treatment.

4. PATHOGENESIS AND IMMUNOLOGY

Control of infection is dependant on normally functioning $CD4^+$ T lymphocytes. Studies in patients with AIDS show an increase in the occurrence of *Pneumocystis* pneumonia as $CD4^+$ T lymphocytes drop. For adults and children older than 6 years of age a $CD4^+$ T cell count of 200 cells/µl or lower is a marker of very high risk for development of PCP. Based on the occurrence of PCP in some patients and mouse strains with various immunologic defects that result in defective antibody production, a possible role for $CD4^+$ T lymphocytes could be to provide help for the production of specific antibody. Passively administered antibody has been shown to aid in the clearance of *Pneumocystis* in mouse models. Thus antibody could be involved in the clearance of organisms through interaction with complement, phagocytes, and/or T lymphocytes.

The mechanism by which *Pneumocystis* damages the lung is not yet fully defined. Animal models have been valuable in helping us understand the immunopathogenesis of PCP *(11)*. Infection of severe combined immunodeficiency (SCID) mice with *Pneumocystis* produces very little alteration in lung histology or function until very late in the course of the disease. However, if *Pneumocystis*-infected SCID mice are immunologically reconstituted with normal splenocytes there is a rapid onset of an inflammatory response that results in an intense cellular infiltrate, markedly reduced lung compliance, and significant hypoxia, all changes seen in humans with PCP. These inflammatory changes are associated with marked disruption of surfactant function. T-cell subset analysis has shown that $CD4^+$ T lymphocytes produce an inflammatory response that clears the organisms but also results in lung injury. In contrast, $CD8^+$ T lymphocytes are ineffective in the eradication of *Pneumocystis*, but do produce a marked injurious inflammatory response, especially in the absence of $CD4^+$ T lymphocytes.

Immune reconstitution inflammatory syndrome (IRIS), also called immune restitution disease or immune reconstitution syndrome, is a recently described manifestation of pulmonary infection in AIDS patients with *Pneumocystis*, *Mycobacterium tuberculosis*, and other pulmonary pathogens who are experiencing rapid reconstitution of their immune system due to administration of effective antiretroviral therapy *(12)*. In general, the severity of IRIS is directly related to the degree and rapidity of T-cell recovery. Mouse models of PCP suggest that $CD8^+$ T lymphocytes help modulate the inflammation produced by $CD4^+$T lymphocytes, but as mentioned in the preceding text, their ineffectual inflammatory response can also contribute significantly to lung injury. These various T-cell effects may be responsible for the variations in presentation and outcome of *Pneumocystis* pneumonia observed in different patient populations.

The inflammatory processes taking place during PCP do not appear to result in major long-term damage to the lung in those who recover. A long-term follow up of 23 children with cancer and PCP showed a return to normal lung function by 6 months in all 18 survivors. Similar studies in adults are complicated by the fact that adult patients, especially those with AIDS, might have multiple pulmonary insults. While some studies, primarily of adult AIDS patients, suggest long-term pulmonary damage after PCP, other studies of renal transplant recipients have shown pulmonary function returned to nearly normal after recovery from PCP.

5. CLINICAL MANIFESTATIONS

5.1. Pneumocystis *Pneumonia*

There are at least three distinct clinical presentations of PCP. In patients with profound immunodeficiency, such as young infants with congenital immunodeficiency, severe malnutrition, or in AIDS patients with very few $CD4^+$ T lymphocytes, the onset of hypoxia and symptoms is subtle, with cough, dyspnea on exertion, or tachypnea, often without fever. Infants may show progression to nasal flaring and intercostal, suprasternal, and infrasternal retractions. As the disease progresses, patients develop hypoxia, with cyanosis in severe cases. In the sporadic form of PCP, occurring in children and adults with underlying immunodeficiency, the onset of hypoxia and symptoms is usually more abrupt, with fever, tachypnea, dyspnea, and cough, progressing to severe respiratory compromise. This latter type accounts for the majority of cases, although the severity of clinical expression may vary. Rales are usually not detected on physical examination. The third pattern of disease is that associated with rapid restoration of immune function referred to as IRIS. It has been best described in newly diagnosed AIDS patients who are severely immunocompromised and present with PCP as their initial manifestation of AIDS *(12)*. These patients appear to respond well to therapy for PCP but 3 to 6 weeks after beginning treatment they experience an unexpected recurrence of pulmonary symptoms and chest x-ray abnormalities that coincide with return of immune function. IRIS may also occur in bone marrow transplant patients who engraft while infected with *Pneumocystis*.

5.2. Extrapulmonary Infections

Extrapulmonary infection with *Pneumocystis* is rare. The incidence is not well defined, but is estimated to be 1000-fold less likely than PCP itself *(13)*. The most commonly reported sites of infection include the ear and eye. Why these two sites seem to predominate is unclear but may reflect the fact that infection at these sites may quickly produce readily apparent signs and symptoms. Other sites of involvement are the thyroid gland, liver, kidney, bone marrow, lymph nodes, spleen, muscle, and gastrointestinal tract. How the organism arrives at these sites is unknown. Response to treatment is usually good when extrapulmonary infections occur in the absence of pulmonary infection.

6. DIAGNOSIS

Pulmonary symptoms in at risk patients should always raise the suspicion of PCP. The classic chest radiograph reveals bilateral diffuse alveolar disease with a granular pattern (see Fig. 5.7, Chapter 5). The earliest densities are perihilar, and progression proceeds peripherally, typically sparing the apical areas until last. Less common chest radiograph appearances in PCP include cystic lesions, pneumothorax, or isolated focal infiltrates. In patients receiving aerosolized pentamidine for prophylaxis there may be a predisposition for upper lobe infiltrates. The arterial oxygen tension (Pao_2) is invariably decreased.

A clinical pearl is that an elevated lactate dehydrogenase (LDH) may be a hint that one is dealing with PCP, because LDH is a useful marker of alveolar and inflammatory cell damage. Because *Pneumocystis* is a diffuse alveolar infection it tends to result in higher and more often elevated levels of LDH than some other opportunistic pulmonary infections. For example, a recent analysis of LDH and pulmonary opportunistic infections in AIDS patients showed that about 90% of those with definite PCP had elevated serum LDH *(14)*. Thus while not specific for PCP, very high LDH levels should raise one's suspicion for PCP, and normal levels make the diagnosis of PCP much less likely.

PCP can be definitively diagnosed only by demonstrating *Pneumocystis* in the lungs of a patient with compatible pulmonary signs and symptoms. Appropriate specimens for analysis include bronchoalveolar lavage, tracheal aspirate, transbronchial lung biopsy, bronchial brushings, percutaneous transthoracic needle aspiration, and open lung biopsy. Induced sputum samples are gaining popularity, but are helpful only if positive; the absence of *Pneumocystis* in an induced sputum sample does not exclude infection. The open lung biopsy is the most reliable method, although bronchoalveolar lavage is generally more practical. Estimates of the diagnostic yield of the various specimens are as follows: induced sputum 20% to 40%, tracheal aspirate 50% to 60%, bronchoalveolar lavage 75% to 95%, transbronchial biopsy 75% to 95%, and open lung biopsy 90% to 100%. Once obtained, the specimens are typically stained with one of four commonly used stains: Gomori methenamine silver (GMS) and toluidine blue stain only cyst forms; polychrome stains such as Giemsa stain for both trophozoites and sporozoites; and the fluorescein-labeled monoclonal antibody stains for both trophozoites and cysts. *Pneumocystis* can also be visualized by Papanicolaou stain. Polymerase chain reaction (PCR) analysis of respiratory specimens offers promise as a rapid diagnostic method, but a standardized system for clinical use has not been established.

7. TREATMENT

The clear drug of choice for the treatment of PCP is trimethoprim-sulfamethoxazole (TMP-SMX) (Table 13.1). Generally TMP-SMX is administered intravenously, but it may be given orally if disease is mild and no malabsorption or diarrhea is present. The duration of treatment is generally 3 weeks for patients with AIDS and 2 weeks for other patients. Adverse reactions occur frequently, more so in adults than children, with TMP-SMX. These include rash, fever, and neutropenia in patients with AIDS. These side effects are less common in non-AIDS patients. For patients who cannot tolerate or fail to respond to TMP-SMX after 5 to 7 days, pentamidine isethionate may be used. Adverse reactions are frequent with pentamidine and include renal and hepatic dysfunction, hyperglycemia or hypoglycemia, rash, and thrombocytopenia. Atovaquone is an alternative treatment that has been used primarily in adults with mild to moderate disease. For adults and adolescents atovaquone is given twice a day with food. Less information is available for the treatment of younger children with this agent.. Other effective therapies include trimetrexate glucuronate or combinations of trimethoprim plus dapsone and of clindamycin plus primaquine.

Administration of corticosteroids in addition to anti-*Pneumocystis* drugs increases the chances for survival in moderate and severe cases of PCP *(15)*. The recommended regimen of corticosteroids for adolescents older than 13 years of age and for adults is oral prednisone, 80 mg/day divided in two doses on days 1 to 5, 40 mg/day once daily on days 6 to 10, and 20 mg/day once daily on days 11 to 21. Although specific studies of adjunctive corticosteroid therapy in young children are not available, a reasonable regimen for children is oral prednisone, 2 mg/kg per day for the first 7 to 10 days, followed by a tapering regimen for the next 10 to 14 days.

Table 13.1
Recommended treatment for *Pneumocystis* pneumonia[a]

	Adults	Children
	Treatment of first choice	
Trimethoprim-sulfamethoxazole (TMP-SMX)	TMP 15–20 mg/kg/d with SMX 75–100 mg/kg per day IV divided into 3 or 4 doses; PO for mild disease	TMP 15–20 mg/kg per day with SMX 75–100 mg/kg per day IV divided into 4 doses; PO for mild disease
	Alternate treatment regimens	
Pentamidine	4 mg/kg per day IV as single dose	4 mg/kg per day as single dose
Atovaquonc	750 mg PO bid	3–24 mo of age: 45 mg/kg per day PO divided into 2 doses; 1–3 mo and over 24 mo: 30 mg/kg per day in 2 divided doses (max. daily dose 1500 mg)
Dapsone plus trimethoprim	Dapsone 100 mg, PO once daily;TMP 15 mg/kg per day PO in 3 divided doses	Dapsone 2 mg/kg per day (100 mg max.) PO once daily; TMP 15 mg/kg per day PO in 3 divided doses
Primaquine plus clindamycin	Primaquine 15–30 mg, PO once daily;clindamycin 600 mg IV every 8 hours	Primaquine 0.3 mg/kg (max 30 mg) PO once daily; clindamycin 40 mg/kg per day IV in 4 divided doses (no pediatric data)
	Trimetrexate	
Trimetrexate plus leucovorin	<50 kg: 1.5 mg/kg per day IV once daily 50–80 kg: 1.2 mg/kg per day IV once daily> 80 kg: 1.0 mg/kg per day IV once daily	45 mg/m^2 IV once daily
	Leucovorin (continue 3 days beyond trimetrexate)	
	<50 kg: 0.8 mg/kg per day IV or PO every 6 hours >50 kg: 0.5 mg/kg per day IV or PO every 6 hours	20 mg/m^2 IV or PO every 6 hours

IV, intravenous; PO, orally; mg/kg, milligrams/kilogram; mg/kg perday, milligrams/kilogram per day; mo, months of age; bid, twice daily.

[a]Duration of therapy is typically 3 weeks in patients with AIDS and 2 weeks in other immunosuppressed patients.

8. PREVENTION

PCP is effectively prevented by the use of antimicrobial prophylaxis; thus all patients at high risk for PCP should be placed on chemoprophylaxis. As noted in the preceding text, $CD4^+$ T-cells are the key cell in determining susceptibility to PCP. However, defining the risk for PCP is not always clear. In AIDS patients there is clear-cut correlation between cell number and function so that firm cutoffs can be given. In adults with AIDS, prophylaxis is indicated at $CD4^+$ T-cell counts of below 200 cells/μl. Because of rapid changes in $CD4^+$ T-cell counts in young infants prophylaxis is recommended for all HIV-infected children during their first year of life. Thereafter prophylaxis is started at $CD4^+$T-cell counts drop below 750 cells/μl for infants 12 to 23 months of age, 500 cells/μl for children from 2 to 6 years of age, and 200 cells/μl for those 6 years of age and older. Prophylaxis is also recommended for all ages if $CD4^+$T-cell percentages drop below 15%. In other disease states in which patients are placed at risk of PCP from being on immunosuppressive drugs, both lymphocyte number and function will be affected. Thus while a patient may have a lymphocyte count above the threshold for susceptibility to develop PCP, suppressed function of remaining lymphocytes may place him or her at risk for PCP. Because of the demonstrated increased risk of PCP with increasing intensity of chemotherapy in patients with cancer, it would seem prudent, in our opinion, to consider prophylaxis for patients receiving prolonged (more than 6 to 8 weeks) therapy with two immunosuppressive agents and to give prophylaxis to all patients receiving three or more immunosuppressive agents.

Table 13.2
Recommended antibiotic prophylaxis for *Pneumocystis* pneumonia

Drug	Adults	Children
Trimethoprim-sulfamethoxazole (TMP-SMX)	1 single or double strength tablet daily or 3 days/week	TMP 5 mg/kg per day with SMX 25 mg/k per day given once daily or divided into 2 doses
Dapsone	100 mg daily or twice weekly	2 mg/kg per day as single dose (max. 100 mg/dose)
Atovaquone	1500 mg once daily	30 mg/kg per day as single dose for children aged 1–3 months and older than 24 mo; 45 mg/kg per day as single dose for children 4–23 mo
Aerosolized pentamidine	300 mg monthly given by Respigard II nebulizer	For children ≥ 5 years—same as for adults

IV, intravenous; PO, orally; mg/kg per day, milligrams/kilogram per day; mo, months of age.

TMP-SMX is the drug of choice for *Pneumocystis* prophylaxis and may be given for 3 days each week, or, alternatively, each day (Table 13.2). The original study testing less than daily administration of TMP-SMX used a schedule of 3 consecutive days on TMP-SMX and 4 days off with the idea of reducing potential bone marrow suppression from the TMP-SMX. Subsequent studies have used alternate day schedules such as dosing on Monday, Wednesday, and Friday. The double strength tablet is preferred for adults receiving 3-days-a-week dosing. Alternatives for prophylaxis, all of which are inferior to TMP-SMX, include dapsone, atovaquone, and aerosolized pentamidine Prophylaxis must be continued as long as the patient remains immunocompromised. Studies in adult AIDS patients who reconstitute adequate immune response during antiretroviral therapy show that prophylaxis may be withdrawn without risk of developing PCP. Small studies in children have provided similar results. Criteria of maintaining the $CD4^+$ T-cell count at or above 200 cells/μl for at least 3 months have been established for discontinuation of both primary and secondary prophylaxis *(16)*.

REFERENCES

1. Masur H, Michelis MA, Greene JB, et al. An outbreak of community-acquired *Pneumocystis carinii* pneumonia: initial manifestation of cellular immune dysfunction. N Engl J Med 1981;305:1431–1438.
2. Gottlieb MS, Schroff R, Schanker HM, et a. *Pneumocystis carinii* pneumonia and mucosal candidiasis in previously healthy homosexual men: evidence of a new acquired cellular immunodeficiency. N Engl J Med 1981;305:1425–1431.
3. Gigliotti F. Host species-specific antigenic variation of a mannosylated surface glycoprotein of *Pneumocystis carini*. J Infect Dis 1992;165:329–336.
4. Gigliotti F, Haidaris PJ, Haidaris CG, Wright TW, Van der Meid KR. Further evidence of host species-specific variation in antigens of *Pneumocystis carinii* using the polymerase chain reaction. J Infect Dis 1993;168:191–194.
5. Wakefield AE. Genetic heterogeneity in *Pneumocystis carinii*: an introduction. FEMS Immunol Med Microbiol 1998;22:5–13.
6. Gigliotti F, Harmsen AG, Haidaris CG, Haidaris PJ. *Pneumocystis carinii* is not universally transmissible between mammalian species. Infect Immun 1993;61:2886–2890.
7. Stringer JR, Cushion MT, Wakefield AE. New nomenclature for the genus Pneumocystis. J Eukaryot Microbiol 2001;Suppl:184S–189S.
8. Gigliotti F. *Pneumocystis carinii*: has the name really been changed? Clin Infect Dis 2005;41:1752–1755.
9. Vargas SL, Hughes WT, Santolaya ME, et al. Search for primary infection by *Pneumocystis carinii* in a cohort of normal, healthy infants. Clin Infect Dis 2001;32:855–861.
10. Gigliotti F, Harmsen AG, Wright TW. Characterization of transmission of *Pneumocystis carinii* f. sp. *muris* through immunocompetent BALB/c mice. Infect Immun 2003;71:3852–3856.
11. Wright TW, Gigliotti F, Finkelstein JW, McBride JT, An CL, Harmsen AG. Immune-mediated inflammation directly impairs pulmonary function, contributing to the pathogenesis of *Pneumocystis carinii* pneumonia. J Clin Invest 1999;104:1307–1317.
12. Cheng VC, Yuen KY, Chan WM, Wong SS, Ma ES, Chan RM. Immunorestitution disease involving the innate and adaptive response. Clin Infect Dis 2000;30:882–892.
13. Ng VL, Yajko DM, Hadley WK. Extrapulmonary pneumocystosis. Clin Microbiol Rev 1997;10:401–418.

14. Butt AA, Michaels S, Kissinger P. The association of serum lactate dehydrogenase level with selected opportunistic infections and HIV progression. Int J Infect Dis 2002;6:178–181.
15. Briel M, Bucher HC, Boscacci R, Furrer H. Adjunctive corticosteroids for *Pneumocystis jiroveci* pneumonia in patients with HIV-infection. Cochrane Database Syst Rev 2006:3:CD006150.
16. Centers for Disease Control and Prevention. Guidelines for preventing opportunistic infections among HIV-infected persons - 2002. Recommendations of the U.S. Public Health Service and the Infectious Diseases Society of America. MMWR 2002;51 (RR-8):1–52.

SUGGESTED READINGS

Gigliotti F, Wright TW. Immunopathogenesis of *Pneumocystis carinii* pneumonia. Exp Rev Molec Med 2005;7:1–16, www.expertreviews.org.

Steele C, Shellito JE, Kolls JK. Immunity against the opportunistic fungal pathogen *Pneumocystis*. Med Mycol 2005;43:1–19.

Thomas CF, Limper AH. *Pneumocystis* pneumonia. N Engl J Med 2004;350:2487–2498.

Walzer PD, Cushion MT. *Pneumocystis* pneumonia. 3rd ed. New York: Marcel Dekker, 2005.

14
Cryptococcosis

Methee Chayakulkeeree, MD and John R. Perfect, MD

1. INTRODUCTION

Cryptococcosis is an infectious disease caused by pathogenic encapsulated yeasts in the genus *Cryptococcus*. Currently, two species of these fungi commonly cause disease in humans: *C. neoformans* which cause cryptococcosis in both immunocompetent and immunocompromised hosts, and *C. gattii* , which is primarily a pathogen in apparently immunocompetent patients. *C. neoformans* was identified as a human pathogen in 1894 by two German physicians, Otto Busse and Abraham Buske, when they described a circular yeastlike microorganism in a lesion on the tibia of a woman; the microorganism was initially named *Saccharomyces hominis (1)*. The name *Cryptococcus neoformans* has been consistently adopted in both the mycology and medical literature since 1950 *(2)*. In the mid-1970s, when Kwon-Chung discovered two mating types of *C. neoformans* that produced fertile basidiospores, the organisms were subsequently separated into two varieties, var. *neoformans* (serotypes A and D) and var. *gattii* (serotypes B and C). These two varieties were recently separated into two species, *C. neoformans* and *C. gattii*, based on their genetic background and phylogenetic diversity, as proposed by Kwon-Chung in 2002 *(3)*. It is possible, as more molecular information is gathered from genome sequencing, that *C. neoformans* var. *neoformans* (serotype D) and *C. neoformans* var. *grubii* (serotype A) will be divided into separate species as well.

The incidence of cryptococcosis began to rise by the late 1970s. Early case reports of cryptococcal infections were primarily associated with cancer, autoimmune diseases, organ transplantation, and receipt of corticosteroids as these immunocompromised populations enlarged *(4)*. A major surge in new cases of cryptococcosis occurred in the mid-1980s to 1990s. In the first two decades of the human immunodeficiency virus (HIV) infection pandemic, cryptococcal infection was an important opportunistic infection in all parts of the world. Further, *C. gattii* has recently caused a localized outbreak of cryptococcosis in apparently immunocompetent individuals on Vancouver Island *(5)*. As a result, these fungi are not only major pathogens in immunocompromised patients such as those with acquired immune deficiency syndrome (AIDS), cancer, and

From: *Infectious Disease: Diagnosis and Treatment of Human Mycoses*
Edited by: D. R. Hospenthal and M. G. Rinaldi © Humana Press Inc., Totowa, NJ

immunosuppressive therapies, but also cause disease in apparently immunocompetent hosts. Despite the development of highly active antiretroviral therapy (HAART), which has decreased the rate of HIV-related cryptococcosis in developed countries, its prevalence is still very high in developing countries and in individuals without access to healthcare.

2. ETIOLOGIC AGENTS

Cryptococcus is a genus of basidiomycetous fungi containing more than 30 species. However, the common pathogenic organisms of cryptococcosis currently consist of two species that can be classified further into three varieties, five serotypes (based on capsular agglutination reactions), and eight molecular types (Table 14.1). *C. neoformans* has been classified into serotype A, D, and the hybrid strain, AD, whereas serotype B and C strains were classified as *C. gattii*. Serotype A strains have also been named *C. neoformans* var. *grubii* and serotype D strains were named *C. neoformans* var. *neoformans*. Recently, both *C. neoformans* and *C. gattii* were further classified into four molecular types for each species, VN I-IV and VG I-IV, respectively.

The life cycle of *C. neoformans* and *C. gattii* involve asexual (yeast) and sexual (basidiospores/hyphae) forms. The asexual stage is the encapsulated yeast form found in clinical specimens, whereas the sexual stage, which exists in one of two mating types, "alpha" or "a," is observed only under certain conditions resulting in meiosis to form basidiospores. Since the sexual stage of *C. neoformans* and *C. gattii* has been described, their teleomorphs were named *Filobasidiella neoformans* and *Filobasidiella bacillospora*, respectively. The majority of cryptococcal infections are caused by serotype A strains worldwide. However, cryptococcal diseases caused by serotype B and C strains, mostly VG II molecular type, are endemic in some subtropical areas, and serotype D is commonly found in Europe *(6)*.

C. neoformans and *C. gattii* usually appear as white-to-cream, opaque, and mucoid colonies that grow to several millimeters in diameter on most routine agar within 48 to 72 hours. With some strains, a few colonies occasionally develop sectors with different pigmentation. Both cryptococcal species can readily grow on most fungal culture media without cycloheximide at 30 ° to 37 °C under aerobic conditions. However, *C. neoformans* is generally more thermotolerant to higher temperature than *C. gattii*, and serotype A is generally more tolerant than serotype D. Besides the ability to grow at 37 °C, the yeast can produce a thick shedding polysaccharide capsule, melanin

Table 14.1
Classification of *Cryptococcus neoformans* and *Cryptococcus gattii*

Serotype	Species and varieties	Molecular types
A	*C. neoformans* var. *grubii*	VN I, VN II
B	*C. gattii*	VG I, VG II, VG III, VG IV
C	*C. gattii*	VG I, VG II, VG III, VG IV
D	*C. neoformans* var. *neoformans*	VN IV
AD	*C. neoformans*	VN III

pigments, and the enzymes urease and phospholipase, which are considered to be yeast virulence factors. *Cryptococcus* asexually reproduces by budding, but under specific conditions, it can have sexual reproduction or haploid fruiting in which the formation of the basidium and basidiospores occurs. The vast majority of infections and environmental isolates are caused by mating locus alpha strains.

3. EPIDEMIOLOGY

Cryptococcosis was considered to be an uncommon infection before the AIDS epidemics, most associated with malignancies and immunosuppressive treatments. Since 1981, when HIV was rapidly becoming prevalent, the incidence of cryptococcosis in certain patients increased significantly and between 6% and 10% of AIDS patients developed cryptococcosis *(7,8)*. In fact, HIV/AIDS was found to be associated with cryptococcosis in about 80% of cases worldwide. Cryptococcal infection became a major opportunistic infection in HIV-infected patients as their $CD4^+$ cell count dropped below 100 cells/μl, especially those without access to HAART. Now that antiretroviral treatment has been widely implemented, in many well developed countries the incidence of cryptococcosis has fallen significantly. The incidence of cryptococcal infection in persons not infected with HIV has not changed during this time. Nevertheless, in developing countries with HIV epidemics and limited resources for HAART, cryptococcosis is still associated with a high incidence of disease and death. Besides HIV infection, other risk factors for acquiring cryptococcal infections include many conditions which result in an immunocompromised status (Table 14.2). Although both *C. neoformans* and *C. gattii* can cause cryptococcosis in apparently normal hosts, the

Table 14.2
Predisposing factors of cryptococcosis

HIV infection
Malignancies[a] (e.g., Hodgkin's disease, other lymphomas and chronic lymphocytic leukemia)
Lymphoproliferative disorders[a]
Idiopathic $CD4^+$ T cell lymphopenia
Rheumatologic or immunologic diseases[a]
Sarcoidosis
Systemic lupus erythematosus
Rheumatoid arthritis
Hyper-IgM syndrome or hyper-IgE syndrome
Monoclonal antibodies (etanercept, infliximab, alemtuzumab)
Corticosteroid and/or immunosuppressive therapies
Diabetes mellitus
Solid organ transplantation[a]
Chronic pulmonary diseases
Renal failure and/or peritoneal dialysis
Chronic liver diseases[b]

[a]Immunosuppressive therapies add to the risk.
[b]Poor prognosis.

Table 14.3
Distribution of *C. neoformans* and *C. gattii*

Cryptococcus species	Primary areas of distribution
C. neoformans var. *grubii* serotype A	Worldwide; pigeon guano, tree hollows
C. gattii	Tropical and subtropical regions: southern California, Hawaii, Brazil, Australia, Southeast Asia, and central Africa; Eucalyptus trees, firs, and oak trees
C. neoformans var. *neoformans* serotype D	Europe: Denmark, Germany, Italy, France, Switzerland; less common in the environment than serotype A

percentage of *C. gattii* infections causing disease in such patients is significantly higher than for *C. neoformans*.

C. neoformans is found throughout the world in association with excreta from certain birds such as pigeons and in tree hollows. *C. gattii* has been commonly associated with several species of eucalyptus trees and other trees *(9)*. The link between environmental sources of infection and cryptococcosis cases is not well established although there is some evidence of cryptococcosis and positive serologies associated with intense bird exposures. Recently, there has been a strong link between the *C. gattii* outbreak in humans on Vancouver Island and common environmental yeast exposures. Although these fungi can be detected as endobroncheal colonization in humans without disease, clinicians should be alert for subclinical disease or potential for disease when these yeasts are isolated from any clinical specimens.

Approximately 95% of cryptococcal infections are caused by serotype A strains (*C. neoformans* var. *grubii*) with the remaining 4% to 5% of infections caused by serotype D (*C. neoformans* var. *neoformans*) or serotype B and C strains (*C. gattii*). Whereas *C. neoformans* serotype A is found worldwide, serotypes B and C are found primarily in tropical and subtropical regions such as southern California, Hawaii, Brazil, Australia, Southeast Asia, and central Africa, and the serotype D is predominantly found in European countries (Table 14.3) *(10)*. In Australia and New Zealand, serotypes B and C caused up to 15% of all cryptococcosis cases in one study, but the serotype A was still the predominant serotype *(6)*. Only *C. gattii* strains have been reported to cause a widespread defined outbreak of disease *(5)*.

4. PATHOGENESIS AND IMMUNOLOGY

Cryptococcosis occurs primarily by inhalation of the infectious propagules, either dehydrated (poorly encapsulated) yeasts or basidiospores, into the alveoli within the lungs. Direct inoculation into tissue due to trauma can be a portal of entry in occasional cases, and potentially the yeast might enter through gastrointestinal tract. After the yeasts are inhaled into the lungs of a susceptible host, they come in contact with the alveolar macrophages, and other inflammatory cells are recruited through release of cytokines and chemokines such as interleukin-12 (IL-12), IL-18, monocyte chemotactic protein (MCP)-1, and macrophage inflammatory protein (MIP)-1α. Cryptococcal infection primarily involves granulomatous inflammation which is a result of a helper T-cell (Th1) response with cytokines including tumor necrosis factor, interferon-γ, and IL-2 *(11)*. In many circumstances, the yeasts can remain dormant in hilar lymph nodes or pulmonary foci of an asymptomatic individual for years and then disseminate outside those complexes when the local immunity is suppressed *(10)*. In a patient with a severely compromised cell-mediated immunity, the yeasts reactivate and proliferate at the site of infection and then disseminate to other sites, causing a progression in clinical manifestations.

Recent advances in molecular biologic research into cryptococcal pathogenesis have confirmed several virulence factors in *C. neoformans*. The three classical virulence factors of *C. neoformans* include capsule formation, melanin pigment production, and ability to grow well at 37 °C *(9,11)*. The prominent antiphagocytic polysaccharide capsule, which is composed of glucuronoxylomannan (GXM), is unique to *Cryptococcus* species and is considered an essential virulence factor that has multiple effects on host immunity. In addition, *C. neoformans* possesses an enzyme that catalyzes the conversion of diphenolic compounds to form melanin, which may have a biological role in protecting the yeasts from host oxidative stresses. Finally, its ability to grow at 37°C is a basic part of the virulence composite for most of the human pathogenic fungi including *Cryptococcus*, as high-temperature growth has been shown to be linked with certain signaling pathways and enzymes through molecular studies. Other virulence factors include phospholipase and urease production and enzymes associated with protection against oxidative stresses.

5. CLINICAL MANIFESTATIONS

Infections caused by *C. neoformans* and *C. gattii* have a predilection for establishing clinical disease in the lungs and central nervous system (CNS). Other organs that may be involved in cryptococcosis include skin, prostate, eyes, bone, and blood *(2,8,10,12)*. In fact, this yeast may cause disease in any organ of the human body, and widely disseminated cryptococcal infection may affect multiple organs in severely immunosuppressed patients (Table 14.4).

5.1. Pulmonary Infection

The respiratory tract serves as the most important portal of entry for this yeast and thus there are many clinical manifestations of pulmonary cryptococcosis, ranging from asymptomatic colonization of the airway or nodule on radiograph to a life-threatening fungal pneumonia *(2,8)*. In a normal host with cryptococcal infection, asymptomatic pulmonary cryptococcosis can occur in about one third of patients with pulmonary infection, and patients may present to healthcare with only an abnormal chest radiograph. The most common radiologic findings of cryptococcosis include well-defined single or multiple nodules (Fig. 14.1) and pulmonary infiltrates (Fig. 14.2), but other less frequent radiographic findings include pleural effusions, hilar lymphadenopathy, and lung cavitation. Patients with pulmonary cryptococcosis can present with symptoms of acute onset of fever, productive cough, respiratory distress, chest pain, and weight

Table 14.4
Clinical manifestations of cryptococcosis

Organs	Common clinical manifestations
Central nervous system	Acute/subacute/chronic meningoencephalitis
	Cryptococcomas
Lung	Asymptomatic with abnormal chest radiographs; pulmonary nodule(s), hilar lymphadenopathy, lobar/interstitial infiltrates, lung cavities, miliary infiltrates
	Acute/subacute pneumonia
	Acute respiratory distress syndrome
	Endobronchial lesions
	Pleural effusion/pneumothorax
Skin	Papules with central ulceration (molluscum contagiosum-like)
	Abscesses
	Nodules/papules
	Cellulitis
	Draining sinuses
	Ulcers
Eyes	Papilledema
	Endophthalmitis
	Optic nerve atrophy
	Chorioretinitis
Genitourinary tract	Prostatitis
	Cryptococcuria
	Renal abscess
Bones and joints	Osteolytic lesions
	Arthritis
Cardiovascular system	Cryptococcemia
	Endocarditis
	Mycotic aneurysm
Other organs	Peritonitis
	Myositis
	Hepatitis
	Thyroiditis
	Adrenal mass

loss *(13)*. The outbreak of *C. gattii* infections in Vancouver Island had involved several cases of severe symptomatic pulmonary cryptococcosis in apparently immunocompetent individuals. In an immunocompromised patient, especially with HIV infection, cryptococcal pneumonia is usually symptomatic and can progress rapidly to an acute respiratory distress syndrome. However, most immunocompromised patients with cryptococcal infection usually present with CNS rather than pulmonary symptoms. In fact, more than 90% of HIV/AIDS patients with cryptococcal infection already have CNS cryptococcosis at the time of diagnosis. The findings in chest radiographs of immunocompromised patients with pulmonary cryptococcosis are the same as those in

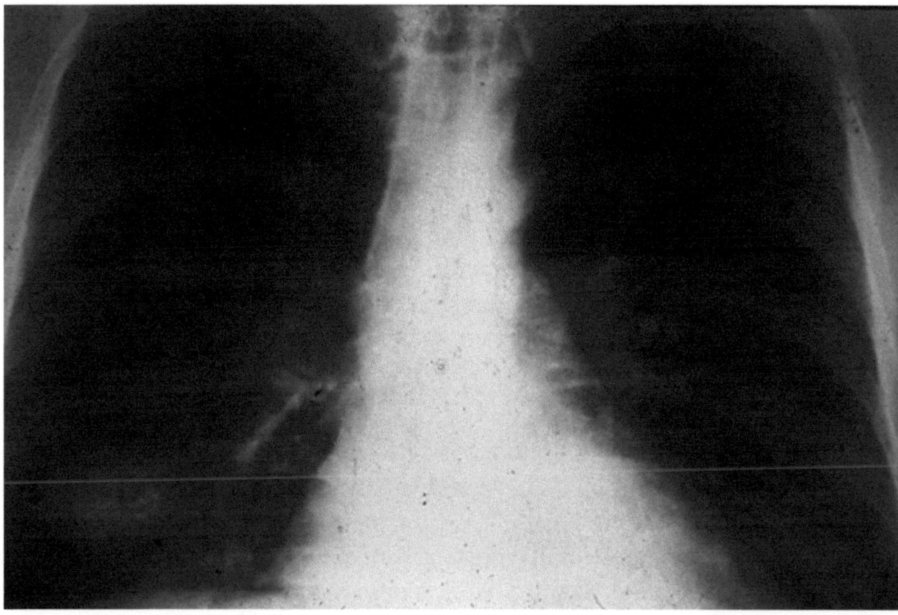

Fig. 14.1. Chest radiograph of pulmonary cryptococcosis presents as a single nodule in the lung at right lower lung field. (Reproduced with permission from A. Casadevall and J.R. Perfect, *Cryptococcus neoformans*, ASM Press, Washington, DC, 1998.).

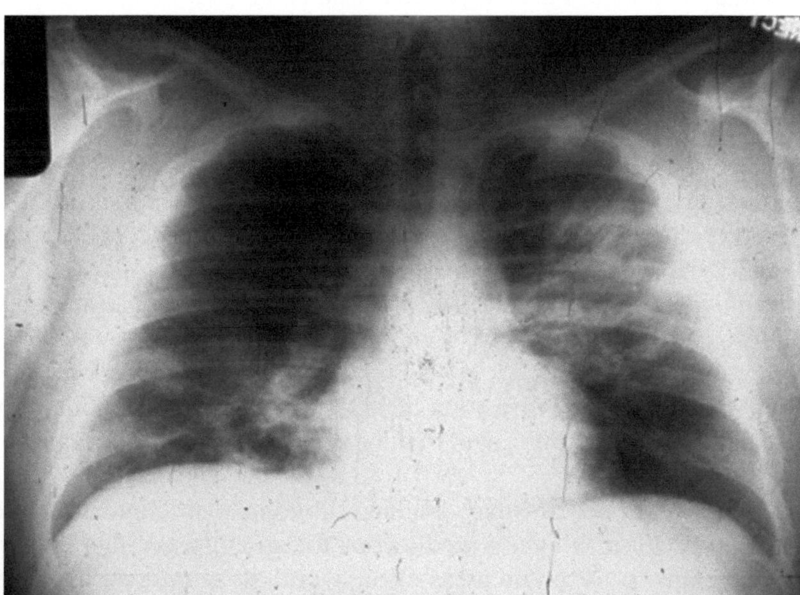

Fig. 14.2. Chest radiograph of pulmonary cryptococcosis presents as a left lobar infiltrates. (Reproduced with permission from A. Casadevall and J.R. Perfect, *Cryptococcus neoformans*, ASM Press, Washington, DC, 1998.).

immunocompetent patients, but alveolar and interstitial infiltrates tend to be more frequent and can mimic *Pneumocystis* pneumonia. In pulmonary cryptococcosis, if the infection is confined to the lung, serum cryptococcal polysaccharide antigen is usually negative and a positive serum polysaccharide antigen may indicate the dissemination of the yeast from the lung and therefore a lumbar puncture needs to be considered to rule out CNS cryptococcosis without symptoms. In immunocompromised individuals with pulmonary cryptococcosis, a lumbar puncture to rule out CNS disease is suggested regardless of the patient's symptoms or serum polysaccharide antigen test results. The only setting in which a screening lumbar puncture may not necessarily need to be performed is in asymptomatic, immunocompetent patients with disease that appears limited to the lungs.

5.2. *CNS Infection*

Clinical manifestations of CNS cryptococcosis include headache, fever, cranial neuropathy, alteration of consciousness, lethargy, memory loss, and meningeal irritation signs *(2,8)*. These findings are usually present for several weeks and therefore cause a clinical syndrome of subacute meningitis or meningoencephalitis. However, on some occasions, patients can present with acute and/or intermittent headaches, or even with an altered mental status without headache. In HIV-infected patients with CNS cryptococcosis, the burden of fungal organisms in the CNS is usually higher. Therefore, these patients may have a shorter onset of signs and symptoms, higher CSF polysaccharide antigen titers, higher intracranial pressures, and slower CSF sterilization after starting antifungal treatment. Further, patients who receive antiretroviral treatment can have a syndrome called immune reconstitution inflammatory syndrome (IRIS) with cryptococcal infections *(14)*. This syndrome usually develops in the few months after HAART is introduced and when the $CD4^+$ cells rise and the immune status improves. This syndrome can also occur in patients with solid organ transplants associated with allograft loss or altered immunosuppression *(15)*. It has been hypothesized that cryptococcal infections are made clinically apparent as inflammation is mobilized to interact with yeasts and/or their capsular antigen. Patients with cryptococcal IRIS can present with signs and symptoms that are indistinguishable from progressive cryptococcal meningitis/meningoencephalitis (i.e., worsening headaches, new inflammation noted on magnetic resonance imaging [MRI] scan, increased intracranial pressure). However, cultures from clinical specimens are always negative for cryptococci although yeasts may be present on a smear. Identification of IRIS has major implications for treatment strategies because it is not an antifungal treatment failure but a host immunity response issue.

Different cryptococcal species may produce differences in clinical manifestations. For instance, one species may have a predilection to cause disease in brain parenchyma rather than the meninges. In certain areas of the world, *C. gattii* tend to cause cerebral cryptococcomas (Fig. 14.3) and/or hydrocephalus with or without large pulmonary mass lesions in immunocompetent hosts more frequently than *C. neoformans*. These patients with brain parenchymal involvement usually have high intracranial pressure, cranial neuropathies, and a poor response to antifungal therapy.

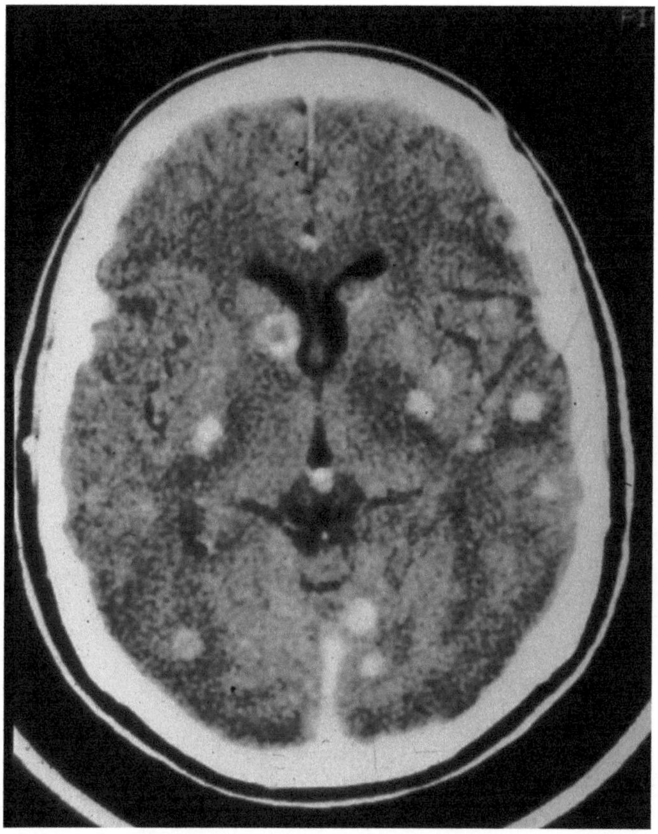

Fig. 14.3. CT scan of the brain showing multiple cryptococcomas in an apparently normal host. (Reproduced with permission from A. Casadevall and J.R. Perfect, *Cryptococcus neoformans*, ASM Press, Washington, DC, 1998.).

5.3. Skin Infection

Cutaneous infections are the third most common clinical manifestations of cryptococcosis. Patients can manifest several types of skin lesions. One common skin lesion is a papule or maculopapular rash with central ulceration that may be described as "molluscum contagiosum-like" lesions. These lesions cannot be distinguished from those found in other fungal infections caused by *Histoplasma capsulatum*, *Coccidioides*, and *Penicillium marneffei*. Other cutaneous lesions of cryptococcosis include acneiform lesions, purpura, vesicles, nodules, abscesses, ulcers (Fig. 14.4), granulomas, pustules, plaques, draining sinus, and cellulitis. Because there are many skin manifestations in cryptococcosis that mimic other infections, skin biopsy with culture and histopathology are essential for definitive diagnosis. Skin lesions of cryptococcosis usually occur as a sign of disseminated cryptococcal infection. Primary cutaneous cryptococcosis is very rare and is usually associated with skin injury and direct inoculation of the yeasts. Patients with solid organ transplants receiving tacrolimus seem to be more likely to develop skin, soft tissue, and osteoarticular cryptococcal infections *(16)*. Tacrolimus

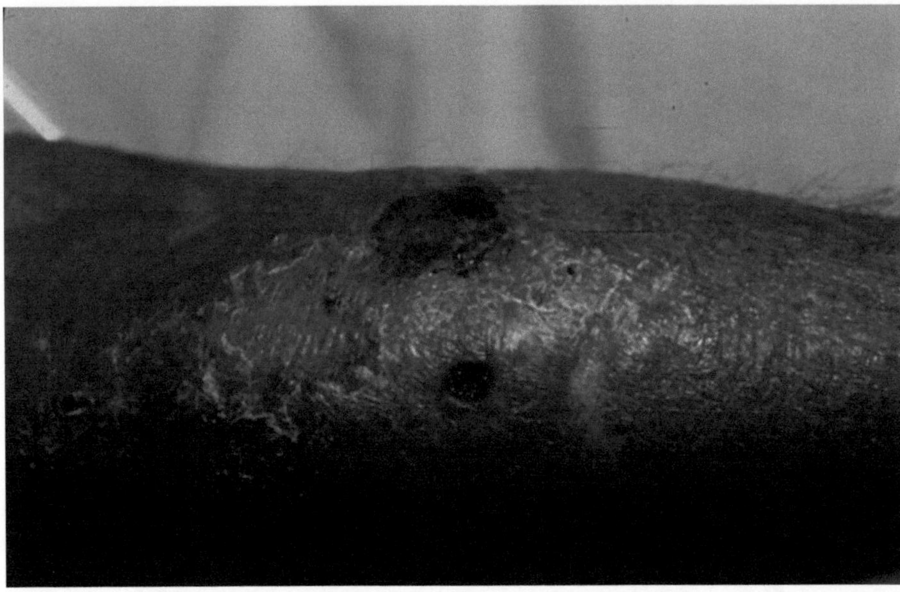

Fig. 14.4. Skin ulceration and cellulitis as cutaneous cryptococcosis. [Figure in color on CD-ROM].

has anticryptococcal activity at high temperatures, but loses this activity as environmental temperatures decrease, which potentially explains the increased frequency of cutaneous cryptococcosis in these solid organ transplant recipients. Despite this series of patients, the most common site of disseminated infection in solid organ transplant recipients still remains the CNS, including in patients receiving tacrolimus.

5.4. Prostate Infection

Prostatic cryptococcosis is usually asymptomatic and, in fact, the prostate gland is considered to be a sanctuary site for this yeast from the full impact of antifungal treatment. It may be an important reservoir for relapse of cryptococcosis in patients with a high burden of yeasts *(17)*. A latent *C. neoformans* infection has even been recognized to spread into the blood during urological surgery on the prostate *(18)*. Cultures of urine or seminal fluid may still be positive for *Cryptococcus* after initial antifungal treatment of cryptococcal meningoencephalitis in AIDS patients *(19)*, strongly supporting a need for prolonged antifungal treatment to clear the prostate in these severely immunocompromised patients.

5.5. Eye Infection

In the early reports of cryptococcal meningoencephalitis before the AIDS epidemic, ocular signs and symptoms were noted in approximately 45% of cases *(20)*. The most common manifestations are ocular palsies and papilledema. However, in the present HIV era, several other manifestations of ocular cryptococcosis have been identified, including the presence of extensive retinal lesions with or without vitritis which can lead to blindness. Further, catastrophic loss of vision without evidence of endophthalmitis has also been reported *(21)*. Visual loss may be due to one of two pathogenic processes.

The first is caused by infiltration of the optic nerve with the yeasts, producing rapid visual loss with few effective treatments. The second is due to increased intracranial pressure. In this setting patients have slower visual loss, and treatment with serial lumbar punctures or ventricular shunts can prevent or slow down visual loss.

5.6. *Infection at Other Body Sites*

In addition to lung, CNS, skin, prostate, and eye, *C. neoformans* can cause disease in many other organs (Table 14.4). Cryptococcemia can occur in severely immunosuppressed patients but rarely causes endocarditis. Bone involvement of cryptococcosis typically presents as one or more circumscribed osteolytic lesions in any bone of the body and can be associated with sarcoidosis. Cryptococcal peritonitis *(22)* and cryptococcuria are also reported in several case series. Any organ of the human body can be a site of cryptococcal infections.

6. DIAGNOSIS

Several methods are used for diagnosis of cryptococcosis, including direct examination of the fungus in body fluids, histopathology of infected tissues, serological studies, and culture of body fluids or tissues.

6.1. *Direct Examination*

The most rapid method for diagnosis of cryptococcal meningitis is direct microscopic examination for encapsulated yeasts by an India ink preparation of cerebrospinal fluid (CSF). *Cryptococcus* can be visualized as a globular, encapsulated yeast cell with or without budding, ranging in size from 5 to 20 μm in diameter. It is easily distinguished in a colloidal medium of India ink when mixed with CSF (Fig. 14.5). Approximately 1 to 5 ml of specimen is recommended for use in the India ink preparation. India ink examination can detect encapsulated yeasts in a CSF specimen with a threshold between 10^3 and 10^4 colony-forming units of yeasts per milliliter of fluid. The sensitivity of India ink preparation technique is 30% to 50% in non-AIDS-related cryptococcal meningitis and up to 80% sensitive in AIDS-related cryptococcal meningitis. Some false-positive results can be found from intact lymphocytes, myelin globules, fat droplets, and other tissue cells. Also, dead yeast cells can remain in the CSF and bc visualized via India ink preparation for varying periods of time during and after appropriate antifungal treatment. This is a limitation of direct microscopy of CSF during the management of cryptococcal meningitis *(23)*.

6.2. *Cytology and Histopathology*

Cryptococcus can be prominently identified by histological stains of tissues from lung, skin, bone marrow, brain, or other organs *(24)*. Histopathological staining of a centrifuged CSF sediment has proven to be more sensitive for rapid diagnosis of cryptococcal meningitis than the India ink method *(25)*. Peritoneal fluid from chronic ambulatory peritoneal dialysis (CAPD), seminal fluid, bronchial wash, or bronchoalveolar lavage fluid can also be used for cytology preparations in the diagnosis of cryptococcal infections *(26,27)*. Fine-needle aspiration (FNA) for cytology of peripheral lymph nodes, adrenal glands; or vitreous aspiration, percutaneous transthoracic biopsy under real-time ultrasound guidance; or video-assisted thorascopic lung

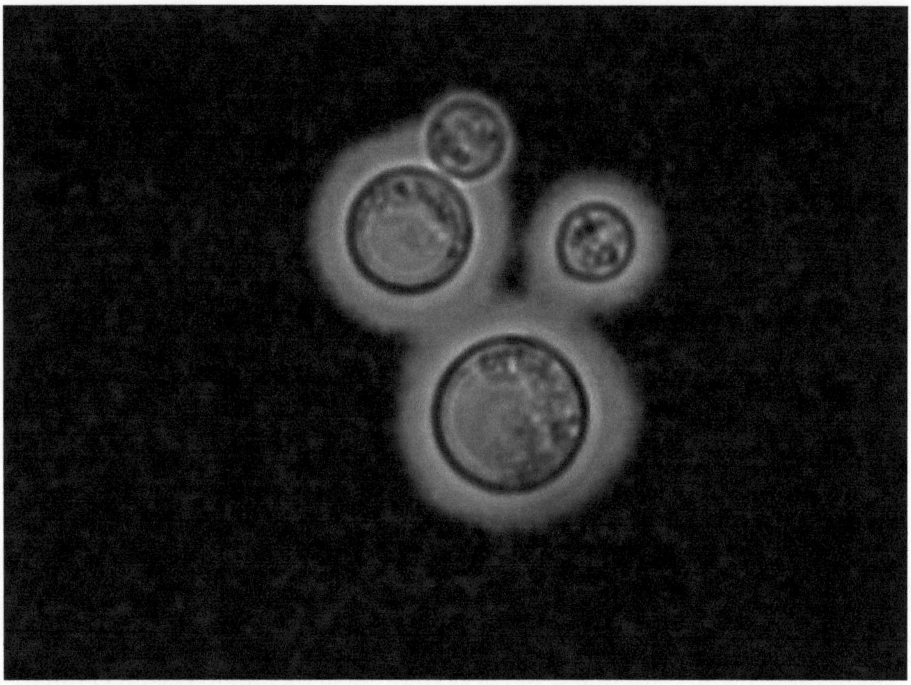

Fig. 14.5. India ink preparation showing budding encapsulated yeasts of *C. neoformans*. [Figure in color on CD-ROM].

biopsy on pulmonary nodules, masses, or infiltrative lesions can be used to obtain tissues for cytology/histopathology *(28)*.

A variety of positive staining methods have been described to demonstrate the yeast cells in tissue or fluids; ranging from the nonspecific Papanicolaou or hematoxylin and eosin stains, to the more specific fungal stains such as Calcofluor, which binds fungal chitin, or Gomori methenamine silver (GMS), which stains the fungal cell wall *(2,26)* (Fig. 14.6). Several stains can identify the polysaccharide capsular material surrounding the yeasts. These stains can be especially useful in presumptively identifying *Cryptococcus* when cultures do not grow or are not obtained. They include Mayer's mucicarmine, periodic acid-Schiff (PAS), and alcian blue stains *(2)* (Fig. 14.6) (also see Fig. 3.4, Chapter 3). The Fontana-Masson stain appears to identify melanin in the yeast cell wall. The fungus is observed as a yeast that reproduces by formation of narrow-based budding with a prominent capsule. Gram stain is not optimal for identification of this yeast, but may show *C. neoformans* as a poorly stained gram positive budding yeast (Fig. 14.7) *(2)*. The recognition of *C. neoformans* in Gram-stained smears of purulent exudates may be hampered by the presence of the large gelatinous capsule, which apparently prevents definitive staining of the yeast-like cells.

6.3. Serology

Diagnosis of cryptococcosis has been significantly improved over the last several decades by the development of serological tests for cryptococcal polysaccharide antigen and/or antibody. Using serum cryptococcal antibodies as the only diagnostic tool for

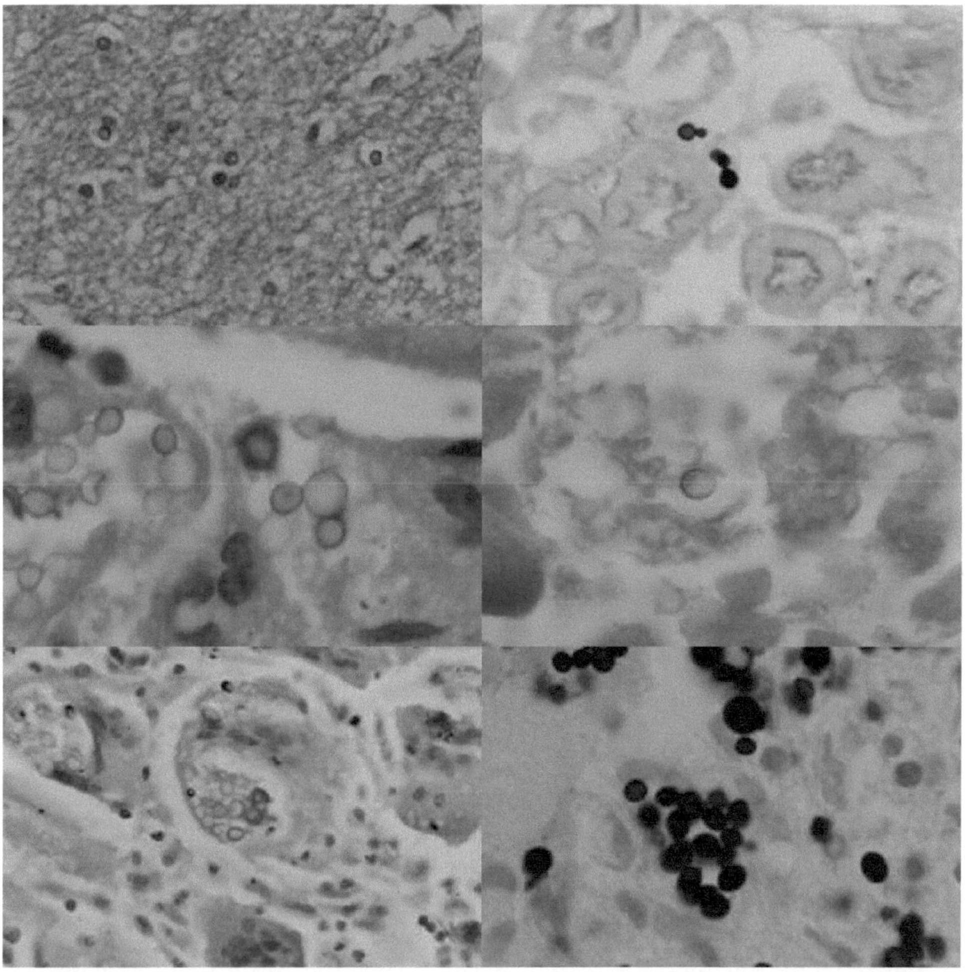

Fig. 14.6. Mouse tissues stained with various stains used to identify cryptococcal infection. Upper left panel is of brain stained with H&E showing meningoencephalitis with encapsulated yeast cells of *C. neoformans*. The upper right panel is of kidney stained with GMS. The middle left panel demonstrates lung stained with Mayer's mucicarmine. Note orange-red staining of polysaccharide capsular material of *C. neoformans*. The middle right panel is liver tissue stained with PAS. Lung stained with Alcian blue stain is seen in the bottom left panel. Lung stained by Fontana-Masson method is seen in the bottom right. Melanin pigment in the cell wall of *C. neoformans* stains dark with this stain. (Courtesy of Dr. W.A. Schell.). [Figure in color on CD-ROM].

cryptococcosis has not been adopted for early diagnosis of cryptococcosis. In contrast, detection of cryptococcal capsular polysaccharide antigen in serum or body fluids via a latex agglutination technique has been robust in its performance and is the most useful diagnostic serological test available for cryptococcosis. This test uses latex particles coated with polyclonal cryptococcal capsular antibodies or antiglucuronoxylomannan monoclonal antibodies and has overall sensitivities and specificities of 93% to 100%

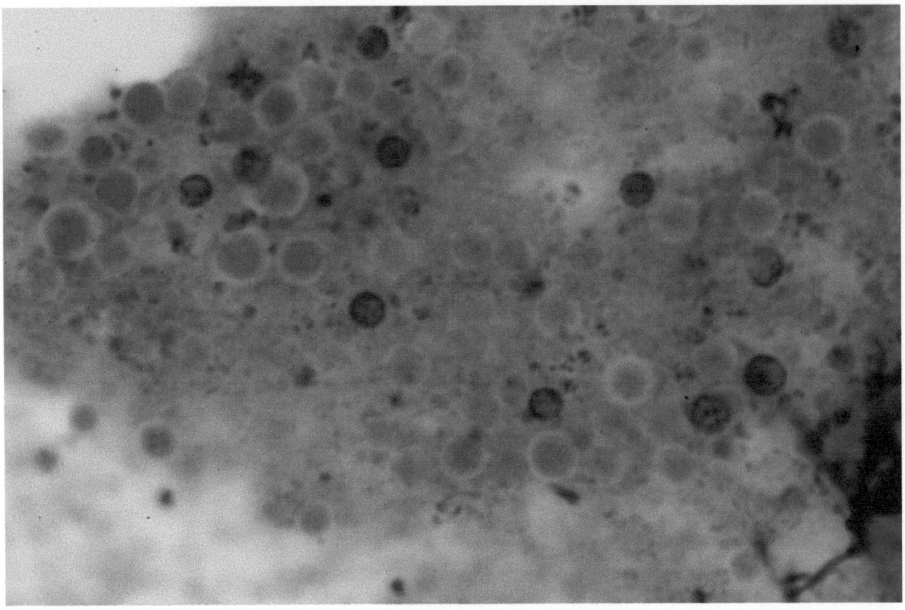

Fig. 14.7. Gram stain of sputum of a patient with pulmonary cryptococcosis. *C. neoformans* appears as poorly stained gram-positive budding yeasts. (Courtesy of Dr. W.A. Schell, Duke University Medical Center.). [Figure in color on CD-ROM].

and 93% to 98%, respectively *(29,30)*. The false-positive rate of cryptococcal capsular polysaccharide antigen testing is only 0% to 0.4% *(31)*. These can be caused by technical error, presence of rheumatoid factor or interference proteins, and infections with *Trichosporon beigelii* or some bacterial species. However, most of the false-positive results of latex agglutination testing for cryptococcal polysaccharide antigen have initial reciprocal titers of 8 or less *(29)*. Therefore results of such low titers must be carefully interpreted within the clinical context. False-negative results of latex agglutination test for cryptococcal polysaccharide antigen in cryptococcal meningitis are unusual but can be due to prozone effect and therefore high-risk negative specimens may need to be diluted and retested *(32)*. Low fungal burden, as in chronic low-grade cryptococcal meningitis or in a very early stage of cryptococcal infection, and improper storage of patient sera can also cause false-negative results in latex cryptococcal polysaccharide antigen agglutination tests *(33)*.

Enzyme immunoassay (EIA) for detection and quantification of cryptococcal polysaccharide antigen of all four serotypes of *C. neoformans* in sera and CSF has been developed to detect the major component of the polysaccharide capsule, glucuronoxylomannan (GXM), with sensitivities and specificities of 85.2% to 99% and 97%, respectively *(29,34)*. Previous studies compared EIA and latex cryptococcal polysaccharide antigen agglutination tests and revealed that there was no significant difference between these tests. EIA for cryptococcal polysaccharide antigen did not give discrepant results with rheumatoid factor, syneresis fluid, or serum macroglobulins, and is not affected by prozone reactions.

Although the presence of cryptococcal polysaccharide antigen in serum is undoubtedly suggestive for dissemination of cryptococcal infection outside the lung, the precise value of cryptococcal polysaccharide antigen for diagnosis of nondisseminated pulmonary cryptococcosis remains less certain. Generally, a positive or negative serum cryptococcal polysaccharide antigen will not prove or disprove limited pulmonary disease, but detectable antigen in serum should make clinicians consider that infection is now also located outside the lung. In a high-risk patient with meningitis, identification of cryptococcal antigen in CSF or serum is rapid, specific, noninvasive, and is virtually diagnostic of meningoencephalitic or disseminated cryptococcosis even when the India ink examination or culture is negative *(35,36)*. The latex agglutination test for serum cryptococcal polysaccharide antigen is widely used for detecting cryptococcal infection in patients with AIDS, as an initial screening test for those with fever of unclear etiologies or neurological symptoms. If financially feasible, this test has become a part of routine clinical practice for suspected cases of cryptococcal infections in geographical areas where a high density of cryptococcal disease is present. In some patients, it may represent the only means of achieving an etiologic diagnosis of invasive cryptococcosis or an early diagnosis prior to CNS involvement.

Likely because of its sensitivity, the detection of cryptococcal polysaccharide antigen in the serum may precede clinically obvious disseminated cryptococcal disease ("isolated cryptococcal polysaccharidemia") in severely immunosuppressed patients *(37,38)*. The management of these cases, in which there is a positive serum antigen and other nonspecific clinical findings in HIV-infected patients with negative fluid or tissue cultures, is uncertain. Isolated cryptococcal antigenemia in persons in high-risk groups probably do benefit from antifungal therapy given to prevent or delay the development of overt cryptococcosis *(37)*. Generally, positive serum antigen tests at titers of 1:4 or more strongly suggest cryptococcal infections in these patients.

Baseline cryptococcal polysaccharide antigen titers in serum and CSF have been shown to be factors that may be used to predict outcome of patients with cryptococcal meningitis *(39)*. A study in HIV-related acute cryptococcal meningitis indicated that a baseline titer of CSF cryptococcal polysaccharide antigen of 1:1024 or greater was a predictor of death during systemic antifungal treatment *(40)*. After initiation of systemic antifungal therapy, patients may respond to treatment and titers of cryptococcal polysaccharide antigen fall. Similarly, a rise in CSF cryptococcal polysaccharide antigen titers during suppressive therapy has been associated with relapse of cryptococcal meningitis *(41)*. However, it is important to emphasize that the use of changing antigen titers to make therapeutic decision is not precise and should be done with caution. The kinetics of polysaccharide elimination remains unclear and despite the accuracy of commercial kits for general diagnosis, the accuracy of specific titers can vary from kit to kit even with the same specimen.

6.4. Culture and Identification

Cryptococcus can be easily grown from biologic samples such as CSF, sputum, and skin biopsy specimens on routine fungal and bacterial culture media. Colonies can usually be observed on solid agar plates after 48 to 72 hours incubation at 30° to 35°C in aerobic conditions. Antibacterial agents, preferably chloramphenicol, can be added to the media when bacterial contamination is considered. The yeasts, however, do not grow in the presence of cycloheximide at the concentration used in selective fungal isolation media (25 μg/ml). Despite relatively rapid growth for most strains, cultures should be held for 3 to 4 weeks before discarding, particularly for patients already receiving antifungal treatment. On the other hand, there may be negative cultures despite positive microscopic examinations (India ink) due to nonviable yeast cells which may have prolonged persistence at the site of infection. Positive blood cultures are frequently reported in AIDS patients, and this may actually be the first positive test for this infection in a febrile high-risk patient.

C. neoformans colonies appear on routine fungal media as opaque, white, creamy colonies that may turn orange-tan or brown after prolonged incubation. The mucoid appearance of the colony is related to the capsule size around the yeasts. *Cryptococcus* does not routinely produce hyphae or pseudohyphae, or ferment sugars, but is able to assimilate inositol and hydrolyze urea *(42)*. *C. neoformans* and *C. gattii* do not assimilate nitrate but have the ability to use galactose, maltose, galactitol, and sucrose *(42)*. There are special media such as canavanine–glycine–bromthymol blue (CGB) agar which can be used to differentiate *C. gattii* strains from *C. neoformans* strains *(43)*.

7. TREATMENT

The 2000 practice guidelines for the management of cryptococcal disease from the Infectious Diseases Society of America (summarized in Table 14.5) provide a good starting point for therapeutic decision making *(44)*. Patients with pulmonary cryptococcosis with or without HIV infection can be treated with an oral regimen of fluconazole. However, in patients with severe symptoms, treatment similar to cryptococcal meningitis is recommended *(44)*.

In brief, amphotericin B deoxycholate remains the drug of choice for disseminated cryptococcosis. A standard induction dose for amphotericin B is 0.7 to 1 mg/kg per day. Liposomal amphotericin B (AmBisome) at 4 mg/kg per day can be used as an alternative treatment with a similar outcome to that of amphotericin B deoxycholate but with less nephrotoxicity *(45)*. Flucytosine (5-FC) is primarily used in combination therapy with amphotericin B for first-line therapy in cryptococcal meningitis or severe pulmonary cryptococcosis at the dosage of 100 mg/kg per day in divided doses in patients with normal renal function *(46,47)*. The combination of amphotericin B and 5-FC represents the most potent fungicidal regimen which produces consistently negative CSF cultures at 2 weeks of treatment in non-AIDS patients. 5-FC levels should be monitored to keep 2-hour postdose levels under 100 μg/ml to reduce its primary side effect of bone marrow suppression.

A three-stage approach is employed in the treatment of cryptococcal meningitis in HIV-infected patients; this can be also followed in non-HIV patients *(46)*. Initial induction treatment usually begins with amphotericin B plus 5-FC for 2 weeks, followed by clearance treatment with fluconazole 400 to 800 mg/day for a minimum of 10 weeks. Finally, a long-term suppressive/maintenance therapy (secondary prophylaxis) usually begins with oral fluconazole, 200 to 400 mg given once daily. Secondary prophylaxis can be discontinued after 2 years in patients who respond to HAART with rise in $CD4^+$ cell counts to greater than 100 cells/μl and decline in viral load (HIV RNA)

Table 14.5
Treatments for cryptococcal disease

Cryptococcal disease in HIV-negative patients
Pulmonary
Mild-to-moderate symptoms:
Fluconazole, 200–400 mg/day for 6–12 months
Itraconazole, 200–400 mg/day for 6–12 months
Amphotericin B, 0.5–1 mg/kg per day (total 1–2 g)
Severe symptoms and immunocompromised hosts:
Treat like CNS disease
Central nervous system
Induction/consolidation or clearance therapy:
Amphotericin B, 0.7–1 mg/kg per day (preferably 0.7 mg/kg per day) plus flucytosine, 100 mg/kg per day (assuming normal renal function) for 2 weeks, then fluconazole, 400–800 mg/day for minimum 10 weeks
Alternative regimens:
Amphotericin B, 0.3 mg/kg per day plus flucytosine, 100 mg/kg per day for 6–10 weeks
Amphotericin B, 0.4–1 mg/kg per day for 6–10 weeks
Lipid formulation of amphotericin B, 4–6 mg/kg per day for 6–10 weeks with or without 2 weeks of flucytosine
Suppressive therapy:
Fluconazole 200–400 mg/day for completion of 1 year of therapy.
Cryptococcal disease in HIV-infected patients
Pulmonary
Mild-to-moderate symptoms
Fluconazole, 200–400 mg/day, for 1–2 years depending on response to HAART
Alternative regimen:
Itraconazole, 200–400 mg/day, for 1–2 years depending on response to HAART
Severe symptoms:
Treat like CNS disease
Central nervous system[a]
Induction/consolidation or clearance therapy:
Amphotericin B, 0.7–1 mg/kg per day (preferably 0.7 mg/kg per day) plus flucytosine, 100 mg/kg per day for 2 weeks, then fluconazole, 400–800 mg/day for a minimum of 10 weeks
Alternatives regimens:
Fluconazole, 400–800 mg/d ay for 10–12 weeks
Fluconazole, 400–800 mg/day plus flucytosine, 100–150 mg/kg per day for 6–10 weeks
Lipid formulation of amphotericin B, 4–6 mg/kg per day for 6–10 weeks with or without flucytosine
Maintenance or suppressive therapy: 1–2 years and may consider stopping if response to HAART
Fluconazole, 200–400 mg/day
Alternatives regimens:
Itraconazole, 200 mg/day
Amphotericin B, 1 mg/kg IV 1–3 times/week

Adapted from the 2000 IDSA Practice Guideline for the Management of Cryptococcal Diseases with personal suggestions *(44)*.
[a]Start HAART 8–10 weeks after beginning antifungal regimen. Control IRIS with corticosteroids.

to undetectable levels for at least 3 months *(48,49)*. Criteria for stopping treatment in non-AIDS patients with cryptococcal meningitis include resolution of symptoms, at least two negative CSF cultures, and a normal CSF glucose; generally following at least 1 year of suppressive therapy. Patients may have prolonged positive cryptococcal polysaccharide antigen tests and/or slightly abnormal CSF findings for months during successful therapy.

Itraconazole can be used as an alternative azole treatment for cryptococcosis, but first-line therapy is with fluconazole. Itraconazole has poor CSF penetration and inconsistent oral bioavailability but has been successfully used in the treatment of cryptococcal meningitis *(50)*. It has been shown to have efficacy inferior to fluconazole during suppressive therapy *(51)*.

In patients with HIV-associated cryptococcal diseases, HAART has a major impact on the patient's long-term prognosis. However, treatment with HAART can cause cryptococcal IRIS. There are limited data for formal recommendations in prevention and treatment of cryptococcal IRIS in AIDS. However, at present, a delay in initiation of HAART for 8 to 10 weeks after starting antifungal therapy for cryptococcal diseases is generally recommended to reduce the complexity of dealing with IRIS and the increased intracranial pressure that may occur during induction therapy. Interruption of HAART and/or corticosteroids treatment may be used to control symptoms if severe cryptococcal IRIS occurs. IRIS in cryptococcosis is not limited to HIV and HAART, although it has been reported in up to 30% of these patients *(14)*. It can occur in any patient in whom immune status changes rapidly; IRIS has been reported in 5% of solid organ transplantations with cryptococcosis *(52)*.

Along with the use of antifungal therapy, management of increased intracranial pressure is also important. An intracranial pressure of 250 mm H_2O or more is considered elevated intracranial pressure (ICP). HIV-infected patients with cryptococcal meningitis and high ICP after 2 weeks of treatment have been shown to have poorer clinical responses *(44)*. Attempts to control increased ICP generally occur after development of symptoms (increasing headache, mental status changes, and new neurological findings). Treatment options recommended for managing acutely elevated ICP include repeated lumbar punctures, lumbar drain insertion, ventriculostomy, or ventriculoperitoneal shunt (Table 14.6). Medical treatments such as corticosteroids (unless there is a component of IRIS linked to the increased ICP), mannitol, or acetazolamide have some clinical data, but are generally not recommended for use in management of increased ICP pressure in cryptococcal meningitis *(53)*. Some patients may develop symptoms of obstructive hydrocephalus requiring a permanent ventriculoperitoneal shunt during the first 1 to 2 years of treatment, and sometimes at initial presentation. The shunt can be put in once a patient is receiving appropriate antifungal therapy; delaying placement until cultures are sterile is not required.

8. PREVENTION

Prevention of cryptococcal diseases can be definitely achieved by use of HAART in HIV-infected patients to improve their immunity. Fluconazole prophylaxis has been shown to be effective for preventing cryptococcosis in AIDS patients who have

Table 14.6
Management of elevated intracranial pressure in HIV-infected patients with cryptococcosis

Initial lumbar puncture
Positive focal neurological signs or altered conscious status
Radiographic imaging before lumbar puncture is indicated
Normal opening pressure
Initiate medical therapy, with follow-up lumbar puncture at 2 weeks
Opening pressure $\geq$ 250 mmH_2O with signs or symptoms
Lumbar drainage sufficient to achieve closing pressure <200 mm H_2O or 50% of initial opening pressure[a]
Follow-up for elevated pressure
Repeated drainage daily until opening pressure <200 mm H_2O and symptoms/signs are stable
If elevated pressure persists, consider
Lumbar drain
Ventriculoperitoneal shunt

This table based on the 2000 IDSA Practice Guideline for the Management of Cryptococcal Diseases *(44)*.
[a]Recommendations are not evidence-based and provided as a guide only.

persistently low CD4$^+$ cell counts (below 100 cells/μl), but this is not currently recommended, and HAART remains the best strategy for prevention in HIV infection. Although cryptococcal GXM-tetanus toxoid conjugate vaccine and specific monoclonal antibodies to cryptococci have been developed, clinical trials have not been initiated to determine their usefulness.

REFERENCES

1. Knoke M, Schwesinger G. One hundred years ago: the history of cryptococcosis in Greifswald. Medical mycology in the nineteenth century. Mycoses 1994;37:229–233.
2. Casadevall A, Perfect JR. *Cryptococcus neoformans*. Washington, DC: ASM Press, 1998.
3. Kwon-Chung KJ, Boekhout T, Fell JW, Diaz M. Proposal to conserve the name *Cryptococcus gattii* against *C. hondurianus* and *C. bacillisporus*. Taxon 2002;51:804–806.
4. Mitchell TG, Perfect JR. Cryptococcosis in the era of AIDS—100 years after the discovery of *Cryptococcus neoformans*. Clin Microbiol Rev 1995;8:515–548.
5. Kidd SE, Hagen F, Tscharke RL, et al. A rare genotype of *Cryptococcus gattii* caused the cryptococcosis outbreak on Vancouver Island (British Columbia, Canada). Proc Natl Acad Sci USA 2004;101:17258–17263.
6. Chen S, Sorrell T, Nimmo G, et al. Epidemiology and host- and variety-dependent characteristics of infection due to *Cryptococcus neoformans* in Australia and New Zealand. Australasian Cryptococcal Study Group. Clin Infect Dis 2000;31:499–508.
7. Hajjeh RA, Conn LA, Stephens DS, et al. Cryptococcosis: population-based multistate active surveillance and risk factors in human immunodeficiency virus-infected persons. Cryptococcal Active Surveillance Group. J Infect Dis 1999;179:449–454.
8. Perfect JR, Casadevall A. Cryptococcosis. Infect Dis Clin North Am 2002;16:837–874.

9. Hull CM, Heitman J. Genetics of *Cryptococcus neoformans*. Annu Rev Genet 2002;36: 557–615.
10. Perfect JR. *Cryptococcus neoformans*. In: Mandell GL, Bennett JE, Dolin R, eds. Mandell, Douglas, and Bennett's principles and practice of infectious diseases. 6th ed. Philadelphia: Elsevier Churchill Livingstone, 2005:2997–3012.
11. Perfect JR. *Cryptococcus neoformans*: a sugar-coated killer with designer genes. FEMS Immunol Med Microbiol 2005;45:395–404.
12. Lewis JL, Rabinovich S. The wide spectrum of cryptococcal infections. Am J Med 1972;53:315–322.
13. Warr W, Bates JH, Stone A. The spectrum of pulmonary cryptococcosis. Ann Intern Med 1968;69:1109–1116.
14. Shelburne SA, Darcourt J, White AC, et al. The role of immune reconstitution inflammatory syndrome in AIDS-related *Cryptococcus neoformans* disease in the era of highly active antiretroviral therapy. Clin Infect Dis 2005;40:1049–1052.
15. Singh N, Lortholary O, Alexander BD, et al. Allograft loss in renal transplant recipients with *Cryptococcus neoformans* associated immune reconstitution syndrome. Transplantation 2005;80:1131–1133.
16. Singh N, Gayowski T, Wagener MM, Marino IR. Clinical spectrum of invasive cryptococcosis in liver transplant recipients receiving tacrolimus. Clin Transplant 1997;11:66–70.
17. Larsen RA, Bozzette S, McCutchan JA, Chiu J, Leal MA, Richman DD. Persistent *Cryptococcus neoformans* infection of the prostate after successful treatment of meningitis. California Collaborative Treatment Group. Ann Intern Med 1989;111:125–128.
18. Allen R, Barter CE, Chachoua LL, Cleeve L, O'Connell JM, Daniel FJ. Disseminated cryptococcosis after transurethral resection of the prostate. Aust NZ J Med 1982;12: 296–299.
19. Staib F, Seibold M, L'Age M. Persistence of *Cryptococcus neoformans* in seminal fluid and urine under itraconazole treatment. The urogenital tract (prostate) as a niche for *Cryptococcus neoformans*. Mycoses 1990;33:369–373.
20. Okun E, Butler WT. Ophthalmologic complications of cryptococcal meningitis. Arch Ophthalmol 1964;71:52–57.
21. Rex JH, Larsen RA, Dismukes WE, Cloud GA, Bennett JE. Catastrophic visual loss due to *Cryptococcus neoformans* meningitis. Medicine (Baltimore) 1993;72:207–224.
22. Albert-Braun S, Venema F, Bausch J, Hunfeld KP, Schafer V. *Cryptococcus neoformans* peritonitis in a patient with alcoholic cirrhosis: case report and review of the literature. Infection 2005;33:282–288.
23. Diamond RD, Bennett JE. Prognostic factors in cryptococcal meningitis. A study in 111 cases. Ann Intern Med 1974;80:176–181.
24. Shibuya K, Coulson WF, Wollman JS, et al. Histopathology of cryptococcosis and other fungal infections in patients with acquired immunodeficiency syndrome. Int J Infect Dis 2001;5:78–85.
25. Sato Y, Osabe S, Kuno H, Kaji M, Oizumi K. Rapid diagnosis of cryptococcal meningitis by microscopic examination of centrifuged cerebrospinal fluid sediment. J Neurol Sci 1999;164:72–75.
26. Kanjanavirojkul N, Sripa C, Puapairoj A. Cytologic diagnosis of *Cryptococcus neoformans* in HIV-positive patients. Acta Cytol 1997;41:493–496.
27. Malabonga VM, Basti J, Kamholz SL. Utility of bronchoscopic sampling techniques for cryptococcal disease in AIDS. Chest 1991;99:370–372.
28. Lee LN, Yang PC, Kuo SH, Luh KT, Chang DB, Yu CJ. Diagnosis of pulmonary cryptococcosis by ultrasound guided percutaneous aspiration. Thorax 1993;48:75–78.

29. Tanner DC, Weinstein MP, Fedorciw B, Joho KL, Thorpe JJ, Reller L. Comparison of commercial kits for detection of cryptococcal antigen. J Clin Microbiol 1994;32: 1680–1684.
30. Wu TC, Koo SY. Comparison of three commercial cryptococcal latex kits for detection of cryptococcal antigen. J Clin Microbiol 1983;18:1127–1130.
31. Kauffman CA, Bergman AG, Severance PJ, McClatchey KD. Detection of cryptococcal antigen. Comparison of two latex agglutination tests. Am J Clin Pathol 1981;75: 106–109.
32. Stamm AM, Polt SS. False-negative cryptococcal antigen test. JAMA 1980;244:1359.
33. Bloomfield N, Gordon MA, Elmendorf DF. Detection of *Cryptococcus neoformans* antigen in body fluids by latex particle agglutination. Proc Soc Exp Biol Med 1963;114:64–67.
34. Gade W, Hinnefeld SW, Babcock LS, et al. Comparison of the PREMIER cryptococcal antigen enzyme immunoassay and the latex agglutination assay for detection of cryptococcal antigens. J Clin Microbiol 1991;29:1616–1619.
35. Chuck SL, Sande MA. Infections with *Cryptococcus neoformans* in the acquired immunodeficiency syndrome. N Engl J Med 1989;321:794–799.
36. Shih CC, Chen YC, Chang SC, Luh KT, Hsieh WC. Cryptococcal meningitis in non-HIV-infected patients. QJM 2000;93:245–251.
37. Feldmesser M, Harris C, Reichberg S, Khan S, Casadevall A. Serum cryptococcal antigen in patients with AIDS. Clin Infect Dis 1996;23:827–830.
38. Tassie JM, Pepper L, Fogg C, et al. Systematic screening of cryptococcal antigenemia in HIV-positive adults in Uganda. J Acquir Immune Defic Syndr 2003;33:411–412.
39. Bindschadler DD, Bennett JE. Serology of human cryptococcosis. Ann Intern Med 1968;69:45–52.
40. Saag MS, Powderly WG, Cloud GA, et al. Comparison of amphotericin B with fluconazole in the treatment of acute AIDS-associated cryptococcal meningitis. The NIAID Mycoses Study Group and the AIDS Clinical Trials Group. N Engl J Med 1992;326:83–89.
41. Powderly WG, Cloud GA, Dismukes WE, Saag MS. Measurement of cryptococcal antigen in serum and cerebrospinal fluid: value in the management of AIDS-associated cryptococcal meningitis. Clin Infect Dis 1994;18:789–792.
42. Viviani MA, Tortorano AM, Ajello L. *Cryptococcus*. In: Anaissie EJ, McGinnis MR, Pfaller MA, eds. Clinical mycology. Philadelphia: Churchill Livingstone, 2003:240–259.
43. Min KH, Kwon-Chung KJ. The biochemical basis for the distinction between the two *Cryptococcus neoformans* varieties with CGB medium. Zentralbl Bakteriol Mikrobiol Hyg [A] 1986;261:471–480.
44. Saag MS, Graybill RJ, Larsen RA, et al. Practice guidelines for the management of cryptococcal disease. Infectious Diseases Society of America. Clin Infect Dis 2000;30: 710–718.
45. Leenders AC, Reiss P, Portegies P, et al. Liposomal amphotericin B (AmBisome) compared with amphotericin B both followed by oral fluconazole in the treatment of AIDS-associated cryptococcal meningitis. AIDS 1997;11:1463–1471.
46. van der Horst CM, Saag MS, Cloud GA, et al. Treatment of cryptococcal meningitis associated with the acquired immunodeficiency syndrome. National Institute of Allergy and Infectious Diseases Mycoses Study Group and AIDS Clinical Trials Group. N Engl J Med 1997;337:15–21.
47. Dismukes WE, Cloud G, Gallis HA, et al. Treatment of cryptococcal meningitis with combination amphotericin B and flucytosine for four as compared with six weeks. N Engl J Med 1987;317:334–341.
48. Vibhagool A, Sungkanuparph S, Mootsikapun P, et al. Discontinuation of secondary prophylaxis for cryptococcal meningitis in human immunodeficiency virus-infected patients

treated with highly active antiretroviral therapy: a prospective, multicenter, randomized study. Clin Infect Dis 2003;36:1329–1331.
49. Mussini C, Pezzotti P, Miro JM, et al. Discontinuation of maintenance therapy for cryptococcal meningitis in patients with AIDS treated with highly active antiretroviral therapy: an international observational study. Clin Infect Dis 2004;38:565–571.
50. Denning DW, Tucker RM, Hanson LH, Hamilton JR, Stevens DA. Itraconazole therapy for cryptococcal meningitis and cryptococcosis. Arch Intern Med 1989;149:2301–2308.
51. Saag MS, Cloud GA, Graybill JR, et al. A comparison of itraconazole versus fluconazole as maintenance therapy for AIDS-associated cryptococcal meningitis. National Institute of Allergy and Infectious Diseases Mycoses Study Group. Clin Infect Dis 1999;28: 291–296.
52. Singh N, Lortholary O, Alexander BD, et al. An immune reconstitution syndrome-like illness associated with *Cryptococcus neoformans* infection in organ transplant recipients. Clin Infect Dis 2005;40:1756–1761.
53. Newton PN, Thai le H, Tip NQ, et al. A randomized, double-blind, placebo-controlled trial of acetazolamide for the treatment of elevated intracranial pressure in cryptococcal meningitis. Clin Infect Dis 2002;35:769–772.

SUGGESTED READINGS

Casadevall A, Perfect JR. *Cryptococcus neoformans*. Washington, DC: ASM Press, 1998.

Kidd SE, Hagen F, Tscharke RL, et al. A rare genotype of *Cryptococcus gattii* caused the cryptococcosis outbreak on Vancouver Island (British Columbia, Canada). Proc Natl Acad Sci USA 2004;101:17258–17263.

Mitchell TG, Perfect JR. Cryptococcosis in the era of AIDS–100 years after the discovery of *Cryptococcus neoformans*. Clin Microbiol Rev 1995;8:515–548.

Mussini C, Pezzotti P, Miro JM, et al. Discontinuation of maintenance therapy for cryptococcal meningitis in patients with AIDS treated with highly active antiretroviral therapy: an international observational study. Clin Infect Dis 2004;38:565–571.

Perfect JR. *Cryptococcus neoformans*. In: Mandell GL, Bennett JE, Dolin R, eds. Mandell, Douglas, and Bennett's principles and practice of infectious diseases. 6th Ed. Philadelphia, PA: Elsevier Churchill Livingstone, 2005:2997–3012.

Perfect JR, Casadevall A. Cryptococcosis. Infect Dis Clin North Am 2002;16:837–874.

Powderly WG, Cloud GA, Dismukes WE, Saag MS. Measurement of cryptococcal antigen in serum and cerebrospinal fluid: value in the management of AIDS-associated cryptococcal meningitis. Clin Infect Dis 1994;18:789–792.

Saag MS, Graybill RJ, Larsen RA, et al. Practice guidelines for the management of cryptococcal disease. Infectious Diseases Society of America. Clin Infect Dis 2000;30:710–718.

Saag MS, Powderly WG, Cloud GA, et al. Comparison of amphotericin B with fluconazole in the treatment of acute AIDS-associated cryptococcal meningitis. The NIAID Mycoses Study Group and the AIDS Clinical Trials Group. N Engl J Med 1992;326:83–89.

15
Blastomycosis

Stanley W. Chapman, MD and Donna C. Sullivan, PhD

1. INTRODUCTION

Blastomycosis is the systemic mycosis, primarily involving the lungs, caused by the thermally dimorphic fungus *Blastomyces dermatitidis*. First described by Gilchrist as a cutaneous disease *(1)*, later analysis showed that the lung was the primary route of infection *(2)* and that skin disease or other organ involvement was secondary to hematogenous dissemination. Blastomycosis of the lung may be asymptomatic or manifest as acute or chronic pneumonia. Hematogenous spread of the organism frequently results in extrapulmonary disease. Blastomycosis has been reported in North America, Africa, India, and parts of Europe, but the majority of cases are from the endemic region around the Mississippi and Ohio Rivers and in areas of southern Canada near the Great Lakes *(3–5)*.

2. ETIOLOGIC AGENT

Blastomyces dermatitidis is the imperfect (asexual) stage of *Ajellomyces dermatitidis*, which exhibits thermal dimorphism growing as a mould (mycelial) form at 25° to 30°C and as a yeast form at 37°C (Fig. 15.1). The mycelia produce terminal conidia, which, when disturbed in the environment, easily become airborne. Human and animal infections typically occur after the inhalation of conidia, which convert to large budding yeast cells inside the lungs associated with the temperature shift to 37°C *(6)*.

Primary isolation of *B. dermatitidis* from clinical specimens is most reliable when grown as the mycelial form at 30°C. Mycelial colonies, which are white to brown in color, grow on agar in 1 to 3 weeks. Positive identification of *B. dermatitidis*, however, generally requires conversion to the yeast form at 37°C or nucleic acid amplification methods that allow early identification of mycelial phase growth. Yeast-like colonies are wrinkled and cream to tan in color. Asexual reproduction is by budding of single, broad-based, thick-walled, multinucleated daughter cells (Fig. 15.1). The same morphologic characteristics are observed in tissue samples from infected individuals, and in the right clinical situation can be used to make a presumptive diagnosis of blastomycosis *(6)*.

From: *Infectious Disease: Diagnosis and Treatment of Human Mycoses*
Edited by: D. R. Hospenthal and M. G. Rinaldi © Humana Press Inc., Totowa, NJ

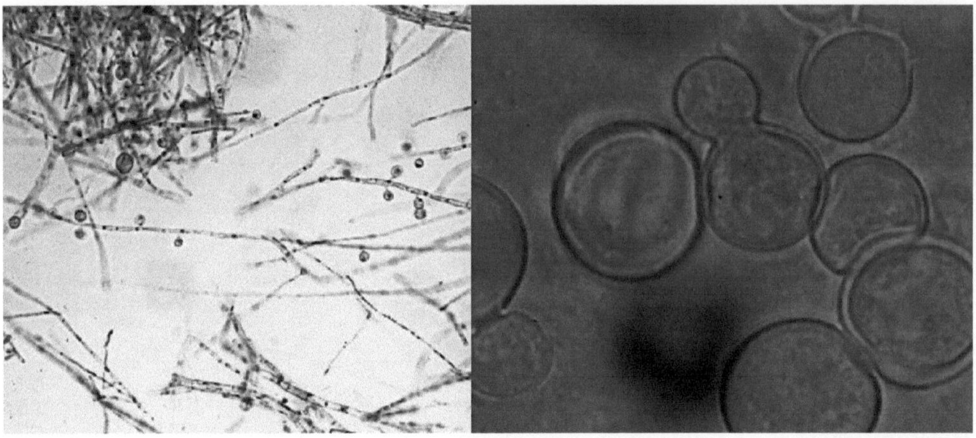

Fig. 15.1. The mycelial phase of *B. dermatitidis* **(left)** produces no unique characteristics that allow organism identification. As a yeast **(right)**, *B. dermatitidis* has characteristic thick-walled, multinucleated cells with single broad-based daughter cells. [Figure in color on CD-ROM].

Two serotypes of *B. dermatitidis* have been identified based on the presence or absence of the A exoantigen *(7)*; A antigen deficient serotypes are restricted to Africa *(8)*. Recent serologic differences in *B. dermatitidis* isolates from different regions of the United States and Africa have been noted via an enzyme-linked immunoassay *(9)*. Restriction fragment length polymorphism analysis of isolates from different geographic regions of North America reveals a high degree of genetic similarity among isolates *(10,11)*. Using a polymerase chain reaction (PCR)-based typing system, three major groups have been identified. These results indicate that different genotypic groups may exist *(10,11)*. These methods of analysis may be useful in future epidemiological studies.

3. EPIDEMIOLOGY

The ecological niche of *B. dermatitidis* has been difficult to conclusively establish. Environmental isolations of the organism associated with disease outbreaks indicate that the organism grows as microfoci in warm, moist soil in wooded areas that is enriched in organic material *(12,13)*. Analysis of sporadic cases in humans and dogs, point source outbreaks, and infrequent environmental isolations has provided the major basis for the definition of endemic regions in North America *(5,6)*. *B. dermatitidis* is endemic to the eastern United States, the Mississippi and Ohio River valleys, extending northward to the Great Lakes and southern Canada. Most cases have been reported in Mississippi, Arkansas, Kentucky, Tennessee, and Wisconsin. Within these endemic regions are hyperendemic areas with exceptionally high attack rates *(14–16)*.

Dogs are the most commonly infected animal although infection in other mammals also occurs *(16–18)*. Although early studies of endemic cases indicated middle-aged men with outdoor occupations were at greatest risk for blastomycosis, subsequent review of reported outbreaks indicate no predilection for sex, age, race, occupation, or seasonal exposure *(6)*. Exposure to soil at work and at play appears to be a common factor associated with both endemic and epidemic disease.

4. PATHOGENESIS AND IMMUNOLOGY

Blastomycosis is initiated by the inhalation of the conidia of *B. dermatitidis*. After inhalation, the infectious conidia may be nonspecifically phagocytosed and killed by polymorphonuclear leukocytes (PMNs), monocytes, and alveolar macrophages. This phagocytic response represents natural or innate immunity and may in part explain the asymptomatic cases in analysis of outbreaks. Conidia that escape the initial phagocytic response rapidly convert to a yeast form that is more resistant to phagocytosis and killing. Several virulence factors have been associated with the pathogenicity of *B. dermatitidis*. The thick cell wall of the yeast has been proposed to have antiphagocytic properties while higher concentrations of lipids and phospholipids have been associated with increased virulence in some strains *(19,20)*. Conversion of *B. dermatitidis* to the yeast form also induces the expression of a yeast phase specific gene designated BAD-1 (formerly WI-1). BAD-1 (WI-1) is a 120-kDa glycoprotein adhesion and immune modulator that has a number of essential properties, including CR3 and $CD14^+$ binding and an epidermal growth factor (EGF)-like domain *(21–24)*.

Cellular immunity in humans, as monitored by antigen-induced lymphocyte proliferation, has been documented using whole yeast phase organisms, an alkali-soluble, water-soluble yeast extract, and BAD-1 *(25–27)*. As with other endemic fungi, *B. dermatitidis* seems to require type 1-dependent cell mediated immunity (CMI) *(28–31)*. Recent vaccine studies in animal models have shown that CMI can be mediated by both vaccine-induced $CD4^+$ *(30)* and $CD8^+$ T cells *(32)* which produce type 1 cytokines such as interferon-gamma (IFN-γ) and tumor necrosis factor-alpha (TNF-α). In addition, the $CD28^+$ T cell receptor has been shown to be required for the induction of protective T cell responses to *B. dermatitidis* infection *(33)*. $CD4^+$ cells require interleukin-12 (IL-12) for the development of CMI while $CD8^+$ cells were less dependent on IL-12 for this process *(34)*. These animal studies are promising and indicate that the development of a vaccine to prevent disease in humans is possible.

5. CLINICAL MANIFESTATIONS

The clinical manifestations of blastomycosis are varied and include asymptomatic infection, acute or chronic pneumonia, and extrapulmonary disease. Extrapulmonary disease results from the hematogenous spread of the fungus from a primary pulmonary infection. Although *B. dermatitidis* infection has been reported to involve almost every organ of the human body, the skin, bones, and genital urinary system are most common (Table 15.1). It is important to note that blastomycosis mimics many other disease processes whether acute or chronic *(35)*. For example, acute pulmonary blastomycosis may be diagnosed as bacterial community-acquired pneumonia or influenza. Chronic pulmonary blastomycosis most commonly mimics a malignancy or tuberculosis. Skin lesions are often misdiagnosed as pyoderma gangrenosa or keratoacanthoma. Blastomycosis of the larynx is frequently misdiagnosed as carcinoma. Thus, a high index of suspicion and a careful histologic evaluation of secretions or biopsy material should be performed in difficult cases.

Table 15.1
Organ involvement in blastomycosis

Organ system involved	No. involved/total patients (%)
Pulmonary	369/534 *(69)*
Cutaneous	306/534 *(57)*
Osseous	116/534 *(22)*
Genitourinary	92/534 *(17)*
Central nervous system	29/534 *(5)*

Modified from ref. 6. Data obtained from clinical and autopsy findings compiled from seven studies *(35–41)*.

5.1. Pulmonary Blastomycosis

5.1.1. Acute Infection

Initial infection occurs after inhalation of conidia into the lungs. Unless associated with an outbreak or group exposure, acute infection is frequently unrecognized. Clinical

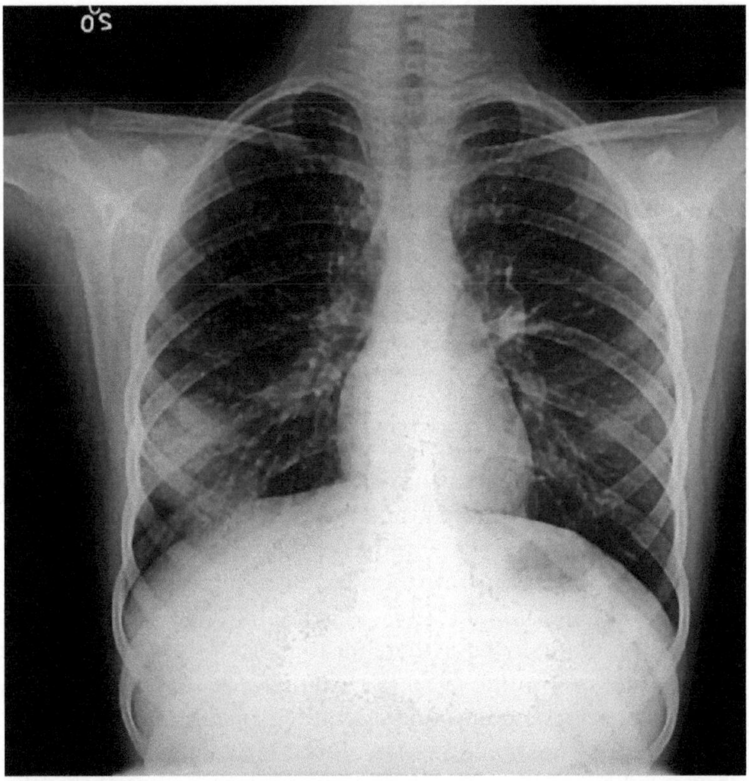

Fig. 15.2. Acute pulmonary blastomycosis. Chest radiograph reveals peripheral alveolar infiltrate that appear to be pleural based. Although this patient clinically improved with antibiotics sputum culture grew *B. dermatitidis*.

studies involving point source outbreaks of infection indicate that symptomatic acute pulmonary disease occurs in only 50% of individuals, usually after an incubation period of 30 to 45 days *(12–14)*. Signs and symptoms of acute pulmonary blastomycosis are similar to those of influenza or bacterial pneumonia. Fever, chills, pleuritic chest pain, arthralgias, and myalgias usually occur abruptly. Cough begins as nonproductive but frequently becomes purulent as disease progresses. Chest radiographs usually reveal alveolar infiltrates with consolidation (Fig. 15.2) *(42,43)*. Pleural effusions are uncommon and, if present, are typically small in volume. Hilar adenopathy is uncommon and is a useful sign in distinguishing acute blastomycosis from acute histoplasmosis. Spontaneous cures of symptomatic acute infection have been documented, but the exact frequency of these cures has not been clearly established *(44,45)*.

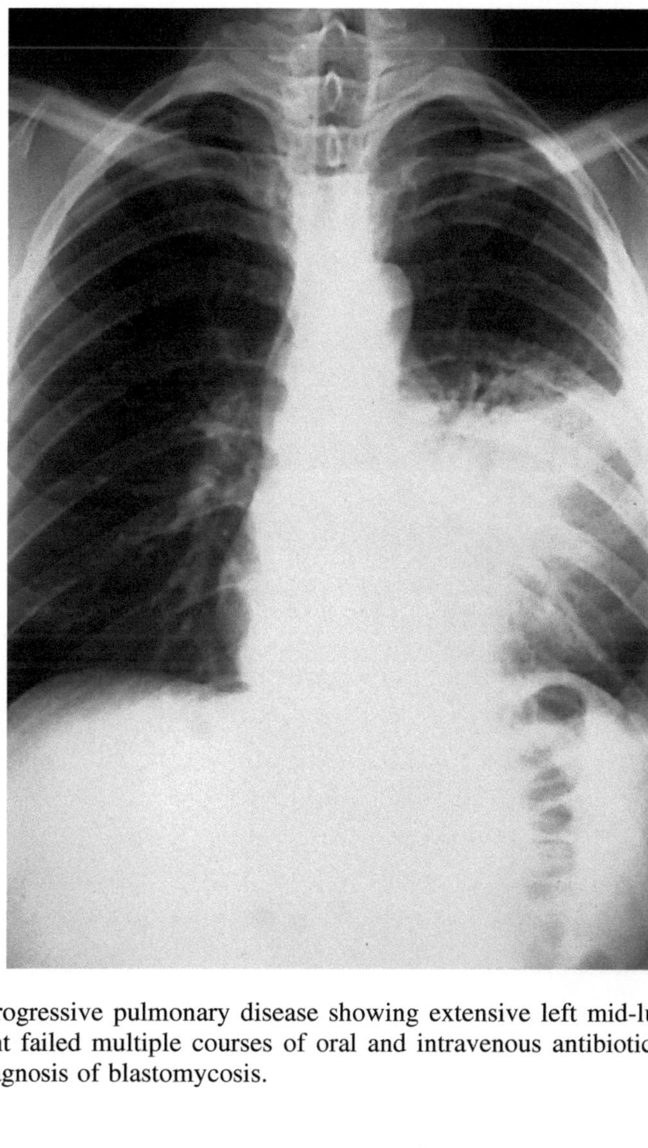

Fig. 15.3. Progressive pulmonary disease showing extensive left mid-lung alveolar infiltrate. This patient failed multiple courses of oral and intravenous antibiotics over a 2-month period before diagnosis of blastomycosis.

5.1.2. Chronic Infection

Most patients diagnosed with pulmonary blastomycosis have a chronic pneumonia that is clinically similar to tuberculosis, other fungal infections, and cancer. Symptoms include fever, weight loss, chronic productive cough, and hemoptysis. The most frequent radiologic findings are alveolar infiltrates (Fig. 15.3) with or without cavitation, mass lesions that mimic bronchogenic carcinoma (Fig. 15.4), and fibronodular infiltrates *(46,47)*. Although small pleural effusions have been reported, large pleural effusions (Fig. 15.5) are distinctly uncommon and, when present, have been associated with poor outcome *(48)*.

5.1.3. Acute Respiratory Distress Syndrome

Patients may occasionally present with acute respiratory distress syndrome (ARDS) associated with miliary disease or diffuse pneumonitis (Fig. 15.6). Mortality exceeds 50% in these patients, and most deaths occur within the first few days of therapy *(46)*. Diffuse pulmonary infiltrates and respiratory failure are more likely to occur in immunocompromised patients, especially those with late stage acquired immunodeficiency syndrome (AIDS) *(45)*.

5.2. Extrapulmonary Blastomycosis

Extrapulmonary disease has been reported in as many as two-thirds of patients with chronic blastomycosis. This high frequency probably reflects selection bias as these

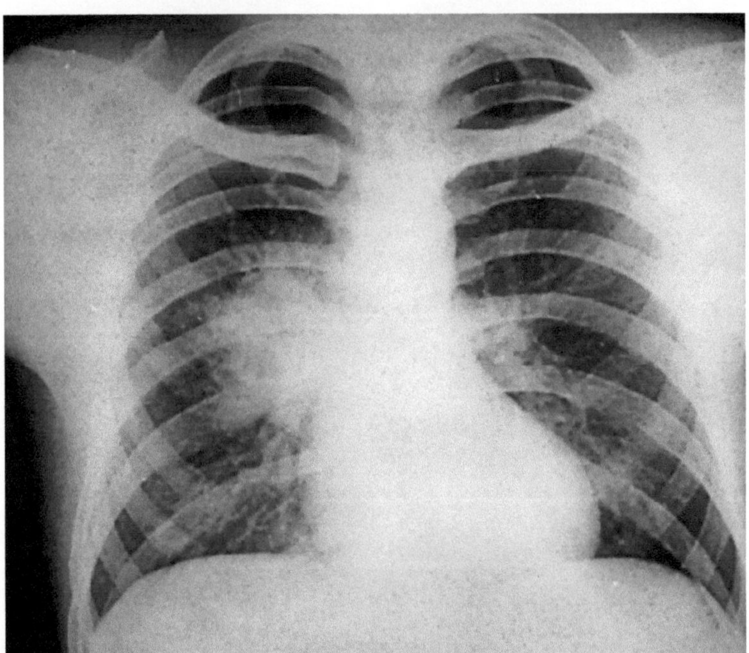

Fig. 15.4. Chest radiograph with right hilar infiltrate that mimics bronchogenic carcinoma. Bronchoscopy with biopsy and pulmonary cytology should be performed in these patients presenting with this radiographic finding to rule out concomitant disease.

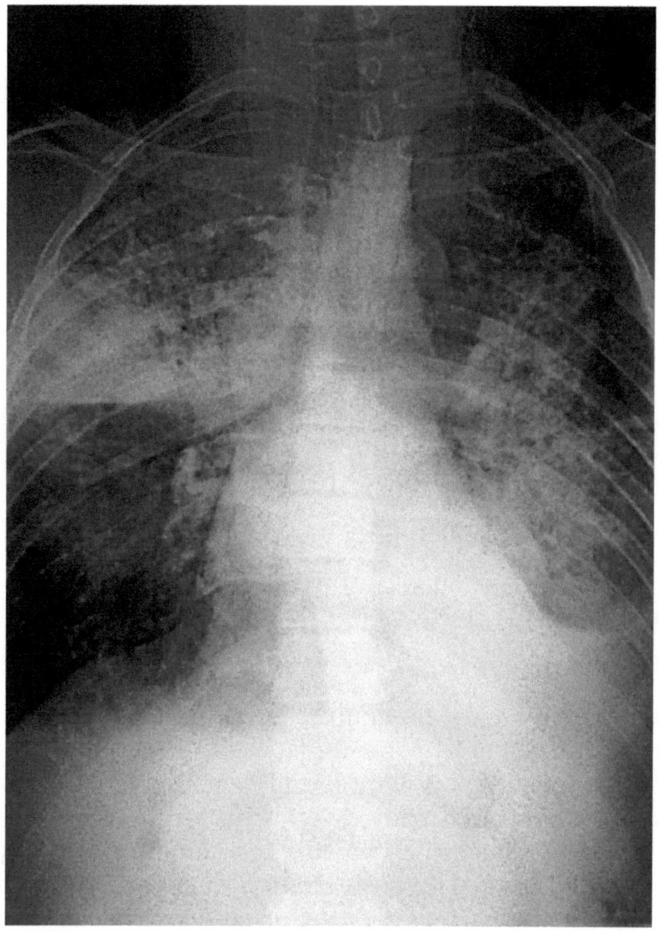

Fig. 15.5. Patient with life-threatening pulmonary disease whose chest radiograph reveals bilateral alveolar infiltrates and large left-sided pleural effusion.

figures were reported in earlier studies before effective therapy was available and were autopsy based *(6)*. More recent studies have documented extrapulmonary disease in only 25 to 40 percent of patients with blastomycosis *(15,47)*. Extrapulmonary disease is usually seen in conjunction with active pulmonary disease.

5.2.1. Skin Disease

Skin disease is the most common extrapulmonary manifestation of blastomycosis. Two types of skin lesions occur, verrucous and ulcerative (Fig. 15.7). The verrucous lesion is most common, typically with well-demarcated borders and color from gray to violaceous hues. These lesions often mimic squamous cell carcinoma. Microabscesses develop at the periphery of these lesions, and specimen samples taken from the margins usually reveal the diagnostic yeast form on wet preparation (Fig. 15.8). The second type of lesion is ulcerative. These ulcers, which bleed easily, usually have well-demarcated,

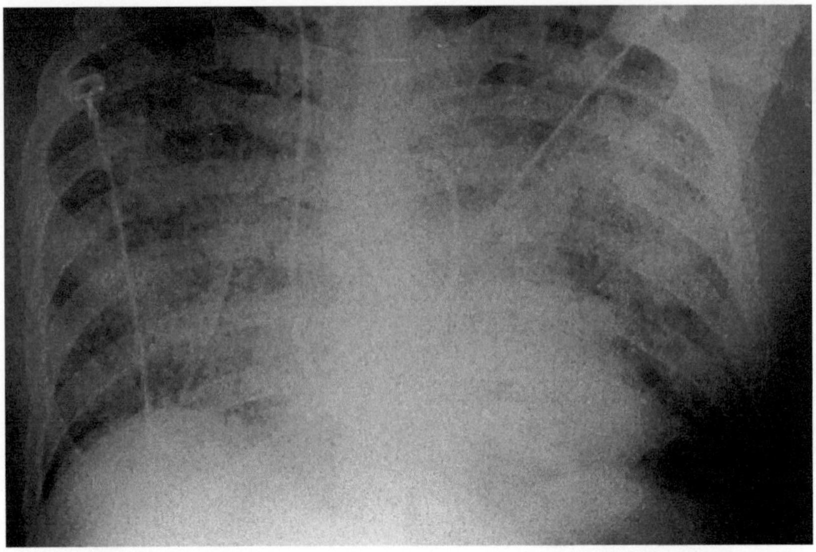

Fig. 15.6. Diffuse pulmonary infiltrates in a patient with ARDS. Patients presenting with this syndrome have a mortality rate greater than 50%.

heaped up borders. The ulcers of blastomycosis develop from subcutaneous pustular lesions that spontaneously drain.

Regional lymphadenopathy is usually not present in cases of pulmonary dissemination. Patients with inoculation blastomycosis occurring after dog bite or autopsy accidents often have lymphadenopathy/adenitis as a prominent feature *(49,50)*. Lesions may also appear on the mucosa of the nose, mouth, and larynx. Laryngeal blastomycosis mimics well differentiated squamous cell carcinoma both clinically and histopatholog-

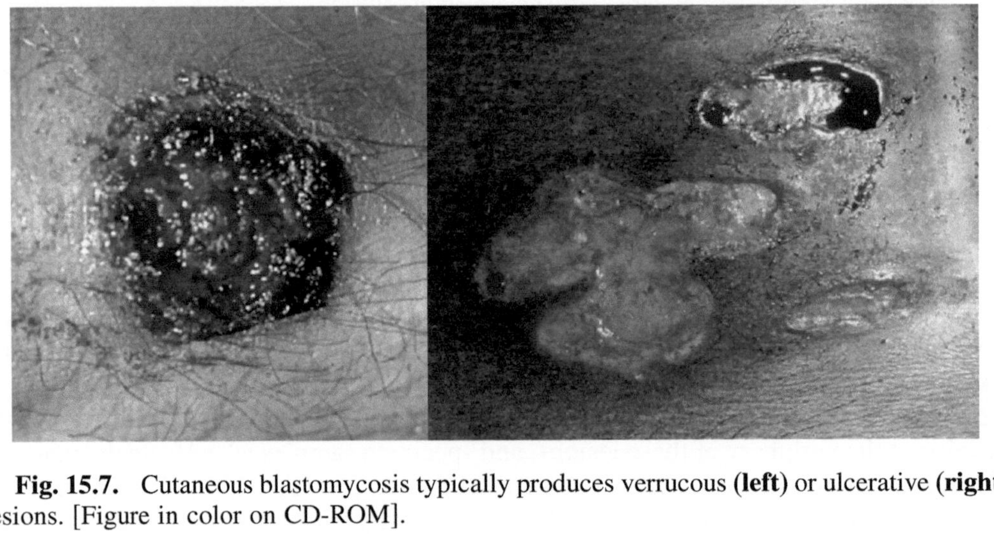

Fig. 15.7. Cutaneous blastomycosis typically produces verrucous **(left)** or ulcerative **(right)** lesions. [Figure in color on CD-ROM].

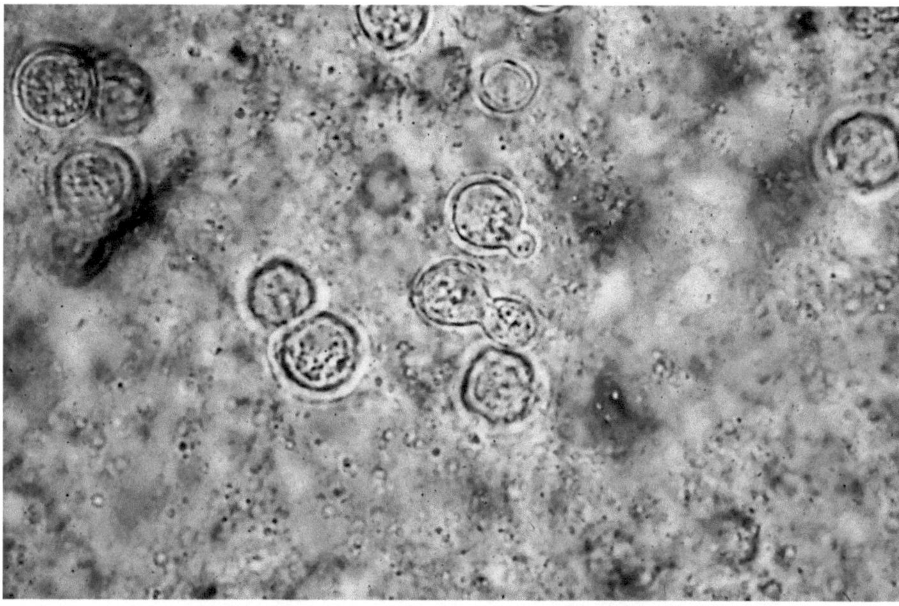

Fig. 15.8. Diagnosis of blastomycosis. This figure shows the characteristic yeast forms in a wet preparation of a skin scraping. Scraping of the edges of the verrucous and ulcerative lesions yield the best diagnostic results. [Figure in color on CD-ROM].

ically *(35)*. Subcutaneous nodules or cold abscesses are usually seen in patients with multiorgan disease.

5.2.2. Osseous

Osteomyelitis is associated with as many as one-fourth of *B. dermatitidis* infections *(51)*. The vertebrae, pelvis, sacrum, skull, ribs, or long bones are most frequently involved, although any bone may be infected. Granuloma, suppuration, or necrosis may be observed in biopsy specimens. A well-circumscribed osteolytic lesion may be observed on x-ray examination, although such lesions cannot be distinguished from other fungal, bacterial, or neoplastic disease. Patients with *B. dermatitidis* osteomyelitis usually present with contiguous soft tissue abscesses or chronic draining sinuses. Although most bone lesions resolve with prolonged antifungal therapy, some may require surgical débridement for cure.

5.2.3. Genitourinary

In men, 10% to 30% of blastomycosis involves the genitourinary tract, primarily the prostate and epididymis *(52)*. Prostatic involvement is frequently associated with symptoms of obstruction, an enlarged tender prostate, and pyuria. Urine cultures obtained following prostate massage are frequently positive.

5.2.4. Central Nervous System

Central nervous system (CNS) involvement normally occurs in fewer than 5% of cases in immunocompetent patients. Persons with AIDS have been reported to have

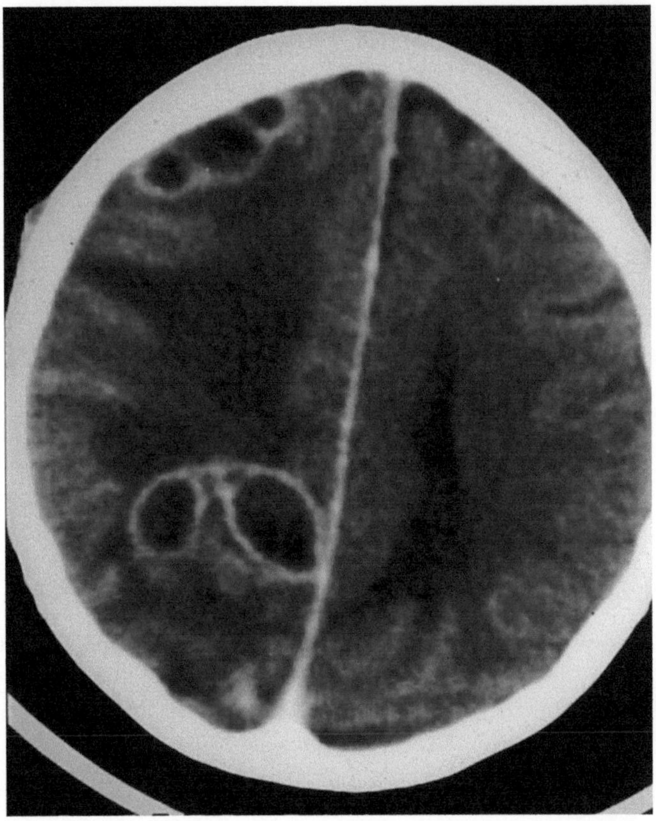

Fig. 15.9. CNS blastomycosis in an AIDS patient. Diagnosis may require aspiration of the abscesses if no active pulmonary or cutaneous disease is present.

rates of CNS involvement of 40% *(53)*. CNS blastomycosis may present as an abscess (epidural, cranial, or spinal) or as meningitis (Fig. 15.9) *(54–56)*. Surgical intervention may be necessary for both diagnosis and to prevent progression of neurologic deterioration *(57)*.

6. DIAGNOSIS

Definitive diagnosis of blastomycosis requires the growth of the organism from sputum, pus, or biopsy material. Mycelial phase cultures grown at 30°C are the most reliable method for isolation of *B. dermatitidis* from clinical specimens and usually become positive within 1 to 3 weeks of incubation (Fig. 15.1). Sputum cultures in pulmonary blastomycosis have a high positive yield (75% per single sample, 86% per patient), but bronchoscopy yields an even higher positive rate (92% of patients).

A presumptive diagnosis is often made by visualization of the characteristic large broad-based budding yeast in sputum, pus, or histopathologic specimens (Fig. 15.8). Because colonization with *B. dermatitidis* does not occur, observation of yeast forms in clinical specimens may prompt empiric therapy in the appropriate clinical presentation. Although direct examination of wet preparations have been reported to have relatively low diagnostic yield *(58)*, the simplicity of the procedure, low cost, and potential for rapid diagnosis warrant the use of this method. Cytology has been shown to have a higher diagnostic yield *(59)*.

Serologic diagnosis of blastomycosis is of limited usefulness. Complement fixation antibodies have been used for epidemiologic purposes, but are severely limited in their specificity because of cross-reactivity to antigens of other fungi, particularly *Histoplasma capsulatum* and *Coccidioides immitis*. Immunodiffusion tests for precipitating antibodies to *B. dermatitidis* are more specific than complement fixation but lack sensitivity in early disease *(60)*. Commercial radioimmunoassays, enzyme immunoassays, and enzyme-linked immunosorbent assays have been developed which offer the promise of higher sensitivity but with specificities similar to complement fixation *(61,62)*. Immunoassays employing the BAD-1 yeast phase specific protein discussed in the preceding text are not currently commercially available.

A commercially available *Blastomyces* assay that detects antigen in urine and serum has been developed by MiraVista Diagnostics (Indianapolis, IN; www.miravistalabs.com). Antigenemia is detected in 70% to 80% of patients with disseminated disease. Antigen detection in the urine was higher than serum, approaching 100%. However, specificity is reduced by the presence of cross-reactive antigens present in specimens obtained from patients with other fungal infections, especially histoplasmosis. Antigen levels are reported to decline with successful treatment and increase in treatment failure or relapse of disease.

Nucleic acid detection techniques, both target and signal amplification methods, have been developed *(63–65)*, including the GEN-PROBE® AccuProbe® culture identification test. These facilitate early identification of *B. dermatitidis* in mycelial cultures without the requirement of conversion to the yeast form. PCR amplification of the rRNA gene along with specific probe hybridization has been used to identify yeast phase organisms in tissue specimens. These molecular techniques offer great promise for the rapid diagnosis of blastomycosis, but have not yet been evaluated in large prospective studies.

7. TREATMENT

Most patients who have blastomycosis require therapy. Before the availability of azoles, amphotericin B was the mainstay of treatment. However, a series of clinical trials performed by the NIAID Mycoses Study Group have shown ketoconazole, itraconazole, and fluconazole to be effective, relatively nontoxic agents when compared to amphotericin B for treatment of patients with mild to moderate non-CNS disease *(66–68)*. Other than its use in diagnosis, the role of surgery is limited. Along with specific antifungal therapy, surgery may be helpful for the drainage of large abscesses, resection of cerebral blastomycomas, and débridement of devitalized bone.

Selection of an appropriate therapeutic regimen must be based on three major considerations: the clinical form and severity of the disease, the immune status of the patient, and the toxicity of the antifungal agent. Specific recommendations of dose and duration of therapy in defined clinical settings are listed in Table 15.2 *(69,70)*. For more detail concerning drug interactions, toxicities, adverse reactions and pharmacokinetics

Table 15.2
Treatment guidelines for *Blastomyces dermatitidis* infections

Type of disease	Primary therapy	Alternate therapy
Pulmonary		
Severe	Amphotericin B 0.7–1.0 mg/kg per day;[a] total dose of 1.5–2.5 g	Switch to itraconazole 200–400 mg/day once patient stabilized
Mild to moderate	Itraconazole 200–400 mg/day	Ketoconazole 400–800 mg/day, or fluconazole 400–800 mg/day
Disseminated		
CNS	Amphotericin B, 0.7–1.0 mg/kg per day; total dose of at least 2 g	If intolerant to full course of amphotericin B, fluconazole 800 mg/day
Non-CNS disease		
Serious	Amphotericin B 0.5–0.7 mg/kg per day; total dose of 1.5–2.5 g	Switch to itraconazole 200–400 mg/day once patient stabilized
Mild to moderate	Itraconazole 200–400 mg/day	Ketoconazole 400–800 mg/day, or fluconazole 400–800 mg/day
Immunocompromised	Amphotericin B 0.3–0.6 mg/kg per day;[a] total dose of 1.5–2.5 g	Selected patients with non-CNS disease may be switched to itraconazole, 200–400 mg/day, once clinically improved. Suppressive therapy with itraconazole should be considered in patients whose immunocompromised state continues. For patients with CNS disease or intolerant to itraconazole, consider fluconazole, 800 mg/day

Modified from ref. 69.
[a]A lipid formulation of amphotericin B (3.0–5.0 mg/kg per day) may be substituted for conventional amphotericin B.

about individual antifungal agents, the reader is referred to the chapter discussing individual agents in this text (Chapter 6).

Amphotericin B (including lipid-based formulations) is currently reserved for the initial treatment of patients with life-threatening disease, immunocompromised patients, and those with CNS disease. In selected patients initially presenting with life-threatening disease, itraconazole has been successfully substituted following an induction course of amphotericin B *(70)*. Patients with CNS disease and severely immunocompromised patients should be treated with a full course of amphotericin B. Most experts recommend a total dose of 1.5 to 2.5 grams.

Fluconazole has been used in only a limited number of patients, but appears efficacious at doses of 400 to 800 mg/day. Two factors may eventually lead to more extensive use of fluconazole: it has fewer side effects and adverse drug interactions and it has excellent penetration into the CNS, suggesting a role for this drug in the treatment of CNS blastomycosis. Voriconazole and posaconazole have activity against *B. dermatitidis* in vitro and have been shown to be effective in murine models of blastomycosis *(71,72)*. The authors are aware of anecdotal cases of patients failing itraconazole therapy, including cases of cerebral blastomycosis, successfully treated with voriconazole as salvage therapy. Caspofungin and micafungin have shown variable activity against *B. dermatitidis* and have not been studied extensively in animal models or in human cases of blastomycosis *(72)*.

In some immunocompetent patients with acute pulmonary blastomycosis, the difficult and controversial decision to withhold therapy has been proposed following the description of self-limiting infections. When the decision to withhold therapy is made, patients should be evaluated for the presence of extrapulmonary disease and carefully monitored for progression of pulmonary infection. These patients should be followed for many years for evidence of reactivation of pulmonary or extrapulmonary disease.

In contrast, all patients with progressive pulmonary infection or extrapulmonary disease and all immunocompromised patients should be treated *(69,70)*. In immunologically normal patients with mild to moderate pulmonary or extrapulmonary disease that does not involve the CNS, the azole antifungal agents, itraconazole, ketoconazole, and fluconazole, administered for 6 months have proven to be effective, less toxic alternatives to amphotericin B. Although no randomized, blinded studies have been performed to compare different azoles, and only a few comparative trials for blastomycosis therapy have been reported, itraconazole appears to be the best tolerated and most effective azole. Itraconazole is considered the drug of choice for patients with non-life-threatening, non-CNS blastomycosis *(69,70)*.

Amphotericin B is the drug of choice for blastomycosis occurring during pregnancy. Azoles are contraindicated *(69)*. The clinical spectrum of blastomycosis in pediatric patients is similar to that seen in adults. Recent reports indicate blastomycosis in children is more difficult to diagnosis and less likely to respond to oral therapy. Children with life-threatening disease should be treated with amphotericin B. Itraconazole has been used successfully at a dosage of 5 to 7 mg/kg per day in a small cohort of pediatric patients *(69)*. CNS disease occurs in approximately 40% of patients with AIDS or other diseases or therapies associated with immunosuppression. Likewise, disseminated disease and life-threatening pulmonary disease also appear more common in the clinical setting of immunosuppression. Hence, the recommendation that amphotericin B is the drug of choice for treatment of immunocompromised patients. Frequent relapses have been reported in patients whose immunosuppression persists and chronic suppressive therapy with an oral azole has been recommended by some experts *(69,70)*.

Relapse rates of 10% to 14% have been reported in patients treated with ketoconazole. Patients should be followed for many years for evidence of relapse, especially in the CNS. Relapse rates of less than 5% are reported in patients treated with amphotericin B and itraconazole. Owing to the problems with bioavailability of oral itraconazole and ketoconazole, serum blood levels may be clinically useful in guiding treatment of patients whose disease progresses on either of these azoles *(69)*.

REFERENCES

1. Gilchrist TC. Protozoan dermatitis. J Cutan Gen Dis 1894;12:496–499.
2. Schawartz J, BaumGL. Blastomycosis. Am J Clin Pathol 1951;21:999–1029.
3. Bradsher RW. Clinical features of pulmonary blastomycosis. Semin Respir Infect 1997;12:229–234.
4. DiSalvo AF. The epidemiology of *Blastomyces dermatitidis*. In: Al-Doory Y, DiSalvo AF, eds. Blastomycosis. New York: Plenum Press, 1992:83–90.
5. DiSalvo AF. The ecology of *Blastomyces dermatitidis*. In: Al-Doory Y, DiSalvo AF, eds. Blastomycosis. New York: Plenum Press, 1992:43–69.
6. Chapman SW. *Blastomyces dermatitidis*. In: Mandell GL, Bennett JE, Dolin R, eds. Mandell, Douglas, and Bennett's principles and practices of infectious diseases. 6th ed. Philadelphia: Elsevier Churchill Livingstone, 2005:3026–3040.
7. Kaufman L, Standard PG, Weeks RJ, et al. Detection of two *Blastomyces dermatitidis* serotypes by exoantigen analysis. J Clin Microbiol 1983;18:110–114.
8. Turner S, Kaufman L. Immunodiagnosis of blastomycosis. Semin Respir Infect 1986;1:22–28.
9. Axtell RC, Scalarone GM. Serological differences in two *Blastomyces dermatitidis* isolates from different geographic regions of North America. Mycopathologia 2002;153:141–144.
10. Yates-Ciilata KE, Sander DM, Keith EJ. Genetic diversity in clinical isolates of the dimorphic fungus *Blastomyces dermatitidis* detected by PCR based random amplified polymorphic DNA assay. J Clin Microbiol 1995;33:2171–2175.
11. McCullough MJ, DiSalvo AF, Clemons KV, Park P, Stevens DA. Molecular epidemiology of *Blastomyces dermatitidis*. Clin Infect Dis 2000;30:328–335.
12. Klein BS, Vergeront JM, Weeks RJ, et al. Isolation of *Blastomyces dermatitidis* in soil associated with a large outbreak of blastomycosis in Wisconsin. N Engl J Med 1986;314:529–534.
13. Klein BS, Vergeront JM, DiSalvo AF, et al. Two outbreaks of blastomycosis along rivers in Wisconsin: Isolation of *Blastomyces dermatitidis* from riverbank soil and evidence of its transmission along waterways. Am Rev Respir Dis 1987;136:1333–1338.
14. Klein BS, Vergeront JM, Davis JP. Epidemiologic aspects of blastomycosis, the enigmatic systemic mycosis. Semin Respir Infect 1986;1:29–39.
15. Proctor ME, Klein BS, Jones JM, Davis JP. Cluster of pulmonary blastomycosis in a rural community: evidence for multiple high-risk environmental foci following a sustained period of diminished precipitation. Mycopathologia 2002;153:113–120.
16. Bumgardner DM, Buggy BP, Mattson BJ, Ludwig D. Epidemiology of blastomycosis in a region of high endemicity of north central Wisconsin. Clin Infect Dis 1992;15:629–635.
17. Baumgardner DJ, Paretsky DP, Yopp AC. The epidemiology of blastomycosis in dogs: north central Wisconsin, USA. J Med Vet Mycol 1995;33:171–176.
18. Legendre AM. Blastomycosis in animals. In: Al-Doory Y, DiSalvo AF, eds. Blastomycosis. New York, NY: Plenum Medical Books, 1992:249–266.
19. DiSalvo AF, Denton JF. Lipid content of four strains of *Blastomyces dermatitidis* of different mouse virulence. J Bacteriol 1963;85:927–931.

20. Cox RA, Best GK. Cell Wall composition of two strains of *Blastomyces dermatitidis* exhibiting differences in virulence for mice. Infect Immunol 1972;5:449–453.
21. Rooney PJ, Sullivan TD, Klein BS. Selective expression of the virulence factor BAD1 upon morphogenesis to the pathogenic yeast form of *Blastomyces dermatitidis*: evidence for transcriptional regulation by a conserved mechanism. Mol Microbiol 2001;39:875–889.
22. Brandhorst TT, Wuthrich M, Warner T, Klein B. Targeted gene disruption reveals an adhesin indispensable for pathogenicity of Blastomyces dermatitidis. J Exp Med 1999;189:1207–1216.
23. Newman SL, Chaturvedi S, Klein BS. The WI-1 antigen of *Blastomyces dermatitidis* yeast mediates binding to human macrophage CD11b/CD18(CR3) and CD14. J Immunol 1995;154:753–761.
24. Hogan LH, Josvai S, Klein BS. Genomic cloning, characterization and functional analysis of the major surface adhesion WI-1 on *Blastomyces dermatitidis* yeast. J Biol Chem 1995;270:30725–30732.
25. Klein BS, Sondel PM, Jones JM. WI-1, a novel 120 kilodalton surface protein on *Blastomyces dermatitidis* yeast cells, is a target antigen of cell-medicated immunity in human blastomycosis. Infect Immunol 1992;60:4291–4300.
26. Bradsher RW. Live *Blastomyces dermatitidis* yeast induced responses of immune and non-immune human mononuclear cells. Mycopathologia 1984;87:159–166.
27. Klein BS, Bradsher RW, Vergeront JM, et al. Development of long-term specific cellular immunity after acute *Blastomyces dermatitidis* infection: assessments following a large point-source outbreak in Wisconsin. J Infect Dis 1990;161:97–101.
28. Cozad GC. Experimental blastomycosis. In Al-Doorey Y, DiSalvo AF, eds. Blastomycosis. New York: Plenum Press, 1992:221–236.
29. Cozad GC, Change CT. Cell mediated immunoprotection in blastomycosis. Infect Immun 1980;28:398–403.
30. Wuthrich M, Filutowicz HI, Klein BS. Mutation of the WI-1 gene yields an attenuated *Blastomyces dermatitidis* strain that induces host resistance. J Clin Invest 2000;106: 1381–1389.
31. Wuthrich M, Filutowicz Warner T, Klein BS. Requisite elements in vaccine immunity to *Blastomyces dermatitidis*: plasticity uncovers vaccine potential in immune-deficient hosts. J Immunol 2002;169:6969–6976.
32. Wuthrich M, Filutowicz HI, Warner T, Deepe GS, Klein BS. Vaccine immunity to pathogenic fungi overcomes the requirements for CD4 help in exogenous antigen presentation to CD8+ T cells: implications for vaccine development in immune-deficient hosts. J Exp Med 2003;197:1405–1416.
33. Wuthrich M, Warner T, Klein BS. CD28 is required for optimal induction, but not maintenance, of vaccine-induced immunity to *Blastomyces dermatitidis*. Infect Immun 2005;73:7436–7441.
34. Wuthrich M, Warner T, Klein BS. IL-12 is required for induction but not maintenance of protective, memory responses to *Blastomyces dermatitidis*: implications for vaccine development in immune-deficient hosts. J Immunol 2005;175:5288–5297.
35. Bradsher RW, Chapman SW, Pappas PG. Blastomycosis. Infect Dis Clin N Am 2003;17:21–40.
36. Cherniss EI, Waisbren BA. North American blastomycosis: a clinical study of 40 cases. Ann Intern Med 1956;44:169–123.
37. Abernathy RS. Clinical manifestations of pulmonary blastomycosis. Ann Intern Med 1959;51:707–727.

38. Blastomycosis Cooperative Study of the Veterans Administration. Blastomycosis I: a review of 198 collected cases in Veterans Administration hospitals. Am Rev Respir Dis 1964;89:659–672.
39. Witorsch P, Utz JP. North American blastomycosis: a study of 40 patients. Medicine (Baltimore) 1968;47:169–200.
40. Lockwood WR, Allison F, Batson BE, et al. The treatment of North American blastomycosis: ten years experience. Am Rev Respir Dis 1969;100:314–320.
41. Duttera MJ, Osterhout S. North American blastomycosis: a survey of 63 cases. South Med J 1969;62:295–301.
42. Sheflin JR, Campbell JA, Thompson GP. Pulmonary blastomycosis: findings on chest radiographs in 63 patients. AJR Am J Roentgenol 1990;154:1177–1180.
43. Brown LR, Sweasen SJ, VanScovy RE, et al. Roentgenologic features of pulmonary blastomycosis. Mayo Clin Proc 1991;66:29–38.
44. Sarosi GA, Davies SF, Phillips JR. Self-limited blastomycosis: a report of 39 cases. Semin Respir Infect 1986;1:40–44.
45. Sarosi GA, Hammerman KJ, Tosh FE, et al. Clinical features of acute pulmonary blastomycosis. N Engl J Med 1974;290:540–543.
46. Meyer KC, McManus EJ, Maki DG. Overwhelming pulmonary blastomycosis associated with the adult respiratory distress syndrome. J Engl J Med 1993;329:1231–1236.
47. Chapman SW, Lin AC, Hendricks DA, et al. Endemic blastomycosis in Mississippi: epidemiological and clinical studies. Semin Respir Infect 1997;12:219–228.
48. Kinasewitz GT, Penn RL, George RB. The spectrum and significance of pleural disease in blastomycosis. Chest 1984;86:580–584.
49. Larson DM, Eckman MR, Alber RL, et al. Primary cutaneous (inoculation) blastomycosis: an occupational hazard to pathologists. Am J Clin Pathol 1983;79:253–255.
50. Gnann JW, Bressler GS, Bodet CA, et al. Human blastomycosis after a dog bit. Ann Intern Med 1983;98:48–49.
51. Moore RM, Green NE. Blastomycosis of bone. J Bone Joint Surg 1982;64:1094–1101.
52. Sarosi GA, Davies SF. Blastomycosis: state of the art. Am Rev Respir Dis 1979;120:911–938.
53. Pappas PG, Pottage JC, Powderly WG, et al. Blastomycosis in patients with acquired immunodeficiency syndrome. Ann Intern Med 1992;116:847–853.
54. Gonyea EF. The spectrum of primary blastomycotic meningitis: a review of central nervous system blastomycosis. Ann Neurol 1978;3:26–39.
55. Kravitz GR, Davies SF, Eckman MR, et al. Chronic blastomycotic meningitis. Am J Med 1981;71:501–505.
56. Roos KL, Bryan JP, Maggio WW, et al. Intracranial blastomycoma. Medicine (Baltimore) 1987;66:224–235.
57. Ward BA, Parent AD, Raila F. Indications for the surgical management of central nervous system blastomycosis. Surg Neurol 1995;43:379–388.
58. Martynowicz MA, Prakash UBS. Pulmonary blastomycosis: an appraisal of diagnostic techniques. Chest 2002;121:768–773.
59. Lemos LB, Guo M, Baliga M. Blastomycosis: organ involvement and etiologic diagnosis. A review of 123 patients from Mississippi. Ann Diagn Pathol 2000;4:391–406.
60. Klein BS, Vergeront JM, Kaufman L, et al. Serological test for blastomycosis: assessments during a large point-source outbreak in Wisconsin. J Infect Dis 1987;155: 262–268.
61. Bradsher RW, Pappas PG. Detection of specific antibodies in human blastomycosis by enzyme immunoassay. South Med J 1995;88:1256–1259.

62. Sekhorn AS, Kaufman L, Kobayashi AS, et al. The value of the Premier enzyme immunoassay for diagnosing *Blastomyces dermatitidis* infections. J Med Vet Mycol 1995;33:123–125.
63. Yeo SF, Wong B. Current status of nonculture methods for diagnosis of invasive fungal infections. Clin Microbiol Rev 2002;15:465–484.
64. Walsh TJ, Larone DH, Schell WA, Mitchell TG. *Histoplasma, Blastomyces, Coccidioides,* and other dimorphic fungi causing systemic mycoses. In: Murray PR, Barron EJ, Jorgensen JH, Pfaller MA, Yolken RH, eds. Manual of clinical microbiology. 8th Ed. Washington, DC: ASM Press, 2003:1781–1797.
65. Lindsey MD, Hurst SF, Iqbal NJ, Morrison CJ. Rapid identification of dimorphic and yeast-like fungal pathogens using specific DNA probes. J Clin Microbiol 2001;39:3505–3511.
66. Treatment of blastomycosis and histoplasmosis with ketoconazole. Results of a prospective randomized clinical trial. National Institute of Allergy and Infectious Diseases Mycoses Study Group. Ann Intern Med 1985;103:861–872.
67. Dismukes WE, Bradsher RW, Cloud GC, et al. Itraconazole therapy for blastomycosis and histoplasmosis. Am J Med 1992;93:489–497.
68. Pappas PG, Bradsher RW, Kauffman CA, et al. Treatment of blastomycosis with higher dose fluconazole. Clin Infect Dis 1997;25:200–205.
69. Chapman SW, Bradsher RW, Campbell GD, Pappas PG, Kauffman CA. Practice guidelines for the management of patients with blastomycosis. Clin Infect Dis 2000;30:679–683.
70. Bradsher RW. Histoplasmosis and blastomycosis. Clin Infect Dis 1996;22:S102–S111.
71. Sugar AM, Liu XP. Efficacy of voriconazole in treatment of murine pulmonary blastomycosis. Antimicrob Agents Chemother 2001;45:601–604.
72. Espinel-Ingroff A. Comparison of in vitro activities of the new triazole SCH56592 and the echinocandins MK-0991 (L-743,872) and LY303366 against opportunistic filamentous dimorphic fungi and yeasts. J Clin Microbiol 1998;36:2950–2956.

SUGGESTED READINGS

Bradsher RW. Blastomycosis. In: Dismukes WE, Pappas PG, Sobel JD, eds. Clinical mycology. New York: Oxford University Press, 2003:299–310.

Bradsher RW, Chapman SW, Pappas PG. Blastomycosis. Infect Dis Clin N Am 2003;17:21–40.

Chapman SW. *Blastomyces dermatitidis*. In: Mandell GL, Bennett JE, Dolin R, eds. Mandell, Douglas, and Bennett's principles and practices of infectious diseases. 6th Ed. Philadelphia: Elsevier Churchill Livingstone, 2005:3026–3040.

16
Coccidioidomycosis

Royce H. Johnson, MD and Shehla Baqi, MD

1. INTRODUCTION

Coccidioidomycosis was first described in 1892, in Buenos Aires by Posadas and Wernicke *(1,2)*. They thought that the individual in their case report suffered from a malignant disease with a likely infectious cause. Organisms seen microscopically were mistakenly thought to be parasites. The disease was next described in San Francisco in 1896 by Rixford and Gilchrist, whose paper was the first extensive study of coccidioidomycosis *(3)*. They better understood that this was an infectious illness and were the first to appreciate the importance of the parasite as the agent of a new and distinctive disease. In 1900, Williams Ophuls began his work on coccidioidal disease. Although he noted the "protozoa" of Rixford and Gilchrist in pathological sections, he discovered that culture of the organism always produced colonies of a mould, what we now know to be the mycelial (saprobic) growth of *Coccidioides*. The life cycle was roughly outlined in a preliminary report and the fungus given the name of *Coccidioides immitis (4)*. During 1925–1936, the early pathologic, epidemiologic, and mycologic studies were completed. Montenegro reported the first recovery of *Coccidioides immitis* from blood *(5)*. Coccidioidal infection in farm animals was described by Beck *(6)*. Meningitis was described first pathologically and subsequently clinically in the early part of the 20th century *(7,8)*. Two important observations were also made during this period; that the lung is the portal of entry and that *Coccidioides immitis* can be isolated from soil *(9,10)*.

Coccidioidomycosis was considered to be a rare and fatal infection until an accidental laboratory exposure of a medical student at Stanford University resulted in only a transient pulmonary infection. This led to a reassessment of the natural history of coccidioidal infection. The work in Kern County by Dr. Myrnie Gifford on a local respiratory illness in the San Joaquin Valley of California, known as Valley Fever, eventually elucidated the primary infection as being predominantly pulmonary *(11)*. During the latter part of the 1930s and 1940s, the natural history of the primary illness and the utility of the skin test and serology were developed by Charles E. Smith and co-workers. William Winn and Hans Einstein made further contributions to disease description and therapy with amphotericin B deoxycholate, both intravenously and intrathecally

From: *Infectious Disease: Diagnosis and Treatment of Human Mycoses*
Edited by: D. R. Hospenthal and M. G. Rinaldi © Humana Press Inc., Totowa, NJ

for meningitis. By the 1950s, the clinical spectrum of coccidioidal infection was well described, with the publication of an excellent monograph by Fiese *(12)*.

2. ETIOLOGIC AGENTS

Kingdom: Fungi

Phylum: Ascomycota

Class: Euascomycetes

Order: Onygenales

Family: Onygenaceae

Genus: *Coccidioides*

Coccidioides was originally described as noted above as one species, *C. immitis*. More recently, two genetically distinct populations of *Coccidioides* have been described, *Coccidioides immitis* and *Coccidioides posadasii*, correlating to separate endemic regions. Currently the *C. immitis* is maintained as the name of isolates that are

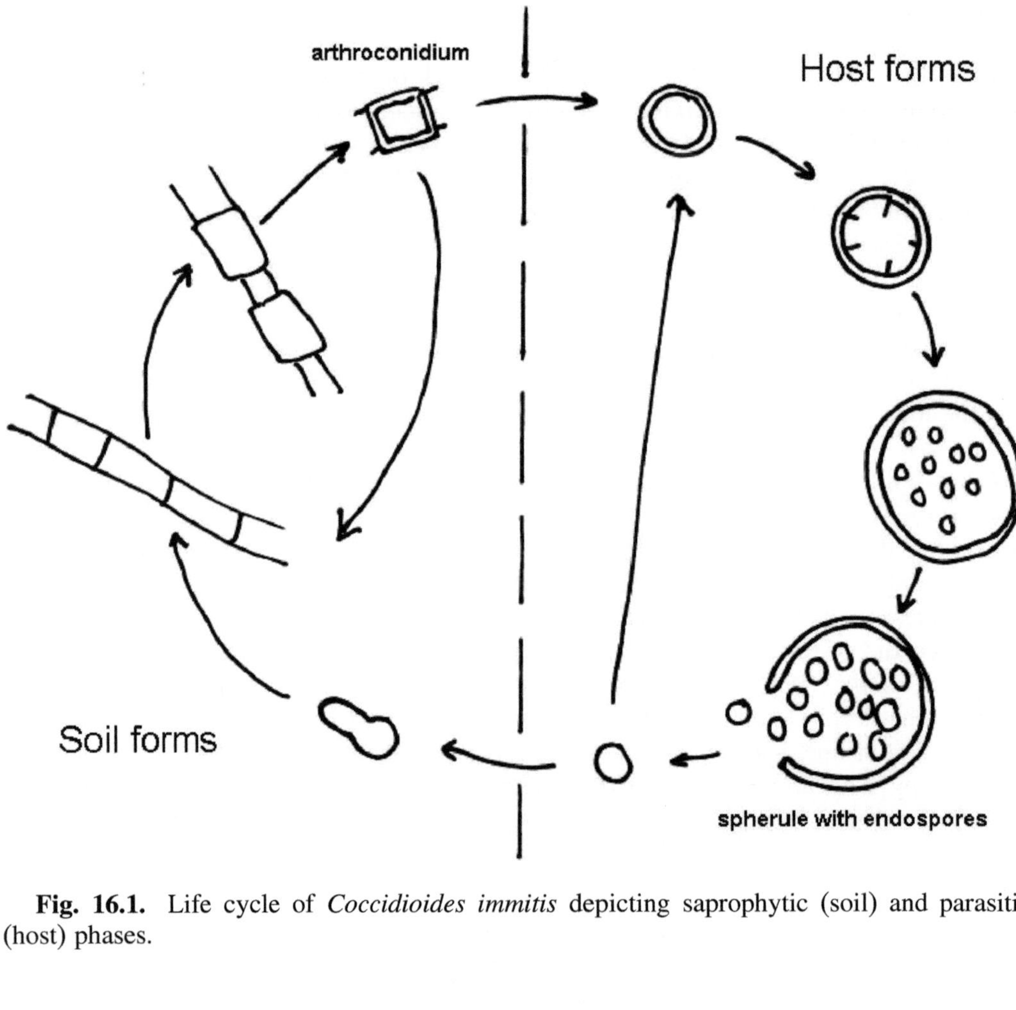

Fig. 16.1. Life cycle of *Coccidioides immitis* depicting saprophytic (soil) and parasitic (host) phases.

predominately found in California. The new species, *C. posadasii*, is predominately found in Texas, Mexico, Central America, and South America. Both species are found in Arizona *(13)*. *Coccidioides* of both species, however, show few phenotypic differences and are mycologically and clinically indistinguishable. *Coccidioides* is a thermal dimorphic fungus that exists either as a mycelium or a spherule. The fungus is found as far North as the northern central valley in California and as far South as Argentina, the place of its original description. The fungus grows in conditions where the soil has a relatively high salinity, and in a climate that has mild winters with few freezes and hot dry summers *(14)*. Under these ideal conditions, the fungus grows in isolated pockets as a mycelium by apical extension. These mycelia produce specialized aerial hyphae that segment and form arthroconidia. The connecting links between arthroconidia are quite fragile and separate easily with minimal mechanical force or air turbulence. The arthroconidia become airborne in a form capable of deposition in the lungs if inhaled, and can travel substantial distances, perhaps as far as 75 miles or more. These arthroconidia, if they find an appropriate soil niche, can reestablish the saprophytic phase. However, if they are inhaled by an appropriate host, they undergo transformation from arthroconidia into spherules. Spherules reproduce by endosporulation, a process whereby the growing spherule is subdivided into numerous subcompartments, each of which become viable daughter cells or endospores. The spherule eventually ruptures, releasing endospores, each of which may continue to propagate in tissue or revert to mycelial growth in soil or on growth media (Fig. 16.1).

3. EPIDEMIOLOGY

The disease was first described in Argentina, but other foci of infection in South America and Central America also exist. *Coccidioides* species are found solely in the Western Hemisphere, in the "lower Sonoran life zone" *(15)*. The majority of the soils that support the organism are found in North America, particularly in the southwestern United States and northwestern Mexico. The areas of greatest endemicity are in the Southern San Joaquin Valley and south central Arizona. The disease extends to the Northern Central Valley in California and as far as Utah in the Great Plains *(16)*. The total number of infections per year is not known, but prevalence surveys in the 1950s of school-age children in California's central valley suggested an annual risk of infection of 15%. More recent estimates from California and Arizona have indicated that the risk has declined to 3% or less *(17,18)*. It has been estimated that in the United States there are approximately 100,000 infections annually *(19)*. There has been a recent increase in the reported number of patients per year that is believed to be due to changes in demographics and medicine. Regions in which coccidioidomycosis is endemic have experienced a tremendous increase in their population. In 2005, it was estimated the populations of southern Arizona and southern California increased by greater than 7 million inhabitants. In addition, there is greater recognition of the disease in patients with compromised cellular immunity and in the elderly, who are more likely to have more severe disease. It appears, however, that the absolute incidence of disease has also increased, particularly during the epidemics described in the 1990s and in the first 2 years of the new millennium *(20–23)*.

4. PATHOGENESIS AND IMMUNOLOGY

Virtually all infections result from inhalation of arthroconidia. Inhaled arthroconidia transform into spherules, an inflammatory response ensues, and a local pulmonary lesion develops. In some infections, the *Coccidioides* species gain access to the vascular space, leaving the lungs and disseminating to other parts of the body. Control of coccidioidomycosis is predominantly cell mediated, with more severe infections seen in T-cell deficient patients *(24–26)*. In addition, in vitro observations have shown that innate cellular responses, mediated by mononuclear cells or natural killer cells, may slow fungal proliferation after infection *(27)*. It is conceivable that interleukin (IL)-12, IL-23, and interferon gamma may play an important role in protective immunity in coccidioidomycosis as recently demonstrated in paracoccidioidomycosis and histoplasmosis *(28,29)*.

5. CLINICAL MANIFESTATIONS

5.1. Pulmonary

Coccidioidomycosis most commonly presents as primary pulmonary disease. The first symptoms of primary infection usually appear 7 to 21 days after infection, although infection is asymptomatic 60% of the time. In patients presenting with symptomatic disease, the majority present with an influenza-like syndrome. Of the 40% of total infections with symptoms, only one out of four is diagnosed; the majority of these present with pneumonic or pleural disease. There are a number of pulmonary complications of primary coccidioidomycosis. The most common is severe and persistent pneumonia, with radiographic and clinical findings of pneumonic disease for greater than 6 weeks. Progressive primary coccidioidomycosis is a syndrome in which the patient has resolution of his or her pulmonary parenchymal disease with persistence of his or her hilar and mediastinal lymphadenitis. Rare cases of progressive fibrocavitary coccidioidomycosis, which often resembles pulmonary tuberculosis, are also described. Solitary thin-walled pulmonary cavities are a frequent complication (see Fig. 5.11, Chapter 5). Residual nodules are often confused with a neoplasm, particularly when individuals with unrecognized primary coccidioidomycosis present with a residual nodule on routine chest radiograph long after the time of infection *(30)*. Modest amounts of pleural fibrosis, a residual of the primary infection, may also be seen. Cavitary disease may rupture into the pleural space causing coccidioidal empyema, not to be confused with simple pleural effusions which may occur as part of the primary disease process. Symptoms prevalent in primary coccidioidomycosis include fever (76%), cough (73%), chest pain (44%), fatigue (38%), erythema nodosum (26 %), myalgias (23%), shortness of breath (22%), sputum production (22%), chills (21%), headache (21%), night sweats (21%), and other rashes (14%) *(31)*. Radiographic findings in primary coccidioidomycosis typically include infiltrate only (70%), infiltrate with hilar adenopathy (10%), or infiltrate with effusion (10%) (Figs. 16.2 through 16.5). Lung cavities are present in about 8% of adults, but are less common in children. Approximately 10% of individuals will have a negative chest radiograph at diagnosis. Skin manifestations develop as part of the primary illness, most often as a transient nonpruritic fine papular rash. Erythema nodosum is

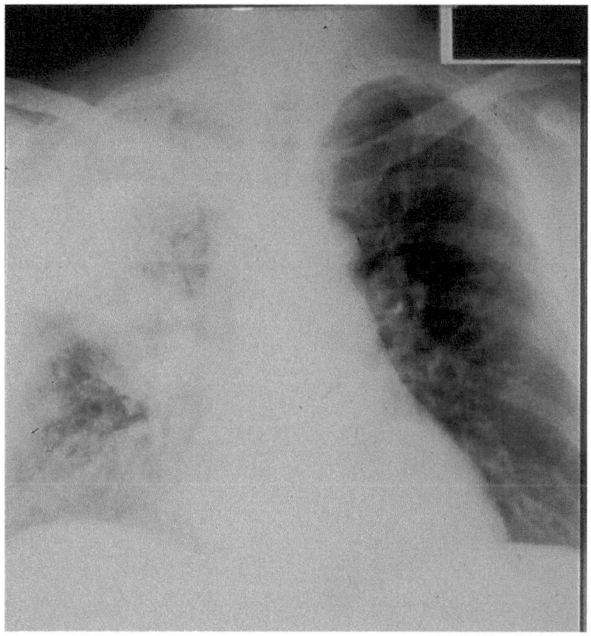

Fig. 16.2. Right upper lobe dense consolidation with associated right hilar adenopathy.

fairly common in primary coccidioidal infection, with a strong predilection for women (Fig. 16.6). Less commonly, erythema multiforme and erythema sweetobullosum are seen *(32,33)*. Migratory arthralgias are common; the triad of fever, erythema nodosum, and arthralgias has been referred to as "desert rheumatism." Rarely, pulmonary coccidioidomycosis may present as a bronchial mass found on bronchoscopy. Chronic fibrocavitary pneumonia can occur, commonly in association with diabetes or preexisting pulmonary fibrosis *(34)*. Miliary disease with coccidioidomycosis is seen with significant frequency in the endemic area, where miliary coccidioidomycosis may be 10 times as frequent as miliary tuberculosis. Overwhelming miliary and/or alveolar coccidioidomycosis can result in respiratory failure. Human immunodeficiency virus (HIV)-infected patients often have a fulminant presentation, particularly when $CD4^+$ T lymphocyte counts are less than 100 cells/μl. Probably the most common cause of death in the endemic area from pulmonary coccidioidomycosis is respiratory failure, although most coccidioidal respiratory infections resolve within several weeks to months without complications.

5.2. Disseminated Disease

The rate of dissemination of coccidioidomycosis is highly dependent on the infected host. The majority of disseminated disease occurs in individuals with antecedent symptomatic pulmonary infection. However, in a minority of patients disseminated disease presents without obvious primary pulmonary infection. Risk factors for dissemination include the extremes of age, male sex, African American or Filipino ancestry, tobacco smoking, and low social economic status *(35,36)*. Persons with

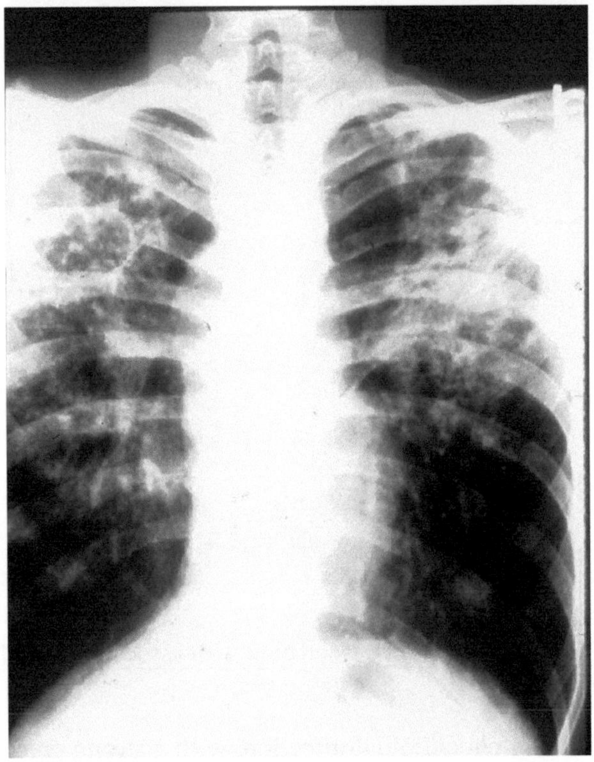

Fig. 16.3. Fibrocavitary changes involving both upper lobes. Right upper lobe cavity with airfluid level.

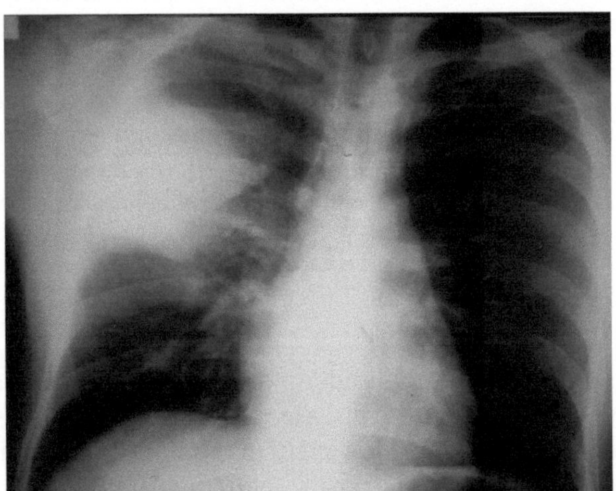

Fig. 16.4. Right upper lobe pleural-based mass with surrounding infiltrate.

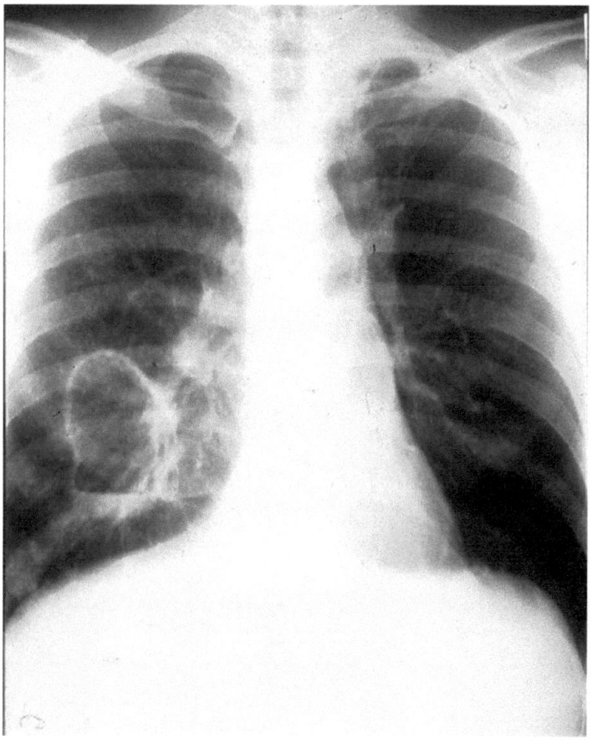

Fig. 16.5. Right middle lobe giant cavity with air-fluid level and associated infiltrate.

immunodeficiency, including that seen with advanced HIV infection, high-dose corticosteroid therapy, Hodgkin's lymphoma and solid organ or bone marrow transplantation, are at greater risk of dissemination *(26,37–41)*. Pregnancy also predisposes to individuals to disseminated disease *(42,43)*. The majority of dissemination is to skin, subcutaneous tissue, bone and joints. These sites taken together represent more than 50% of disseminated disease. Unfortunately, the single most common site of dissemination is the meninges. Cutaneous dissemination has a variable clinical appearance; perhaps the most characteristic is one or more verrucous lesions, which may vary in size from a few millimeters to a few centimeters (Fig. 16.7). Subcutaneous tissue infection, which usually presents as a cold abscess, is also seen with some frequency. Infections of virtually all joints have been described. Infections of the knee, elbow, wrist, and ankle are seen, with the knee most commonly involved *(44–46)*. Dissemination similarly has been described in almost every bone. Particularly common are infections of the axial skeleton, the pelvic bones, tibia, and femur. It is not unusual to see osteomyelitis and joint involvement in the same patient. Single bone or joint infections are most common but multiple sites may be involved, particularly in African American males. The most severe disseminated manifestation of coccidioidomycosis is meningitis. This is the single most common dissemination site in Caucasian and Latino males. Untreated, meningitis is fatal within a few months, although there are rare reports of survival for 2 or more years *(47)*. Meningitis usually develops within

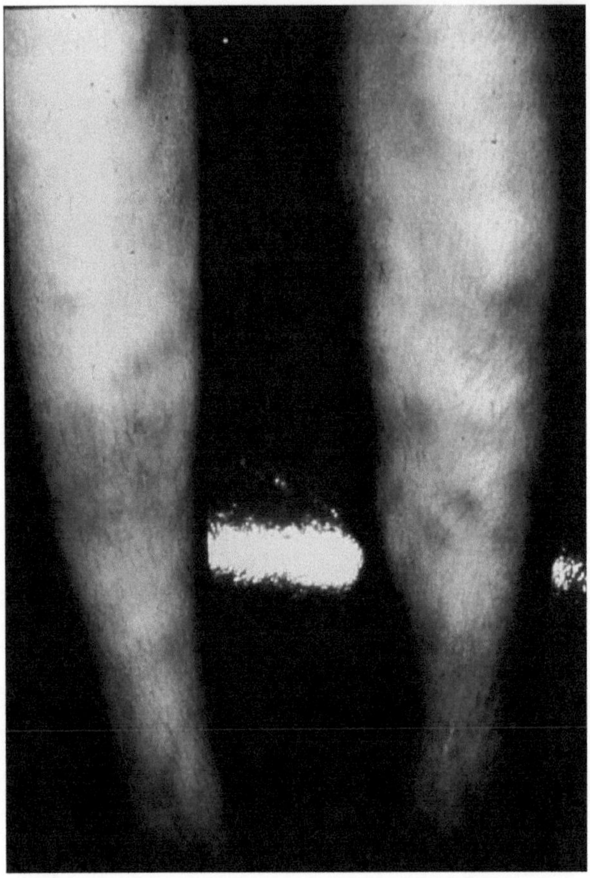

Fig. 16.6. Erythema nodosum affecting the lower extremities. [Figure in color on CD-ROM].

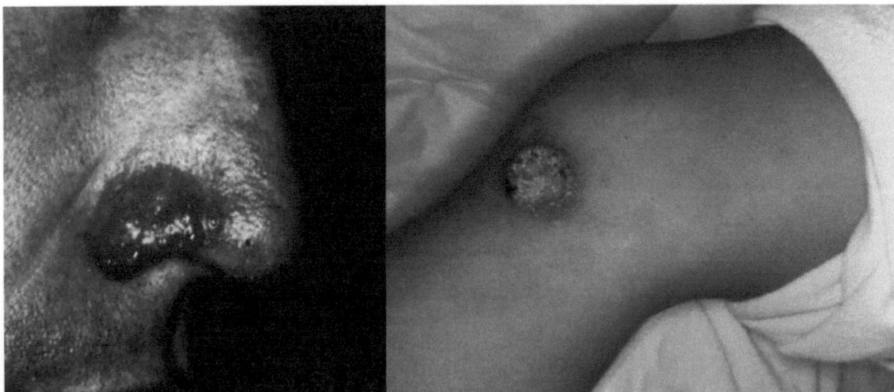

Fig. 16.7. Characteristic lesions of cutaneous coccidioidomycosis. [Figure in color on CD-ROM].

6 months of the initial infection *(48)*. The cerebrospinal fluid has an elevated white blood cell count and protein, with depressed glucose. Eosinophils are not common but when present are highly suggestive of the diagnosis of coccidioidal meningitis *(49)*. Finally, *Coccidioides* may disseminate to virtually any site in the body. Coccidioidal endophthalmitis, peritonitis, and prostatitis have all been described.

6. DIAGNOSIS

The diagnosis of coccidioidomycosis is dependent on a compatible clinical illness with positive laboratory confirmation by culture, histopathology, or serology. It is essential to obtain a detailed travel history for exposure to an endemic area. Exposure does not need to be over a prolonged period of time and infection has occurred after only briefly passing through an endemic area.

6.1. Culture

Suitable material for culture is sputum, tissue aspirates, or biopsy specimens. *Coccidioides* species grow well on most culture media after 5–7 days of incubation in aerobic conditions at 25°, 30°, or 35°C. Typically these fungi produce a white mould, although more pigmented strains have been observed. Laboratory cultures are highly infectious when mature and arthroconidia have formed (see Fig. 2.14, Chapter 2). Typically it takes about 10 to 20 days for *Coccidioides* to mature and produce arthroconidia. Because of their size, the arthroconidia are easily dispersed in the air and inhaled; therefore *Coccidioides* presents an extreme hazardous when cultured in the laboratory. At a minimum, Biosafety Level 2 practices and facilities are recommended for handling and processing of clinical specimens. When working with known *Coccidioides*, Biosafety Level 3 is required *(50)*. Accidental percutaneous inoculation of the spherule form may result in local granuloma formation. Clinical specimens, prior to culture, however, are not infectious to personnel. The much larger size spherules are considerably less effective as airborne pathogens. *Coccidioides* will grow in most of the media used in the microbiology laboratories including 5% sheep blood agar, chocolate agar, Sabouraud dextrose agar, Mycosel agar, and brain heart infusion agar with or without blood. Growth on 5% sheep blood agar and chocolate agar incubated at 35°C can be seen in as little as 24 hours. Growth on Sabouraud dextrose agar and Mycosel agar incubated at 25°C (room temperature) can be seen after 3 to 4 days. Accidental recovery of *Coccidioides* on 5% sheep blood agar and chocolate agar from respiratory, tissue, aspirates and biopsy specimens can be extremely hazardous to laboratory personnel. Specimens from known or suspected cases should not be cultured on unsealed plated media. Tubed media must be used (Fig. 16.8). Presumptive identification may be made based on colony morphology, growth rate, and the production of alternating arthroconidia. Care must be taken when attempting to identify *Coccidioides* because other mycoses may have similar macroscopic and microscopic morphologies, especially if arthroconidia are not abundant (Fig. 16.9). Laboratories that are not experienced with working with *Coccidioides* should refer these suspected isolates to qualified reference laboratories. *Coccidioides* species are dimorphic fungi that have the ability to grow vegetatively at 25°C as moulds, and at 37°C in tissue or in special medium (Converse liquid medium) in 10% CO_2 incubator as spherules. Confirmation

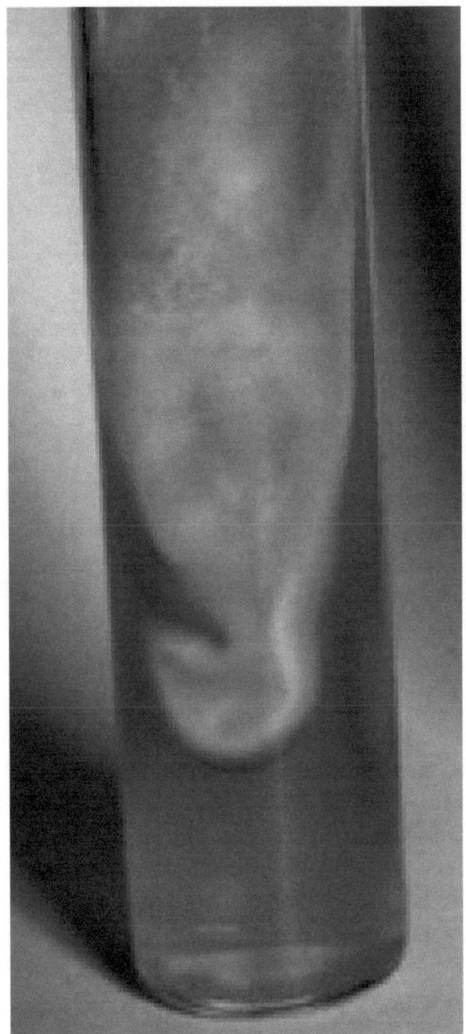

Fig. 16.8. Growth of *Coccidioides* in tubed fungal medium. [Figure in color on CD-ROM].

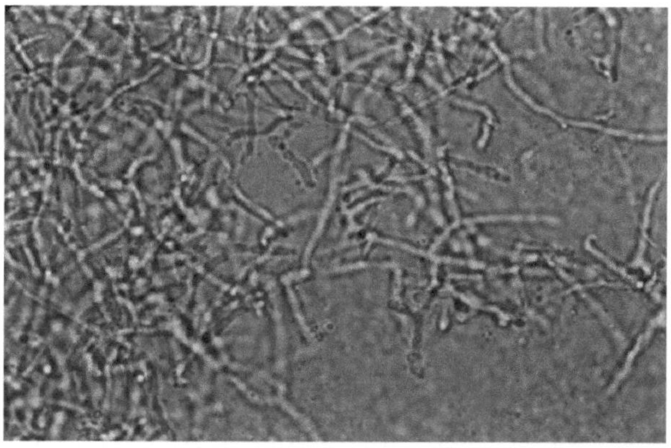

Fig. 16.9. Mycelial form of *Coccidioides immitis*. [Figure in color on CD-ROM].

traditionally was performed by animal inoculation with identification of endosporulating spherules on histopathology. Exoantigen tests and the production of spherules in Converse liquid medium could also be used. These methods have now been supplanted by molecular testing; a DNA probe is available commercially.

6.2. *Histopathology*

Diagnosis may also be confirmed histopathologically with the demonstration of endosporulating spherules usually in the setting of granulomatous inflammation (see Fig. 3–9, Chapter 3).

6.3. *Serologic Testing*

The most common method of diagnosis is serologic testing in individuals who have typical clinical features or based on suspicion. Correctly performed serologic tests are both sensitive and specific for the disease. A negative serologic test, however, does not exclude the presence of infection, especially if recently acquired, and should be repeated over the course of several weeks to months. Serologic tests for *Coccidioides* are many. The most commonly used currently are enzyme immunoassay (EIA), immunodiffusion (ID), and complement fixation (CF) antibody tests. The EIA allows the detection of immunoglobulin M (IgM) antibodies for the determination of recent infection. Although this test suffers from many false positives, it is probably the most sensitive test for early infection. The ID IgM test has somewhat less sensitivity but a better specificity than the EIA test. The EIA IgG test appears to have a significant number of false negatives, which limit its utility in the diagnosis of severe and advanced disease. The ID IgG test, while somewhat less sensitive, has a high degree of specificity and fewer false negatives in individuals with significant or disseminated disease. Complement fixation tests are both sensitive and specific in the diagnosis of coccidioidal infections. The quantitative CF test is expressed as a titer and has the additional advantage of being not only diagnostic, but prognostic. There is an inverse relationship of the IgG antibody titer to prognosis. Individuals with low amounts of IgG antibodies tend to have modest primary infections. Individuals with high amounts of IgG antibodies are more likely to have extensive primary infection or disseminated disease. It must be understood, however, that this holds true for a population of patients. In a given individual, the extent and severity of disease cannot be accurately predicted solely on the measurement of IgG antibodies.

The majority of patients with disseminated disease will eventually have a titer greater than or equal to 1:16. At present, EIA results should be confirmed with the more established immunodiffusion or complement fixation tests *(51,52)*. Immunodiffusion and complement fixation IgG tests will have a false-negative rate of approximately 1% in disseminated disease. The majority of individuals with disseminated disease who have falsely negative *Coccidioides* serology are HIV infected. The complement fixation titer in individuals with meningitis is higher than in individuals with primary disease but lower than in those with other forms of disseminated disease *(53)*.

6.4. Skin Testing

Skin test antigens derived from both mycelia and spherules have been marketed in the past. No skin testing reagents are currently commercially available. Skin testing detects the delayed-type hypersensitivity reaction to *Coccidioides (54)*. Because skin tests commonly remain positive for life in most people, a positive result may not be related to current illness, analogous to tuberculin skin testing. The diagnosis of coccidioidomycosis can be made by demonstrating the conversion of the skin test from negative to positive. False-negative skin tests can occur in immunocompromised individuals and in the setting of overwhelming infection. Thus a negative skin test cannot exclude a diagnosis of current or past coccidioidal infection. Skin testing therefore is limited as a screening procedure for recent infection, but may be useful in epidemiologic studies.

6.5. Other Laboratory Findings

Nonspecific laboratory tests such as the complete blood count and chemistry tests occasionally offer clues to coccidioidal infection. In an endemic area, an individual presenting with what appears to be community-acquired pneumonia who has an absolute eosinophilia (greater than 350 cells/μl) is more likely to have primary coccidioidal infection. It has also been noted that individuals who present with coccidioidomycosis and elevated alkaline phosphatase may also have liver involvement.

6.6. Radiologic Imaging

Radiographic imaging may be of great help in defining the extent and severity of both pleural pulmonary and disseminated disease. Chest radiograph is mandatory in evaluation of primary disease. Computed tomography of the chest may be helpful in selected cases, especially with cavitary disease. Bone scan is the most frequently utilized test for osteomyelitis and plain radiograph is frequently utilized (see Figs. 5.13 and 5.14, Chapter 5). Magnetic resonance imaging (MRI) of bone and joint will help define problematic cases. Approximately 50% of patients with meningitis will have a normal study, but neuroimaging of the brain and spinal cord with MRI may reveal meningeal enhancement, hydrocephalus, or vasculitic infarction *(55)* (see Fig. 5.3, Chapter 5).

7. TREATMENT

7.1. General Approach

The treatment of coccidioidomycosis is both complex and at times controversial. A treatment guideline published by the Infectious Disease Society of America (IDSA) in 2005 gives a consensus framework *(56)*. It is clear that many individuals infected with *Coccidioides* species recover. This is especially true when one notes that 60% of infections are asymptomatic and, by definition, go undiagnosed and untreated. Of symptomatic individuals, large numbers also go undiagnosed and most recover uneventfully. There is some controversy as to whether individuals who are diagnosed with symptomatic primary disease need to be treated. Some experts believe that the majority of these persons will recover without treatment and therefore treatment ought not to be offered. Other authorities note that a small but significant percentage of individuals with primary disease will have either pulmonary or disseminated complications and it is difficult to predict with certainty who these individuals might be; thus the majority should be treated. Unfortunately, there is no evidence-based study of primary disease that has examined whether improvement in the primary symptom complex, rate of pulmonary complications, or frequency of dissemination, is affected by treating or not treating. What is generally agreed upon is that individuals with significant risk factors for dissemination or poor outcome should receive treatment for primary disease (Table 16.1). Thus advanced age; male sex; vulnerable race; presence of associated comorbid diseases such as diabetes, liver disease, and underlying lung disease; and elevated complement fixation titers should favor treatment of primary disease. HIV infection and other conditions associated with immunodeficiency, such as lymphoma, cancer chemotherapy, and organ transplantation, mandate early and aggressive therapy of primary disease. Pregnancy represents a special circumstance. The development of primary disease during the middle trimester through the early postpartum period puts an otherwise low-risk group of individuals at much higher risk. Coccidioidomycosis had been the leading cause of maternal mortality in Kern County, California for more than 50 years *(57)*. Despite the risk, many women will have favorable outcomes without drug treatment, and abortions or early delivery in subjects with active infection is rare *(58)*.

7.2. Primary Coccidioidomycosis

Most individuals with uncomplicated acute coccidioidal pneumonia, if treated, are initiated on oral azole therapy (Fig. 16.10). Fluconazole 400 mg daily has been prescribed most often. Alternatively, itraconazole 200 mg twice daily is also commonly prescribed *(59)*. Some institutions are initiating higher doses as primary therapy. This has especially been true with the recent availability of generic fluconazole. It should be noted that fluconazole and itraconazole are not approved for coccidioidomycosis by the Food and Drug Administration (FDA), nor are doses greater than 400 mg daily, in any disease. Despite lack of an FDA indication, these two drugs have become the mainstay in treatment of primary disease. Duration of recommended treatment ranges from 3 to 6 months, although longer courses may be prescribed in diabetics, persons

Table 16.1
Antifungal therapy of coccidioidomycosis

Disease	Primary therapy	Alternate therapy	Duration
Acute pulmonary infection			
Uncomplicated			3–6 months
Low risk	Observation	Oral azole[a]	
High risk[b]	Oral azole[c]	Amphotericin B	
Diffuse/severe	Amphotericin B[d]	High dose fluconazole[e]	≥12 months
Chronic infection			
Chronic infection Pneumonia	Oral azole	Surgical resection (cavitary disease only)	≥12 months
Disseminated Nonmeningeal	Oral azole	Amphotericin B	Years
Meningeal	Oral fluconazole[e,f]	Voriconazole, or itraconazole, or intrathecal amphotericin B	Life-long
Other			
Nodule	Observation		
Cavity			
Asymptomatic	Observation		
Symptomatic	Oral azole		
Ruptured	Surgery and antifungal therapy		≥12 months

Modified from Infectious Diseases Society of America guidelines *(56)*.
[a]Oral azoles include fluconazole and itraconazole, typically 400 mg or more daily.
[b]See text for description of patients at high risk.
[c]Amphotericin B should be used in pregnant patients due to the teratogenicity of azoles.
[d]Typically replaced with azole therapy once patient is clinically improving and stable.
[e]High-dose fluconazole (800–1200 mg daily) is often used in severe disease, at least initially.
[f]Consider early shunting if hydrocephalus is present and corticosteroids if vasculitis is present.

of African American or Filipino descent, and in immunocompromised patients. In individuals presenting with severe, diffuse pulmonary coccidioidomycosis or miliary disease with respiratory failure, azoles are not the initial drugs of choice. In this circumstance, amphotericin B deoxycholate, liposomal amphotericin B, or amphotericin B lipid complex continue to be preferred. It appears that there is a more rapid response to the amphotericin than to the azole drugs. There does not seem to be a difference in efficacy between amphotericin B compounds, albeit in other diseases there has been a demonstrable difference in toxicity *(60)*. Several weeks of therapy with amphotericin B are often required for improvement, after which oral azole therapy is employed. A brief initial course of corticosteroids is considered beneficial by some in case of fulminant diffuse pneumonia with hypoxia *(61)*.

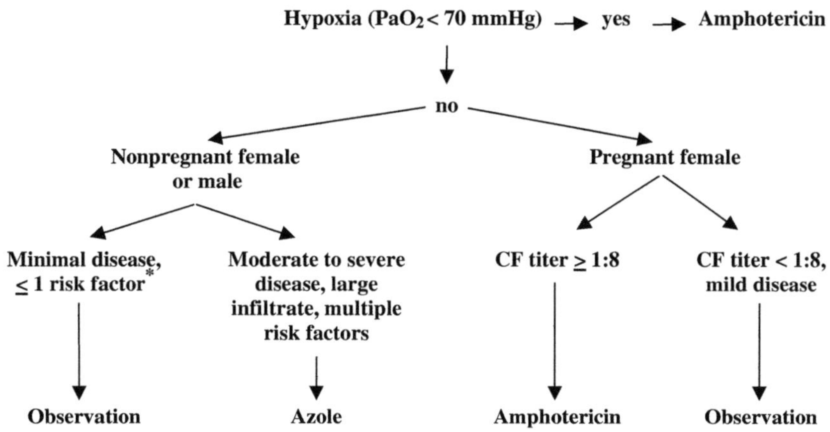

Fig. 16.10. Approach to the patient with acute pulmonary coccidioidomycosis. CF, complement fixation antibody. See text for listing of the risk factors associated with poorer prognosis. These include age greater than 40, African or Asian ancestry, and immunodeficiency..

7.3. *Pulmonary Nodule*

Antifungal therapy or resection is unnecessary for stable pulmonary nodules with an established diagnosis. If enlargement of the nodule occurs, reevaluation with sputum cultures and measurement of serum coccidioidal antibodies should be done to determine if the infection is active and warrants treatment.

7.4. *Pulmonary Cavity*

Asymptomatic, cavitary disease caused by *Coccidioides* seldom requires intervention. Symptomatic solitary cavity coccidioidomycosis may benefit from azole therapy. A course of varying duration until symptoms are resolved is appropriate. Resolution of fever, cough and hemoptysis, improvement in appetite, and decrease in complement fixation titers, if any, may be used to guide therapy. Approximately one-half of cavities smaller than 3 cm will resolve in 6 to 12 months. If the cavity persists but the symptoms abate, a trial of withdrawal of azole therapy can be undertaken. If symptoms recrudesce, reinstitution of therapy for a longer period of time is suggested. Indications for resection of the cavity include recurrent bacterial superinfections and recurrent or life-threatening hemoptysis. Rupture of the cavity into the pleural space, with development of empyema often requires surgical as well as medical therapy.

7.5. *Chronic Progressive Fibrocavitary Pneumonia*

Fibrocavitary pneumonia of coccidioidomycosis in the pre-azole era often resulted in death from respiratory failure and pulmonary hypertension. Since the advent of azoles, death is less common. Fluconazole or itraconazole at 400 mg or more per day is the most common therapy. At this time, amphotericin has little role in the management of this subacute illness.

7.6. Coccidioidomycosis in Pregnancy

Because of demonstrated concerns of teratogenicity of azole compounds, amphotericin is the drug of choice in pregnancy for those requiring therapy. Pregnant females with mild disease of limited extent and with low complement fixation titers are usually followed very closely, as often as weekly, without initiation of any therapy. Those with greater extent of disease or with high complement fixation titers are immediately placed on amphotericin. This should be done in concert with an obstetrician who deals with high-risk pregnancies.

7.7. Disseminated Disease (Extrapulmonary)

Therapy of disseminated disease requires more expertise and judgment than does uncomplicated pulmonary disease (Fig. 16.11). It has been noted that minimal cutaneous disseminated disease may remit without specific antifungal therapy. At this time however, no expert recommends that treatment of disseminated disease not include antifungal therapy. Disseminated disease of the skin, soft tissue, joints and bones that is limited and not life or limb threatening is usually treated with azole therapy. Some experts prefer itraconazole for disseminated disease, particularly bony dissemination, because of a trend toward superior resolution at 1 year with itraconazole 200 mg every 12 hours when compared with fluconazole 400 mg daily *(59)*. However, both drugs are used, albeit fluconazole is now commonly used at doses greater than 400 mg per day. A duration of therapy substantially longer than a year is frequently recommended. Some experts are recommending therapy for 3 years for significant disseminated disease. Severe multifocal osseous disease that affects the axial skeleton or a major long bone may be treated with azole therapy, though many experts prefer to use amphotericin initially in this circumstance. If the disease is amenable to surgical debridement, this may be a valuable adjunct. After individuals undergo treatment with amphotericin, secondary therapy with azoles is undertaken for protracted periods. Doses higher than 400 mg of fluconazole or itraconazole are frequently administered.

In coccidioidal meningitis, fluconazole is the preferred drug, given at doses of 800–1200 mg daily as a single dose *(62,63)*. Itraconazole is not as commonly used

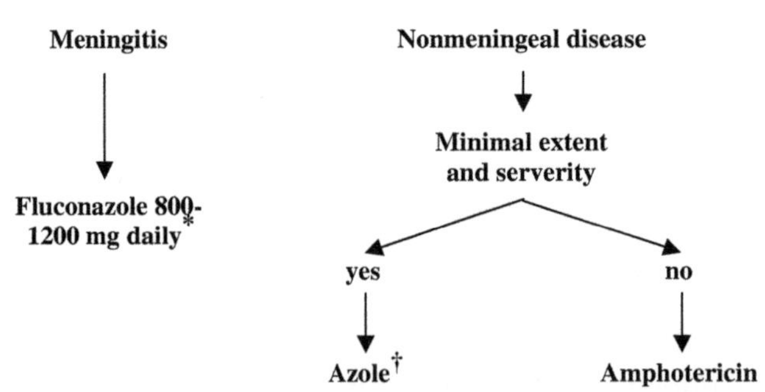

Fig. 16.11. Approach to the patient with disseminated coccidioidomycosis. * Alternatives for treatment failure include voriconazole, itraconazole, and intrathecal amphotericin B. † Fluconazole 400 to 1000 mg daily (as one dose) or itraconazole 400 to 800 mg daily (in divided doses). Voriconazole and posaconazole may also have a role.

as fluconazole but has had reported success. In patients failing high dose fluconazole therapy, voriconazole has been used and has significant theoretical appeal as rescue therapy at a dose of 4 mg/kg every 12 hours *(64,65)*. Intrathecal amphotericin B was the primary therapy of CNS coccidioidomycosis until supplanted by azole therapy. This therapy can and has been given by direct cisternal injection, via ventricular or cisternal reservoir, or via intrathecal lumbar injection or reservoir. It is now used primarily in those failing other initial or secondary therapies. Coccidioidal meningitis is often complicated by hydrocephalus (Fig. 16.12), which is treated by ventriculoperitoneal shunting *(66)*. Therapy for coccidioidal meningitis is usually life-long.

7.8. Monitoring Therapy

Patients with primary coccidioidomycosis should be monitored at 1- to 3-month intervals, both with laboratory and radiologic studies. If there is suspicion for dissemination by history or on examination, biopsy and culture of suspected sites of infection should be performed. Lumbar puncture should be performed in patients who develop headaches after the initial primary infection or other neurologic signs at any time. Bone scan is indicated to evaluate bony or joint involvement.

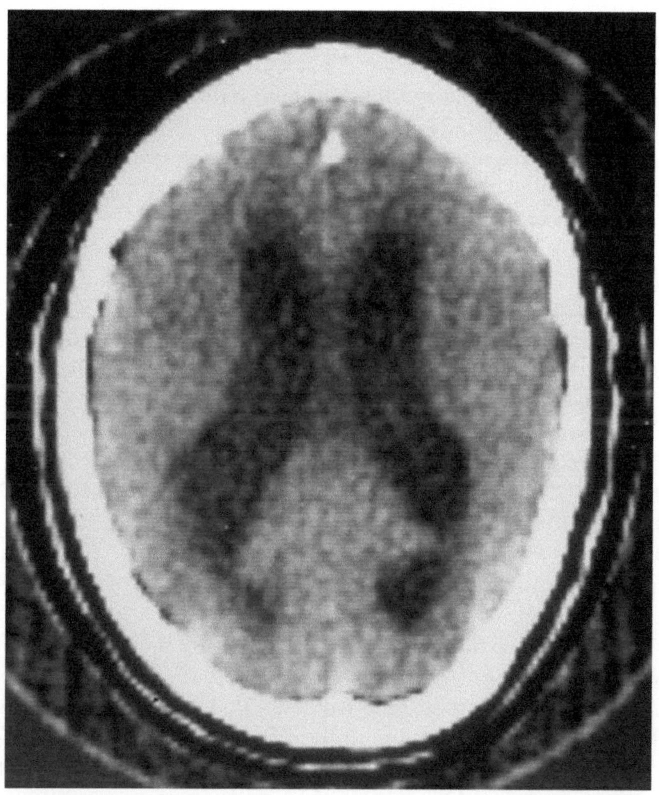

Fig. 16.12. Hydrocephalus in coccidioidal meningitis.

8. PREVENTION

Developing a vaccine has been a goal for many years. A formalin-killed, whole-cell spherule vaccine was used in a human field trial but was not found to be protective *(67)*. New research on a subcellular vaccine has been initiated and is ongoing.

ACKNOWLEDGMENT

The authors wish to thank D. Caldwell, H. Einstein, J. Pusavat, and C. Burke for their help and/or advice in the preparation of this chapter.

REFERENCES

1. Posadas A. Un nuevo caso de micosis fungoidea con psorospermias. Annales del Circulo Medico Argentina 1892;5:585–597.
2. Wernicke R. Ueber einen Protozoenbefund bei Mycosis fungoides. Zentralb Bakt 1892;12:859–861.
3. Rixford E, Gilchrist TC. Two cases of protozoan (coccidioidal) infection of the skin and other organs. John Hopkins Hosp Rep 1896;1:209–268.
4. Ophuls W, Moffitt HC. A new pathogenic mould (formerly described as a protozoan: *Coccidioides immitis*): preliminary report. Phila Med J 1900;5:1471–1472.
5. Montenegro J. Septicemia por Coccidioides immitis. Brasil-med 1925;1:69–70.
6. Beck MD. Occurrence of Coccidioides immitis in lesions of slaughtered animals. Proc Soc Exper Biol Med 1929;26:534–536.
7. Rand CW. Coccidioidal granuloma: report of two cases simulating tumor of the spinal cord. Arch Neurol Psychiat 1930;23:502–511.
8. Abbott KH, Cutler OI. Chronic coccidioidal meningitis: review of the literature and report of seven cases. Arch Path 1936;21:320–330.
9. Pulford DS, Larson EE. Coccidioidal granuloma; report of a case treated by intravenous dye, colloidal lead, and colloidal copper, with autopsy observations. JAMA 1929;93:1049–1056. (Discussed by William Ophuls)
10. Stewart RA, Meyer KF. Isolation of *Coccidioides immitis* (Stiles) from the soil. Proc Soc Exper Biol Med 1932;29:937–938.
11. Gifford MA. San Joaquin Fever. Kern County Dept Public Health Annu Rep 1936:22–23.
12. Fiese MJ. Coccidioidomycosis. Springfield, IL: Charles C Thomas, 1958.
13. Fisher MC, Koenig GL, White TJ, Taylor JW. Molecular and phenotypic description of *Coccidioides posadasii* sp. nov., previously recognized as the non-California population of *Coccidioides immitis*. Mycologia 2002;94:73–84.
14. Centers for Disease Control and Prevention. Coccidioidomycosis in workers at an archeologic site–Dinosaur National Monument, Utah, June–July 2001. MMWR Morb Mortal Wkly Rep 2001;50:1005–1008.
15. Abuodeh RO, Orbach MJ, Mandel MA, Das A, Galgiani JN. Genetic transformation of *Coccidioides immitis* facilitated by *Agrobacterium tumefaciens*. J Infect Dis 2000;181:2106–2110.
16. Smith CE. Diagnosis of pulmonary coccidioidal infections. California Med 1951;75: 385–391.
17. Dodge RR, Lebowitz MD, Barbee RA, Burrows B. Estimates of *C. immitis* infection by skin test reactivity in an endemic community. Am J Public Health 1985;75:863–865.
18. Larwood TR. Coccidioidin skin testing in Kern County, California: decrease in infection rate over 58 years. Clin Infect Dis 2000;30:612–613.
19. Stevens DA. Current concepts: coccidioidomycosis. N Engl J Med 1995;332:1077–1082.

20. Centers for Disease Control and Prevention. Coccidioidomycosis-United States, 1991–1992. MMWR Morb Mortal Wkly Rep 1993;42:21–24.
21. Leake JA, Mosley DG, England B, et al. Risk factors for acute symptomatic coccidioidomycosis among elderly persons in Arizona, 1996–1997. J Infect Dis 2000;181: 1435–1440.
22. Komatsu K, Vaz V, McRill C, et al. Increase in coccidioidomycosis-Arizona, 1998–2001. JAMA 2003;289:1500–1502 (Reprinted from MMWR Morb Mortal Weekly Rep 2003;52:109–112).
23. Park BJ, Sigel K, Vaz V, et al. An epidemic of coccidioidomycosis in Arizona associated with climate changes, 1998–2001. J Infect Dis 2005;191:1981–1987.
24. Beaman L, Pappagianis D, Benjamini E. Mechanisms of resistance to infection with *Coccidioides immitis* in mice. Infect Immun 1979;23:681–685.
25. Blair JE, Logan JL. Coccidioidomycosis in solid organ transplantation. Clin Infect Dis 2001;33:1536–1544.
26. Woods CW, McRill C, Plikaytis BD, et al. Coccidioidomycosis in human immunodeficiency virus-infected persons in Arizona, 1994–1997: incidence, risk factors, and prevention. J Infect Dis 2000;181:1428–1434.
27. Ampel NM, Bejarano GC, Galgiani JN. Killing of *Coccidioides immitis* by human peripheral blood mononuclear cells. Infect Immun 1992;60:4200–4204.
28. De Moraes-Vasconcelos D, Grumach AS, Yamaguti A, et al. *Paracoccidioides brasiliensis* disseminated disease in a patient with inherited deficiency in the beta 1 subunit of the interleukin (IL)-12/IL-23 receptor. Clin Infect Dis 2005;41:e31–e37.
29. Zerbe CS, Holland SM. Disseminated histoplasmosis in persons with interferon gamma receptor 1 deficiency. Clin Infect Dis 2005;41:e38–e41.
30. Forseth J, Rohwedder JJ, Levine BE, Saubolle MA. Experience with needle biopsy for coccidioidal lung nodules. Arch Intern Med 1986;146:319–320.
31. Johnson RH, Caldwell JW, Welch G, et al. The great coccidioidomycosis epidemic: clinical features. In: Einstein HE, Catanzaro A, eds. Coccidioidomycosis. Proceedings of the Fifth International Conference. Washington DC: National Foundation for Infectious Diseases; 1996;77–87.
32. Quimby SR, Connolly SM, Winkelmann RK, Smilack JD. Clinicopathologic spectrum of specific cutaneous lesions of disseminated coccidioidomycosis. J Am Acad Dermatol 1992;26:79–85.
33. Elbaum DJ. Erythema sweetobullosum: the missing link in San Joaquin Valley Fever. Proceedings of the 42nd Annual Coccidioidomycosis Study Group Meeting, Visalia, CA, April 4, 1998.
34. Sarosi GA, Parker JD, Doto IL, Tosh FE. Chronic pulmonary coccidioidomycosis. N Engl J Med 1970;283:325–329.
35. Pappagianis D. Epidemiology of coccidioidomycosis. Curr Top Med Mycol 1988;2: 199–238.
36. Louie L, Ng S, Hajjeh R, et al. Influence of host genetics on the severity of coccidioidomycosis. Emerg Infect Dis 1999;5:672–680.
37. Ampel NM. Coccidioidomycosis among persons with human immunodeficiency virus infection in the era of highly active antiretroviral therapy (HAART). Semin Respir Infect 2001;16:257–262.
38. Deresinski SC, Stevens DA. Coccidioidomycosis in compromised hosts: experience at Stanford University Hospital. Medicine (Baltimore) 1974;54:377–395.
39. Rutala PJ, Smith JW. Coccidioidomycosis in potentially compromised hosts: the effect of immunosuppressive therapy in dissemination. Am J Med Sci 1978;275:283–295.
40. Blair JE, Logan JL. Coccidioidomycosis in solid organ transplantation. Clin Infect Dis 2001;33:1536–1544.

41. Logan JL, Blair JE, Galgiani JN. Coccidioidomycosis complicating solid organ transplantation. Semin Respir Infect 2001;16:251–256.
42. Walker MP, Brody CZ, Resnik R. Reactivation of coccidioidomycosis in pregnancy. Obstet Gynecol 1992;79:815–817.
43. Peterson CM, Schuppert K, Kelly PC, Pappagianis D. Coccidioidomycosis and pregnancy. Obstet Gynecol Surv 1993;48:149–156.
44. Bisla RS, Taber TH. Coccidioidomycosis of bone and joints. Clin Orthop 1976;121: 196–204.
45. Bried JH, Galgiani JN. *Coccidioides immitis* infections in bones and joints. Clin Orthop 1986;211:235–243.
46. Lund PJ, Chan KM, Unger EC, Galgiani JN, Pitt MJ. Magnetic resonance imaging in coccidioidal arthritis. Skeletal Radiol 1996;25:661–665.
47. Rosen E, Belber JP. Coccidioidal meningitis of long duration: report of a case of four years and eight months duration, with necropsy findings. Ann Intern Med 1951;34:796–808.
48. Vincent T, Galgiani JN, Huppert M, Salkin D. The natural history of coccidioidal meningitis: VA-Armed Forces cooperative studies, 1955–1958. Clin Infect Dis 1993;16:247–254.
49. Ragland AS, Arsura E, Ismail Y, Johnson RH. Eosinophilic pleocytosis in coccidioidal meningitis: frequency and significance. Am J Med 1993;95:254–257.
50. Biosafety in Microbiological and Biomedical Laboratories. CDC. Fourth ed, May 1999.
51. Kaufman L, Sekhon AS, Moledina N, Jalbert M, Pappagianis D. Comparative evaluation of commercial Premier EIA and microimmunodiffusion and complement fixation tests for *Coccidioides immitis* antibodies. J Clin Microbiol 1995;33:618–619.
52. Wieden MA, Lundergan LL, Blum J, Jalbert M, Pappagianis D. Detection of coccidioidal antibodies by 33-kDa spherule antigen, *Coccidioides* EIA, and standard serologic tests in sera from patients evaluated for coccidioidomycosis. J Infect Dis 1996;173:1273–1277.
53. Smith CE, Saito MT, Beard RR, Keep RM, Clark RW, Eddie BU. Serological tests in the diagnosis and prognosis of coccidioidomycosis. Am J Hyg 1950;52:1–21.
54. Drutz DJ, Catanzaro A. Coccidioidomycosis: Part 1. Am Rev Respir Dis 1978;117:559–585.
55. Penrose J, Johnson R, Einstein H, et al. Neuroimaging in coccidioidal meningitis. Proceedings of the 39th Annual Coccidioidomycosis Study Group Meeting, Bakersfield, CA, April 1, 1995.
56. Galgiani JN, Ampel NM, Blair JE, et al. Coccidioidomycoses. Clin Infect Dis 2005;41: 1217–1223.
57. Vaughn JE, Ramirez H. Coccidioidomycosis as a complication of pregnancy. Calif Med J 1951;74:121–125.
58. Caldwell JW, Arsura EL, Kilgore WB, Garcia AL, Reddy V, Johnson RH. Coccidioidomycosis in pregnancy during an epidemic in California. Obstet Gynecol 2000;95:236–239.
59. Galgiani JN, Catanzaro A, Cloud GA, et al. Comparison of oral fluconazole and itraconazole for progressive, nonmeningeal coccidioidomycosis: a randomized, double-blind trial. Mycoses Study Group. Ann Intern Med 2000;133:676–686.
60. Walsh TJ, Finberg RW, Arndt C, et al. Liposomal amphotericin B for empirical therapy in patients with persistent fever and neutropenia. National Institute of Allergy and Infectious Diseases Mycoses Study Group. N Engl J Med 1999;340:764–771.
61. Shibli M, Ghassibi J, Hajal R, O'Sullivan M. Adjunctive corticosteroids therapy in acute respiratory distress syndrome owing to disseminated coccidioidomycosis. Crit Care Med 2002;30:1896–1898.
62. Classen DC, Burke JP, Smith CB. Treatment of coccidioidal meningitis with Fluconazole. J Infect Dis 1988;158:903–904.
63. Galgiani JN, Catanzaro A, Cloud GA, et al. Fluconazole therapy for coccidioidal meningitis. Ann Intern Med 1993;119:28–35.

64. Proia LA, Tenorio AR. Successful use of voriconazole for treatment of *Coccidioides* meningitis. Antimicrobial Agents Chemother 2004;48:2341.
65. Cortez KJ, Walsh TJ, Bennett JE. Successful treatment of coccidioidal meningitis with voriconazole. Clin Infect Dis 2003;36:1619–1622.
66. Johnson RH, Einstein HE. Coccidioidal Meningitis. Clin Infect Dis 2006;42:103–107.
67. Pappagianis D. Valley Fever Vaccine Study Group: Evaluation of the protective efficacy of the killed *Coccidioides immitis* spherule vaccine in humans. Am Rev Respir Dis 1993;148:656–660.

SUGGESTED READINGS

Galgiani JN. *Coccidioides* species. In: Mandell GL, Bennett JE, Dolin R, eds. Mandell, Douglas, and Bennett's principles and practice of infectious diseases. 6th ed. Philadelphia: Elsevier Churchill Livingstone, 2005:3040–3051.

Galgiani JN, Ampel NM, Blair JE, et al. Coccidioidomycosis. Clin Infect Dis 2005; 41: 1217–1223.

Johnson RH, Einstein HE. Coccidioidal Meningitis. Clin Infect Dis 2006;43:103–107.

Stevens DA. Current concepts: coccidioidomycosis. N Engl J Med 1995;332:1077–1082.

17
Histoplasmosis

L. Joseph Wheat, MD and Nicholas G. Conger, MD

1. INTRODUCTION

Histoplasma capsulatum is a dimorphic fungus primarily found in the Americas, Africa, and Asia, but may be found worldwide, particularly in travelers and immigrants from the endemic areas *(1)*. Among the endemic mycoses, histoplasmosis is the leading cause of hospitalization and death in the United States *(2)*. Darling first described the organism in 1906, believing it to be *Leishmania*. First thought to cause a progressive and fatal disseminated disease, subsequently histoplasmosis was shown to be very common and usually asymptomatic or clinically self-limited.

2. ETIOLOGIC AGENT

Histoplasma is a dimorphic fungus, defined by its ability to grow as a mould in the environment and yeast at 37°C. Clinical specimens viewed via potassium hydroxide (KOH) preparation, calcofluor white, Giemsa, or hematoxylin and eosin (H&E) stains may demonstrate the 2 to 4 μm budding yeast cells (Fig. 17.1). *Histoplasma capsulatum* var. *capsulatum* causes the vast majority of clinical disease, while its closely related variant *Histoplasma capsulatum* var. *duboisii* is the etiologic agent of African histoplasmosis.

3. EPIDEMIOLOGY

Histoplasmosis is most commonly reported to occur in and around the Mississippi and Ohio River valleys of the United States, South and Central America, and less so in parts of Africa and Asia. This is thought to be due to factors such as the climate, humidity, and soil acidity. Large amounts of bird and bat excreta enrich the soil in which the fungi are found, facilitating growth and accelerating sporulation. When disturbed,

Dr. Wheat is the president of MiraVista Diagnostics, the company that developed and performs *Histoplasma* antigen testing. The views expressed herein are those of the authors and do not reflect the official policy of the Department of the US Air Force, Department of Defense, or other departments of the US Government.

From: *Infectious Disease: Diagnosis and Treatment of Human Mycoses*
Edited by: D. R. Hospenthal and M. G. Rinaldi © Humana Press Inc., Totowa, NJ

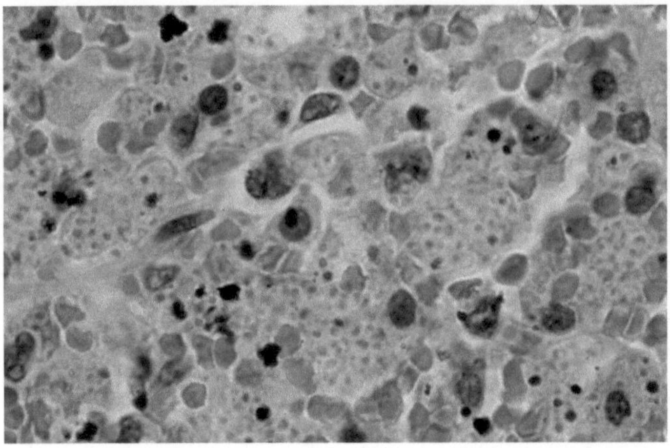

Fig. 17.1. Hematoxylin and eosin stain of yeast in macrophages. [Figure in color on CD-ROM].

microfoci or niches harboring a large number of infective particles may lead to high infectivity rates or large outbreaks. In most cases, however, the exposure is small and usually unrecognized. Cases outside the endemic area usually occur in individuals who have traveled or previously lived in endemic area *(3)*. However, microfoci containing the organism can sometimes be found outside the endemic area and may be the source for exposures.

4. PATHOGENESIS AND IMMUNOLOGY

Infection occurs when aerosolized microconidia (spores) are inhaled (Fig. 17.2). Infection usually is asymptomatic in healthy individuals after low-level exposure. Further, infection usually is self-limited except after heavy exposure or in patients with

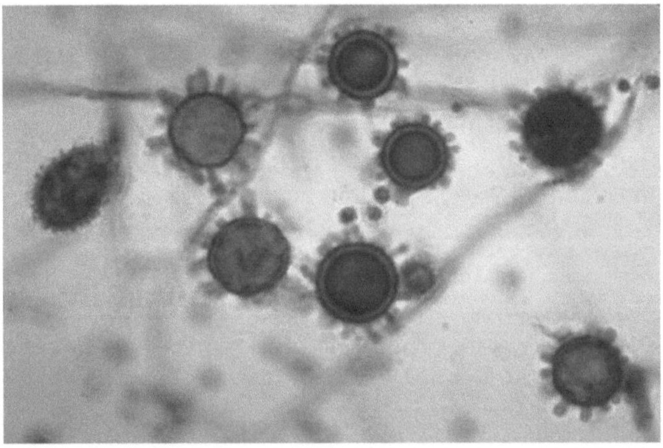

Fig. 17.2. Lactophenol cotton blue stain of the mould grown at 25°C. Note microconidia and tuberculate macroconidia. [Figure in color on CD-ROM].

underlying diseases that impair immunity. In addition, pulmonary infection may be progressive in patients with underlying obstructive lung disease. Also, for unknown reasons, pulmonary infection may rarely elicit exuberant mediastinal fibrosis.

In the alveoli, the conidia attract phagocytic cells including macrophages, neutrophils, and dendritic cells *(4)*. Within a few days the conidia transform to yeast, which multiply within the nonactivated macrophages and disseminate via the bloodstream to extrapulmonary organs. Neutrophils and dendritic cells inhibit proliferation of the organism, and dendritic cells present antigen to T lymphocytes as the initial step in development of specific cell-mediated immunity. Consequently, tumor necrosis factor-α and interferon-γ are induced, which activate macrophages to inhibit the growth of the organism, leading to spontaneous recovery and immunity against reinfection in most individuals *(5)*. Traditionally, humoral immunity is not believed to be important, but recent studies using monoclonal antibodies suggest otherwise.

Reactivation of latent infection has been proposed as the mechanism for progressive disseminated histoplasmosis (PDH) in immunocompromised patients. However, the rarity of PDH in immunosuppressed patients (0.1% to 1%) argues against reactivation. Among more than 600 patients undergoing solid organ or bone marrow transplantation in Indianapolis, a hyperendemic area in which three outbreaks occurred between 1978 and 1993, none developed PDH during the year after transplantation *(6)*. More likely, PDH in this population occurs because low-grade histoplasmosis was present at the time immunosuppression was initiated, or infection was acquired exogenously. In endemic areas, repeated exposure to *Histoplasma* spores probably occurs, permitting reinfection in immunosuppressed individuals whose immunity to *H. capsulatum* has waned.

5. CLINICAL MANIFESTATIONS

5.1. Asymptomatic Infection

The infection is asymptomatic in most otherwise healthy individuals who experience low inoculum exposure, as indicated by skin test positivity rates above 50% to 80% in the endemic areas *(7)*. Asymptomatic infection also may be identified via radiographic findings of pulmonary nodules or mediastinal lymphadenopathy, which eventually calcify, by splenic calcifications, or via positive serologic tests performed during screening for organ or bone marrow transplantation or epidemiologic investigation. In endemic areas about 5% of healthy subjects have positive complement fixation tests for anti-*Histoplasma* antibodies.

5.2. Acute Pulmonary Histoplasmosis

Healthy individuals who experience a heavy exposure usually present with acute diffuse pulmonary disease 1 to 2 weeks after exposure. Fever, dyspnea, and weight loss are common, and physical examination may demonstrate hepatomegaly or splenomegaly as evidence of extrapulmonary dissemination. In most cases after heavy exposure the illness is sufficiently severe to require hospitalization, with some individuals experiencing respiratory failure. Chest radiographs usually show diffuse infiltrates, which may be described as reticulonodular or miliary (Fig. 17.3).

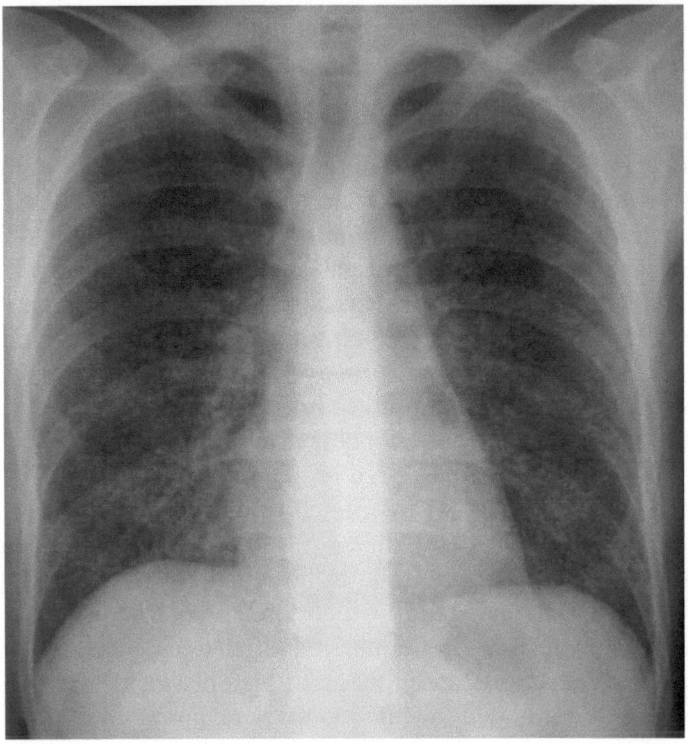

Fig. 17.3. Chest radiograph showing diffuse infiltrate seen in acute pulmonary or disseminated histoplasmosis.

5.3. *Subacute Pulmonary Histoplasmosis*

In symptomatic cases the most common syndrome is a subacute pulmonary infection manifested by respiratory complaints and fever lasting for several weeks, then resolving spontaneously over 1 or 2 months. The chest radiograph or computed tomography (CT) scan usually shows focal infiltrates with mediastinal or hilar lymphadenopathy (Fig. 17.4). Symptoms caused by a mediastinal adenopathy may prevail, and in some cases persist for months to years (granulomatous mediastinitis). In some cases respiratory symptoms may be mild or absent, and findings of pericarditis or arthritis/arthralgia may be prominent. Pericarditis and this rheumatologic syndrome represents inflammatory reactions to the acute infection, rather than infection of the pericardium or joints.

5.4. *Chronic Pulmonary Histoplasmosis*

Patients with underlying obstructive pulmonary disease develop chronic pulmonary disease after infection with *H. capsulatum*. The underlying lung disease prevents spontaneous resolution of the infection. Chest radiographs reveal upper lobe infiltrates with cavitation, often misdiagnosed as tuberculosis (Fig. 17.5). The course is chronic and gradually progressive, highlighted by systemic complaints of fever and sweats, associated with shortness of breath, chest pain, cough, sputum production, and

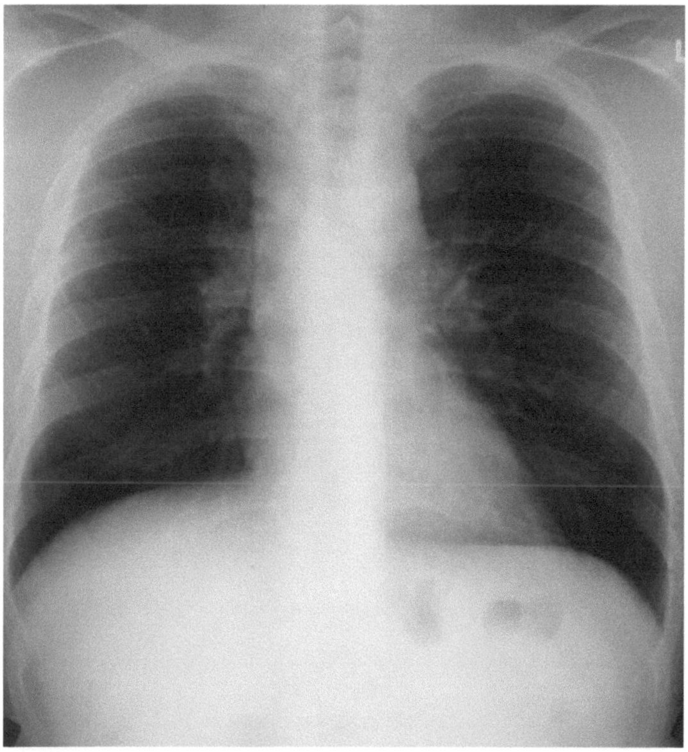

Fig. 17.4. Chest radiograph showing hilar lymphadenopathy seen in subacute pulmonary histoplasmosis.

occasional hemoptysis. Patients often experience repeated bacterial respiratory tract infections, and occasionally superinfection with mycobacteria or *Aspergillus*.

5.5. *Progressive Disseminated Histoplasmosis (PDH)*

Hematogenous dissemination is common during acute pulmonary histoplasmosis, but is nonprogressive *(8)*. With the development of specific cell-mediated immunity, the infection resolves in the lung and extrapulmonary tissues. In contrast, disease is progressive in individuals with defective cell-mediated immunity. In many cases the cause for immune deficiency is easily identified, and often includes the extremes of age, solid organ transplantation *(9)*, treatment with immunosuppressive medications *(10)*, acquired immunodeficiency syndrome (AIDS) *(11)*, idiopathic $CD4^+$ T-lymphocytopenia *(12)*, deficiency in the interferon-γ/interleukin-12 pathway *(13)*, or malignancy *(14)*. In other cases the cause for immunodeficiency remains unknown, awaiting a more complete understanding of immunity in histoplasmosis and development of better tests for diagnosis of immunodeficiency.

Clinical findings in PDH include progressive fever and weight loss, often associated with hepatomegaly or splenomegaly, and laboratory abnormalities including anemia, leukopenia, from the cytopenia, liver enzyme elevation, and ferritin elevation *(8)*. An elevation in serum lactate dehydrogenase has been associated with disseminated

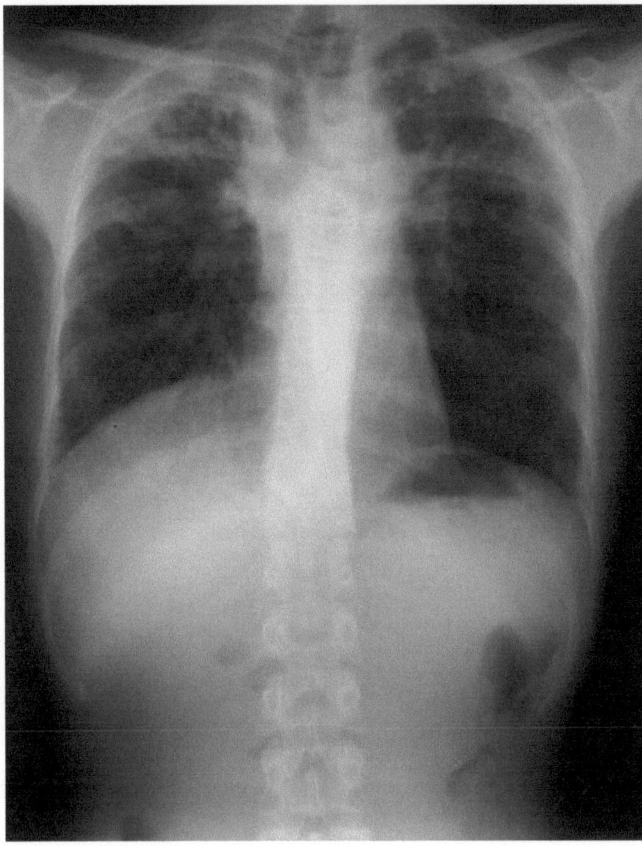

Fig. 17.5. Chest radiograph showing upper lobe infiltrates with cavitation seen in chronic pulmonary histoplasmosis.

histoplasmosis, particularly levels greater than 600 IU/liter. Other less frequent sites of involvement include the central nervous system, gastrointestinal tract, skin, and adrenal glands.

5.6. *Fibrosing Mediastinitis and Mediastinal Granuloma*

Fibrosing mediastinitis is a rare complication of pulmonary histoplasmosis *(7)*. The mechanism for this manifestation appears to be an excessive fibrotic response to antigens released into the mediastinal tissues rather than progressive infection. It is unclear why the immune response from subclinical histoplasmosis can lead to either mediastinal granuloma formation (with inflammation and caseating necrosis) or this fibrotic process. Genetic influences, inoculum size, and host immunity are all likely factors. The clinical findings of fibrosing mediastinitis are caused by obstruction of mediastinal structures and may include involvement of the superior vena cava, airways, or pulmonary vessels. Infiltrative inflammatory mediastinal masses that do not respect fat or fascial planes are characteristic CT findings of fibrosing mediastinitis. Fibrosing mediastinitis most commonly involves the right hemithorax, although bilateral involvement may occur. In most patients obstruction does not progress, but mild to moderate symptoms persist indefinitely. In fewer than one quarter of patients the illness is progressive, highlighted by repeated bouts of pneumonia, hemoptysis, respiratory failure, or pulmonary hypertension. No proven medical therapy exists for fibrosing mediastinitis due to histoplasmosis, including antifungal and corticosteroid therapy. Because the pathogenesis involves fibrosis rather than inflammation or infection, antifungal or anti-inflammatory therapy is not effective. Because fibrosis infiltrates adjacent mediastinal structures, surgical therapy has been of little benefit and is associated with a high risk for surgical morbidity and mortality. Surgical therapy is rarely indicated, and should be considered only after careful consideration of the risks and benefits by experts in the management of patients with fibrosing mediastinitis. Various procedures to relieve compression of vascular structures, and airway and esophageal compression are often employed with mixed results.

Distinguishing fibrosing mediastinitis from mediastinal granuloma is key. Mediastinal granuloma represents persistent inflammation in mediastinal or hilar lymph nodes. Enlarged, inflamed nodes may cause chest pain with or without impingement upon soft mediastinal structures, such as the esophagus or superior vena cava. Fistulae may develop between the lymph nodes, airways, or esophagus. Improvement may occur spontaneously or following antifungal therapy. The enlarged lymph nodes are usually encased in a discrete capsule, which can be dissected free from the adjacent tissues with a low risk for surgical morbidity or mortality. Thus, surgery may be appropriate in patients with persistent symptoms despite antifungal therapy, weighing the risk of surgery with the severity of the clinical findings. However, studies establishing the effectiveness of surgery for mediastinal granuloma are scant, and surgical therapy is rarely necessary in such cases.

Often mediastinal lymphadenopathy is asymptomatic, identified on chest radiographs or CT scans performed for other reasons. In such cases concern arises if the mass may represent malignancy. Differentiation of mediastinal lymphadenopathy caused by histoplasmosis or other granulomatous infection from that caused by a malignancy is best deferred to pulmonary disease consultants *(7)*. The presence of calcification strongly suggests that lymphadenopathy is caused by granulomatous infection, but cannot rule out concomitant neoplasm. Conversely, the absence of calcification does not exclude granulomatous infection, and is quite typical of histoplasmosis during the first year or two after infection. Positron emission tomography (PET) scan has been suggested as a method to distinguish malignancy from nonmalignant causes for mediastinal or pulmonary masses, but PET scan is often positive in patients with histoplasmosis. For most patients lacking risk factors for malignancy, follow-up CT scan at 3- to 6-month intervals for 1 year is appropriate; lack of progressive enlargement supports the diagnosis of histoplasmosis. In others, especially those with risk factors for malignancy, biopsy may be necessary for definitive diagnosis. Choices include surgical excision or mediastinoscopy, although many recommend avoiding the latter because of risk of excessive bleeding.

5.7. *African Histoplasmosis*

In addition to infection with *Histoplasma capsulatum* var. *capsulatum*, *Histoplasma capsulatum* var. *duboisii* causes disease in Africa. Bony abscesses, more commonly involving the axillary skeleton, and skin lesions are much more common with African histoplasmosis. Pulmonary disease is rare, although infection with this variant also likely occurs via inhalation of spores. Disseminated African histoplasmosis resembling PDH as described in the preceding text has been reported, with fever, multi-organ involvement, and a progressive course. The yeasts of *H. capsulatum* var. *duboisii* are 10 to 15 μm in diameter (much larger than var. *capsulatum*) and can be seen within giant cells. This can be easily confused with *Blastomyces dermatitis* or *Coccidioides immitis* on histopathological examination. DNA and antigen tests with the African variant should react similarly to *H. capsulatum* var. *capsulatum*. Likewise, therapy is similar with the exception that isolated cutaneous disease, or "cold abscesses" may heal spontaneously or with excisional surgery. Disseminated African histoplasmosis, especially with HIV coinfection, has a poor prognosis.

6. DIAGNOSIS

6.1. *Culture*

The only test specific for histoplasmosis is culture, but the sensitivity is low, and delays up to 1 month may be required to isolate the organism *(15)*. Identification as *H. capsulatum* can be determined by conversion from the mould to the yeast, exoantigen detection, or through use of the commercially available DNA probe. Despite these limitations, culture should be performed unless the patient is already improving at the time the diagnosis is suspected. In patients with pulmonary disease, bronchoscopy may be required if patients are unable to produce sputum. In those with suspected PDH, fungal blood cultures should be obtained, but cultures of tissues requiring invasive procedures may be deferred if tests for antigen are positive. In such cases, failure to improve within 2 weeks after initiation of therapy would raise question about the diagnosis and support additional testing.

6.2. *Antigen Detection*

Antigen detection is most useful method for rapid diagnosis of the more severe histoplasmosis syndromes, including acute diffuse pulmonary histoplasmosis and PDH *(15)*. The Histoplasma antigen assay has been revised to reduce false-positive *(16)* and false-negative results *(17)*. Antigen may be detected in any body fluid, but urine and serum testing is recommended in all cases. In some patients with pulmonary histoplasmosis, antigen may be detected in the bronchoalveolar lavage fluid but not in urine or serum *(18)*. Antigen may also be detected in the cerebrospinal fluid in patients with central nervous system histoplasmosis *(19)*, in pleural fluid, synovial fluid, peritoneal fluid, or in pericardial fluid in patients with infection localized to those tissues. Antigen levels decline with effective therapy, persist with ineffective therapy, and rebound in patients who relapse during or following treatment *(15)*.

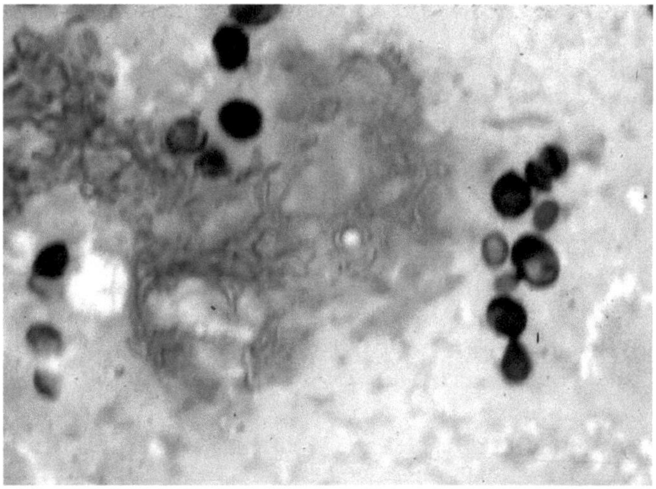

Fig. 17.6. Gomori methenamine silver (GMS) stain of yeast showing narrow neck budding. [Figure in color on CD-ROM].

6.3. Histopathology

Demonstration of yeast-like structures in body fluids or tissues may provide a rapid diagnosis in some cases *(7)* (Fig. 17.6) (see also Fig. 3.6, Chapter 3). Limitations of histopathology include the need for performance of an invasive procedure and low sensitivity. Histopathology may be falsely negative or falsely positive when performed by pathologists inexperienced with recognition of fungal pathogens. If histopathology is inconsistent with clinical findings or other laboratory tests, the specimens should be reviewed by a pathologist experienced with recognition of fungal pathogens.

6.4. Serologic Tests

Serologic tests for antibodies are most useful in patients with subacute pulmonary histoplasmosis, chronic pulmonary histoplasmosis, granulomatous mediastinitis, pericarditis, or rheumatologic syndromes *(15)*. Immunodiffusion and complement fixation tests should be performed in all cases of suspected histoplasmosis. Serologic tests may be falsely negative during the first 2 months after acute exposure, limiting their usefulness in acute pulmonary histoplasmosis. Also, these tests may be falsely negative in immunosuppressed patients, limiting their role in PDH. Further, positive serologic tests persist for several years after recovery from histoplasmosis, and thus may provide misleading information in patients with other diseases.

6.5. Conclusions

Accurate diagnosis of histoplasmosis requires skilled use of all of these laboratory methods. Except for culture, none of the tests are specific, and physicians must consider that the positive result may be falsely positive. Further, none of the tests are positive in all cases, and the physician must consider the possibility that the test is falsely negative.

In cases in which the diagnosis is uncertain, or the laboratory tests are inconsistent, additional testing should be performed, including repetition of the antigen test or serology, and in some cases, invasive procedures to obtain tissues for histopathology and culture; expert advise should be sought.

7. TREATMENT

Practice guidelines, published in 2000 *(20)*, are currently being updated. Treatment is indicated in patients with acute diffuse pulmonary histoplasmosis, chronic pulmonary histoplasmosis, and PDH (Table 17.1). Adjunctive treatment with methyl prednisolone or prednisone may hasten recovery in otherwise healthy individuals with respiratory distress caused by acute pulmonary histoplasmosis, and can be administered safely if patients also receive antifungal therapy.

Treatment also should be considered in patients with subacute pulmonary histoplasmosis or granulomatous mediastinitis who are not improving within a month

Table 17.1
Primary and alternate therapy for treatment for histoplasmosis

Presentation	Primary therapy	Alternate therapy
Acute pulmonary Mild	Itraconazole 200 mg qd or bid for 6–12 weeks	Posaconazole 400 mg bid, or voriconazole 200 mg bid, or fluconazole 800 mg qd
Moderately severe or severe	Liposomal amphotericin B 3–5 mg/kg per day for 1–2 weeks followed by itraconazole 200 mg bid for 12 weeks;[a] methyl prednisolone or prednisone 0.5–1 mg/kg per day for 1–2 weeks[b]	Amphotericin B lipid complex 3–5 mg/kg per day, or amphotericin B deoxycholate 0.7–1.0 mg/kg per day
Chronic pulmonary	Itraconazole 200 mg bid for at least 12 months	Posaconazole 400 mg bid, or voriconazole 200 mg bid, or fluconazole 800 mg qd
Disseminated	Liposomal amphotericin B 3–5 mg/kg per day for 1–2 weeks followed by itraconazole 200 mg bid at least 12 months[a]	Amphotericin B lipid complex 3–5 mg/kg per day, or amphotericin B deoxycholate 0.7–1.0 mg/kg per day

qd, once daily; bid, twice daily; tid, three times daily; mg/kg per day, milligram/kilogram per day.
[a]Itraconazole may be given 200 mg tid × 3 days as a loading dose to achieve steady-state levels more quickly. The capsule formulation should be administered with food whereas the solution should be administered on an empty stomach. Measurement of drug concentrations is recommended because itraconazole drug exposure is highly variable. The intravenous formulation of itraconazole would be an alternative in a hospitalized patient with moderately severe or severe disease who cannot be treated with any amphotericin formulation.
[b]Adjunctive treatment with methyl prednisolone or prednisone may hasten recovery in otherwise healthy individuals with respiratory distress caused by acute pulmonary histoplasmosis.

or two of the onset of symptoms; however, the effectiveness of therapy for these manifestations remains uncertain. Treatment for fibrosing mediastinitis is ineffective, and is not indicated except in cases in which granulomatous mediastinitis cannot be reasonably excluded. Treatment is not indicated in patients with calcified or noncalcified pulmonary nodules or as prophylaxis before immunosuppression in patients without evidence of active histoplasmosis within the last 2 or 3 years.

Liposomal amphotericin B is the treatment of choice for patients with severe manifestations of histoplasmosis requiring hospitalization *(21)*. In some cases, however, because of intolerance or cost, other lipid formulations may be used. In children, deoxycholate amphotericin B is well tolerated and preferred over the lipid formulations because of cost. Itraconazole is recommended for mild cases not requiring hospitalization and for continued therapy after response to liposomal amphotericin B. Treatment should be continued for 6 to 12 weeks in patients with acute pulmonary histoplasmosis and 1 year or longer in patients with chronic pulmonary histoplasmosis or PDH. In patients with AIDS who achieve a good immunologic response to antiretroviral therapy, itraconazole may be stopped after 1 year if the $CD4^+$ T lymphocyte count is above 200 cells/μl and the antigen concentration in urine and serum are below 4 ng/ml *(22)*. However, in those with persistent immune deficiency, or who relapse after stopping an appropriate course of therapy, lifelong maintenance therapy may be required. Itraconazole blood levels should be monitored to ensure adequate drug exposure, and the dosage should be increased or the capsule formulation should be replaced with the solution if random concentrations are below 2 μg/ml.

If the antigen test is positive, treatment should be continued until antigen levels become undetectable or below 4 ng/ml. Further, antigen levels should be monitored during the first year following discontinuation of therapy, and at the time of recurrence of symptoms suggesting relapse of histoplasmosis.

The best alternative oral therapy in patients unable to take itraconazole is posaconazole, which is highly active in vitro *(23)*, in animal models *(23)*, and in patients *(24)*. Fluconazole is less active in histoplasmosis, and relapse associated with development of resistance has been observed in patients with AIDS *(25)*. Voriconazole is more active in vitro than fluconazole, but less active than itraconazole or posaconazole. Although minimum inhibitory concentrations (MICs) are lower to voriconazole than fluconazole, higher drug exposure with fluconazole offsets the lower MICs. Further, prior exposure to fluconazole or voriconazole may induce resistance to voriconazole *(26)*. Voriconazole has not been studied in animal models or patients with histoplasmosis, and offers no clear advantage over fluconazole. Measurement of voriconazole or posaconazole blood levels is recommended because of the wide variation in drug levels. Voriconazole exhibits a short half-life (approximately 6 hours) and concentrations decline in at least twofold from the peak to the trough time after administration. Accordingly, trough concentrations of voriconazole of at least 0.5 μg/ml are recommended. Posaconazole exhibits a long half-life, similar to that of itraconazole (approximately 24 hours), supporting a similar target random concentration of 2 μg/ml. The echinocandins are not active in histoplasmosis and should not be used *(27)*.

REFERENCES

1. Panackal AA, Hajjeh RA, Cetron MS, Warnock DW. Fungal infections among returning travelers. Clin Infect Dis 2002;35:1088–1095.
2. Chu JH, Feudtner C, Heydon K, Walsh TJ, Zaoutis TE. Hospitalizations for endemic mycoses: a population-based national study. Clin Infect Dis 2006;42:822–825.
3. Antinori S, Magni C, Nebuloni M et al. Histoplasmosis among human immunodeficiency virus-infected people in Europe: report of 4 cases and review of the literature. Medicine (Baltimore) 2006;85:22–36.
4. Newman SL. Interaction of *Histoplasma capsulatum* with human macrophages, dendritic cells, and neutrophils. Methods Mol Med 2005;118:181–191.
5. Deepe GS. Modulation of infection with *Histoplasma capsulatum* by inhibition of tumor necrosis factor-alpha activity. Clin Infect Dis 2005;41 (Suppl 3):S204–S207.
6. Vail GM, Young RS, Wheat LJ, Filo RS, Cornetta K, Goldman M. Incidence of histoplasmosis following allogeneic bone marrow transplant or solid organ transplant in a hyperendemic area. Transpl Infect Dis 2002;4:148–151.
7. Wheat LJ, Conces DJ, Allen S, Blue-Hnidy D, Loyd J. Pulmonary histoplasmosis syndromes: recognition, diagnosis, and management. Semin Respir Crit Care Med 2004;25:129–144.
8. Wheat LJ, Kauffman CA. Histoplasmosis. Infect Dis Clin North Am 2003;17:1–19.
9. Freifeld AG, Iwen PC, Lesiak BL, Gilroy RK, Stevens RB, Kalil AC. Histoplasmosis in solid organ transplant recipients at a large Midwestern university transplant center. Transpl Infect Dis 2005;7:109–115.
10. Wood KL, Hage CA, Knox KS, et al. Histoplasmosis after treatment with anti-TNF-alpha therapy. Am J Respir Crit Care Med 2003;167:1279–1282.
11. Wheat J. Histoplasmosis in the acquired immunodeficiency syndrome. Curr Top Med Mycol 1996;7:7–18.
12. Duncan RA, Von Reyn CF, Alliegro GM, Toossi Z, Sugar AM, Levitz SM. Idiopathic CD4+ T-lymphocytopenia—four patients with opportunistic infections and no evidence of HIV infection. N Engl J Med 1993;328:393–398.
13. Zerbe CS, Holland SM. Disseminated histoplasmosis in persons with interferon-gamma receptor 1 deficiency. Clin Infect Dis 2005;41:e38–e41.
14. Adderson EE. Histoplasmosis in a pediatric oncology center. J Pediatr 2004;144:100–106.
15. Wheat LJ. Current diagnosis of histoplasmosis. Trends Microbiol 2003;11:488–494.
16. Wheat LJ, Connolly P, Durkin M, et al. False-positive Histoplasma antigenemia caused by antithymocyte globulin antibodies. Transpl Infect Dis 2004;6:23–27.
17. Wheat LJ, Connolly P, Durkin M, Book BK, Pescovitz MD. Elimination of false-positive Histoplasma antigenemia caused by human anti-rabbit antibodies in the second generation Histoplasma antigen test. Transpl Infect Dis 2006;8:219-221.
18. Hage CA, Davis TE, Egan L, et al. Diagnosis of pulmonary histoplasmosis and blastomycosis by detection of antigen in bronchoalveolar lavage fluid using an improved second-generation enzyme-linked immunoassay. Respir Med 2007;101:43–47.
19. Wheat LJ, Musial CE, Jenny-Avital E. Diagnosis and management of central nervous system histoplasmosis. Clin Infect Dis 2005;40:844–852.
20. Wheat J, Sarosi G, McKinsey D, et al. Practice guidelines for the management of patients with histoplasmosis. Infectious Diseases Society of America. Clin Infect Dis 2000;30: 688–695.
21. Johnson PC, Wheat LJ, Cloud GA, et al. Safety and efficacy of liposomal amphotericin B compared with conventional amphotericin B for induction therapy of histoplasmosis in patients with AIDS. Ann Intern Med 2002;137:105–109.

22. Goldman M, Zackin R, Fichtenbaum CJ, et al. Safety of discontinuation of maintenance therapy for disseminated histoplasmosis after immunologic response to antiretroviral therapy. Clin Infect Dis 2004;38:1485–1489.
23. Connolly P, Wheat LJ, Schnizlein-Bick C, et al. Comparison of a new triazole, posaconazole, with itraconazole and amphotericin B for treatment of histoplasmosis following pulmonary challenge in immunocompromised mice. Antimicrob Agents Chemother 2000;44: 2604–2608.
24. Restrepo A, Tobon A, Clark B, et al. Salvage treatment of histoplasmosis with posaconazole. J Infect 2007;54:319–327.
25. Wheat LJ, Connolly P, Smedema M, Brizendine E, Hafner R. Emergence of resistance to fluconazole as a cause of failure during treatment of histoplasmosis in patients with acquired immunodeficiency disease syndrome. Clin Infect Dis 2001;33:1910–1913.
26. Wheat LJ, Connolly P, Smedema M, et al. Activity of newer triazoles against *Histoplasma capsulatum* from patients with AIDS who failed fluconazole. J Antimicrob Chemother 2006;57:1235–1239.
27. Kohler S, Wheat LJ, Connolly P, et al. Comparison of the echinocandin caspofungin with amphotericin B for treatment of histoplasmosis following pulmonary challenge in a murine model. Antimicrob Agents Chemother 2000;44:1850–1854.

SUGGESTED READINGS

Goldman M, Zackin R, Fichtenbaum CJ, et al. Safety of discontinuation of maintenance therapy for disseminated histoplasmosis after immunologic response to antiretroviral therapy. Clin Infect Dis 2004;38:1485–1489.

Johnson PC, Wheat LJ, Cloud GA, et al. Safety and efficacy of liposomal amphotericin B compared with conventional amphotericin B for induction therapy of histoplasmosis in patients with AIDS. Ann Intern Med 2002;137:105–109.

Lee JH, Slifman NR, Gershon SK, et al. Life-threatening histoplasmosis complicating immunotherapy with tumor necrosis factor alpha antagonists infliximab and etanercept. Arthritis Rheum 2002;46:2565–2570.

Limaye AP, Connolly PA, Sagar M, et al. Transmission of *Histoplasma capsulatum* by organ transplantation. N Engl J Med 2000;343:1163–1166.

Vail GM, Young RS, Wheat LJ, Filo RS, Cornetta K, Goldman M. Incidence of histoplasmosis following allogeneic bone marrow transplant or solid organ transplant in a hyperendemic area. Transpl Infect Dis 2002;4:148–151.

Wheat LJ. Histoplasmosis: a review for clinicians from non-endemic areas. Mycoses 2006;49:274–282.

Wheat LJ, Conces DJ, Jr., Allen S, Blue-Hnidy D, Loyd J. Pulmonary histoplasmosis syndromes: recognition, diagnosis, and management. Semin Respir Crit Care Med 2004;25:129–144.

Wheat LJ, Musial CE, Jenny-Avital E. Diagnosis and management of central nervous system histoplasmosis. Clin Infect Dis 2005;40:844–852.

Woods JP. *Histoplasma capsulatum* molecular genetics, pathogenesis, and responsiveness to its environment. Fungal Genet Biol 2002;35:81—97.

18
Paracoccidioidomycosis

Angela Restrepo, PhD, Angela M. Tobón, MD, and Carlos A. Agudelo, MD

1. INTRODUCTION

Paracoccidioidomycosis (PCM), formerly known as South American blastomycosis, was first described by Lutz in Brazil in 1906. Lutz and Splendore described the etiologic agent but considered it to be a strain of *Coccidioides immitis*. It was not until 1930 when the de Almeida properly differentiated its etiologic agent and designated it *Paracoccidioides brasiliensis*. The Brazilian disease was soon diagnosed in other Latin American countries and its peculiar geographic limitation to Latin American countries recognized *(1)*.

PCM is an endemic and systemic disease caused by the thermally dimorphic fungus, *Paracoccidioides brasiliensis,* a microorganism exogenous to humans that has an as yet undiscovered habitat. The infection is acquired by the inhalation of mycelial form structures (conidia, mycelial fragments) that settle into the lungs where they convert into the tissue yeast form structure that characteristically reproduces by multiple budding. PCM exists in two forms, subclinical infection and the clinically manifested disease. The latter is usually chronic with involvement of the primary target, the lungs, and of other organs and systems (including the mucosa, skin, adrenal glands, and lymph nodes). The mycosis afflicts men more frequently than women and is more common in adults. Latency is known to exist and is frequently prolonged *(2)*.

2. ETIOLOGIC AGENT

P. brasiliensis is a thermally dimorphic fungus that at temperatures between 4°C and 25°C grows as a white mould, microscopically composed of thin septated hyphae, occasional chlamydospores, and rare conidia; the latter are infectious. At 35° to 37°C the colony is soft and wrinkled and microscopically is comprised of oval to round yeast cells of varying sizes (4 to 40 μm) that reproduce by budding. The key distinguishing feature is that of multiple budding yeast cells with a larger mother cell surrounded by multiple daughter cells (blastoconidia), a structure thought to resemble the pilot wheel of a ship. A thick refractive cell wall and prominent intracytoplasmic vacuoles

From: *Infectious Disease: Diagnosis and Treatment of Human Mycoses*
Edited by: D. R. Hospenthal and M. G. Rinaldi © Humana Press Inc., Totowa, NJ

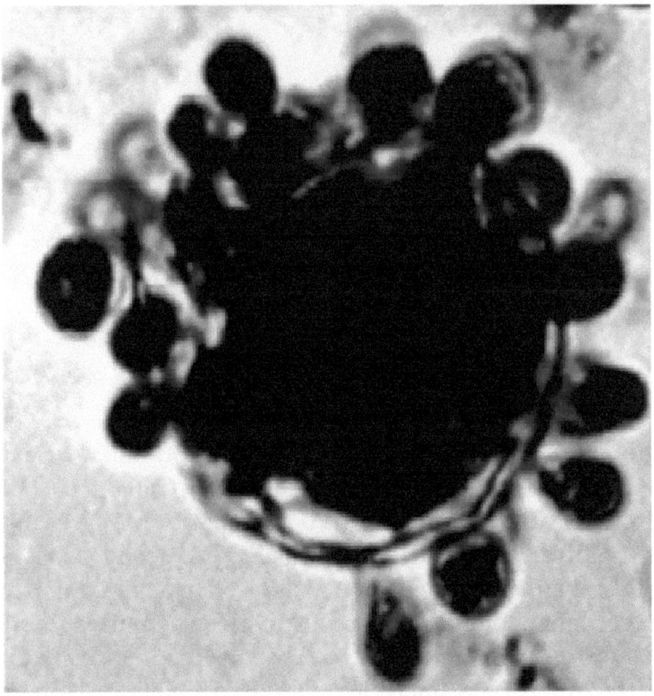

Fig. 18.1. *P. brasiliensis* yeast cell surrounded by multiple budding daughter blastoconidia ("pilot's wheel"). [Figure in color on CD-ROM].

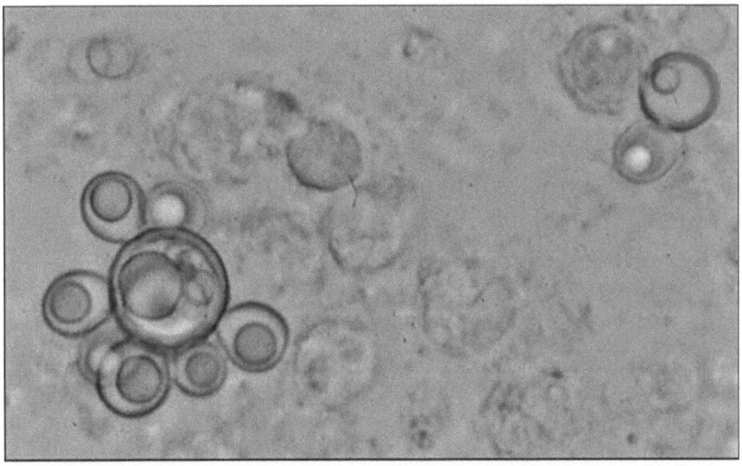

Fig. 18.2. *P. brasiliensis* in sputum sample. Note multiple budding yeast cell and single yeasts with prominent lipid vacuoles. KOH and blue ink. [Figure in color on CD-ROM].

further characterize the organism at these temperatures (Fig. 18.1). The aforementioned morphologic characteristics are also observed in clinical specimens (Fig. 18.2) *(1,3)*.

Despite the absence of a sexual stage or teleomorph, *P. brasiliensis* has been classified in the phylum Ascomycota, order Onygenales, family Onygenaceae on the basis of phylogenetic studies and on its sharing certain characteristics with other dimorphic fungi (e.g., *Blastomyces dermatitidis, Histoplasma capsulatum*) exhibiting teleomorphic stages, genus *Ajellomyces (4)*.

3. EPIDEMIOLOGY

Demographic data indicate that clinically manifested PCM predominates in adults, 80% to 95% of cases. In highly endemic areas, skin testing with paracoccidioidin has indicated that among healthy populations the prevalence of infection is close to 10%. The prevalence of disease in other areas of Latin America has been estimated to be much lower, 0.33 to 3 cases per 100,000 inhabitants *(1,3)*. The disease is more often diagnosed in males than in females (ratio of 15:1), even though similar infection rates are demonstrated by paracoccidioidin skin testing. Most patients (73%) have or have had agriculture-related occupations *(2,5–8)*.

One of the most relevant characteristics of PCM is its restricted geographic limitation to Central and South America from Mexico (23° North) to Argentina (34° South), sparing certain countries within these latitudes (Chile, Surinam, the Guyana, Nicaragua, Belize, most of the Caribbean Islands) *(3)*. Also of note is the fact that within endemic countries the mycosis is not diagnosed everywhere, but in areas with relatively well-defined ecologic characteristics. These characteristics include the presence of tropical and subtropical forests, abundant watercourses, mild temperatures (<27°C), high rainfall (2000 to 2999 mm), and coffee/tobacco crops *(9)*. Risk factors include living and working in these areas, as well as malnutrition. Alcoholism and smoking may also play a role. A direct relationship with underlying immunosuppressive conditions, including human immunodeficiency virus (HIV) infection, has not been clearly demonstrated although sporadic cases have been reported *(1,3,10)*. In the case of the PCM–HIV coinfection, the total number of reported cases in the endemic areas appears to not have exceeded 200 patients *(1,3,11)*.

Approximately 60 cases of PCM have been reported outside of the endemic areas (North America, Europe, Asia); however all these patients had previously resided in recognized endemic countries *(3,12,13)*. These cases demonstrate that *P. brasiliensis* can remain latent for long periods (mean 13 years) from the time of infection to disease manifestations *(3)*. Latency may explain why the microniche of *P. brasiliensis* has not been precisely demonstrated, as with delay in presentation, the site and type of activities that led to infection are likely forgotten. No outbreaks have been reported and the isolation of the fungus from nature (e.g., soils) has seldom been successful *(14)*.

4. PATHOGENESIS AND IMMUNOLOGY

Lack of data on *P. brasiliensis* habitat and on the characteristics of the primary infection has hindered full understanding of the pathogenesis of PCM. Based on experimental animal studies it is accepted that infection is acquired by inhalation of the conidia produced by the mycelial form, structures that are sufficiently small to reach

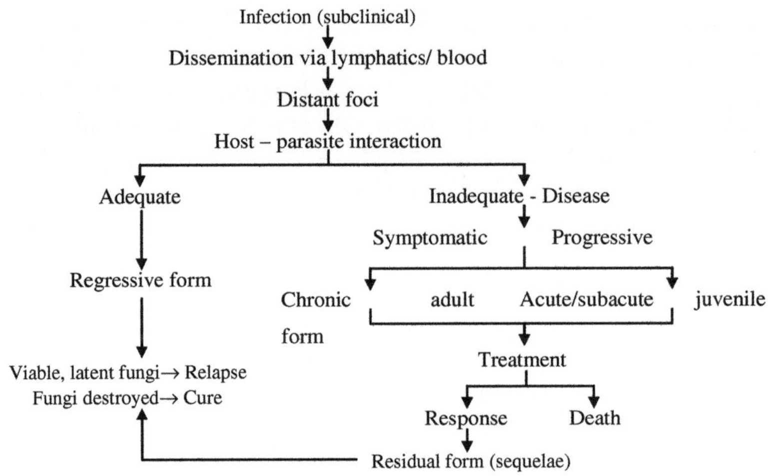

Fig. 18.3. Natural history of paracoccidioidomycosis.

the alveoli, where they soon transform into yeast cells *(15,16)*. The organism then multiplies in the lung parenchyma and disseminates by the venous/lymphatic routes to extrapulmonary organs (Fig. 18.3). Infection gives rise to an intense host response with alveolitis and abundant neutrophils engulfing the fungus, later on replaced by migrating mononuclear cells that convert into epithelial cells initiating granuloma formation and attracting $CD8^+$ T lymphocytes *(1,2,17)*.

The host immune response determines the course of the infection, with subclinical infection predominating in immunocompetent individuals and clinically manifested disease appearing in those whose cellular immunity is deficient. Thus, children and some HIV-infected individuals develop disseminated disease with predominant involvement of the reticuloendothelial system, the acute/subacute juvenile type disease *(18–20)*. Adult patients tend to develop a chronic, progressive disease, marked by more severe pulmonary damage accompanied in most cases by dissemination to the lymphatic system, the mucosa, the adrenals, skin, and other organs *(1–3)*. Lung damage progresses to fibrosis, leaving behind important sequelae *(1–3)*. An efficient T helper 1 (Th1) cellular immune response is required to control fungus invasion while a T helper 2 (Th2) type response is reflected by abundant fungal multiplication and extra-pulmonary dissemination with progression of disease *(21,22)*. Antibodies are detected in most patients with either the acute or the chronic type of disease but their role in protection or dissemination is still unclear *(1,23)*.

5. CLINICAL MANIFESTATIONS

PCM is a disorder characterized by protean manifestations; usually it is a chronic progressive disease involving various organs and systems. In untreated and patients with chronic, advanced disease, mortality rates may be high; 1.4 per one million inhabitants in Brazil *(24)*. Most patients present with constitutional symptoms such as general malaise, asthenia, weight loss and fever, as well as symptoms specific to the organs infected by the fungus. The lungs are the site of primary infection, but often neither the patient nor the clinical examiner will note abnormalities at this site.

On the basis of the clinical presentation and the host immune response to PCM, the disease is categorized as *(1)* subclinical infection or *(2)* symptomatic infection, which is divided into two forms, the acute/subacute juvenile and the chronic adult type. The latter may involve one (unifocal) or various organs (multifocal) with the severity of the symptoms varying with the patient. The acute/subacute juvenile type is always disseminated. A third, residual form characterized by fibrotic sequelae has also been suggested *(1–3)*.

5.1. Subclinical Infection

Subclinical infection has no special characteristics and is detected mostly by a reactive paracoccidioidin skin testing, and sometimes by chest radiograph abnormalities *(25)*. However, *P. brasiliensis* may remain latent in the infected host and give rise to symptomatic paracoccidioidomycosis years after the initial contact, as demonstrated by the cases diagnosed outside of the endemic areas for the mycosis *(2,12,13)*.

5.2. Symptomatic Infection

The clinically manifested disease varies with patient age.

5.2.1. Juvenile Type Disease

The juvenile type disease is a serious disorder that afflicts children and immunocompromised individuals of either sex; it represents fewer that 10% of all cases. Involvement of the reticuloendothelial system with lymphadenopathy, hepatomegaly, and splenomegaly characterize this form. Skin lesions, often multiple, may also be present, along with fever, marked weight loss, and general malaise. Bone involvement is frequent in the subacute severe cases. Respiratory symptoms are minimal but the fungus can be seen in respiratory secretions. High-resolution computed tomography (CT) studies reveal lung abnormalities in a significant proportion of these patients *(8,18–20)*.

5.2.2. Chronic Adult Type Disease

The chronic, adult type disease predominates (80% to 90%) in all case series, typically occurring in patients older 30 years of age with agriculture-related occupations; males are more frequently afflicted than females (15:1). The disease course is characterized by protracted pulmonary and extrapulmonary organ damage, mainly of the mucous membranes and the skin, where the lesions tend to be ulcerative, granulomatous, and infiltrated (Fig. 18.4). Sialorrhea, dysphagia, and dysphonia are common. Regional lymph nodes are hypertrophied and may spontaneously drain forming fistulae. The adrenals glands may also become involved, with associated symptoms of adrenal deficiency. Central nervous system (CNS) involvement is also considered important. Chest radiographs reveal infiltrates, mostly interstitial but at times also alveolar; these are located in the central and lower fields and are bilateral. Sequelae represented mainly by pulmonary fibrosis can be observed in half of the cases (Fig. 18.5) *(1,2,6,7,26–29)*. Usually, at time of the initial consultation, more than one organ is involved.

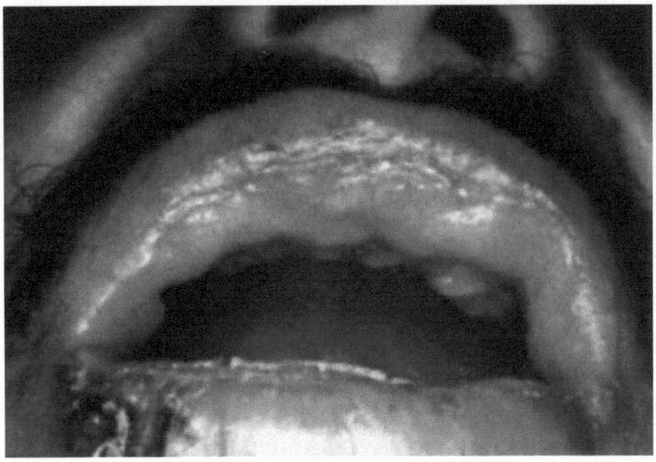

Fig. 18.4. Cutaneous and mucosal lesions in a patient with paracoccidioidomycosis. Note lip edema, ulceration, and scarring. [Figure in color on CD-ROM].

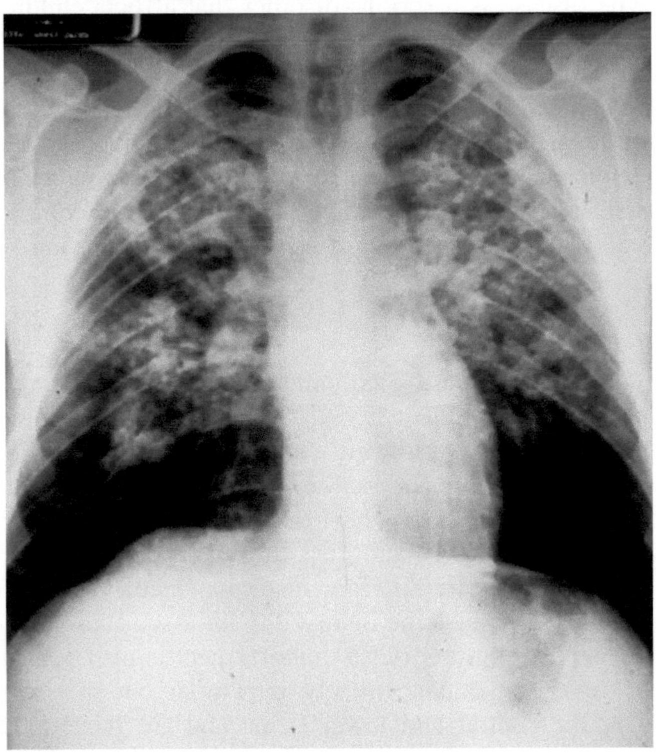

Fig. 18.5. Pulmonary paracoccidioidomycosis. Note abundant fibronodular infiltrates in central fields and basal bullae. [Figure in color on CD-ROM].

6. DIAGNOSIS

Diagnosis is based on directed diagnostic techniques in persons with the relevant symptoms and risk factors/endemic exposures (Table 18.1). Direct potassium hydroxide (KOH) examination of clinical material including sputum, bronchoalveolar lavage (BAL) fluid, exudates, lymph node drainage, and biopsies offer a diagnosis in more than 90% of the cases; the rather large yeast cells with their translucent wall and multiple budding allow prompt identification. Most cases can be diagnosed by the histopathological study of biopsies; although Gomori methenamine silver (GMS) stain is more reliable, hematoxylin and eosin (H&E), may reveal these fungi, especially in and around granulomas (Fig. 18.6).

Isolation of *P. brasiliensis* in culture is evidence of active disease, but mould cultures are positive in only of 80% of the cases and require between 20 to 30 days for growth adequate for microscopic diagnosis. Room temperature incubation is preferred for nonsterile site specimens, but requires a transfer to 36°–37°C for transformation of the fungus into its yeast form (with its multiple budding cells) once growth is noted for confirmation. Primary isolation often requires multiple samples (e.g., sputum) and a variety of culture media *(1,3)*.

Antibody detection is useful not only for diagnosis but also for disease monitoring; antibodies of the immunoglobulin classes G, M, and E are regularly detected. Because of its simplicity, the gel immunodiffusion (ID) test is typically used in endemic countries. This test demonstrates circulating antibodies in 95% of the cases, and is very specific for PCM. Complement fixation (CF) testing allows quantification of antibody levels, and indirectly aids in determination of the severity of illness and response to treatment. CF is reactive in more than 85% of the cases, but cross-reactivity with *H. capsulatum* antigens is seen. Other tests, such as immunofluorescence, counterimmunoelectrophoresis, dot-blot, enzyme-linked immunosorbent assay, and immunoblotting, are also currently used by some centers *(30–32)*. Improvements in serodiagnosis include detection in more than 60% of the cases of circulating fungal antigens in patients'

Table 18.1
Key factors in the consideration of the diagnosis of paracoccidioidomycosis

History of residence in an endemic country (even if many years previous to symptoms/lesions)
History of working in agriculture or related occupation
Being an adult male with a chronic, progressive illness
Complaints related to external manifestations (mucous membrane, skin, and or lymph node lesions)
Pulmonary involvement is often ignored by the patient but is almost always demonstrated by radiographic or other imaging studies
Reticuloendothelial system (RES) involvement is commons in children and young adults. Presence of multiple skin lesions or bone damage may also be observed in these age groups
Coexistence with immunodeficiency states is not a hallmark, but may occur.
Remember: paracoccidioidomycosis is a disease of protean manifestations that may exhibit peculiar clinical aspects hindering proper diagnosis

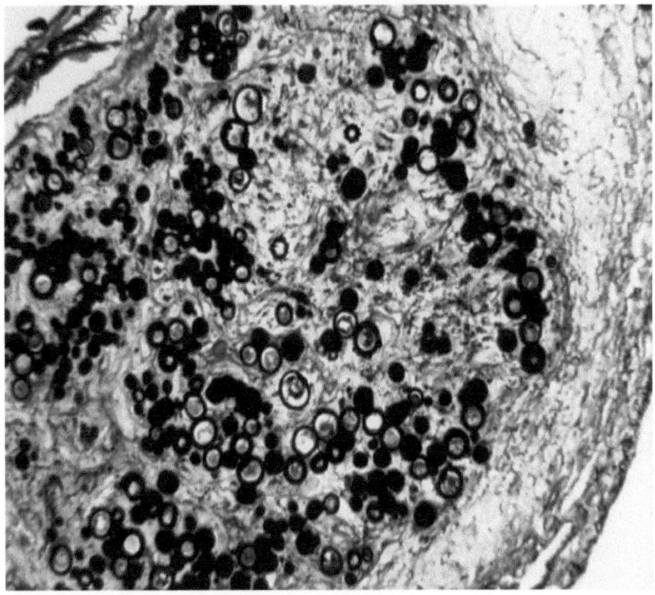

Fig. 18.6. Tissue biopsy with abundant *P. brasiliensis* yeasts enclosed within a granuloma. GMS. [Figure in color on CD-ROM].

sera. Most importantly, immunosupressed patients who do not raise antibodies can be diagnosed by antigen detection, and in addition, decreasing antigen titers correlate with their clinical improvement. Skin tests play no role in diagnosis *(33,34)*.

7. TREATMENT

Antimicrobial agents from three different classes are currently used to treat PCM, with varying success. They include the sulfonamides, the polyene amphotericin B, and certain azoles (Table 18.2). Use of the newer agents, including voriconazole, posaconazole, and caspofungin, has been reported in isolated cases, but all appear promising. It should be stated that additional measures such as adequate nutrition and suspension of alcohol intake and smoking are required to accelerate recovery and diminish fibrous sequelae. In advanced cases (approximately 10%) no response to treatment may occur *(1–3)*.

Sulfonamides are of low cost and appear effective in 70% of patients. They require prolonged periods of treatment (3 to 5 years) to avoid relapses and the development of resistance. Rapidly absorbed sulfonamides such as sulfadiazine are given at a dose of 4 g per day while those characterized by prolonged absorption are administered at half the dose (2 g per day). Trimethoprim–sulfamethoxazole also appears to be effective at a 160/800 mg per tablet, two tablets twice daily. Adverse effects more commonly seen with the sulfonamides include rash, crystalluria photosensitivity, emesis, and diarrhea *(1,18)*.

Amphotericin B is effective in about 70% of cases, but its use is now limited to severely ill patients, to those with CNS or cardiac disease, and those unable to tolerate azole agents. A total cumulative dose of 1 to 2 g, based on clinical response,

Table 18.2
Antifungal use in paracoccidioidomycosis

Antifungals	Dose (daily)	Route	Duration (mean)	Response rate (%)	Relapse rate (%)
Sulfonamides	4 grams	PO	3–5 years	70	20
Amphotericin B	1 gram (cumulative dose)[a]	IV	Based on clinical response	75	20
Ketoconazole	200–400 mg	PO	6–18 months	70	10
Itraconazole					
Capsules	200 mg	PO	6 months	95	5
Suspension	100–200 mg	PO	6 months	95	5
Parenteral	200 mg	IV[b]	Based on clinical response	95	5

PO, oral; IV, intravenous.
[a]To be followed by an oral medication.
[b]To be followed by an oral azole.

is typically given, followed by maintenance therapy with oral medications. Infusional toxicity, electrolyte abnormalities, and renal dysfunction are common adverse effects. Lipid-based formulations of amphotericin B have been used in a few cases, limited likely by their high costs *(1–3)*.

With the exception of fluconazole, most of the systemically absorbed azole antifungals have proven effective in the therapy of PCM. Ketoconazole can be used successfully at a dose of 200 to 400 mg/day in adults or 5 mg/kg per day in children for 6 to 18 months; relapses occur in approximately 10% of the cases. Complications include hepatitis, gonadal dysfunction, and gastrointestinal toxicity. Interactions with several medications that are metabolized through the P450 cytochrome also limit the use of this drug. Since the introduction of itraconazole, now considered as the best option for the treatment of PCM, use of ketoconazole has decreased. Itraconazole is typically administered at a dose of 100 to 200 mg/day for approximately 6 months of therapy, based on clinical response and mycology laboratory data. Itraconazole has been shown to be effective in 95% of the patients with less adverse effects; relapses occur in 5% of the cases. Despite this high response rate, itraconazole has not reduced the fibrous pulmonary sequelae *(35)*. Care should be taken with the administration of antacids and H2 blockers as they hinder proper absorption; ingestion with a cola drink (acid) appears to improve absorption *(1–3)*. Itraconazole is also available as an oral solution with improved absorption compared to the capsular formulation. As for the solution, a loading dose similar to that of capsular itraconazole (200 mg, three times per day for 3–5 days) is administered and followed by a lower 200 mg/day dose. An intravenous formulation has made it possible to treat severely ill patients at 200 mg bid for four doses, followed by 200 mg daily until favorable changes occur in the patient's clinical aspects *(1,2,35,36)*.

8. PREVENTION

Preventive measures are difficult to establish because the source of infection is unknown; the mycosis is not transmissible from person to person. Nonetheless, precaution against aerosols is recommended when falling trees or hunting armadillos in the forest *(1)*.

REFERENCES

1. Lacaz CS, Porto E, Martins JEC, et al. Paracoccidioidomicose. In: Lacaz CS, Porto E, Martins JEC, et al., eds. Tratado de micologia médica lacaz 2002, 9th ed. Sao Paulo: Servier, 2002:639–729.
2. Restrepo A, Tobón AM. Paracoccidioides brasiliensis. In: Mandell GL, Bennett JE, Dolin R, eds. Mandell, Douglas, and Bennett's principles and practice of infectious diseases. 6th ed. Philadelphia: Elsevier Churchill Livingstone, 2005:3062–3068.
3. Restrepo A. Paracoccidioidomycosis. In: Dismukes WE, Pappas PG, Sobel JD, eds. Clinical mycology. New York: Oxford University Press, 2003:328–345.
4. San-Blas G, Niño-Vega G, Iturriaga T. *Paracoccidioides brasiliensis* and paracoccidioidomycosis: molecular approaches to morphogenesis, diagnosis, epidemiology, taxonomy and genetics. Med Mycol 2002;40:225–242.
5. Blotta MH, Mamoni RL, Oliveira SJ, et al. Endemic regions of paracoccidioidomycosis in Brazil: a clinical and epidemiologic study of 584 cases in the southeast region. Am J Trop Med Hyg 1999;61:390–394.
6. Paniagoa AM, Aguiar JI, Aguiar ES, et al. Paracoccidioidomicose: a clinical and epidemiological study of 422 cases observed in Mato Grosso do Soul. Rev Soc Bras Med Trop 2003;36:455–459.
7. Kalmar EM, Alencar FE, Alves FP, et al. Paracoccidioidomycosis: an epidemiologic survey in a pediatric population from the Brazilian Amazon using skin tests. Am J Trop Med Hyg 2004,71:82–86.
8. Rios-Gonçalves AJ, Londero AT, Terra GM, Rozenbaum E, Abreu TF, Nogueira SA. Paracoccidioidomycosis in children in the state of Rio de Janeiro (Brazil). Geographic distribution and the study of a "reservarea". Rev Inst Med Trop Sao Paulo 1998;40:11–13.
9. Calle D, Rosero DS, Orozco LC, Camargo D, Castañeda E, Restrepo A. Paracoccidioidomycosis in Colombia: an ecological study. Epidemiol Infect 2001;126:309–315.
10. Zavascki AP, Bienardt JC, Severo LC. Paracoccidioidomycosis in organ transplant recipient: case report. Rev Inst Med Trop Sao Paulo 2004;46:279–281.
11. Paniagoa AMM, Carli ACF, Aguiar JIA, et al. Paracoccidioidomycosis in patients with human immunodeficiency virus: review of 12 cases observed in an endemic region in Brazil. J Infect 2005;51:248–252.
12. Horre R, Schumacher G, Alpers K, et al. A case of imported paracoccidioidomycosis in a German legionnaire. Med Mycol 2002;40:213–216.
13. Mayr A, Kirchmair M, Rainer J, et al. Chronic paracoccidioidomycosis in a female patient in Austria. Eur J Clin Microbiol Infect Dis 2004;23:916–919.
14. Franco M, Bagagli E, Scapolio S, da Silva Lacaz C. A critical analysis of isolation of *Paracoccidioides brasiliensis* from soil. Med Mycol 2000,38:185–191.
15. McEwen JG, Bedoya V, Patiño MM, Salazar ME, Restrepo A. Experimental murine paracoccidioidomycosis induced by the inhalation of conidia. J Med Vet Mycol 1987;25:165–175.
16. Cock AM, Cano LE, Vélez D, Aristizabal BH, Trujillo J, Restrepo A. Fibrotic sequelae in pulmonary paracoccidioidomycosis: histopathological aspects in BALB/c mice infected

with viable and non-viable *Paracoccidioides brasiliensis* propagule. Rev Inst Med Trop S Paulo 2000;42:59–66.

17. Borges-Walmsley MI, Chen D, Shu X, Walmsley AR. The pathobiology of *Paracoccidioides brasiliensis*. Trends Microbiol 2002:10:80–87.
18. Pereira RM, Bucaretchi F, Barison Ede M, Hessel G, Tresoldi AT. Paracoccidioidomycosis in children: clinical presentation, follow-up and outcome. Rev Inst Med Trop S Paulo 2004;46:127–131.
19. Benard G, Kavakama J, Mendes-Giannini MJ, Kono A, Duarte AJ, Shikanai-Yasuda MA. Contribution to the natural history of paracoccidioidomycosis: identification of the primary pulmonary infection in the severe acute form of the disease–a case report. Clin Infect Dis 2005;40:e1–e4.
20. Benard G, Duarte AJ. Paracoccidioidomycosis: a model for evaluation of the effects of human immunodeficiency virus infection on the natural history of endemic tropical diseases. Clin Infect Dis 2000;31:1032–1039.
21. Marques Mello L, Silva-Vergara ML, Rodrigues V. Patients with active infection with *Paracoccidioides brasiliensis* present a Th2 immune response characterized by high Interleukin-4 and Interleukin-5 production. Hum Immunol 2002;63:149–154.
22. Mamoni RL, Blotta MH. Kinetics of cytokines and chemokines gene expression distinguishes *Paracoccidioides brasiliensis* infection from disease. Cytokine 2005;32:20–29.
23. Souza AR, Gesztesi JL, del Negro GM, et al. Anti-idiotypic antibodies in patients with different clinical forms of paracoccidioidomycosis. Clin Diagn Lab Immunol 2000;7: 175–181.
24. Coutinho ZF, da Silva D, Lazera M, et al. Paracoccidioidomycosis mortality in Brazil (1980–1995). Cad Saude Publica 2002;18:1441–1454.
25. dos Santos JW, Debiasi RB, Miletho JN, Bertolazi AN, Fagundes AL, Michel GT. Asymptomatic presentation of chronic pulmonary paracoccidioidomycosis: case report and review. Mycopathologia. 2004;157:53–57.
26. Fumari K, Kavakama J, Shikanai-Yasuda MA, et al. Chronic pulmonary paracoccidioidomycosis (South American blastomycosis): high resolution CT findings in 41 patients. Am J Roentgenol 1999;173:59–64.
27. Leal AM, Bellucci AD, Muglia VF, Lucchesi FR. Unique adrenal gland imaging features in Addison's disease caused by paracoccidioidomycosis. Am J Roentgenol 2003;181: 1433–1434.
28. Almeida SM, Queiroz-Telles F, Teive HA, Ribeiro CE, Werneck LC. Central nervous system paracoccidioidomycosis: clinical features and laboratorial findings. J Infect 2004;48:193–198.
29. Godoy H, Reichart PA. Oral manifestations of paracoccidioidomycosis. Report of 21 cases from Argentina. Mycoses 2003;46:412–417.
30. San Blas G, Niño-Vega G. *Paracoccidioides brasiliensis*: virulence and host response. In: Cihlar RL, Caldernone RA, eds. Fungal pathogenesis: principles and clinical applications. New York, NY: Marcel Dekker, Inc.; 2000:206–226.
31. Do Valle ACF, Costa RLB, Fialho Monteiro PC, Von Helder J, Muniz MM, Zancopé-Oliveira RM. Interpretation and clinical correlation of serological tests in paracoccidioidomycosis. Med Mycol 2001;39:373–377.
32. Del Negro GMB, Pereira CN, Andrade HF, et al. Evaluation of tests for antibody response in the follow-up of patients with acute and chronic forms of paracoccidioidomycosis. J Med Microbiol 2000;49:37–46.
33. Marques da Silva SH, Colombo AL, Blotta MH, Lopes JD, Queiroz-Telles F, Pires de Camargo Z. Detection of circulating gp43 antigen in serum, cerebrospinal fluid, and bronchoalveolar lavage fluid of patients with paracoccidioidomycosis. J Clin Microbiol 2003;41:3675–3680.

34. Gómez BL, Figueroa JI, Hamilton AJ, et al. Antigenemia in patients with paracoccidioidomycosis: detection of the 87-kilodalton determinant during and after antifungal therapy. J Clin Microbiol 1998;36:3309–3316.
35. Tobon AM, Agudelo CA, Osorio ML, et al. Residual pulmonary abnormalities in adult patients with chronic paracoccidioidomycosis: prolonged follow-up after itraconazole therapy. Clin Infect Dis 2003:37:898–904.
36. Restrepo A, Benard G. Paracoccidioidomycosis. In: Feigin R, Cherry J, Demmler G, Kaplan S, eds. Textbook of pediatric infectious diseases. 5th ed. Philadelphia: WB Saunders, 2004:2592–2601.

SUGGESTED READINGS

Bethlem EP, Capone D, Maranhao B, Carvalho CR, Wanke B. Paracoccidoidiomycosis. Curr Opin Pulm Med 1999;5:319–325.

Bicalho RN, Santo MF, de Aguiar MCF, Santos VR. Oral paracoccidioidomycosis: a retrospective study of 62 Brazilian patients. Oral Dis 2001;7:56–60.

de Camargo ZP, de Franco MF. Current knowledge on pathogenesis and immunodiagnosis of paracoccidioidomycosis. Rev Iberoam Micol 2000;17:41–48.

Franco M, Lacaz CS, Restrepo-Moreno A, del Negro G, eds. Paracoccidioidomycosis. Boca Raton, FL: CRC Press, 1994:1–410.

Hahn RC, Hamdan JS. Effects of amphotericin B and three azole derivatives on the lipids of yeast cells of *Paracoccidioides brasiliensis*. Antimicrob Agents Chemother 2000;44: 1997–2000.

Kashino SS, Fazioli RA, Cafalli-Favati C, et al. Resistance to *Paracoccidioides brasiliensis* infection is linked to a preferential Th1 immune response, whereas susceptibility is associated with absence of IFN-gamma production. J Interferon Cytokine Res 2000;20:89–97.

Manns BJ, Baylis BW, Urbanski SJ, Gibb AS, Rabin HR. Paracoccidioidomycosis: case report and review. Clin Infect Dis 1996;23:1026–1032.

Tobon AM, Orozco B, Estrada S, et al. Paracoccidioidomycosis and AIDS: report of the first two Colombian cases. Rev Inst Med Trop Sao Paulo 1998;40:377–381.

Yamaga LY, Benard G, Hironaka FH, et al. The role of gallium-67 scan in defining the extent of disease in an endemic deep mycosis, paracoccidioidomycosis: a predominant multifocal disease. Eur J Nucl Med Mol Imaging 2003;30:888–894.

19
Sporotrichosis

Carol A. Kauffman, MD

1. INTRODUCTION

Sporotrichosis is a subacute to chronic mycotic infection of skin and subcutaneous tissues. Most cases of sporotrichosis arise from direct inoculation of the organism from soil, vegetation, or wood into the subcutaneous tissues. Subsequent spread along the lymphatics draining the primary lesion is common, but hematogenous spread is rare. The organism is occasionally inhaled from the soil, causing pneumonia. Immunosuppressed hosts can develop disseminated infection, and alcoholism and diabetes mellitus appear to be risk factors for locally invasive osteoarticular sporotrichosis.

The etiologic agent is *Sporothrix schenckii*, named after Dr. Schenck, who described the first case in Baltimore in 1898. The disease has a worldwide distribution, but most cases currently are reported from the Americas and Japan. Early in the twentieth century, the most important work on the mycological and clinical aspects of sporotrichosis was carried out in France by de Beurmann and Gougerot. Their monograph is still timely in its description of the disease *(1)*. In 1903, they also developed the first effective antifungal therapy, potassium iodide, which although now relegated to a secondary role, is still useful for the treatment of lymphocutaneous sporotrichosis.

2. ETIOLOGIC AGENT

S. schenckii is a dimorphic fungus that exists as a mould in the environment and as a yeast in tissues. The dimorphism is temperature dependent. In the environment and in the laboratory, at 25° to 27°C, *S. schenckii* is a mould with thin, septate, branching hyphae that have conidia that can be either dark or hyaline and that tend to arrange themselves along the hyphae in "bouquet-like" arrangements (Fig. 19.1). In the laboratory, on Sabouraud's dextrose agar, growth of a white to cream-colored mould occurs within 1 to 2 weeks. The colony becomes brown or black and assumes a wrinkled appearance over the ensuing weeks (Fig. 19.2).

In tissues and in vitro at 37°C, *S. schenckii* assumes a yeastlike form. The yeasts are 4 to 6 μm in diameter and may show budding; they are classically described as

From: *Infectious Disease: Diagnosis and Treatment of Human Mycoses*
Edited by: D. R. Hospenthal and M. G. Rinaldi © Humana Press Inc., Totowa, NJ

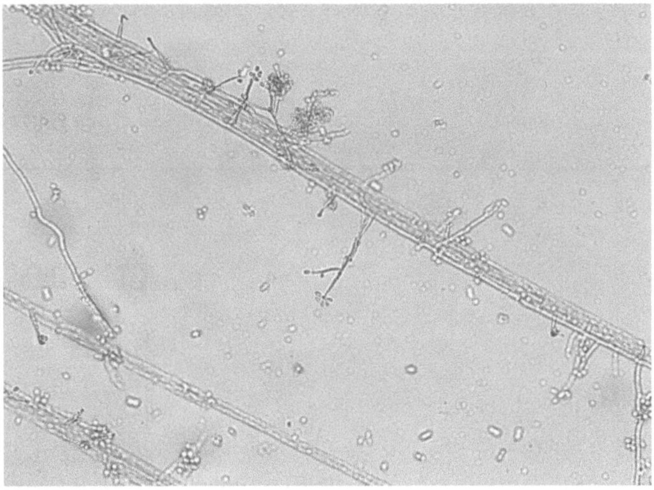

Fig. 19.1. Microscopic view of the mould form of *Sporothrix schenckii* grown at 25°C on Sabouraud dextrose agar. Note the thin septate hyphae with conidiophores that bear oval conidia that appear "bouquet-like." (Courtesy of Dr. D. R. Hospenthal.) [Figure in color on CD-ROM].

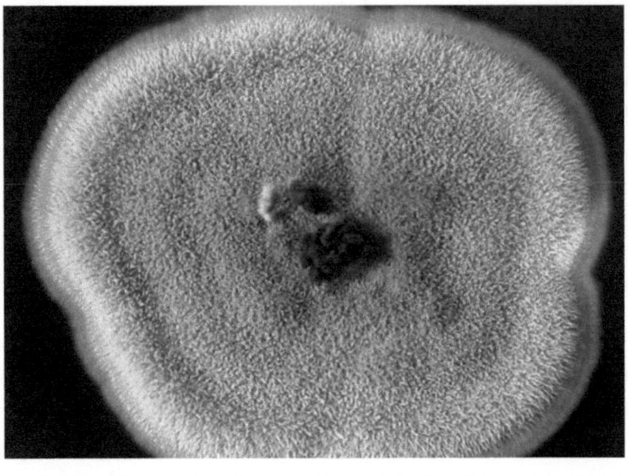

Fig. 19.2. Colony of *Sporothrix schenckii* grown at 25°C on malt extract agar. Initially cream-colored, the colony darkens over time. [Figure in color on CD-ROM].

being cigar-shaped although round and oval forms are also seen (Fig. 19.3). In the laboratory, growth of the yeast phase is accomplished by incubation at 35° to 37°C using enriched media, such as brain heart infusion (BHI) agar. The colony morphology of *S. schenckii* in the yeast phase is usually off-white and wrinkled. Some strains of *S. schenckii* do not grow well at 37°C but do grow at 35°C. These strains are generally found in fixed cutaneous lesions that do not manifest lymphangitic spread *(2)*.

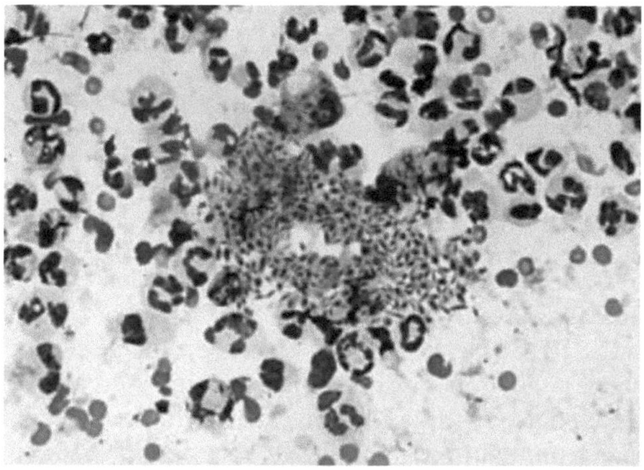

Fig. 19.3. Smear of an ulcerated lesion caused by *Sporothrix schenckii* showing a large number of oval and cigar-shaped yeasts, 4 to 6 μm in diameter. Courtesy of Dr. K. Reed. [Figure in color on CD-ROM].

3. EPIDEMIOLOGY

S. schenckii is found throughout the world. Most cases are reported from the Americas and Japan. In the environment, *S. schenckii* is found in sphagnum moss, decaying wood, vegetation, hay, and soil *(3)*. For infection to occur, one must be exposed to an environmental source, and the organism must be inoculated through the skin. This can occur with motor vehicle accidents, hay baling, landscaping, and in developing countries, just the activities of daily living *(4–7)*.

The typical person who develops sporotrichosis is a healthy man whose occupation or hobby takes him into the out-of-doors. Classically, landscapers and gardeners develop sporotrichosis because they are exposed to contaminated materials and their activities frequently lead to nicks and cuts on their extremities, allowing the organism easy access.

Zoonotic transmission also occurs from infected animals or from soil transferred from the nails of burrowing animals, such as armadillos *(8,9)*. Cats develop ulcerated skin lesions due to sporotrichosis and many die of the infection. These ulcers are teeming with organisms and are highly infectious. The persons most often infected are veterinarians, children, and their household caretakers, who are usually women. Sporotrichosis also has occurred in laboratory workers who, in the course of handling infected animals or culture material, have inoculated themselves or splashed material into their eyes *(10)*.

Outbreaks of sporotrichosis are not uncommon. The largest outbreak involved more than 3000 South African gold miners who were inoculated with *S. schenckii* from contaminated timbers in the mines *(3)*. Other outbreaks have been traced back to contaminated sphagnum moss packed around trees and bushes, contaminated seedlings used in topiary creations, and hay used for Halloween parties *(4,11–13)*. Outbreaks have also been traced back to transmission from cats. A large outbreak of cat-associated sporotrichosis affecting mainly housewives in Rio de Janeiro has been ongoing since 1998 *(14)*.

4. PATHOGENESIS AND IMMUNOLOGY

Infection with *S. schenckii* is almost always initiated when the mould that is present in the environment is inoculated into the skin, usually through minor trauma. Inhalation of the conidia of *S. schenckii* is the presumed method of transmission in the uncommon syndrome of pulmonary sporotrichosis. Virulence factors of *S. schenckii*, other than the ability to grow at 37°C, have not been clarified, but likely include extracellular proteinases and melanin *(15)*. The host response is comprised primarily of neutrophils, monocytes, and macrophages, cells able to ingest and kill the yeast phase of *S. schenckii* *(16)*. Antibody appears unimportant in immunity, but cell-mediated immunity is crucial in containing infection with *S. schenckii (17,18)*. This appears further supported by the clinical observation that *S. schenckii* causes disseminated infection in acquired immunodeficiency syndrome (AIDS) patients, a complication rarely noted in normal hosts *(19)*. It now appears that tumor necrosis factor (TNF) also plays a role in immunity, given the recent clinical observation that treatment with an antagonist for this cytokine has led to disseminated sporotrichosis *(20)*.

5. CLINICAL MANIFESTATIONS

The usual manifestation of sporotrichosis is localized lymphocutaneous infection. Most patients who present with typical lymphocutaneous sporotrichosis are healthy hosts. Extensive disseminated cutaneous lesions and spread to other structures, including joints, meninges, lungs, and other organs almost always occur in those who have certain underlying illnesses. Alcoholism and diabetes mellitus are two consistent risk factors for more severe sporotrichosis *(3)*. Chronic obstructive pulmonary disease is almost always present in patients who have pulmonary sporotrichosis, and disseminated sporotrichosis is rare unless cell-mediated immunity is suppressed (Table 19.1).

5.1. Lymphocutaneous Sporotrichosis

The first manifestation of infection generally occurs several days to weeks after cutaneous inoculation of the fungus when a papule appears at the site of inoculation. This primary lesion becomes nodular, and most will eventually ulcerate. Drainage from the lesion is minimal, is not grossly purulent, and has no odor. Pain is generally mild, and most patients have no systemic symptoms. Over the next few weeks, new nodules, that often ulcerate, appear proximal to the initial lesion along the lymphatic distribution (Fig. 19.4).

The differential diagnosis for this form of sporotrichosis includes infection with *M. marinum* or another atypical mycobacterium, *Leishmania* species, and *Nocardia brasiliensis (21)*. Rarely, other bacterial, fungal, and even viral infections cause a similar lymphocutaneous syndrome *(22)*.

Fixed cutaneous sporotrichosis is uncommon in North America, but common in South America (Fig. 19.5). Patients with this form of sporotrichosis manifest only a single lesion, often on the face, which can be verrucous or ulcerative *(6)*. The lesion

Table 19.1
Clinical manifestations of sporotrichosis

Clinical syndrome	Known risk factors	Initiation of infection
Lymphocutaneous	None	Local inoculation
Fixed cutaneous	None	Local inoculation
Osteoarticular	Alcoholism, diabetes	Local inoculation or hematogenous spread
Pulmonary	COPD, alcoholism	Inhalation
Meningitis	AIDS	Hematogenous spread
Other focal disease (eye, breast, larynx, pericardium, epididymis, rectum, spleen, liver)	None known	Hematogenous spread or local inoculation
Disseminated	AIDS	Hematogenous spread

COPD, chronic obstructive pulmonary disease.

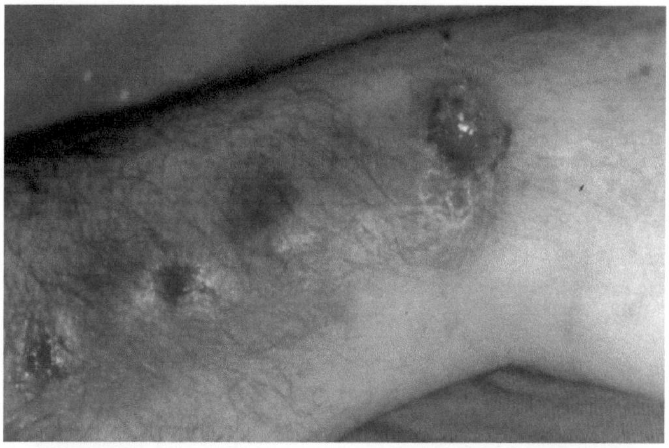

Fig. 19.4. Typical skin lesions in lymphatic distribution seen in a patient who was a horticulturist and had inoculation of *Sporothrix schenckii* in the subcutaneous tissue of the wrist. (Reproduced with permission from C. Watanakunakorn, *Clinical Infectious Diseases*, University of Chicago Press, 1996.) [Figure in color on CD-ROM].

may regress and flare periodically, and can be present for years until it is treated. Pain and drainage are not prominent symptoms.

5.2. Pulmonary Sporotrichosis

Pulmonary sporotrichosis is usually a subacute to chronic illness *(23)*. The symptoms mimic those of reactivation tuberculosis. Patients have fever, night sweats, weight loss, and fatigue; dyspnea, cough, purulent sputum, and hemoptysis also occur frequently. Chest radiography shows unilateral or bilateral fibronodular or cavitary disease; the

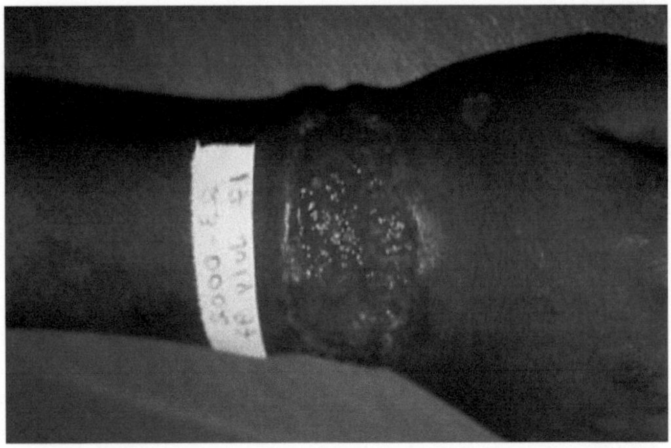

Fig. 19.5. Fixed cutaneous skin lesion of sporotrichosis. In this form of the disease, lymphatic spread does not occur, and the lesion may remain for months to years until treated. (Courtesy of Dr. P. Pappas. Reproduced with permission from C.A. Kauffman, *Clinical Infectious Diseases*, University of Chicago Press, 1999.) [Figure in color on CD-ROM].

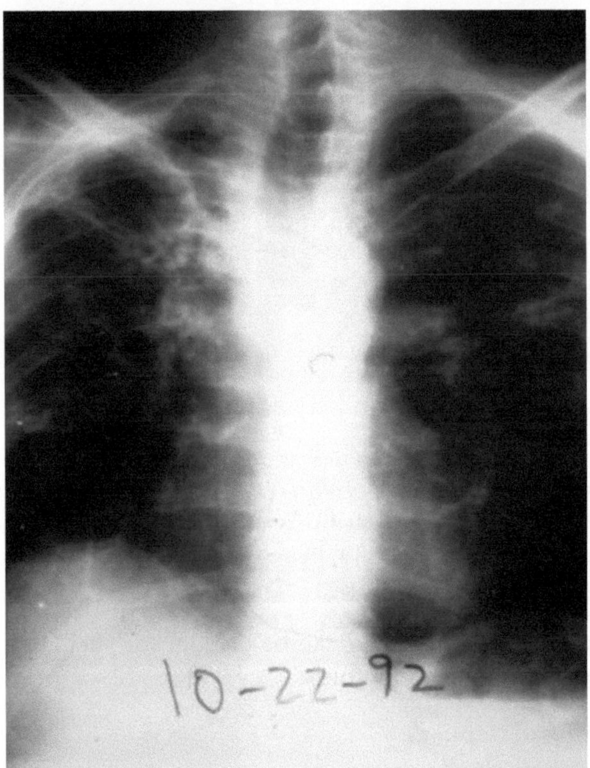

Fig. 19.6. Chest radiograph of a patient with pulmonary sporotrichosis. The patient was an alcoholic who also had diabetes mellitus and chronic obstructive pulmonary disease.

upper lobes are preferentially involved (Fig. 19.6). Sporotrichosis must be differentiated from tuberculosis, chronic cavitary histoplasmosis or blastomycosis, and sarcoidosis. Some, but not all, patients with pulmonary sporotrichosis have disease elsewhere, especially in the skin and osteoarticular structures.

5.3. Osteoarticular Sporotrichosis

Osteoarticular sporotrichosis is an uncommon manifestation of infection with *S. schenckii* that can occur after local inoculation, but more often arises from hematogenous spread. It is found most often in middle-aged men and appears to occur more frequently in alcoholics. Overlying cutaneous lesions may or may not be present, and one or more joints may be involved. Most commonly, the knees, elbows, wrists, and ankles are infected *(24)*. Bone involvement usually occurs contiguous to an infected joint (Fig. 19.7). Bursitis and tenosynovitis, the latter presenting as nerve entrapment, also have been described *(25)*.

5.4. Meningitis and Disseminated Infection

Meningitis, a rare manifestation of sporotrichosis that occurs almost always in those with cellular immune defects, is usually chronic and must be differentiated from tuberculosis or cryptococcosis *(26)*. Fever and headache are prominent symptoms, and the cerebrospinal fluid (CSF) findings are those of a lymphocytic meningitis with mild hypoglycorrhachia. Meningitis may be an isolated finding or a manifestation of widespread dissemination. Disseminated sporotrichosis is very uncommon, with most cases having been reported in patients with AIDS *(27)*. *S. schenckii* has been reported

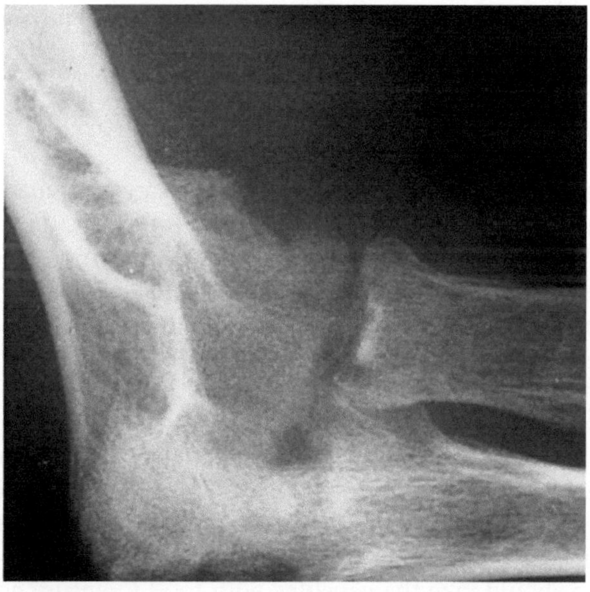

Fig. 19.7. Elbow radiograph of a patient who had osteoarticular sporotrichosis manifested by infection of both elbows and one knee. There is destruction of the joint and adjacent osteomyelitis of the radius, ulna, and humerus.

very rarely to cause infection of eye, larynx, breast, pericardium, spleen, liver, bone marrow, lymph nodes, rectum, and epididymis *(28)*.

6. DIAGNOSIS

Culture of *S. schenckii* is the gold standard for establishing the diagnosis of sporotrichosis. Biopsy or aspiration material from a cutaneous lesion should be sent to the laboratory for both culture and histopathology. Sputum, synovial fluid, or CSF should be obtained, when appropriate, for smear and culture. Material obtained for culture should be inoculated onto Sabouraud's agar or blood agar and incubated at room temperature to allow growth of the mould phase of *S. schenckii*. Growth usually occurs within a week, but can take several weeks. The characteristic arrangement of conidia on the hyphae makes the diagnosis likely, but conversion to the yeast phase at 35° to 37°C, which may take several weeks, allows definitive identification of the organism as *S. schenckii*.

The histopathology of sporotrichosis reveals a mixed granulomatous and pyogenic inflammatory process. The organism is an oval to cigar-shaped yeast, 3 to 5 μm in diameter, and can exhibit multiple buds. However, it is difficult to visualize the organisms within tissues, even with the use of methenamine silver or periodic acid Schiff stains (see Fig. 3.10, Chapter 3). In some cases, a tissue reaction that may represent antigen–antibody complexes, called an asteroid body, can be seen. In an asteroid body, the basophilic yeast is surrounded by eosinophilic material radiating outward like spokes on a wheel. This is also known as the Splendore–Hoeppli phenomenon, which is not specific for sporotrichosis, but can be seen in various parasitic, fungal, and bacterial infections, and may be due to antigen–antibody complexes.

Serology is not useful in the diagnosis of sporotrichosis. In the special case of sporotrichal meningitis, a latex agglutination assay and an enzyme immunoassay on CSF have been reported to be both sensitive and specific, although neither test is readily available *(29)*.

7. TREATMENT

In general, most patients who have sporotrichosis are treated with oral antifungal agents. Those patients who have disseminated infection, meningitis, or severe pulmonary involvement should be treated initially with intravenous amphotericin B. Guidelines for the management of the various forms of sporotrichosis have been updated by the Infectious Diseases Society of America *(30)*. The suggestions that follow are modified from these Guidelines (Table 19.2).

7.1. Lymphocutaneous Sporotrichosis

Itraconazole is the drug of choice for the treatment of this form of sporotrichosis *(30–32)*. The dosage should be 200 mg/day, which is best given as the oral solution to achieve higher serum concentrations. If itraconazole capsules are used the patient cannot be taking any acid-inhibiting drugs, such as antacids, proton pump inhibitors, or H2 blockers, and should take the capsules with food to ensure adequate absorption. Treatment should continue until the lesions have resolved; this usually takes 3 to 6 months.

Saturated solution of potassium iodide (SSKI) has been used successfully to treat lymphocutaneous sporotrichosis for decades. It still is not clear how SSKI inhibits

Table 19.2
Treatment of sporotrichosis

Clinical syndrome	Primary therapy	Alternate therapy	Duration
Lymphocutaneous and cutaneous	Itraconazole 100-200 mg daily	SSKI, titrated dose Fluconazole 400 mg/day Terbinafine 1000 mg/day Hyperthermia	3–6 months
Pulmonary	Itraconazole 400 mg/day	Amphotericin B, 1–2 g total	1–2 years
Osteoarticular	Itraconazole 400 mg/day	Amphotericin B, 1–2 g total	1–2 yr
Meningitis	Amphotericin B 1–2 g total or equivalent dosage of lipid formulation	Itraconazole 400 mg/day	See below[a]
Disseminated	Amphotericin B 1–2 g total or equivalent dosage of lipid formulation	Itraconazole 400 mg/day	See below[b]

[a]Therapy for meningeal sporotrichosis has not been studied. Initial therapy should be with amphotericin B or a lipid formulation of amphotericin B; therapy can be changed to itraconazole after 4–6 weeks if the patient is doing well. The duration of treatment is unknown, and some patients may require life-long suppressive therapy.
[b]In patients with HIV infection and disseminated sporotrichosis, therapy can be changed to itraconazole after the patient's condition has stabilized; life-long suppressive therapy with itraconazole is indicated in these patients.

S. schenckii (33). The initial dose is 5 to 10 drops three times daily, increasing weekly to a maximum of 40 to 50 drops three times daily, as tolerated. Side effects are very common and include nausea, rash, metallic taste, fever, and salivary gland swelling.

Several other options exist if the patient is unable to tolerate itraconazole or SSKI. Fluconazole at a dosage of 400 mg daily can be used *(34)*. Voriconazole appears to be less active than itraconazole and should not be used to treat sporotrichosis *(35)*. High doses of terbinafine (500 mg twice daily) appear to be effective for lymphocutaneous sporotrichosis *(36)*. However, experience is limited, and this should be tried only in those who fail standard therapy.

Local hyperthermia can be used to treat cutaneous sporotrichosis *(37)*. A variety of different warming devices are available, but each must be used faithfully for months to effect improvement in cutaneous lesions *(38)*.

7.2. *Pulmonary Sporotrichosis*

Pulmonary sporotrichosis can be quite recalcitrant to therapy. If the patient is seriously ill, amphotericin B, preferably as a lipid formulation, should be used initially *(23,30)*. The daily dosage of amphotericin B is 0.7 mg/kg daily, and for the lipid formulations it is 3 to 5 mg/kg daily. When the patient is stable, therapy can be changed to oral itraconazole, 200 mg twice daily. The duration of therapy should be at least 1 year and perhaps longer for some patients. Surgical resection is an option for patients who have a single focal lesion that has not responded to medical management.

7.3. Osteoarticular Sporotrichosis

This form of sporotrichosis, which is almost always chronic and not life-threatening, can be treated with an oral antifungal agent *(24)*. Itraconazole is the agent of choice, and the dosage is 200 mg twice daily *(30)*. Therapy should continue for 1 to 2 years. Although inferior to itraconazole in the treatment of this infection, if the patient cannot tolerate itraconazole, fluconazole at a dosage of 800 mg daily can be tried *(34)*. Amphotericin B (0.7 mg/kg per day) or a lipid formulation of amphotericin B (3 to 5 mg/kg per day) is the only remaining option. Intraarticular, amphotericin B has been reported to be effective, but is not recommended *(39)*. Even if cure occurs, joint function rarely is recovered.

7.4. Meningitis and Disseminated Infection

Amphotericin B is the drug of choice for patients with these life-threatening forms of sporotrichosis *(30)*. For meningitis, it is recommended that a lipid formulation of amphotericin B be given at a dosage of 5 mg/kg daily for 4–6 weeks. Itraconazole can be used after the patient has responded to amphotericin B if long-term suppressive therapy is needed.

REFERENCES

1. de Beurmann L, Gougerot H. Les Sporotrichosis. Paris. Felix Alcan, 1912.
2. Kwon-Chung KJ. Comparison of isolates of *Sporothrix schenckii* obtained from fixed cutaneous lesions with isolates from other types of lesions. J Infect Dis 1979;139:424–431.
3. Kauffman CA. Sporotrichosis. Clin Infect Dis 1999;29:231–237.
4. Dixon DM, Salkin IF, Duncan RA, et al. Isolation and characterization of *Sporothrix schenckii* from clinical and environmental sources associated with the largest U.S. epidemic of sporotrichosis. J Clin Microbiol 1991;29:1106–1113.
5. Zhang X, Andrews JH. Evidence for growth of *Sporothrix schenckii* on dead but not on living sphagnum moss. Mycopathologia 1993;123:87–94.
6. Pappas PG, Tellez I, Deep AE, et al. Sporotrichosis in Peru: description of an area of hyperendemicity. Clin Infect Dis 2000;30:65–70.
7. Lyon GM, Zurita S, Casquero J, et al. Population-based surveillance and a case-control study of risk factors for endemic lymphocutaneous sporotrichosis in Peru. Clin Infect Dis 2003;36:34–39.
8. Conti Diaz IA. Epidemiology of sporotrichosis in Latin America. Mycopathologia 1989;108:113–116.
9. Reed KD, Moore FM, Geiger GE, Stemper ME. Zoonotic transmission of sporotrichosis: case report and review. Clin Infect Dis 1993;16:384–387.
10. Cooper CR, Dixon DM, Salkin IF. Laboratory-acquired sporotrichosis. J Med Vet Mycol 1992;30:169–171.
11. Powell KE, Taylor A, Phillips BJ, et al. Cutaneous sporotrichosis in forestry workers. Epidemic due to contaminated sphagnum moss. JAMA 1978;240:232–235.
12. Hajjeh R, McDonnell S, Reef S, et al. Outbreak of sporotrichosis among tree nursery workers. J Infect Dis 1997;76:499–504.

13. Dooley DP, Bostic PS, Beckius ML. Spook house sporotrichosis. A point-source outbreak of cutaneous sporotrichosis from hay bale props in a Halloween haunted-house. Arch Intern Med 1997;157:1885–1887.
14. Barros MBL, Schubach AAO, Valle ACF, et al. Cat-transmitted sporotrichosis epidemic in Rio de Janeiro, Brazil: description of a series of cases. Clin Infect Dis 2004;38: 529–535.
15. Tsuboi R, Sanada T, Takamori K, Ogawa H. Isolation and properties of extracellular proteinases from *Sporothrix schenckii.* J Bacteriol 1987;169:4104–4109.
16. Cunningham KM, Bulmer GS, Rhoades ER. Phagocytosis and intracellular fate of *Sporothrix schenckii.* J Infect Dis 1979;140:815–817.
17. Shiraishi A, Nakagaki K, Arai T. Role of cell-mediated immunity in the resistance to experimental sporotrichosis in mice. Mycopathologia 1992;120:15–21.
18. Tachibana T, Matsuyama T, Mitsuyama M. Involvement of CD4+ T cells and macrophages in acquired protection against infection with *Sporothrix schenckii* in mice. Med Mycol 1999;37:397–404.
19. Bolao F, Podzamczer D, Ventin M, Gudiol F. Efficacy of acute phase and maintenance therapy with itraconazole in an AIDS patient with sporotrichosis. Eur J Clin Microbiol Infect Dis 1994;13:609–612.
20. Gottlieb GS, Lesser CF, Holmes KK, Wald A. Disseminated sporotrichosis associated with treatment with immunosuppressants and tumor necrosis factor-alpha antagonists. Clin Infect Dis 2003;37:638–640.
21. Kostman JR, DiNubile MJ. Nodular lymphangitis: a distinctive but often unrecognized syndrome. Ann Intern Med 1993;118:883–888.
22. Smego RA, Castiglia M, Asperilla MO. Lymphocutaneous syndrome. A review of non-Sporothrix causes. Medicine (Baltimore) 1999;78:38–63.
23. Pluss JL, Opal SM. Pulmonary sporotrichosis: review of treatment and outcome. Medicine (Baltimore) 1986;65:143–153.
24. Winn RE, Anderson J, Piper J, Aronson NE, Pluss J. Systemic sporotrichosis treated with itraconazole. Clin Infect Dis 1993;17:210–217.
25. Atdjian M, Granda JL, Ingberg HO, Kaplan BL. Systemic sporotrichosis polytenosynovitis with median and ulnar nerve entrapment. JAMA 1980;243:1841–1842.
26. Donabedian H, O'Donnell E, Olszewski C, MacArthur RD, Budd N. Disseminated cutaneous and meningeal sporotrichosis in an AIDS patient. Diagn Microbiol Infect Dis 1994;18:111–115.
27. Al-Tawfiq JA, Wools KK. Disseminated sporotrichosis and *Sporothrix schenckii* fungemia as the initial presentation of human immunodeficiency virus infection. Clin Infect Dis 1998;26:1403–1406.
28. Wilson DE, Mann JJ, Bennett JE, Utz JP. Clinical features of extracutaneous sporotrichosis. Medicine (Baltimore) 1967;46:265–279.
29. Scott EN, Kaufman L, Brown AC, Muchmore HG. Serologic studies in the diagnosis and management of meningitis due to *Sporothrix schenckii.* N Engl J Med 1987;317:935–940.
30. Kauffman CA, Bustamante B, Chapman SW, Pappas PG. Clinical practice guidelines for the management of sporotrichosis: 2007 update by IDSA. Clin Infect Dis (In press).
31. Sharkey-Mathis PK, Kauffman CA, Graybill JR, et al. Treatment of sporotrichosis with itraconazole. Am J Med 1993;95:279–285.
32. Restrepo A, Robledo J, Gomez I, Tabares AM, Gutierrez R. Itraconazole therapy in lymphangitic and cutaneous sporotrichosis. Arch Dermatol 1986;122:413–417.
33. Rex JH, Bennett JE. Administration of potassium iodide to normal volunteers does not increase killing of *Sporothrix schenckii* by their neutrophils and monocytes. J Med Vet Mycol 1990;28:185–189.

34. Kauffman CA, Pappas PG, McKinsey DS, et al. Treatment of lymphocutaneous and visceral sporotrichosis with fluconazole. Clin Infect Dis 1996;22:46–50.
35. McGinnis MR, Nordoff N, Li R-K, Pasarell L, Warnock DW. *Sporothrix schenckii* sensitivity to voriconazole, itraconazole, and amphotericin B. Med Mycol 2001;39:369–371.
36. Chapman SW, Pappas P, Kauffman C, et al. Comparative evaluation of the efficacy and safety of two doses of terbinafine (500 and 1000 mg day^{-1}) in the treatment of cutaneous or lymphocutaneous sporotrichosis. Mycoses 2003;47:62–68.
37. Hiruma M, Kagawa S. The effects of heat on *Sporothrix schenckii* in vitro and in vivo. Mycopathologia 1998;84:21–30.
38. Hiruma M, Kawada A, Noguchi H, Ishibashi A, Conti Diaz IA. Hyperthermic treatment of sporotrichosis: experimental use of infrared and far infrared rays. Mycoses 1992;35:293–299.
39. Downs NJ, Hinthorn DR, Mhatre VR, Liu C. Intra-articular amphotericin B treatment of *Sporothrix schenckii* arthritis. Arch Intern Med 1989;149:954–955

SUGGESTED READINGS

Kauffman CA. Old and new therapies for sporotrichosis. Clin Infect Dis 1995;21:981–985.

Kauffman CA, Bustamante B, Chapman SW, Pappas PG. Clinical practice guidelines for the management of sporotichosis: 2007 update by IDSA. Clin Infect Dis (In press).

Kwon-Chung KJ, Bennett JE. Sporotrichosis. In: Medical Mycology. Philadelphia: Lea & Febiger, 1992:707–729.

20

Dermatophytosis (Tinea) and Other Superficial Fungal Infections

Aditya K. Gupta, MD, PhD and Elizabeth A. Cooper, HBSc

1. INTRODUCTION

Superficial dermatophyte infection has been reported under a variety of different terminologies since the early days of recorded human civilization *(1)*. However, it has only been during the past 200 years with the development of modern science that the contagious nature of the disease could be related to the presence of fungal organisms *(1)*. The current taxonomy of dermatophytes used today, dividing organisms into *Trichophyton*, *Microsporum*, and *Epidermophyton* species, was not developed until 1934 *(1)*. Topical preparations have been the historic method of treatment for dermatophyte infections. The first effective oral medication for dermatophytes, griseofulvin, was not developed until 1958 *(1)*. Thus, although the term "tinea" used for dermatophyte infection has ancient roots *(1)*, the current standards of medical treatment for dermatophyte infection are a recent development, and the field continues to develop as more fungal knowledge and more effective therapies become available.

Dermatophytes require keratin for growth and therefore infect hair, nails, and superficial skin, with clinical manifestations named for the area affected: tinea capitis (scalp); tinea corporis (body); tinea cruris (groin); tinea pedis (feet); tinea manuum (hands); tinea barbae (affecting the beard area, in males); tinea faciei (face); and tinea unguium (nails) *(2)*. Tinea infections have alternately been called "ringworm," because of the lesions that present as a circular or oval clearing surrounded by a red, scaly, elevated border ("ring"). Tinea unguium is the subset of onychomycosis infections caused by dermatophytes, as opposed to nail infections caused by *Candida* or nondermatophyte moulds.

Besides the dermatophytoses, superficial infections may also result from infection with other fungi, including the *Malassezia* species of yeast. *Malassezia* feed on lipids found in areas where sebaceous gland activity is highest and in individuals with high levels of sebaceous secretions. Although first recognized as a pathogen in 1846, laboratory culture was not successful until it was recognized that the organisms had a lipid requirement, in 1927 *(3)*. Initially only two species were described, under the genus

From: *Infectious Disease: Diagnosis and Treatment of Human Mycoses*
Edited by: D. R. Hospenthal and M. G. Rinaldi © Humana Press Inc., Totowa, NJ

name *Pityrosporum*, and only three species were recognized as of 1970 *(3)*. Difficulty in identification was also complicated by the existence of both yeast and mycelial forms; conversion between forms was not induced in the laboratory until 1977. Genetic research in the 1990s confirmed at least seven species of *Malassezia* existed, and more have been discovered since. Because of the issues of species identification, definitive understanding of *Malassezia* infection has been difficult. *Malassezia* is known to cause pityriasis (tinea) versicolor and is associated with seborrheic dermatitis, and thus these superficial conditions will be included here along with the dermatophyte infections.

Other rare superficial fungal infections, including those secondary to *Candida* (Chapter 7), white piedra (caused by *Trichosporon*, Chapter 8), black piedra, and tinea nigra (Chapter 11), are discussed elsewhere in this text, as are the nonsuperficial infections caused by *Malassezia* (Chapter 8).

2. ETIOLOGIC AGENTS

Three fungal genera cause tinea infections: *Microsporum*, *Trichophyton*, and more rarely, *Epidermophyton (2)*. Species may be grouped by their source of human infection, other humans (anthropophilic), animals (zoophilic), or less commonly, soil (geophilic). Infections may be transmitted between humans or, much more rarely, from animals or soil to humans. The major causative species differ geographically and may change in prevalence over time owing to population movements from immigration or travel. Anthropophilic dermatophytes are the most frequent causes of onychomycosis and other superficial dermatophytoses, and the most frequently seen agents of infection are *T. rubrum* and *T. mentagrophytes*. *T. tonsurans* is currently the most frequent cause of tinea capitis in North America. *M. canis* is a zoophilic organism frequently picked up by humans from contact with animals such as dogs and cats.

The *Malassezia* yeast species are associated with the superficial fungal infections pityriasis (tinea) versicolor (PV) and seborrheic dermatitis (SD). The currently recognized species are *M. furfur*, *M. pachydermatis*, *M. sympodialis*, *M. globosa*, *M. slooffiae*, *M. restricta*, and *M. obtusa (4)*. *M. pachydermatis* is typically associated with animal infection rather than human infection *(3)*. Up to five new species have been described in the recent literature: *M. dermatis*, *M. equi*, *M. japonica*, *M. yamatoensis*, and *M. nana (4)*. The most common *Malassezia* species contributing to PV lesions are *M. globosa* (50% to 60%), *M. sympodialis* (3% to 59%), *M. furfur*, and *M. slooffiae* (1% to 10%) *(5)*.

3. EPIDEMIOLOGY

Dermatophytosis is a frequent diagnosis, and it has been estimated that the risk of acquiring such infection is 10% to 20% in an individual's lifetime *(6)*. While some types of infections are well studied (tinea capitis, onychomycosis), other types are less well defined. Overall rates of dermatophyte infection in subjects seeking outpatient treatment in the United States have been measured using the National Ambulatory Medical Care Survey (NAMCS) from 1990 to 1994 *(7)*. This survey modeled an estimated 21.6 million physician office visits for fungal infections during this period, breaking down into types of infection as follows: tinea corporis—27.2%, tinea cruris—16.9%, tinea pedis—16.7%, tinea unguium—15.6%, tinea of hair and beard—6.9%, and tinea manuum—1.0%.

3.1. Tinea Pedis/Manuum

Tinea pedis is estimated to affect 10% of the world population *(8)*. Infections are more frequent in tropical climates and may also be associated with use of occlusive footwear *(8)*. Males are more often affected than females for both tinea pedis and tinea manuum, with most infections affecting the web space between the fourth and fifth toes *(8)*. Children do not often develop tinea pedis. Patients with atopic dermatitis or immunosuppressive disorders may be predisposed to developing tinea pedis. Predisposing factors for tinea manuum include manual work that results in repeated trauma to the hands, hyperhidrosis, and the frequent use of alkaline soaps.

3.2. Tinea Corporis/Cruris

Tinea corporis and tinea cruris are found commonly, with worldwide distribution *(9)*. Little data on prevalence in North America has been published, but tinea corporis was found to be the most common dermatophytosis for which patients sought treatment during the National Ambulatory Medical Care Survey from 1990 to 1994 (27.2% of all dermatophytoses, with an estimated 2.3 million physician visits made) *(7)*. A subset of tinea corporis affecting only the nonbearded regions of the face, tinea faciei, makes up 3% to 4% of tinea corporis cases, and is more frequently seen in warm, humid climates *(10)*.

3.3. Tinea Capitis

In North America, the genus *Trichophyton*, particularly *T. tonsurans*, is the predominant cause of tinea capitis infection *(1)*. In Western Europe, *M. canis* and *T. violaceum* are the most common pathogens of tinea capitis; *T. tonsurans* is dominant in the Caribbean and South America; *M. canis*, *T. mentagrophytes*, and *T. violaceum* dominate in the Middle East *(1)*.

Tinea capitis is most prevalent in children older than 6 months of age and before puberty *(1)*. African Americans develop tinea capitis at much higher frequencies than the general US population *(1)*. *Trichophyton* species affect males and females equally, although *M. audouinii* and *M. canis* affect males more than females *(1)*. Infection spread may increase in conditions of overcrowding, poverty, and poor hygiene.

3.4. Onychomycosis

Onychomycosis has an estimated prevalence of 6.5% to 12.8% in North America, accounting for up to 50% of all nail disease *(11,12)*. It is more common in males than females, and in people older than 60 years of age. Other risk factors include trauma to the nail, diabetes, peripheral arterial disease, and immunocompromised status *(12)*. Tinea pedis may be present in patients with toenail onychomycosis *(12)*.

3.5. Pityriasis Versicolor

Pityriasis versicolor (PV) has worldwide distribution. Prevalence in tropical climates has been reported at 30% to 40%, compared to 1% to 4% in temperate climates *(3,13)*.

PV does not typically affect prepubescent children, but is more frequent in adults when sebaceous gland activity is most active *(5,13)*. Equal prevalence between the sexes has been noted *(5)*.

3.6. *Seborrheic Dermatitis*

Seborrheic dermatitis (SD) is a chronic, recurrent disorder affecting between 1% and 5% of immunocompetent adults *(3,13,14)*. Typically referred to as dandruff, the mild form affects a large proportion of the North American population, but reported numbers are likely underestimated as people to do not tend to seek medical advice for dandruff. Males are more frequently affected than females, and the disease is more severe in winter, improving with summer sun exposure *(15)*. SD chiefly affects adolescents, young adults, and adults older than age 50 *(16)*. Incidence may increase in immunocompromised populations such as in persons infected with human immunodeficiency virus (HIV), in whom estimates of incidence of SD are as high as 83% *(3)*.

4. PATHOGENESIS AND IMMUNOLOGY

The dermatophytes colonize keratinized tissue of the stratum corneum; invasion by anthropophilic species usually result in less inflammation than that of zoophilic or geophilic species *(17)*. The epidermis functions as a barrier to microorganisms, and commensal flora may also help reduce infection by pathogens *(3)*. Entry into the stratum corneum may result from trauma to the skin or some other breach of the skin barrier. Excessive sweating and occlusive clothing/footwear aid in providing a warm, moist environment conducive to tinea infection. Infection may be transferred from one area of the body to another. Infection may also be transmitted between individuals by direct or indirect contact with scales containing fungal arthroconidia from infected individuals, such as seen in individuals participating in contact sports including wrestling and rugby *(9)*.

Fungicidal proteins are present in the epidermis, and some skin lipids in the scalp and hair are fungicidal to certain, but not all, dermatophyte species *(3)*. Dermatophyte glycopeptides prompt development of delayed hypersensitivity, although patients with inflammatory infection are more likely to demonstrate such a reaction than patients with noninflammatory chronic infection *(18)*. Dermatophytes and other microorganisms can activate the alternate pathway of the complement cascade of immune response, causing production of molecules that prompt the chemotactic activity of neutrophils into the skin *(3)*. Immunoglobulins are secreted onto the skin surface via sweat, and commensal organisms including *Malassezia* species have been found to be coated with such immunoglobulins *(3)*.

Malassezia organisms are a normal part of human commensal skin flora, found particularly in sebaceous skin such as the chest, back, and head, and in the yeast form rather than the mycelial form *(3)*. *Malassezia* species vary in the antigens presented, and can alter their expressed antigens throughout the growth cycle *(3)*. The ability of *Malassezia* to elicit activities of the human immune system is not clear *(3)*.

People and animals, though uninfected, may still be asymptomatic pathogen carriers. Fomites also play a significant role in transmission. Autoinoculation may also occur, for example, tinea pedis spreading to tinea cruris, tinea capitis to tinea corporis, or onychomycosis to tinea pedis *(19)*. High levels of perspiration may be predisposing to infection, as fungal arthroconidia persist to a greater extent on the scalp with higher levels of oils *(9)*.

5. CLINICAL MANIFESTATIONS

Clinical presentations and differential diagnoses for the various superficial infections are summarized in Table 20.1.

Table 20.1
Clinical presentations and differential diagnoses of common dermatophyte and superficial fungal infections

Condition	Presentation	Differential diagnosis
Tinea pedis	*Interdigital*: Scaling, fissuring, maceration, erosions, hyperhidrosis, pruritus, odor *Moccasin*: Fine silvery scales with underlying pink or red skin on soles, heels, sides of feet *Vesicobullous*: Inflammatory vesicular or bullous lesions, particularly at in-step	Candidiasis, erythrasma, bacterial infection, psoriasis, contact dermatitis, dyshidrotic eczema, Reiter's syndrome
Tinea manuum	Dry, scaly, hyperkeratotic skin particularly of the palmar area, minimal erythema	Contact dermatitis, atopic dermatitis, pompholyx, psoriasis, lamellar dyshidrosis
Tinea corporis	Annular erythematous plaques with raised leading edges and scaling, over glabrous skin of trunk; may be central clearing	Impetigo, nummular dermatitis, secondary or tertiary syphilis, psoriasis, lichen planus, seborrheic dermatitis, pityriasis rosea, pityriasis rubra pilaris, candidal intertrigo, atopic dermatitis, cutaneous lupus, pityriasis versicolor
Tinea cruris	Annular erythematous plaques with raised leading edges and scaling, over pubic area, perineal and perianal skin, typically not affecting the scrotum or labia majora	Psoriasis, seborrheic dermatitis, candidiasis, erythrasma, lichen simplex chronicus, Darier's disease, pemphigus vegetans
Tinea capitis	*Noninflammatory*: Erythematous papules around hair shaft spreading out with fine scaling in noticeable patches and partial or complete alopecia	Seborrheicdermatitis, psoriasis, atopic dermatitis, tinea amiantacia, alopecia areata, trichotillomania, lupus erythematosus, lichen planopilaris, traction folliculitis, bacterial pyoderma

(Continued)

Table 20.1
(Continued)

Condition	Presentation	Differential diagnosis
	Black dot: Noticeable black dots where hair breakage at scalp level occurs, scaling with little inflammation (particularly with *T. tonsurans* or *T. violaceum*) *Inflammatory*: Kerion with pustules, loose hair, discharge of pus *Favic*: Large yellow crusts on the scalp	
Onychomycosis	*Distal lateral subungual (DLSO)*: Infection at the distal end of nail plate; discoloration and thickening of nail plate, onycholysis, subungual debris *Superficial white (SWO)*: White spots or patches on the surface of the nail plate *Proximal subungual (PSO)*: Infection of the proximal nail fold, and extending distally, typically whitish in color *Endonyx:* Milky white discoloration of the nail plate without hyperkeratosis, onycholysis; may show lamellar splitting of the nail plate (typically caused by *T. soudanense* or *T. violaceum*)	Psoriasis, chronic onycholysis, chronic paronychia, trauma, hemorrhage, onychogryphosis, lichen planus, alopecia areata, subungual malignant melanoma, subungual squamous cell carcinoma
Ptyriasis versicolor	Well-defined, hyperpigmented or hypopigmented lesions of areas with high concentrations of sebaceous glands such as scalp, chest, back, upper arms and face; showing fine scaling in most cases (caused by *Malassezia* species)	Vitiligo, chloasma, tinea corporis, pityriasis rotunda, erythrasma
Seborrheic dermatitis	Red, flaky, greasy-looking patches of skin on scalp, nasolabial folds, eyebrows and ears: "dandruff" of the scalp; may also affect groin, axillae, anterior chest; pruritus, irritation may be associated (associated with *Malassezia* infection)	Psoriasis, atopic dermatitis, tinea capitis, rosacea, lupus erythematosus

5.1. Tinea Pedis/Manuum

Also known as "athlete's foot," there are three common presentations recognized in tinea pedis: interdigital, moccasin, and vesicobullous *(8)*.

Interdigital is the most common presentation, and typically infects the toe webs, particularly between the fourth and fifth toes (Fig 20.1) *(8)*. Interdigital infection may show fissuring, scaling, maceration, and erosions. Hyperhidrosis, pruritus, and foul odor may also be present. Dermatophytosis simplex is an uncomplicated form of interdigital tinea pedis, contrasted with dermatophytosis complex which is associated with concomitant bacterial infection showing inflammation, maceration and odor, and may be facilitated by breakdown of the skin in preliminary infection stages *(8)*.

Moccasin tinea pedis manifests as fine silvery scales with underlying pink to red skin, on the soles, heels and sides of feet (Fig. 20.2) *(8)*. More severe cases may show cracked, inflamed skin, erythema, and odor. This infection is most commonly produced by *T. rubrum*.

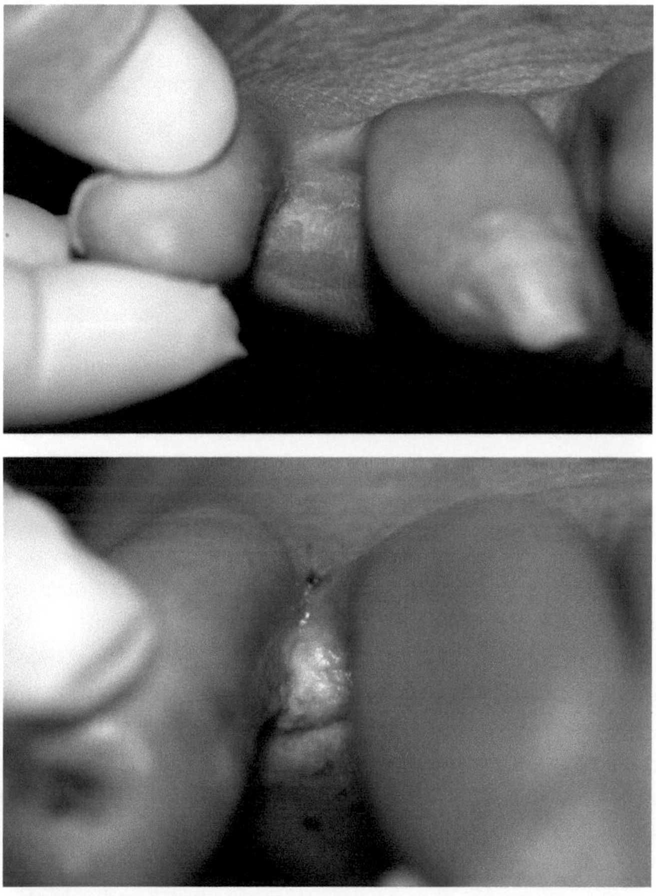

Fig. 20.1. Interdigital tinea pedis. [Figure in color on CD-ROM].

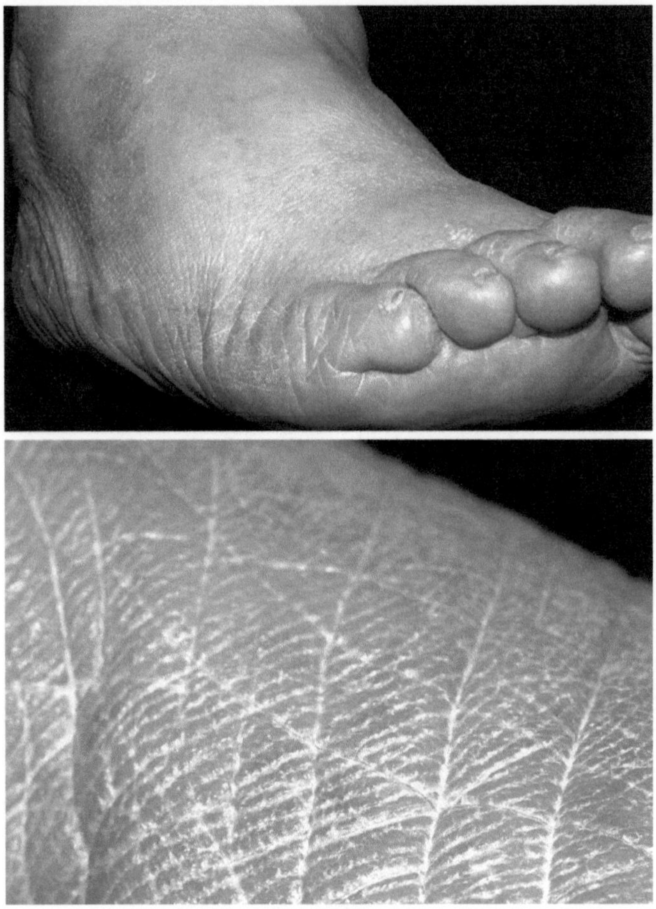

Fig. 20.2. Moccasin tinea pedis, with close-up of fine scaling. [Figure in color on CD-ROM].

Vesicobullous tinea pedis is the least common type, and shows as acute and highly inflammatory vesicular or bullous lesions, typically at the in-step, but inflammation may spread over the whole sole *(8)*. This type of infection is associated with *T. mentagrophytes* infection.

Tinea manuum is a rare form that primarily affects the palmar areas of the hands, and presents as chronic, dry, scaly, hyperkeratotic skin with minimal erythema *(8)*. Infections are most frequently caused by *T. rubrum*. Tinea manuum may accompany tinea pedis or onychomycosis, and a two feet–one hand syndrome has been noted to occur *(20)*. This syndrome consists of development of tinea manuum from excoriation of infected soles (tinea pedis) and/or toenails (onychomycosis). Typically one hand is dominant in the excoriation, leading to infection in that hand which may also lead to fingernail onychomycosis.

5.2. *Tinea Corporis/Cruris*

Tinea corporis is a superficial dermatophyte infection of the glabrous skin, excluding the scalp, beard, face, hands, feet, and groin (Fig. 20.3) *(9)*. It is more common in men than in women, and is also common in children *(9)*. Tinea faciei is a subset of tinea corporis affecting only the facial area, excluding the beard region *(10)*.

Also known as "jock itch," tinea cruris is a dermatophyte infection of the genitalia, pubic area, perineal skin, and perianal skin (Fig. 20.4). The scrotum and labia majora are typically not affected. Infection is more common in men than in women *(9)*.

Tinea cruris and tinea corporis present as annular erythematous plaques with raised leading edges and scaling; central clearing of the lesion may be noticed, but nodules may remain present throughout the lesion *(9)*. Infection is typically associated with pruritus. Infection may also present as an erythematous papule or series of vesicles. Significant inflammation may result from infection with zoophilic organisms such as *T. verrucosum*, producing large pustular lesions or a kerion or associated with formation of frank bullae causing tinea corporis bullosa *(9)*. Infection may also spread down the hair shaft into the dermis producing inflammatory papules and pustules *(9)*.

Tinea faciei has a broad range of presentations. Infection may begin as flat, scaly macules that develop into a raised border advancing outward in all direction, with or without development of papules, vesicles, and crusts (Fig. 20.5) *(10)*. Lesions may not be annular. The central area may become either hypopigmented, or hyperpigmented. Lesions may occur singly or in multiple patches, and may extend to other parts of the body *(10)*.

Tinea imbricata or Tokelau is a chronic infection of glabrous skin caused by the anthropophilic dermatophyte *T. concentricum* , presenting as distinctive scaly, concentric, overlapping plaques that may cover large areas of the body *(21)*. Lesions typically begin on the face, and spread to large areas of the body. The infection is endemic to Polynesia, Central and South America, particularly in rural areas.

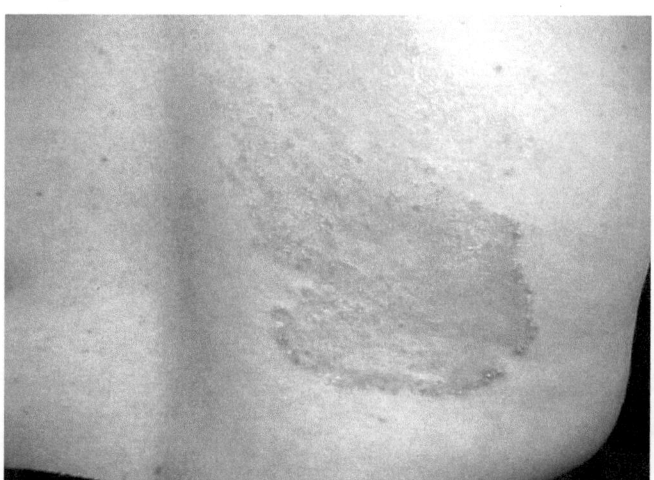

Fig. 20.3. Tinea corporis. [Figure in color on CD-ROM].

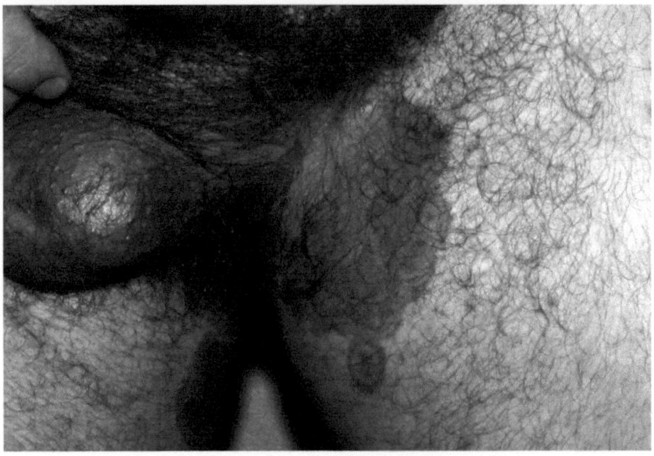

Fig. 20.4. Tinea cruris. [Figure in color on CD-ROM].

5.3. *Tinea Capitis*

Infection of the scalp involves hyphal proliferation in the stratum corneum that extends into the hair follicle orifice and hair shaft *(1)*. Exposure of the scalp to the inoculum from an infected individual, animal, or other source of organism may result in infection where trauma or some other factor (tight braiding exposing the scalp, application of hair oil that facilitates adherence of arthroconidia) aids arthroconidia implantation *(1)*. Inflammatory tinea capitis is associated with zoophilic or geophilic species such as *M. canis* or *M. gypseum*, but may also occur with *T. verrucosum*, *T. schoenleinii*, *T. tonsurans*, and *M. audouinii (1)*. A kerion may be produced: an oozing

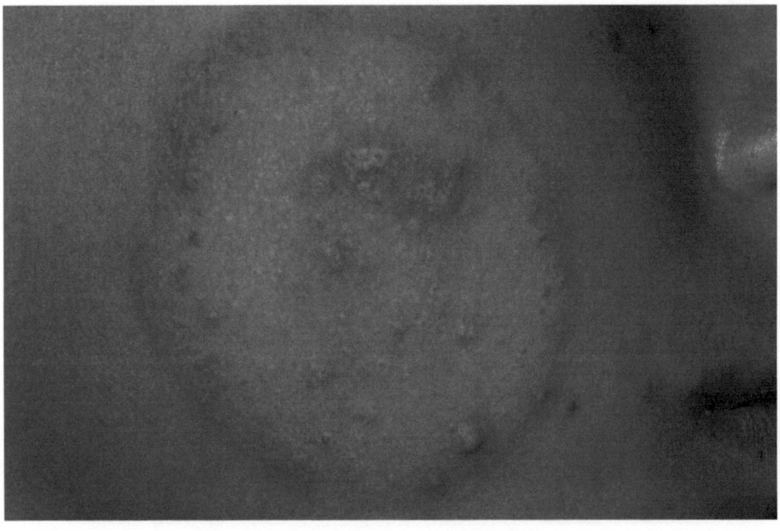

Fig. 20.5. Tinea faciei. [Figure in color on CD-ROM].

mass with pustules, loose hair and discharge of pus. Signs of systemic illness may be present, including fever and lymphadenopathy.

Noninflammatory or epidemic tinea capitis may begin as a small erythematous papule around the hair shaft which spreads outwards, developing fine scaling in noticeable patches (Fig. 20.6) *(1)*. Partial or complete alopecia may result where brittle hair breaks off a few millimeters from the scalp. Affected hair may appear grey due to coating with arthroconidia. Non-inflammatory infection is associated with *M. audouinii* and *M. ferrugineum*; however *T. tonsurans* and *M. canis* may infrequently cause noninflammatory infection.

Black dot tinea capitis is most frequently associated with *T. tonsurans* or *T. violaceum* infection, and results from hair breakage at the level of the scalp, showing diseased hair in the follicle as a "black dot" *(1)*. Scaling is typically present with little inflammation, although inflammatory kerions are possible *(1)*.

Favic infection is rare in North America and most often caused by *T. schoenleinii*, leading to large yellow crusts *(1,22)*.

5.4. Onychomycosis

The most common presentation of onychomycosis is distal lateral subungual onychomycosis (DLSO), which presents as a nail with discoloration and varying degrees of hyperkeratosis, onycholysis (separation of nail from nail bed), subungual

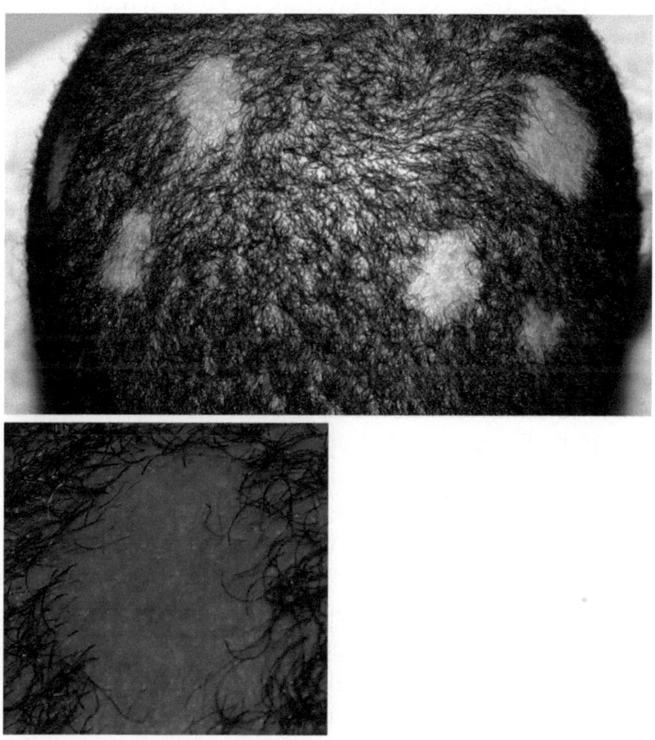

Fig. 20.6. Noninflammatory tinea capitis. [Figure in color on CD-ROM].

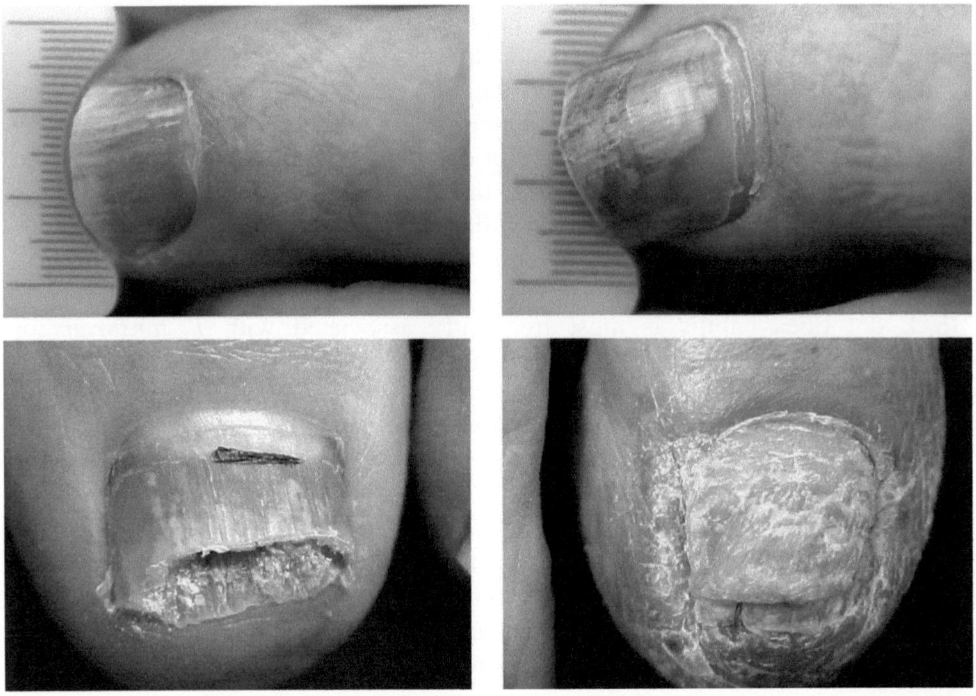

Fig. 20.7. Top left and right: onychomycosis; bottom left:onycholysis; bottom right: psoriasis. [Figure in color on CD-ROM].

debris, and thickening *(23,24)* (Fig. 20.7). DLSO begins at the distal edge of the nail (hyponychium) and travels proximally through the stratum corneum of the nail bed and involving the nail plate (Fig. 20.8). The most severe grades of DLSO may progress to total dystrophic onychomycosis (TDO), where the nail plate becomes friable and crumbles away to varying degree, leaving exposed thickened nail bed and subungual debris. Within the spectrum of DLSO presentations, infections may spread relatively evenly across the nail plate. Alternatively, infection may penetrate only the lateral edge or edges of the nail plate (lateral infection), or may penetrate longitudinally in a "spike" formation *(25)*. Infection may also develop as a dermatophytoma, where debris and fungus clump densely to form a thick, hyperkeratotic mass *(25)*. These presentations may not respond as well to therapy as a more diffuse DLSO presentation.

Infrequently, infection may present as superficial white onychomycosis (SWO), proximal subungual onychomycosis (PSO), or endonyx onychomycosis *(23,24)*. SWO involves infection of the superficial nail plate, showing patches of white discoloration on the nail surface. Multiple nails may be affected, and varying degrees of nail plate area may be covered (Fig. 20.9). The rare presentation PSO results from invasion of the proximal nail fold and extending distally along the underside of the nail plate as a white patch of infection (Fig. 20.10). PSO is more common in HIV-infected persons than in the healthy population, and may serve as a marker for degree of immunodeficiency *(26)*. Endonyx infection presents as a diffuse milky white discoloration of the nail in

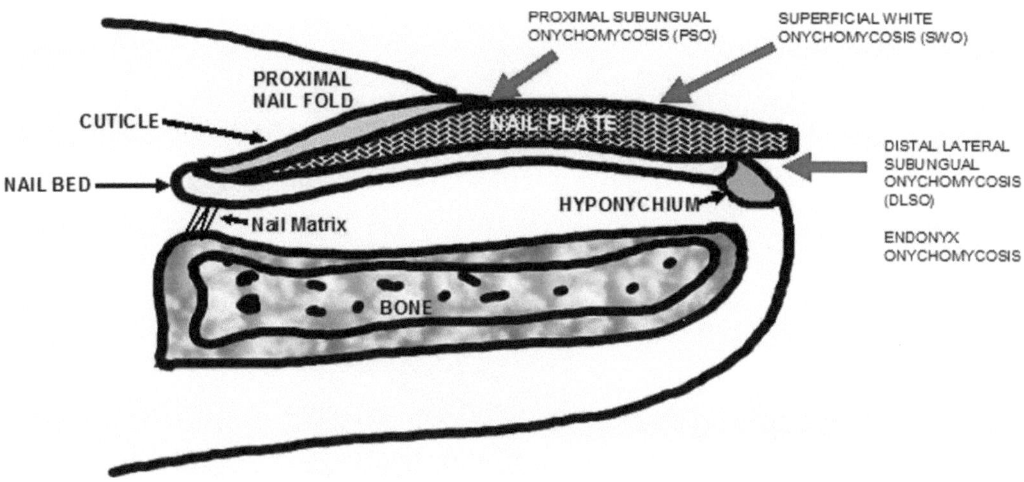

Fig. 20.8. Routes of infection causing the typical presentations of onychomycosis. [Figure in color on CD-ROM].

the absence of hyperkeratosis and onycholysis, with nail plate surface and thickness remaining normal *(23)*. Alternately, the nail may show lamellar splitting of the nail plate, with invasion of superficial and deeper layers of the nail plate, without excessive thickening or discoloration of the nail unit *(24)*. Endonyx infections are usually caused by *T. soudanense* or *T. violaceum (23,24)*.

5.5. Pityriasis Versicolor

Pityriasis versicolor presents as well-defined lesions, with a fine scale from desquamation, that are either hyperpigmented (pink, tan, dark brown, or black) or hypopigmented (white, or lighter than normal skin). Hypopigmentation may not always exhibit

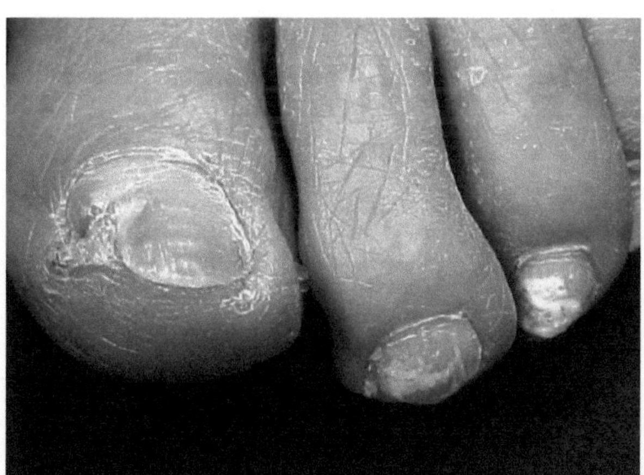

Fig. 20.9. Typical presentation of superficial white onychomycosis (SWO) on the third toenail with DLSO presented in the great toenail. [Figure in color on CD-ROM].

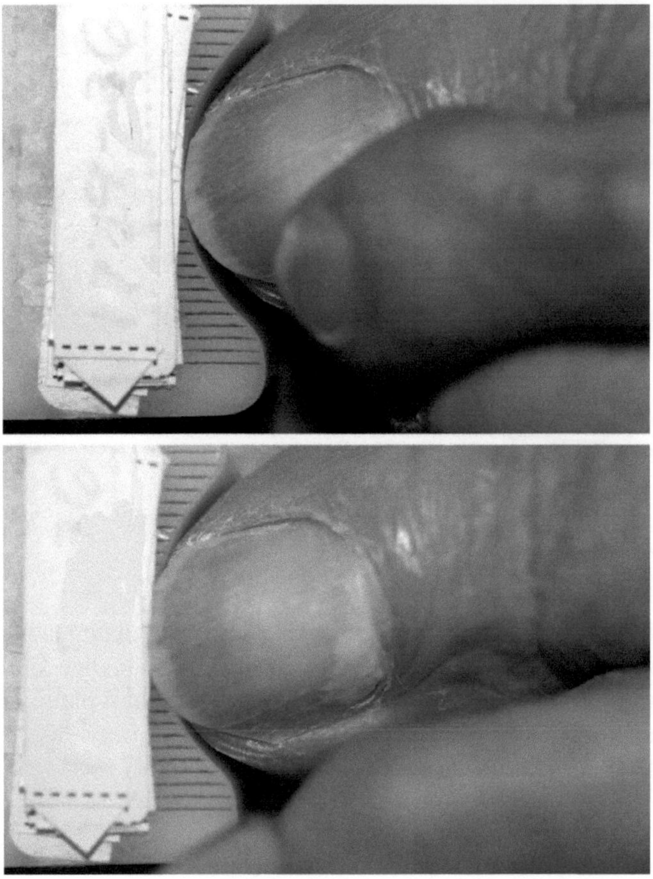

Fig. 20.10. Proximal subungual onychomycosis (PSO) developed during occlusion by the neighboring digit. [Figure in color on CD-ROM].

scaling (Fig. 20.11) *(27)*. It is a cosmetic disorder that is largely asymptomatic, with the exception of possible mild pruritus *(5)*. There is a large variation in lesion size from macules to entire trunk coverage *(28)*. Lesions are predominant in areas with a high number of sebaceous glands such as the scalp, chest, and back, as well as upper arms and face *(5,27)*. Facial lesions are more common in children than adults *(3)*. Hypopigmentation may occur independently or following the hyperpigmented stage *(27)*.

5.6. Seborrheic Dermatitis

Seborrheic dermatitis presents as red, flaking, greasy-looking patches of skin on the scalp and hair-bearing areas of the face such as the nasolabial folds, eyebrows, and ears (Fig. 20.12) *(15)*. SD is a more severe form of dandruff involving body sites of abundant sebaceous gland activity. It may occur on the groin, axillae, anterior chest, or inside/behind the ears *(15,29)*. Dandruff can appear as loosely adherent white or gray flakes, while severe SD may be thick, oily, yellow-brown crusts. Pruritus, irritation, and

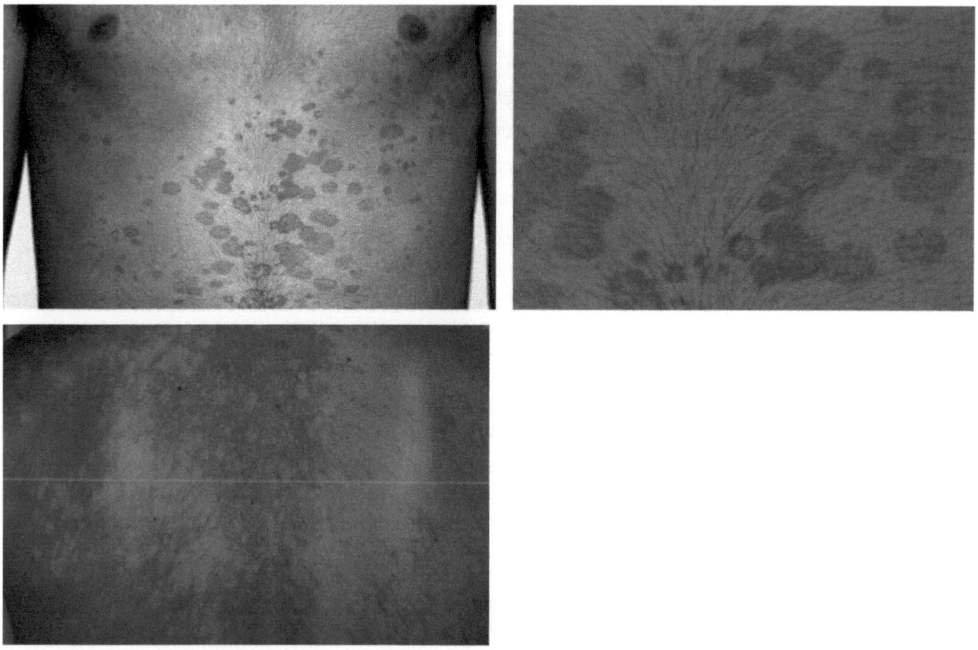

Fig. 20.11. Tinea versicolor showing hyperpigmentated lesions (upper photos) and hypopigmented lesions (lower photo). [Figure in color on CD-ROM].

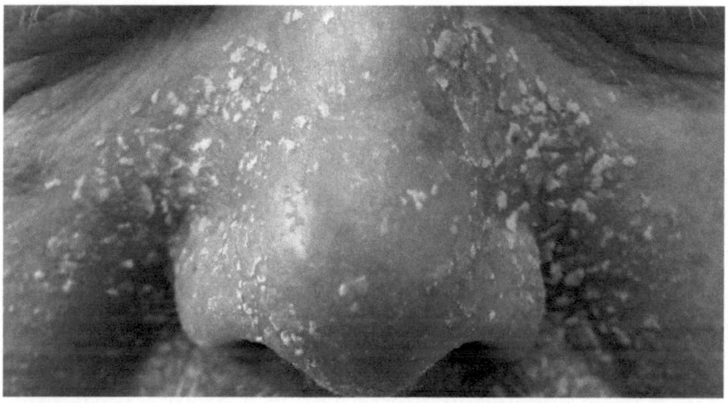

Fig. 20.12. Seborrheic dermatitis—severe presentation. [Figure in color on CD-ROM].

a tight, dry feeling may be associated with the afflicted area *(30)*. Some cases present with little erythema, while others present as a sore scalp with occasional pustules *(14)*.

6. DIAGNOSIS

Definitive diagnosis of tineas require confirmation of dermatophyte organisms by microscopic examination and laboratory fungal culture methods. For skin infections, scrapings or swabs can be taken from the leading edge of a lesion *(1,29)*. Nail clippings and subungual debris can similarly be investigated. Potassium hydroxide (KOH) is added to the samples to dissociate hyphae from keratinocytes, and the samples are examined by microscopy *(1,31)*. Microscopy can indicate the presence of dermatophytes via the presence of hyphae, however dermatophyte species cannot be distinguished by microscopy, thus cultures are required to confirm the causative species. *Malassezia* species may show a distinctive "spaghetti and meatball" form (mixture of yeasts and short hyphae) on microscopic examination *(3)*.

Microscopic examination of hairs may help differentiate types of tinea capitis infection: ectothrix infection can be distinguished from endothrix infection where arthroconidia appear as chains of the surface of the hair shaft or as a mosaic sheath around the hair *(1)*. Inspection under the Wood's light (filtered ultraviolet light with a peak of 365 nm) may aid in diagnosis *(1)*. Ectothrix infections with *M. audouinii, M. canis,* and *M. ferrugineum* show bright green fluorescence under the Wood's light. *T. schoenleinii* shows dull green fluorescence. *T. tonsurans*, however, does not fluoresce, and the utility of the Wood's lamp for diagnosis is currently limited in countries where this is the major infecting agent.

7. TREATMENT

Treatment for superficial fungal infections varies widely, although the antifungal medications used typically belong to either the azole or allylamines drug classes (Table 20.2). Topical use of these drugs can be effective in infections of limited area. Some of the newer topical antifungals exhibit anti-inflammatory and antibacterial activities as well as antifungal activity, and may therefore be a suitable choice for infections showing inflammation or concomitant bacterial infection. Five main systemic agents are available: terbinafine, itraconazole, fluconazole, griseofulvin, and ketoconazole. Oral formulations may be required for infections of more severe or more widespread presentation. Oral therapy may alternately be preferred for immunocompromised patients, in whom prompt, thorough resolution of infection is mandatory. Oral therapy may also be a more convenient choice for the patient than daily topical therapy applications.

Safety of therapy is more of a concern for oral treatment than topical treatment, as serum absorption tends to be minimal with topical drug use for dermatophytosis. With topical agents, most adverse events are skin reactions at the application site that are mild and transient. Owing to the large number of topical medications, adverse events will not be discussed here. Adverse events with oral medications are discussed where relevant. The oral antifungal medications are commonly associated with the potential for severe hepatic toxicity, rare serious skin events such as Stevens–Johnson syndrome, and possible drug–drug interactions due to metabolism through the cytochrome P-450 system. Current country-specific prescribing information for any dermatophytosis medication should be consulted before providing any medication.

Relapse of therapy has been noted with most types of dermatophyte infection. Patients must be encouraged to complete a full treatment cycle, as infection can be present without visible symptoms. Treatment must include microscopic examination and culture to confirm elimination of the pathogen. Infection transmission from symptom-free carriers such as family members and pets may need to be controlled with adjunct therapies and techniques; fomites such as hats and combs must also be treated.

Table 20.2
Treatment options available for dermatophytoses and other superficial fungal infections[a]

	Terbinafine	Itraconazole	Fluconazole	Ketoconazole	Griseofulvin	Topicals	
Tinea pedis/ manuum[a]	Cream[b]: Apply twice daily × 1–4 weeks 1% Solution[b]: Apply twice daily × 1 week Oral: 250 mg/day × 2 weeks	Oral: 200 mg bid × 1 week	Oral: 150 mg once weekly × 2–6 weeks	2% Cream[b]: Apply once daily × 6 weeks Oral[b]: 200–400 mg/day × >4 weeks	Microsize[b]: 1 g/day Ultramicrosize: 660 or 750 mg/day × 4–8 weeks	Cipclopiro 0.77% cream or gel[b]: Twice daily × 4 weeks Antifungal powder for prevention	Clotrimazole[b] Miconazole[b] Butenafine[b] Econazole[b]
Tinea corporis/cruris	Cream[b]: Apply twice daily × 1–4 weeks 1% Solution[b]: Apply twice daily × 1 week Oral: 250 mg/day × 2–4 weeks	Oral: 200 mg/day × 1 week	Oral:150–300 mg once weekly × 2–4 weeks	2% Cream[b]: Apply once daily × 2 weeks Oral[b]: 200–400 mg/day × 4 weeks	Microsize[b]: 500 mg/day Ultramicrosize: 330–375 mg/day × 2–4 weeks	Cipclopiro 0.77% cream or gel[b]: Twice daily × 4 weeks	Clotrimazole Miconazole Butenafine Econazole
Tinea capitis	See Table 20.3 for pediatric dosing	See Table 20.3 for pediatric dosing	See Table 20.3 for pediatric dosing	Only effective against *Trichophyton*. 2% shampoo used as adjunct therapy	See Table 20.3 for pediatric dosing	Selenium sulfide shampoo 1% as adjunct therapy	Corticosteroid adjunct therapy for severe inflammatory varieties

(Continued)

Table 20.2
(Continued)

	Terbinafine	Itraconazole	Fluconazole	Ketoconazole	Griseofulvin	Topicals	
Onychomycosis	Oral[b]: 250 mg/day *Toenail:* 12 weeks *Fingernail:* 6 weeks	Oral[b]: Continuous therapy[b]: 200 mg/day × 12 weeks Pulse therapy: 200 mg bid for 1 week, followed by 3 itraconazole–free weeks *Toenails:* 3 pulses *Fingernails*[b] *only:* 2 pulses	Oral: 150mg once weekly *Toenail:* 9–15 months *Fingernail:* 4–9 months	Oral: 200–400 mg/day × 6 months-*Not recommended due to hepatotoxicity risk*	Microsize[b] 1 g/day Ultramicrosize 660 or 750 mg/day× 4–12 months	† Cipclopiro 8% lacquer: once daily × 48 weeks	Amorolfine 5% lacquer – *Not approved in North America*
Pityriasis versicolor	1% Solution[b]: Apply twice daily × 1 week Oral: not effective	Oral: 200 mg/day × 5–7 days	2% Shampoo: 5 days Oral: 300 mg once weekly × 2 weeks	†2% Cream[b]: Apply once daily × 2 weeks Oral: 200 mg/day × 2 weeks, 10 days or 5 days; 400 mg per week × 2 weeks; 400 mg per day × 3 days; 3 doses of 400 mg given every 12 hours	Not effective	Cipclopiro[b] 0.77% cream Selenium sulfide[b]	Clotrimazole[b] Miconazole[b] Butenafine[b] Econazole[b]

Seborrheic dermatitis	1% Solution: Once daily × 4 weeks Oral: 250 mg/day × 4 weeks	Oral: 200 mg/day × 1 week	2% Shampoo: Twice a week × 4 weeks	2% Cream[b]: Apply twice daily × 4 weeks Shampoo[b]: Twice a week × 4 weeks Oral[b]: 200–400 mg/day × 4 weeks	Not effective	Cipclopirox[b]: 0.77% cream, shampoo, or gel Selenium sulfide[b] Coal tar[b] Hydrocortisone[b]	Zinc pyrithione[b] Metronidazole Bifonazole Miconazole

bid, twice daily.

[a]There are no approved treatments specifically for tinea manuum; treatments shown are for tinea pedis which are effective in the treatment of tinea manuum.

[b]FDA-approved indications.

7.1. Tinea Pedis/Manuum

Griseofulvin and topical terbinafine, butenafine, miconazole, econazole, ketoconazole, clotrimazole, and ciclopirox are US Food and Drug Administration (FDA)-approved treatments (Table 20.2) *(6,17)*. Studies have shown that oral terbinafine and itraconazole may be the most effective treatments, and a higher cure rate has been shown with topical allylamines than with topical azoles *(17,32)*. Topical formulations may be used for milder, limited presentations. For widespread or more severe presentations, oral formulations may be required. There is a higher relapse rate when using topical agents *(32)*.

Broad-spectrum topical agents may be useful, and agents with antibacterial activity may be preferred for presentations where it is suspected bacterial infection is superimposed on fungal infection (e.g., miconazole nitrate 1%, ciclopirox olamine 1%, naftifine hydrochloride 1%, sulconazole nitrate 1%). Formulations allowing once daily application may be preferred to twice daily usage, to aid patient compliance (e.g., naftifine 1% cream, bifonazole 1%, ketoconazole cream 2%). Chronic infection may warrant the use of oral antifungals, particularly if previous topical regimens have failed. Oral itraconazole, terbinafine, and fluconazole have been used successfully in the treatment of tinea pedis, although none of these agents is currently approved by the FDA for use in tinea pedis. These oral agents are preferred over ketoconazole, owing to the potential for hepatic side effects with ketoconazole use. Oral griseofulvin has lower efficacy than the newer antifungals, poor keratin adherence and has activity limited to dermatophytes, which may be a limitation where superimposed bacterial infection is present *(8)*. There are no approved treatments specifically for tinea manuum; treatments for tinea pedis are effectively used to treat tinea manuum.

Tinea pedis may frequently recur. Proper foot hygiene may help prevent reinfection. Patients should avoid walking barefoot in communal areas such as bathrooms, showers, or swimming areas, and ensure that feet are dried thoroughly after bathing, showering, or swimming *(33)*. In addition, patients should avoid occlusive footwear or alternate shoes every 2 to 3 days, and change socks often *(33)*.

7.2. Tinea Corporis/Cruris

Griseofulvin and topical terbinafine, butenafine, econazole, miconazole, ketoconazole, clotrimazole, and ciclopirox are FDA-approved treatments (Table 20.2) *(19)*. Topical formulations may be used for infections of smaller areas. (e.g., sulconazole, oxiconazole, miconazole, clotrimazole, econazole, ketoconazole) *(9)*. Oral therapy may be required where larger areas are involved, or where infection is chronic/recurrent. Topical corticosteroid use is not recommended, as it may lead to suppression of physical signs of infection, with lack of symptoms being wrongly associated with clearance of infection, leading to treatment relapse *(9)*. Oral itraconazole, terbinafine, and fluconazole have been used successfully in the treatment of tinea corporis/cruris, although none of these agents is currently approved by the FDA for use in these indications. These oral agents are preferred over ketoconazole, owing to the potential for hepatic side effects with ketoconazole use, and griseofulvin is not recommended as it does not adequately bind the keratin in the stratum corneum, reducing efficacy *(9)*.

Tinea faciei are typically cleared with topical treatment. Topical ciclopirox and terbinafine may provide good anti-inflammatory effects as well as antifungal activity *(10)*. Miconazole or similar azoles may also be effective. Azoles should be used for 3 to 4 weeks, or at least 1 week after resolution of lesions. Resistant lesions, cases of extensive disease, or more severe cases of infection may require oral therapy *(10)*.

Tinea imbricata is best treated with oral terbinafine or griseofulvin, although a high rate of recurrence has been noted *(21)*. Itraconazole and fluconazole have not been effective. Adjunctive therapy with keratolytic creams such as Whitfield's ointment (benzoic and salicylic acids) may increase treatment efficacy *(21)*.

7.3. Tinea Capitis

Oral therapy is required to adequately treat tinea capitis. Topical antifungals such as antifungal shampoos (selenium sulfide, povidone iodine, zinc pyrithione) may be used as adjunct therapy with or without oral antifungals to prevent reinfection or to treat asymptomatic carriers *(1,33)*. As most infections occur in children, dosing regimens are modified from the typical adult regimens provided in other indications, and are usually given on a weight-based schedule (Table 20.3). Further, infections with *Microsporum* may require higher dosing than infections with *Trichophyton*, or longer regimens of therapy *(1,34)*. Griseofulvin is the only FDA-approved oral treatment; however, terbinafine, itraconazole, and fluconazole have frequently been used in the successful resolution of tinea capitis. Shorter treatment durations are required for itraconazole, terbinafine, and fluconazole than for griseofulvin *(1)*. Liquid formulations are available for griseofulvin, itraconazole, and fluconazole, and may aid in pediatric dosing, although dosing regimens may vary from that suggested for tablet/capsule formulations.

Infected children do not need to be kept out of school once treatment is initiated, particularly children in higher grades *(33,35)*. Infection transmission from symptom-free carriers such as family members and pets may need to be controlled by using adjunct therapies and objects which may carry fomites such as hats, combs, pillows, blankets, and scissors may need to be disinfected with bleach *(33)*.

An "id" reaction has been observed with tinea capitis patients after initiation of drug therapy, and can be confused with allergic drug reaction *(1)*. An "id" reaction may present as symmetrical, skin colored, or erythematous papules and plaques on the face, neck, and upper body, but can be generalized. The reaction may also be present before initiation of treatment.

7.4. Onychomycosis

Onychomycosis is difficult to cure and has a high rate of recurrence *(6,11)*. Typically, oral therapy is required to adequately treat onychomycosis infections (Table 20.2). Following successful treatment of infection, the infected nail area must be grown out, gradually becoming replaced by normal healthy nail material. This process may take from 9 to 18 months, depending on nail growth rate. Fingernails may show better treatment success rates than toenails, as they grow faster *(36)*. Where the nail has been injured or shows other abnormal growth patterns, nail outgrowth may be slow, and the nail may never regain a normal appearance. Further, relapse of infection is

Table 20.3
Pediatric tinea capitis dosing regimens

	Regimen	Duration[a]	Weight (kg)				
			10–20	21–30	31–40	41–50	50+
Terbinafine (continuous)	5 mg/kg per day[b]	2-4 weeks	62.5 mg/day	125 mg/day	125 mg/day	250 mg/day	250 mg/day
Itraconazole (continuous)	5 mg/kg per day	2-4 weeks	100 mg every other day	100 mg/day	100 mg once daily alternating with twice daily	200 mg/day	200 mg/day
Itraconazole (pulse)[c]	Capsules: 5 mg/kg per day	1–3 pulses	100 mg every other day	100 mg/day	100 mg once daily alternating with twice daily	200 mg/day	200 mg bid[d]
	Oral suspension: 3 mg/kg per day	1–3 pulses					
Fluconazole (continuous)	Oral suspension: 6 mg/kg per day	20 days					
Fluconazole (pulse)[e]	Oral suspension: 6 mg/kg per day	8–12 weeks					
Griseofulvin (continuous)	Microsize: 20–25 mg/kg per day	6–12 weeks					
	Ultramicrosize: 10–15 mg/kg per day	6–12 weeks					
	Oral suspension: 15–25 mg/kg perday[f]	6–12 weeks					

bid, twice daily.
[a]Durations of treatment are for *Trichophyton tonsurans* infection. Longer durations are often required for *Microsporum canis* infections.
[b]Drugs are given by once daily dosing unless otherwise specified.
[c]Itraconazole pulses are given for 1 week, with 3 weeks "off" before starting the next pulse.
[d]Itraconazole adult dose 200 mg bid (approved for pulse use in fingernail onychomycosis). No standard has been established in clinical trials for tinea capitis for children >50 kg, and use varies from once-daily as with continuous regimen to twice-daily 200-mg dosing.
[e]Fluconazole pulses are 1 day on, 6 days off, before beginning next pulse.
[f]Dosing based on Grifulvin V suspension 125 mg/5 ml.

frequently noted. Patient expectations should be discussed, so the patient understands that successful treatment is unlikely to occur quickly, that long-term follow-up is necessary to catch any relapses in the early stages, and that the nail may not return to a normal appearance even though the infection may clear.

Topical therapy may be effective in mild to moderate cases of infection; ciclopirox 8% lacquer is the only topical therapy currently approved for onychomycosis by the FDA. Amorolfine 5% nail lacquer has not been approved for use in North America *(36–38)*. Routine nail débridement may be needed to provide effective delivery of drug to the infected area and to reduce the burden of fungal material needing treatment.

The newer oral agents terbinafine and itraconazole are most frequently used for onychomycosis. Ketoconazole is not often used, owing to the potential for hepatic side effects. Griseofulvin is also not recommended, as the required regimens are significantly longer than those of the itraconazole or terbinafine and efficacy is low *(39)*. Fluconazole has shown high efficacy, low relapse rates, and usefulness with yeast coinfection; however, there have been few studies on this treatment method *(19,36)*.

The approved oral therapy regimens for onychomycosis are as follows: terbinafine 250 mg/day for 12 weeks (toenails) or 6 weeks (fingernails only); itraconazole 200 mg/day for 12 weeks (toenails with or without fingernail involvement); and itraconazole 200 mg twice daily as pulse therapy (one pulse: 1 week of itraconazole followed by 3 weeks without itraconazole) using two pulses (fingernails only). Although only a continuous regimen of itraconazole is FDA-approved for toenail onychomycosis, the current standard of care of toenail onychomycosis for US dermatologists is a pulse itraconazole regimen (one pulse: 1 week of itraconazole followed by 3 weeks without itraconazole; three pulses given).

Both terbinafine and itraconazole are readily taken up in the nail from the nail bed and matrix and may remain in the nail for a significant period after dosing is completed. Itraconazole action tends to be fungistatic, while terbinafine is fungicidal *(39)*. Mycological cure rates (KOH negative and culture negative) for terbinafine use are estimated at 76% in a meta-analysis of clinical trial data from the medical literature *(40)*. By comparison, itraconazole mycological cure rates are 59% (continuous therapy) and 63% (pulse therapy). Clinical response rates (infection cleared or showing marked improvement) were as follows: terbinafine—66%, itraconazole continuous therapy—70%, and itraconazole pulse therapy—70% *(40)*.

Itraconazole may be associated with more drug interactions than terbinafine owing to its metabolism through the CYP 3A4 pathway, limiting its use in some patients. Itraconazole is also prohibited in patients showing ventricular dysfunction such as current or past congestive heart failure *(40)*. A current country-specific product monograph should be consulted for complete listing of known drug interactions, warnings, and monitoring requirements before prescribing. Rare cases of hepatic injury have been reported, and monitoring of hepatic enzymes is recommended for subjects with preexisting hepatic abnormality or a history of liver toxicity with use of other medications *(39)*. Capsules must be taken with a meal or cola beverage to ensure adequate absorption *(39)*.

Terbinafine may interfere with metabolism of CYP 2D6 substrates, and some other drug interactions have been noted. A current country-specific product monograph should be consulted for complete listing of known drug interactions, warnings, and monitoring requirements before prescribing. Rare cases of hepatic injury have been reported with terbinafine. Terbinafine is not recommended for patients with existing liver disease, and all patients should be screened for hepatic enzyme abnormalities (alanine transaminase [ALT] and aspartate transaminase [AST]) before initiating terbinafine *(39)*. Terbinafine may be taken in fasted or fed state without affecting absorption.

Routine nail débridement may be complementary for subjects using oral therapy as well as topical therapy, particularly where the nail is thickened, or where the infection presents as a dermatophytoma, spike, or lateral infection. Caution must be taken not to damage the underlying skin during débridement, particularly in subjects who are vulnerable to severe lower limb complications, such as diabetics or individuals with reduced lower limb profusion.

As with tinea pedis, proper foot and nail hygiene may help prevent reinfection. Patients should avoid walking barefoot in communal areas such as bathrooms, showers, or swimming areas, and ensure that feet are dried thoroughly after bathing, showering, or swimming *(33)*. Nails should be kept short and clean. Shoes should fit properly and socks should be made from absorbent material such as cotton.

7.5. *Pityriasis Versicolor*

A variety of topical agents may be used to treat PV (Table 20.2). Topical azoles (ketoconazole, fluconazole, bifonazole, clotrimazole, miconazole) have been effective in treating *Malassezia*, both in cream formulation or shampoos *(5)*. Terbinafine solution, cream, gel, or spray has also been effective *(5)*. Topical ciclopirox provides both antifungal and anti-inflammatory activity against *Malassezia*.

Systemic therapies may be warranted in severe cases, or cases with widespread body involvement. Patients may also prefer a short-duration oral therapy to frequent application of a topical agent. Oral therapy with ketoconazole, itraconazole, and fluconazole has been effective for PV, and the regimens reported in the literature provide similar, high efficacy rates *(5)*. Oral terbinafine and griseofulvin are not effective for PV *(5)*.

Relapse of PV is common owing to endogenous host factors: recurrence rates have been reported as high as 60% to 90% in 2 years posttreatment *(41)*. Both ketoconazole (single 400-mg dose or 200 mg daily for 3 days once monthly) and itraconazole (single 400-mg dose once monthly for 6 months) have been used in prophylactic regimens for PV *(5)*.

Individual treatments for hyper- and hypopigmented variations of PV do not exist. Although fungal organisms may be eradicated after 2 weeks of therapy, it may take significantly longer before the skin's normal pigmentation is restored, particularly with hypopigmented lesions *(5)*.

7.6. *Seborrheic Dermatitis*

There is no definitive cure for SD; it is a recurrent disease requiring prophylactic treatment *(14)*. Topical corticosteroid lotions have typically been used as treatment but are being replaced by antifungal treatments in the form of shampoos, gels, and creams (Table 20.2).

Topical ketoconazole (cream, shampoo, gel, emulsion) is the most prescribed azole for SD *(42)*. Bifonazole, miconazole, and fluconazole may also be effective. Low-potency corticosteroids may be useful in providing anti-inflammatory treatment, although many newer antifungal agents such as ciclopirox may also provide anti-inflammatory activity comparable to corticosteroids *(42)*. Ciclopirox (cream, gel or shampoo) provides effective antifungal treatment, and also has antibacterial and anti-inflammatory activities *(43,44)*. Zinc pyrithione shampoos are safe and effective in controlling dandruff and SD of the scalp, and exhibit strong keratolytic and antifungal activity against *Malassezia (15,45)*. Some patients benefit as well from non-antifungal, keratolytic agents (selenium sulfide, sulfur, salicylic acid) or antiproliferative (coal tar) shampoos *(14,30)*. Tar shampoos often cause sensitivity of the skin to sunlight and are not as favorable cosmetically *(30)*. Topical 1% terbinafine solution has been effectively used for scalp SD *(42)*.

Oral therapy should be reserved for severe inflammatory SD, widespread SD, or SD that has been refractory to topical treatment *(42)*. Oral ketoconazole and oral itraconazole have been used effectively for SD. Oral itraconazole is safer than ketoconazole and is effective in severe cases that have not responded to other antifungals *(15)*.

REFERENCES

1. Gupta AK, Summerbell RC. Tinea capitis. Med Mycol 2000;38:255–287.
2. Hainer BL Dermatophyte infections. Am Fam Physician 2003;67:101–108.
3. Ashbee RH, Evans EGV. Immunology of diseases associated with *Malassezia* species. Clin Microbiol Rev 2002;15:21–57.
4. Crespo-Erchiga V, Florencio VD. *Malassezia* yeasts and pityriasis versicolor. Curr Opin Infect Dis 2006;19:139–147.
5. Gupta AK, Batra R, Bluhm R, Faergemann J. Pityriasis versicolor. Dermatol Clin 2003;21:413–429.
6. Noble SL, Forbes RC, Stamm PL. Diagnosis and management of common tinea infections. Am Fam Physician 1998;58:163–168.
7. Smith ES, Fleischer AB, Feldman SR, Williford PM. Characteristics of office-based physician visits for cutaneous fungal infections: an analysis of 1990 to 1994 National Ambulatory Medical Care Survey data. Cutis 2002;69:191–204.
8. Gupta AK, Chow M, Daniel CR, Aly R. Treatments of tinea pedis. Dermatol Clin 2003;21:431–462.
9. Gupta AK, Chaudhry M, Elewski B. Tinea corporis, tinea cruris, tinea nigra, and piedra. Dermatol Clin 2003;21:395–400.
10. Lin RL, Szepietowski JC, Schwartz RA. Tinea faciei, an often deceptive facial eruption. Int J Dermatol 2004;43:437–440.
11. Gupta AK, Scher RK. Management of onychomycosis: a North American perspective. Dermatol Ther 1997;3:58–65.
12. Gupta AK, Ryder JE. How to improve cure rates for the management of onychomycosis. Dermatol Clin 2003;21:499–505.
13. Faergemann J. Management of seborrheic dermatitis and pityriasis versicolor. Am J Clin Dermatol 2000;1:75–80.
14. Gupta AK, Kogan N. Seborrhoeic dermatitis: current treatment practices. Expert Opin Pharmacother 2004;5:1755–1765.

15. Gupta AK, Bluhm R. Seborrheic dermatitis. J Eur Acad Dermatol Venereol 2004;18:13–26.
16. Lynch PJ. Dermatologic problems of the head and neck in the aged. Otolaryngol Clin North Am 1982;15:271–285.
17. Padhye AA, Weitzman I. The dermatophytes. In: Collier L, Balows A, Sussman M, Ajello L, Hay RJ, eds. Topley and Wilson's medical mycology. New York: Oxford University Press, 1998:215–236.
18. Kwon-Chung KJ, Bennett JE. Dermatophytoses (ringworm, tinea, dermatomycosis). In: Medical mycology. Malvern, PA: Lea & Febiger, 1992:105–161.
19. Trent JT, Federman D, Kirsner RS. Common viral and fungal skin infections. Ostomy Wound Manage 2001;47:28–34.
20. Daniel CR, Gupta AK, Daniel MP, Daniel CM. Two feet-one hand syndrome: a retrospective multicenter survey. Int J Dermatol 1997;36:658–660.
21. Bonifaz A, Archer-Dubon C, Saul A. Tinea imbricata or Tokelau. Int J Dermatol 2004;43:506–510.
22. Gupta AK, Hofstader SL, Adam P, Summerbell RC. Tinea capitis: an overview with emphasis on management. Pediatr Dermatol 1999;16:171–189.
23. Mahoney JM, Bennet J, Olsen B. The diagnosis of onychomycosis. Dermatol Clin 2003;21:463–467.
24. Baran R, Hay RJ, Tosti A, Haneke E. A new classification of onychomycosis. Br J Dermatol 1998;139:567–571.
25. Gupta AK, Baran R, Summerbell RC. Onychomycosis: strategies to improve efficacy and reduce recurrence. J Eur Acad Dermatol Venereol 2002;16:579–586.
26. Gupta AK, Taborda P, Taborda V, et al. Epidemiology and prevalence of onychomycosis in HIV-positive individuals. Int J Dermatol 2000;39:746–753.
27. Thoma W, Kramer HJ, Mayser P. Pityriasis versicolor alba. J Eur Acad Dermatol Venereol 2005;19:147–152.
28. Mellen LA, Vallee J, Feldman SR, Fleischer Je AB. Treatment of pityriasis versicolor in the United States. J Dermatol Treat 2004;15:189–192.
29. Elewski BE. Clinical diagnosis of common scalp disorders. J Invest Dermatol Symp Proc 2005;10:190–193.
30. Gee BC. Seborrhoeic dermatitis. Clin Evid 2004;2344–2352.
31. Feuilhade de Chauvin M. New diagnostic techniques. J Eur Acad Dermatol Venereol 2005;19(Suppl 1):20–24.
32. Crawford F. Athlete's foot. In: Williams H, Bigby M, Diepgen T, Herxheimer A, Naldi L, Rzany B, eds. Evidence based dermatology. London: BMJ Books, 2003:436–440.
33. Gupta AK, Ryder JE, Chow M, Cooper EA. Dermatophytosis: the management of fungal infections. Skinmed 2005;4:305–310.
34. Lipozencic J, Skerlev M, Orofino-Costa R, et al. A randomized, double-blind, parallel-group, duration-finding study of oral terbinafine and open-label, high-dose griseofulvin in children with tinea capitis due to *Microsporum* species. Br J Dermatol 2002;146:816–823.
35. Roberts BJ, Friedlander SF. Tinea capitis: a treatment update. Pediatr Ann 2005;34: 191–200.
36. Gupta AK, Ryder J, Bluhm R. Onychomycosis. In: Williams H, Bigby M, Diepgen T, Herxheimer A, Naldi L, Rzany B, eds. Evidence based dermatology. London: BMJ Books, 2003:441–468.
37. Gupta AK, Ryder JE, Skinner AR. Treatment of onychomycosis: pros and cons of antifungal agents. J Cutan Med Surg 2004;8:25–30.
38. Lecha M, Effendy I, Feuilhade de Chauvin M, Di Chiacchio N, Baran R. Treatment options-development of consensus guidelines. J Eur Acad Dermatol Venereol 2005;19(Suppl 1):25–33.

39. Gupta AK, Ryder JE. The use of oral antifungal agents to treat onychomycosis. Dermatol Clin 2003;21:469–479.
40. Gupta AK, Ryder JE, Johnson A.M. Cumulative meta-analysis of systemic antifungal agents for the treatment of onychomycosis. Br J Dermatol 2004;150:537–544.
41. Faergemann J. Pityrosporum infections. J Am Acad Dermatol 1994;31:S18–S20.
42. Gupta AK, Bluhm R, Cooper EA, Summerbell RC, Batra R. Seborrheic dermatitis. Dermatol Clin 2003;21:401–412.
43. Aly R, Katz HI, Kempers SE, et al. Ciclopirox gel for seborrheic dermatitis of the scalp. Int J Dermatol 2003;42:19–22.
44. Lebwohl M, Plott T. Safety and efficacy of ciclopirox 1% shampoo for the treatment of seborrheic dermatitis of the scalp in the US population: results of a double-blind, vehicle-controlled trial. Int J Dermatol 2004;42:17–20.
45. Rogers JS, Moore AE, Meldrum H, Harding CR. Increased scalp skin lipids in response to antidandruff treatment containing zinc pyrithione. Arch Dermatol Res 2003;295:127–129.

SUGGESTED READINGS

Baran R, Gupta AK, Pierard GE. Pharmacotherapy of onychomycosis. Expert Opin Pharmacother 2005;6:609–624.

Crespo-Erchiga V, Florencio VD. Malassezia yeasts and pityriasis versicolor. Curr Opin Infect Dis 2006;19:139–147.

Gupta AK, Chaudhry M, Elewski B. Tinea corporis, tinea cruris, tinea nigra, and piedra. Dermatol Clin 2003;21:395–400.

Gupta AK, Chow M, Daniel CR, Aly R. Treatments of tinea pedis. Dermatol Clin 2003;21: 431–462.

Gupta AK, Cooper EA, Ryder JE, Nicol KA, Chow M, Chaudhry MM. Optimal management of fungal infections of the skin, hair, and nails. Am J Clin Dermatol 2004;5:225–237.

Gupta AK, Summerbell RC. Tinea capitis. Med Mycol 2000;38:255–287.

Hay R. Literature review. Onychomycosis. J Eur Acad Dermatol Venereol 2005;19 (Suppl 1):1–7.

Roberts BJ, Friedlander SF. Tinea capitis: a treatment update. Pediatr Ann 2005;34:191–200.

21

Subcutaneous Fungal Infections (Chromoblastomycosis, Mycetoma, and Lobomycosis)

Michael B. Smith, MD and Michael R. McGinnis, PhD

1. INTRODUCTION

Fungal infections involving subcutaneous tissue often develop following a penetrating wound through the skin. The etiologic agents are usually soil fungi or decomposers of plant material and infection typically occurs when woody plant material such as splinters and thorns penetrate the cutaneous barrier. With the exception of *Sporothrix schenckii*, the pathogens that cause infection in subcutaneous tissue are not dimorphic, that is, they do not grow in different morphological forms in vitro and in vivo. In tissue, they may form hyphae, yeast cells, muriform cells, or be organized into microcolonies called sclerotia (syn. grains, granules) *(1)*. The combination of tissue morphology of the fungus, whether or not the fungus contains melanin in its cell wall (dematiaceous), and the clinical presentation, determines the specific type of subcutaneous mycosis (Table 21.1). This information guides management approaches and assists with determining the prognosis for the patient.

Fungal infections involving subcutaneous tissue are frequently grouped as (1) mycetoma, which can be caused by both dematiaceous and nondematiaceous fungi *(2)*; (2) chromoblastomycosis, in which the etiologic agent develops dematiaceous muriform cells with thickened melanized cell walls in subcutaneous microabscesses *(3)*; (3) subcutaneous phaeohyphomycosis, characterized by dematiaceous yeast cells, pseudohyphae, and irregular shaped hyphae to well-developed septate hyphae (may be present in any combination); or (4) hyalohyphomycosis, an infection that is similar to phaeohyphomycosis except that the fungi that cause this disease are not dematiaceous. Sporotrichosis (Chapter 19), subcutaneous hyalohyphomycosis (Chapter 10), subcutaneous phaeohyphomycosis (Chapter 11), and subcutaneous zygomycosis (including entomophthoramycosis; Chapter 12) are discussed elsewhere in this text. Rhinosporidiosis, caused by a protoctistan classified in a Mesomycetozoa clade, is not discussed. Mycetoma and chromoblastomycosis are considered together because these two infections have a number of clinical and pathological

From: *Infectious Disease: Diagnosis and Treatment of Human Mycoses*
Edited by: D. R. Hospenthal and M. G. Rinaldi © Humana Press Inc., Totowa, NJ

Table 21.1
Overview of the major subcutaneous fungal infections

Disease	Etiology	Key histological features	Comments
Chromoblastomycosis	*Cladophialophora, Fonsecaea*[a]	Dematiaceous muriform cells in subcutaneous micro-abscesses	
Hyalohyphomycosis	*Aspergillus, Fusarium*[a]	Hyaline, septate hyphae, yeast cells, pseudohyphae, or any of the above	See Chapter 10
Lobomycosis	*Lacazia*	Hyaline yeast cells in a chain with connectors between the cells	
Mycetoma	*Madurella, Scedosporium*[a]	Sclerotia (grains, granules) composed of dematiaceous or hyaline fungal hyphae	
Phaeohyphomycosis	*Exophiala*[a]	Dematiaceous septate hyphae, yeast cells, pseudohyphae, or any of the above	See Chapter 11
Rhinosporidiosis	*Rhinosporidium*	Hyaline sporangia with sporangiospores of different sizes that are released into the environment through a pore; see Figure 3-3, Chapter 3	Etiologic agent recently proven not to be a fungus
Sporotrichosis	*Sporothrix*	Oval budding yeast cells	See Chapter 19
Zygomycosis (Entomophthoramycosis)	*Basidiobolus, Conidiobolus*	Hyaline, sparsely septate, random branching, irregular diameter hyphae	See Chapter 12
Zygomycosis (not Entomophthoramycosis)	*Apophysomyces, Rhizopus*[a]	Hyaline, sparsely septate, random branching, irregular diameter hyphae	See Chapter 12

[a]Examples of major etiological agents; not inclusive.

aspects in common with each other. Chromoblastomycosis has been referred by some as essentially a "mini mycetoma" because of its pathologic and clinical similarities to mycetoma. Both of these infections demonstrate the presence of tumefaction, draining sinuses, and aggregates of the etiologic agents within the subcutaneous tissue. Lobomycosis, which is caused by *Lacazia loboi*, is an infection that occurs in people living near water in Central and South America. In addition to human cases, this fungus causes cutaneous–subcutaneous infection in some animals (e.g., dolphins) *(4)*.

2. ETIOLOGIC AGENTS

2.1. *Chromoblastomycosis*

Chromoblastomycosis is caused by members of the genera *Cladophialophora, Exophiala, Fonsecaea*, and *Phialophora*, which belong to the ascomycete family Herpotrichiellaceae (Chaetothyriales) (Table 21.2). The genus *Fonsecaea* currently

Table 21.2
Etiologic agents of human chromoblastomycosis, mycetoma, and lobomycosis

Chromoblastomycosis
Cladophialophora carrionii
Exophiala dermatitidis
Exophiala jeanselmei
Exophiala spinifera
Fonsecaea compacta
Fonsecaea pedrosoi
Phialophora verrucosa
Rhinocladiella aquaspersa
Mycetoma
Acremonium kiliense
Acremonium recifei
Aspergillus flavus
Aspergillus hollandicus
Emericella nidulans
Fusarium falciforme
Corynespora cassicola
Curvularia lunata
Cylindrocarpon cyanescens
Cylindrocarpon destructans
Exophiala jeanselmei
Fusarium falciforme
Fusarium solani
Fusarium verticillioides
Leptosphaeria senegalensis
Leptosphaeria tompkinsii
Madurella grisea
Madurella mycetomatis
Neotestudina rosatii
Phaeoacremonium inflatipes
Phialophora verrucosa
Polycytella hominis
Pseudallescheria boydii
Pseudochaetosphaeronema larense
Pyrenochaeta mackinnonii
Pyrenochaeta romeroi
Rhinocladiella atrovirens
Lobomycosis
Lacazia loboi

contains three species, two of which are primary agents of chromoblastomycosis, *F. compacta* and *F. pedrosoi*. *Fonsecaea pedrosoi* is the primary etiologic agent of chromoblastomycosis throughout the world. On the basis of molecular analysis, a new species called *F. monophora* has been proposed for isolates that were previously identified as *F. pedrosoi* which cause CNS infections *(5)*. This latter infection is a phaeohyphomycosis because the fungus grows as dematiaceous hyphae in tissue.

The genus *Cladophialophora* contains a number of species, including *C. bantiana*, the etiologic agent of CNS phaeohyphomycosis. Recently, *Cladosporium carrionii*, an important agent of chromoblastomycosis, was reclassified as *Cladophialophora carrionii*. This species is geographically more localized than *F. pedrosoi*.

2.2. *Mycetoma*

Mycetoma is caused by a variety of genera, the frequency of which vary geographically. The genus *Pseudallescheria* contains a number of species. *Pseudallescheria boydii* (anamorph *Scedosporium apiospermum*) is the major species of medical interest. It is unknown if the other species of *Pseudallescheria* can cause mycetoma. At this time, it is thought that *P. boydii* is the only etiologic agent of this genus that causes mycetoma. *Pseudallescheria* is classified in the order Microascales.

The genus *Madurella* was originally established for sterile dematiaceous fungi causing mycetoma. Based on rDNA small subunit and internal transcribed spacer (ITS) sequence data, *Madurella* has been determined to be a heterogeneous group of fungi *(6)*. *Madurella mycetomatis*, which worldwide is the most common cause of mycetoma, is in the Sordariales, whereas *M. grisea* is in the Pleosporales. The Ascomycetes orders Hypocreales, Eurotiales, and Dothideales contain several etiologic agents of mycetoma.

2.3. *Lobomycosis*

Lacazia loboi (previously named *Loboa loboi*) is a noncultured fungus that resembles *Paracoccidioides brasiliensis* in vivo. It is the sole etiologic agent of lobomycosis, regardless of human or animal origin. Based on its morphology in tissue and its phylogenetic distinctness, the fungus is classified with the dimorphic Ascomycetes in the Onygenales.

3. EPIDEMIOLOGY

Chromoblastomycosis, lobomycosis, and mycetoma have a number of features in common. Infected patients typically live in tropical and subtropical regions. The etiologic agents are introduced by localized trauma to the skin by woody plant material or other injuries such as insect bites. They are more commonly seen in individuals working in agriculture, mining, fishing, farming, and similar occupations where they are in constant contact with the environment. Infections occur more commonly in males, which is likely a reflection of occupational exposure. Mycetoma tends to occur in arid areas with short rainy seasons and a low relative humidity.

Lobomycosis, unlike the other two infections, is not worldwide in occurrence. It is restricted to South and Central America, especially in communities located along rivers. Lobomycosis tends to develop on exposed and cooler areas of the body such as the extremities and the ears. This contrasts with chromoblastomycosis and mycetoma, which most frequently occur on the legs and feet.

4. PATHOGENESIS AND IMMUNOLOGY

The three infections are characterized by chronic, granulomatous, slowly progressing, cutaneous–subcutaneous inflammatory processes resulting in disfiguring lesions. The duration of infection prior to diagnosis can be years. Many patients recall splinters or similar wounds at the infection site prior to the development of the infection. Chromoblastomycosis does not involve bones and it does not usually spread through the lymphatic system. Mycetoma, in contrast, often extends to bone where it causes extensive destruction. Lobomycosis remains localized to the dermis and subcutaneous tissue and does not cause disseminated infections.

5. CLINICAL MANIFESTATIONS

5.1. *Chromoblastomycosis*

Chromoblastomycosis may exhibit a range of different types of lesions that vary depending on the duration and body site of the infection *(7)*. After local injury, small verrucous papules develop. Localized spread or extension of the lesions can occur by autoinoculation. The slow growing lesions can develop into clusters of large hyperkeratotic verrucous plaques that produce ulceration, cystic areas, and eventually, scarring (Fig. 21.1). Scarring can become so extensive that the flexibility of limbs can be compromised. Muriform cells occur in subcutaneous areas of epitheliomatous hyperplasia and microabscesses, and are expelled to the surface by transepithelial elimination. This results in "black dots" on the lesion surface which are accumulations of necrotic tissue and fungal cells. This process is similar to mycetoma, which is characterized by "sclerotia" being transported to the surface by draining sinuses associated with edema (tumefaction). For this reason, chromoblastomycosis has been referred to as a mini-mycetoma.

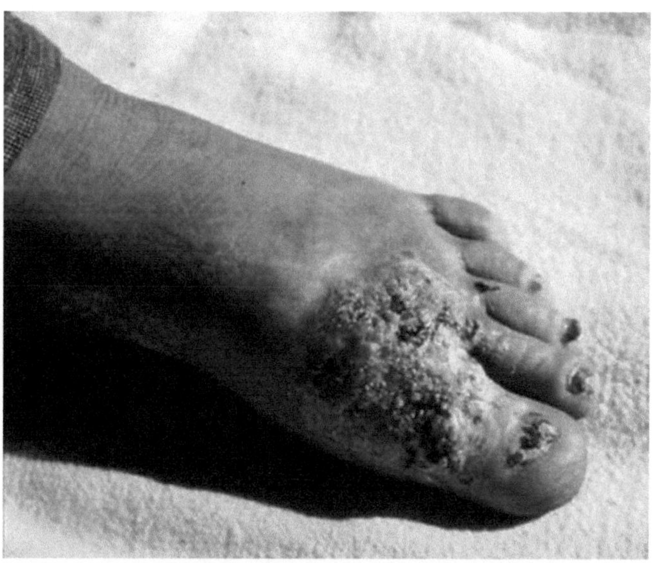

Fig. 21.1. Chromoblastomycosis caused by *Fonsecaea pedrosoi*. (Courtesy of Dr. C. Halde.) [Figure in color on CD-ROM].

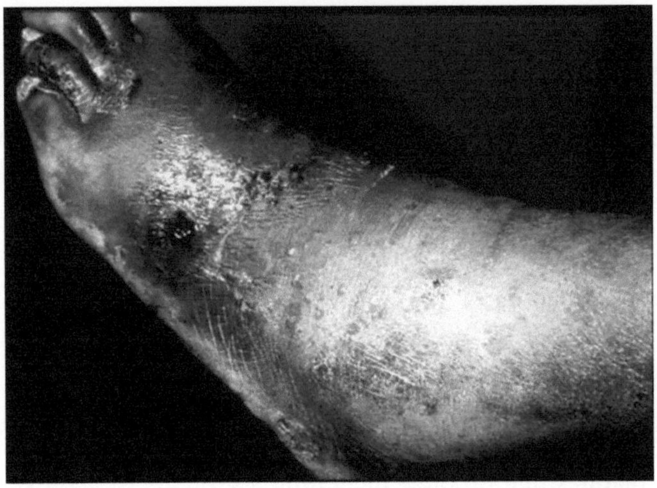

Fig. 21.2. Mycetoma caused by *Madurella mycetomatis*. (Courtesy of Dr. C. Halde.) [Figure in color on CD-ROM].

5.2. *Mycetoma*

Fungal mycetoma develops more slowly than mycetoma caused by bacterial agents (actinomycotic mycetoma) *(8)*. Encapsulated lesions with clearly defined margins slowly develop after introduction of the fungus on a splinter or thorn. A subcutaneous painless swelling develops that is usually soft, firm, and lobate. Additional foci often

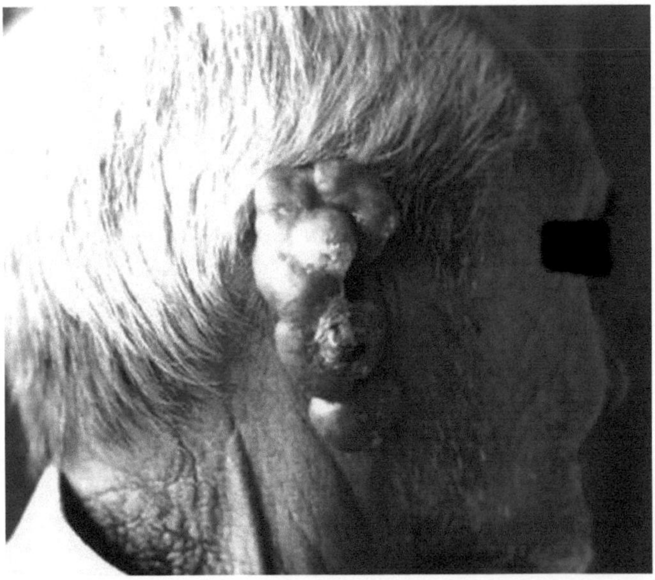

Fig. 21.3. Lobomycosis caused by *Lacazia loboi*. Courtesy of Dr. P. Taborda. [Figure in color on CD-ROM].

develop, suppurate, and drain through multiple sinus tracts. Additional sinuses develop that are interconnected with each other, sterile deep abscesses, and the skin. Sclerotia of different colors (e.g., white grain, black grain) that are formed by specific fungi find their way to the surface. Even though mycetoma is painless owing to anesthetic effect or nerve damage, pain may occur when bone expands due to the fungal sclerotial mass, or when secondary infections develop. Mycetoma can produce functional disability, distortion, and deformity of limbs (Fig. 21.2).

5.3. *Lobomycosis*

Lesions of lobomycosis develop slowing and become cutaneous nodules or plaques that may be smooth, verrucous, or ulcerative, and eventually can become surrounded by keloidal scar tissue *(4)*. The lesions may be solitary or multiple; painless or slightly pruritic; with the fungus spreading contiguously or via lymphatic channels (Fig. 21.3). The lesions contain granulomatous inflammatory tissue and the yeast cells. The fungus does not cause disseminated infection.

6. DIAGNOSIS

The diagnosis of these infections is based primarily on clinical presentation, histopathology, and culture. Culture is not useful in the diagnosis of lobomycosis as *L. loboi* has not yet been cultured. The tissue forms for these infections are distinctive, and can be used to a limited degree for presumptive identification purposes (see Fig. 3.2, Chapter 3). Chains of yeast cells with a narrow connection between each yeast cell are characteristic of *L. loboi (9)*. The architecture of the sclerotia in mycetoma patients can be associated with particular known agents (Fig. 21.4). The structure is especially useful for distinguishing the granules of aerobic actinomycetes composed of 0.5 to 1.0 μm gram-positive filaments from sclerotia of true fungi having hyphal cells. The muriform cells and hyphae in the dermis of chromoblastomycosis cases do

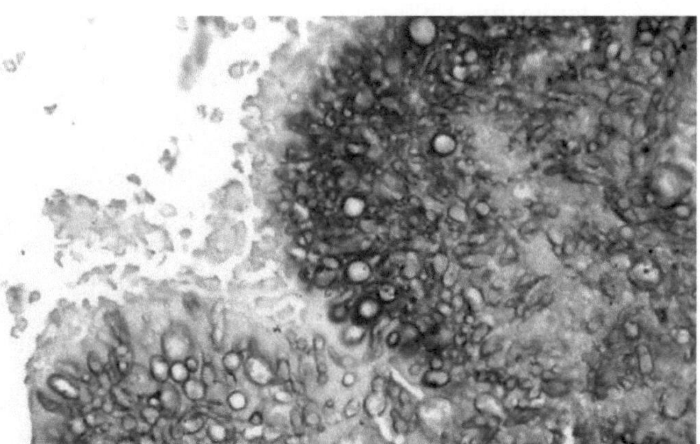

Fig. 21.4. Sclerotia of *Madurella mycetomatis* in a foot. Gridley Fungus Stain. Courtesy of Dr. L. Ajello. [Figure in color on CD-ROM].

not allow for the differentiation of the different etiologic agents, although they are virtually pathognomonic of the disease.

In culture, the agents of chromoblastomycosis and mycetoma are easily identified. *Madurella mycetomatis* represents an interesting challenge because it is defined on the basis of being a typically sterile dematiaceous, slow growing mould isolated from a mycetoma. As mentioned, the fungus appears to be a complex of different phylogenetic members.

7. TREATMENT

Chromoblastomycosis, lobomycosis, and mycetoma are chronic infections without a single treatment of choice. Currently used treatments often have low cure rates and high relapse rates, although these rates vary based on the etiologic agent, affected body area, and health status of the patient (Table 21.3). The dense fibrosis and lymphostasis that occurs in these infections can impede drug penetration into the infected area. Courses of therapy of 6 to 12 months (or more) are not uncommon.

7.1. Chromoblastomycosis

Chromoblastomycosis is often treated with the triazole itraconazole, or terbinafine *(3)*. These antifungal agents are used at high dosage concentrations, typically for 6 to 12 months. Of the azoles, itraconazole has been the most successful antifungal drug,

Table 21.3
Management of chromoblastomycosis, mycetoma, and lobomycosis

Infection	Management
Chromoblastomycosis	Surgery, electrodessication, and cryosurgery are effective in early stages. Local heat can reduce extension of lesions. Disabled or deformed limbs may require amputation. Combination therapy with terbinafine (500 mg daily) plus itraconazole (50–100 mg daily) or terbinafine alone has been successful.
Mycetoma	Historically, surgery has been used for treatment of mycetoma. Mycetomas are well encapsulated, and care must be exercised to avoid rupturing. There are some reports of successful treatment with ketoconazole and itraconazole. The dose for both is 400 mg daily with treatment continuing for a few to many years. A good clinical response has been seen in some patients with ketoconazole, itraconazole, voriconazole, and terbinafine.
Lobomycosis	Wide surgical excision of the affected area. Relapse is common. Electrodessication is useful in early stages of the disease. Clofazimine at 300 mg/d has been used with good results in some patients. Antifungal drugs such as ketoconazole, itraconazole, amphotericin B, and 5-fluorocytosine are generally ineffective, although there is one report of successful treatment with itraconazole.

Modified from Lupi et al.*(4)*

given as long-term continuous or pulse therapy. In one large study, the cure rate was 42% with a mean treatment period of 7.2 months *(2)*. In contrast, a large clinical study with terbinafine had a cure rate of 74.2% after 12 months therapy *(10)*. Overall cure rates for both drugs range from 40% to 70% *(3)*. These two drugs can be used alone to treat small to medium-sized lesions, or they can be combined with localized heat and cryosurgery in one to several sessions. Combined antifungal drug therapy with itraconazole and terbinafine may be a useful approach to consider.

Superficial forms of chromoblastomycosis tend to respond well to antifungal drugs, whereas verrucous or tumorlike forms often do not respond well. These patients often require both chemotherapy and thermotherapy. Because of the high possibility of secondary bacterial infections, prophylactic antibacterial therapy is often given. If surgery is to be used, it is recommended that antifungal agents be given systematically both before the procedure and afterwards.

7.2. *Mycetoma*

It is important to distinguish mycetoma caused by aerobic actinomycetes from cases caused by fungi because their treatment is different. An actinomycetoma is amenable to therapy with antibacterial agents. A fungal mycetoma is more difficult to manage and may require aggressive surgery up to and including amputation in advanced disease. Surgical management may be appropriate after antifungal agents have been used. A good clinical response has been seen in some patients treated with ketoconazole, itraconazole, voriconazole, and terbinafine.

The Mycetoma Research Center (Khartoum, Sudan; www.mycetoma.org) recommends both ketoconazole and itraconazole for first line use. Treatment duration depends upon the severity of the infection and the general health status of the patient. Therapy may be needed for extended periods (years). Itraconazole treatment has been shown to have a high degree of success with a low recurrence rate. Surgery is used to completely excise small, well-encapsulated lesions, or to reduce of the amount of infected tissue. Effective surgery may require aggressive excision, which may lead to permanent disability. Surgery without effective chemotherapeutic treatment has a high rate of recurrence; up to 90% in advanced cases. Surgery is the treatment of choice for early cases, typically well-encapsulated lesions without bone involvement.

7.3. *Lobomycosis*

Lobomycosis is an infection that involves the dermis and subcutaneous tissue that is frequently managed with surgical excision (with wide margins). Surgical excision is curative in most instances *(4)*. Itraconazole may have value in treating this mycosis, but the use of this antifungal agent has been reported in only one patient.

REFERENCES

1. Pang KR, Wu JJ, Huang DB, Tyring SK. Subcutaneous fungal infections. Dermatol Ther 2004;17:523–531.
2. Queiroz-Telles F, McGinnis MR, Salkin I, Graybill JR. Subcutaneous mycoses. Infect Dis Clin North Am 2003;17:59–85.
3. Bonifaz A, Saul A, Paredes-Solis V, Araiza J, Fierro-Arias L. Treatment of chromoblastomycosis with terbinafine: experience with four cases. J Dermatol Treat 2005;16:47–51.

4. Lupi O, Tyring SK, McGinnis MR. Tropical dermatology: fungal tropical diseases. J Am Acad Dermatol 2005;53:931–951.
5. Surash S, Tyagi A, De Hoog GS, Zeng JS, Barton RC, Hobson RP. Cerebral phaeohyphomycosis caused by *Fonsecaea monophora*. Med Mycol 2005;43:465–472.
6. de Hoog GS, Adelmann D, Ahmed AO, van Belkum A. Phylogeny and typification of *Madurella mycetomatis*, with a comparison of other agents of eumycetoma. Mycoses 2004;47:121–130.
7. McGinnis MR. Chromoblastomycosis and phaeohyphomycosis: new concepts, diagnosis, and mycology. J Am Acad Dermatol 1983;8:1–16.
8. McGinnis MR. Mycetoma. Dermatol Clin 1996; 14:97–104.
9. Haubold EM, Cooper CR, Wen JW, McGinnis MR, Cowan DF. Comparative morphology of *Lacazia loboi* (syn. *Loboa loboi*) in dolphins and humans. Med Mycol 2000;38:9–14.
10. Esterre P, Inzan CK, Ramarcel ER, et al. Treatment of chromomycosis with terbinafine: preliminary results of an open pilot study. Br J Dermatol 1996;134 (Suppl 46):33–36.

Instructive Cases

INTRODUCTION

The instructive cases that follow are provided to allow the reader a review of many of the important concepts presented in this book. They may also provide the clinician preparing for subspecialty boards practice cases and questions. Each case is presented as an unknown to test knowledge obtained from reading this book or to emphasize an important or complex topic in the field of medical mycology.

INSTRUCTIVE CASE 1

A 57-year-old patient with acute myelogenous leukemia (AML) and a 3-week history of neutropenia develops fever that is unresponsive to broad-spectrum antimicrobial therapy (piperacillin–tazobactam and levofloxacin). High-resolution computed tomography (HRCT) of the lungs revealed several pleural-based nodular lesions. The patient was empirically started on amphotericin B deoxycholate 1 mg/kg every 24 hours. After 5 days of therapy, the patient's serum potassium begins to drop but the serum creatinine and blood urea nitrogen (BUN) remain stable.

Questions

1. The decrease in serum potassium is most likely due to what amphotericin B toxicity?
   A. Afferent arteriole constriction in the kidney
   B. Distal tubular damage in the kidney
   C. Suppression of erythropoietin synthesis
   D. Damage of the pancreatic islet cells
2. Which of the following approaches should be used if the patient's serum creatinine doubles and he begins to develop azotemia?
   A. Change amphotericin B dosing to every other day.
   B. Change amphotericin B to continuous infusion dosing.
   C. Change amphotericin B to a lipid amphotericin B formulation.
   D. Begin administering 500 ml of normal saline before and after infusion.

INSTRUCTIVE CASE 2

While riding his dirt bike on a vacant lot in southeastern Michigan, a 22-year-old man abraded his right leg on the dirt while rounding a corner. He was taken to the emergency room, where the large abrasion was cleaned and débrided. Because there was extensive loss of skin, a skin graft was placed several weeks later. About 2 weeks after the graft was placed, he noted that a few "bumps" had developed in the grafted area. These "bumps" became larger, broke open, and began to discharge what he

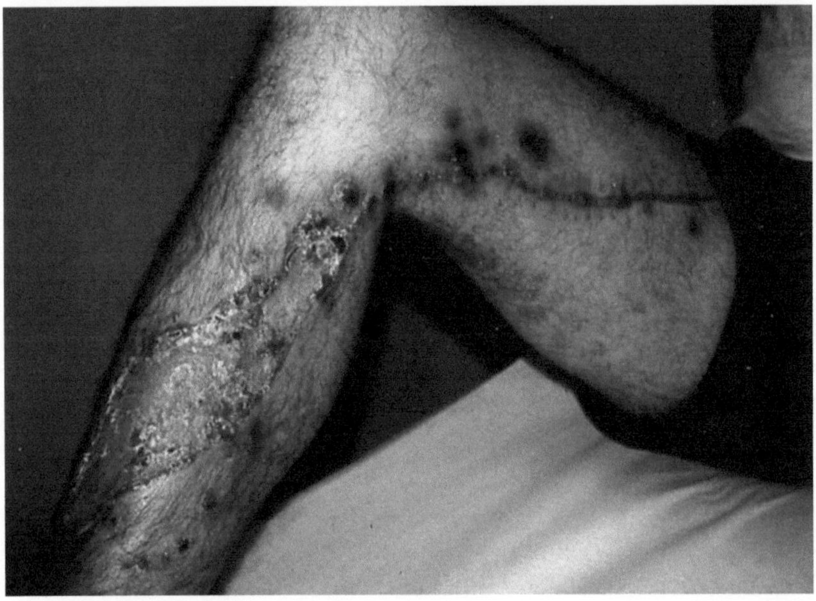

Fig. IC.1. Poor healing and nodular disease about lower extremity scar prior to antifungal therapy (patient later proven to have sporotrichosis). [Figure in color on CD-ROM].

described as a thin fluid with some pink discoloration. Similar lesions then developed in the thigh proximal to the original injury and graft. Several different antimicrobial agents were prescribed (including those with *Staphylococcus aureus* coverage), but the lesions did not respond, and in fact new lesions appeared.

When the patient was seen by an infectious diseases consultant, the graft was beginning to break down and multiple nodules of various sizes were noted in the original abraded area that had been grafted and proximal to the graft into the upper thigh (Fig. IC.1). Some were ulcerated and weeping serosanguinous fluid, and others were crusted. The nodules were not tender to palpation. The patient felt well and specifically denied having chills or fever. Biopsies were taken of several nodules for culture and histopathological examination. The tissue sections showed granulomas, but no organisms were seen. Within 1 week, the cultures held at 25 °C showed growth of an off-white mould that on microscopic examination showed tiny conidia arranged "bouquet-like" on thin hyphae. The diagnosis of sporotrichosis was made and the patient was begun on an experimental protocol using fluconazole, 400 mg daily. The lesions began to resolve by 2 months (Fig. IC.2), and were finally all resolved by 5 months. Therapy was continued for a total of 6 months. No recurrences were noted. The patient was admonished to change hobbies from dirt bike riding to something less dangerous, but he chose to ignore that medical advice.

INSTRUCTIVE CASE 3

A 29-year-old African American man was in his usual state of good health until September, at which time he presented with a nonproductive cough, shortness of breath, back pain, chills, fever, headache, and body aches. Evaluation led to a diagnosis of pneumonia with right hilar and peritracheal adenopathy. He was originally treated

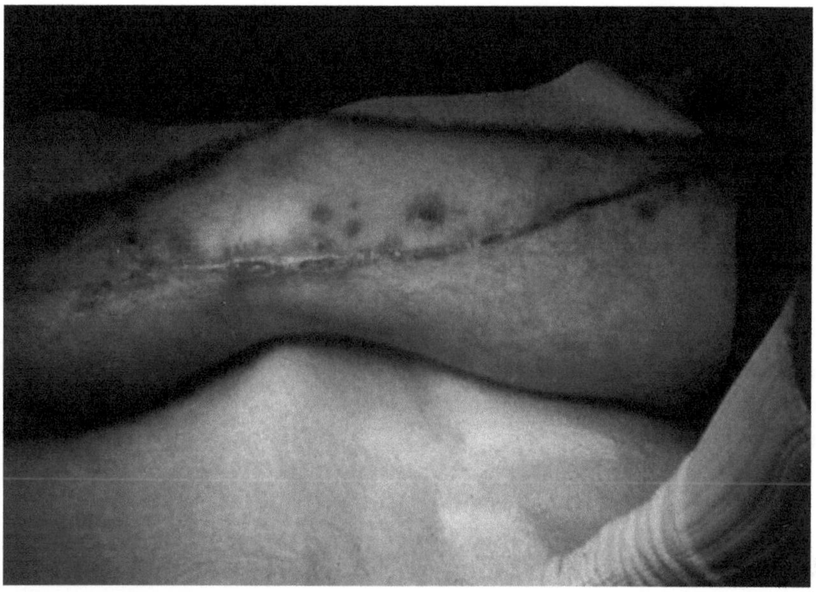

Fig. IC.2. Improvement of sporotrichosis after 2 months of fluconazole therapy. [Figure in color on CD-ROM].

with antimicrobial agents for community-acquired pneumonia without resolution of symptoms. Approximately 2 weeks later, three skin lesions consistent with granulomas were noted. A punch biopsy performed approximately 1 month after his original presentation revealed granulomatous inflammation with endosporulating spherules, thus confirming the diagnosis of cutaneous coccidioidomycosis. Since the patient had complained of intermittent headache, and there was now a diagnosis of pulmonary and cutaneous coccidioidomycosis, it was essential to rule out coccidioidal meningitis. A lumbar puncture was done, which was normal. At this time, the patient was also noted to have subcutaneous nodules in the left preauricular and right submandibular areas as well as over the right humerus and left knee.

The patient was started on oral fluconazole, 800 mg daily. Subsequently the patient developed multiple draining lesions over the anterior chest. A bone scan was positive for disease of multiple ribs and the manubrium as well as the left parietal skull, right frontal skull, right superior orbit, and left hind foot. The positive areas on bone scan were confirmed with plain radiographs, as osteomyelitis. Culture of fluid from the draining sternal lesion grew *Coccidioides immitis.* Given the extensive dissemination to bone and skin in this patient, therapy was intensified to a lipid preparation of amphotericin B at a dose of 5 mg/kg three times per week for approximately 3 months. At the same time, aggressive surgical débridement of the draining thoracic lesions was undertaken, in an attempt to reduce the fungal burden. The patient's original complement fixation titer at presentation was less than 1:2. It subsequently rose to 1:16 and eventually to $\geq$1:512, and stayed at that level despite therapy. The patient continues to have draining lesions of the anterior chest despite repeat surgeries and several courses of amphotericin, and is now being treated with voriconazole 4 mg/kg twice daily. Lifelong therapy is anticipated.

INSTRUCTIVE CASE 4

A-27 year-old male agricultural worker seen in consultation to evaluate an illness of 2 months duration characterized by the presence of rapidly enlarging lymph nodes in both cervical chains, accompanied by pain, and high fever, especially at nights. One of the nodes had drained spontaneously, producing yellow-tinged purulent material. The patient also experienced productive cough without dyspnea. On examination, he was pale, looked frail, and had enlarged cervical, axillary, and inguinal lymph nodes (Fig. IC.3). His spleen and liver were normal by physical examination. Lung auscultation did not reveal altered breath sounds and chest radiographs were normal.

A human immunodeficiency (HIV) test was negative, hemoglobin was 8.8 g/dl, and white blood cell count was 25,700 cells/μl. A direct KOH examination of the discharge from the ruptured nodule showed abundant yeast cells, some with the characteristic multiple budding of *Paracoccidioides brasiliensis;* this fungus was also isolated in culture. Serology with paracoccidioidin proved reactive with one band of precipitate and a complement fixation (CF) titer of 1:1024.

INSTRUCTIVE CASE 5

A 70-year-old man with hypereosinophilic syndrome, non-insulin dependent diabetes mellitus (NIDDM), and long-term prednisone therapy (25 mg/day $\times$ 25 years) was admitted with fatigue, weakness, and shortness of breath. Physician examination was

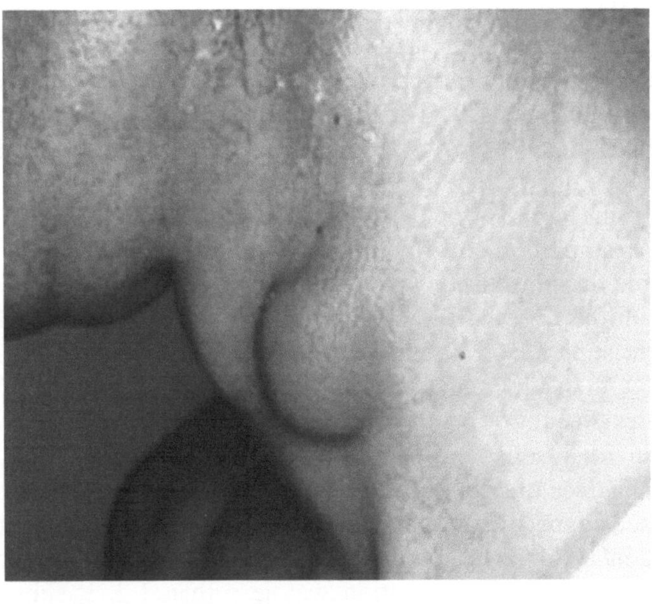

Fig. IC.3. Paracoccidioidomycosis. Hypertrophied cervical lymph node about to rupture. Scarring lesions of a similar process can be seen above. [Figure in color on CD-ROM].

remarkable for a temperature of 99°F, an area of erythema over the left thigh that was tender to palpation and an effusion in the right knee. On admission, he had a hemoglobin of 5.9 g/dl, WBC 8600/mm^3, a serum creatinine 2.7 mg/dl, and a glucose 382 mg/dl. Aspiration of the right knee revealed a WBC of 40,500/mm^3 with 96% neutrophils, Gram stain revealed gram-negative bacilli and budding yeasts. The patient was initially started on imipenem, vancomycin, tobramycin, and fluconazole (FLZ) 400 mg/day.

Within 72 hours, the blood cultures drawn on admission were found to be positive for yeast, later identified as *Trichosporon asahii (beigelii)*. In addition, joint fluid cultures were also positive for*Trichosporon asahii* and *Pseudomonas aeruginosa*. Biopsy and culture of the left thigh area of erythema also grew *P. aeruginosa and T. asahii*.

After 5 days of fluconazole treatment, the blood cultures were still positive and caspofungin (Cancidas) 50 mg IV qd was added to the fluconazole. He also underwent arthroscopic flushing of the right knee. Ten days after admission, the patient had negative blood cultures and had responded well to antimicrobial therapy. He was subsequently transferred to a rehabilitation unit in good condition.

In vitro susceptibilities (MICs) of *T. asahii* revealed fluconazole 8 μg/mg, itraconazole 0.5 μg/ml, and caspofungin 2 μg/ml.

INSTRUCTIVE CASE 6

A 42-year-old black man presented to the University Hospital emergency department with a 1-week history of fever, chills, cough productive of white sputum, night sweats, and malaise. He denied hemoptysis. Risk factors for HIV infection included a blood transfusion in 1985 and heterosexual promiscuity. He denied intravenous drug abuse or homosexual activity. Over the last 8 months he had lost 80 pounds. Past medical history was significant for a prior appendectomy, a perirectal abscess that was surgically drained, and a chronic perirectal fistula for 5 years. There was also a history of venereal disease including primary syphilis associated with a chancre and a positive rapid plasma reagin (RPR) of 1:32. There was no documented therapy and the patient was lost to follow-up.

On admission, the patient was afebrile but cachectic. He was in no acute respiratory distress. On physical examination, he was noted to have dry crusting lesions on the tip of his nose and both cheeks of the face (Fig. IC.4). Similar lesions were noted over the shins and a small draining abscess was noted over the medial aspect of the left foot. Oral hairy leukoplakia was present on the tongue and he was noted to have prominent generalized lymphadenopathy. No rales, rhonchi, or wheezes were heard on auscultation of chest. A fistula-in-ano was also noted. Chest radiograph revealed bilateral reticulonodular infiltrates, which were more prominent in the upper lobes. The patient was lymphopenic with an absolute lymphocyte count of 410 cells/μl. The serum RPR of 1:32 was positive. Skin scrapings of the lesions were performed and wet preparations of the specimens revealed characteristic thick-walled multinucleated yeast forms compatible with *Blastomyces dermatitidis* (Fig. IC.5). Subsequently, the patient underwent bronchoscopy with bronchoalveolar lavage (BAL), and cytology preparations of the washings also revealed *B. dermatitidis*. Cultures of skin scrapings and BAL washings grew this organism. An enzyme-linked immunoassay (ELISA) and Western

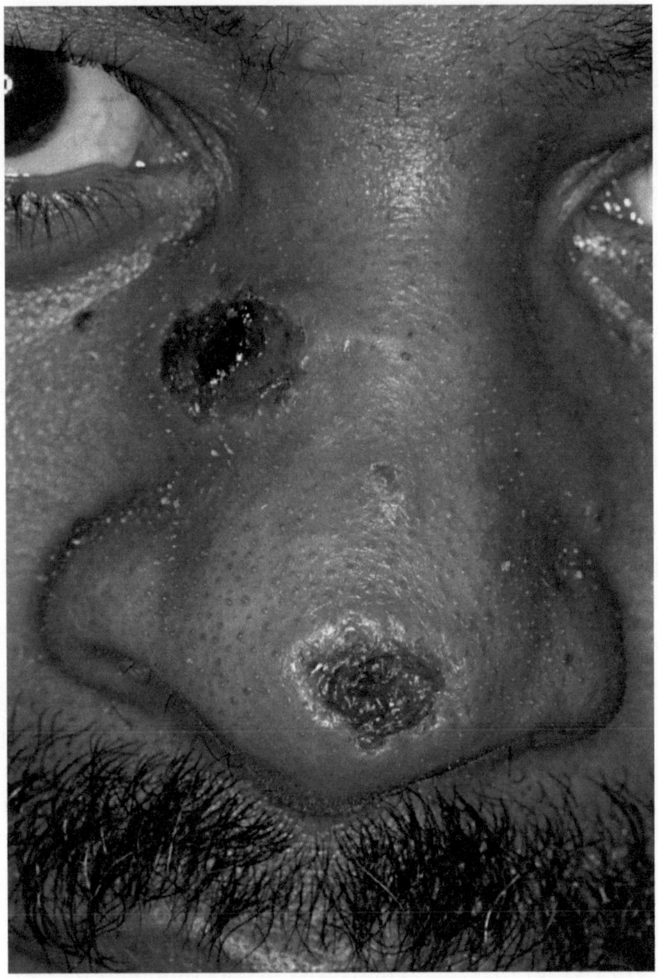

Fig. IC.4. Multiple cutaneous lesions in a patient with end-stage AIDS. Similar lesions were noted on both cheeks of the face and both shins. [Figure in color on CD-ROM].

Blot confirmed HIV infection and total $CD4^{+}$ T lymphocyte count was 8 cells/μl. A computed tomography (CT) scan of the head was performed because of complaints of headache. This study revealed multiple enhancing brain lesions (Fig. IC.6). Owing to concerns of a second opportunistic pathogen, i.e., *Toxoplasma gondii*, the brain lesions were aspirated. Wet preparations again revealed characteristic yeast forms of *B. dermatitidis*.

The patient was begun on highly active antiretroviral therapy (HAART) and amphotericin B deoxycholate therapy at an initial dose of 1 mg/kg per day. Intravenous penicillin, 18 million units per day in divided doses, was administered for 21 days because of concerns of neurosyphilis. During the remainder of the hospitalization, the patient was carefully monitored for evidence of renal insufficiency and 500 ml of normal saline were infused prior to each amphotericin B infusion. During this

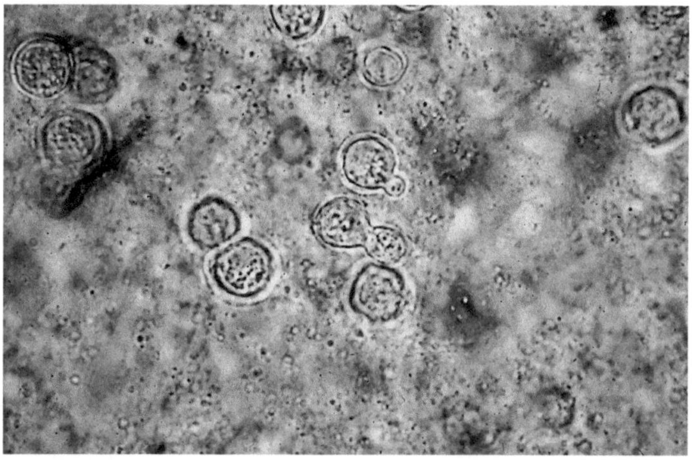

Fig. IC.5. Wet preparation of skin scrapings. This figure shows the characteristic yeast forms in a wet preparation of skin scrapings. Scraping of the edges of the verrucous and ulcerative lesions yield the best diagnostic results. [Figure in color on CD-ROM].

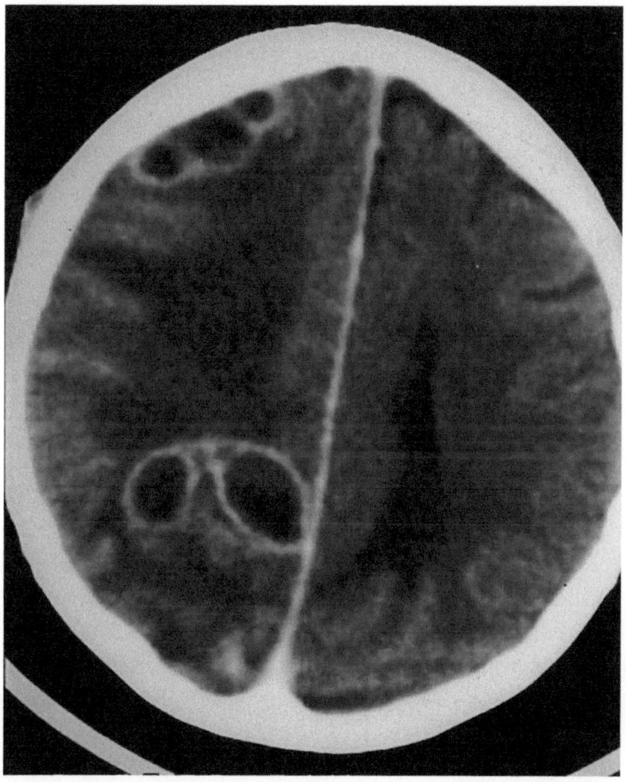

Fig. IC.6. CNS blastomycosis in an AIDS patient. Diagnosis may require aspiration of the abscesses if no active pulmonary or cutaneous disease is present.

hospitalization, he received a total of 1600 milligrams of amphotericin B. Serial CT scans documented progressive improvement of brain abscesses and oral fluconazole was substituted after the full course of amphotericin B and the patient was discharged to home. He completed 8 more weeks of fluconazole therapy at a dose of 800 mg/day. Although the brain abscesses had resolved on CT scan, a maintenance suppressive dose of fluconazole of 400 mg per day was initiated. HAART was continued and a clinical response was documented by a falling HIV viral load and rising $CD4^+$ T lymphocyte count.

INSTRUCTIVE CASE 7

A 45-year-old construction worker presented with a 3-week history of fever, chills, myalgias, headache, and dyspnea. Examination was unremarkable and laboratory tests revealed a white blood cell count of 3300 cells/μl and a platelet count of 94,000 cells/μl. Aspartate transaminase (AST) was 87 units/l, alkaline phosphatase 337 units/l. Angiotensin converting enzyme was elevated at 213 units/l. Chest and abdomen CT showed small nodules in the lungs, enlarged mediastinal lymph nodes, small pleural effusions, and splenomegaly. Transbronchial biopsies of the subcarinal lymph node and right lower lobe and bone marrow biopsy showed noncaseating granuloma. Histopathology was negative for fungi and cultures were negative after 1 week of incubation. Prednisone 60 mg daily was prescribed for presumed sarcoidosis, which resulted in resolution of fever and improvement of dyspnea. The prednisone dosage was tapered over 4 weeks to 10 mg daily, which was maintained.

Two months later the patient complained of recurrent fever, 10-pound weight loss, and worsening dyspnea. Chest CT showed more extensive diffuse interstitial infiltrates and increasing splenomegaly. Hemoglobin was 9.3 g/dl, white blood cell count 2500 cells/μl, and a platelet count of 89,000 cells/μl. Alkaline phosphatase was 987 units/l. Cultures from the lung tissue, lymph nodes, and bone marrow performed during the earlier admission were negative after 4 weeks of incubation. Bronchoscopy was performed and cytology revealed small yeastlike structures resembling *Histoplasma capsulatum*, which was later confirmed by culture. Treatment was started with amphotericin B, and the patient noted progressive improvement.

INSTRUCTIVE CASE 8

A 52-year-old man who underwent renal transplantation 2 years earlier presented with a slightly painful mass above his right knee. This mass began as a small lesion 4 weeks ago and has been slowly enlarging since first noted by the patient. He denies fever, chills, night sweats, or trauma to the area. He is taking tacrolimus and prednisone as his immunosuppressive regimen. The patient was afebrile with stable vital signs, but his physical examination was significant for a 1.5 cm firm nodule above his right knee, which was slightly tender, but without erythema or drainage. Routine laboratory studies are unremarkable.

Surgery was consulted for excision of the nodule, which was performed without complications. Pathology showed chronic inflammation and pigmented fungal elements suggestive of phaeohyphomycosis; margins were clear of infection (Fig. IC.7). Culture of the specimen grew *Exophiala jeanselmei*. He was given itraconazole for 3 months, and no further lesions appeared.

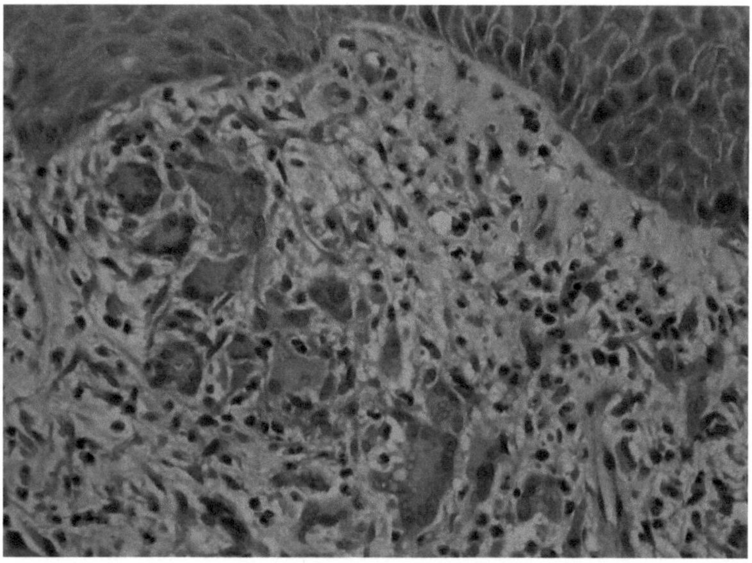

Fig. IC.7. Histopathological examination of subcutaneous nodule showing granulomatous changes and dark-walled fungal elements. Phaeohyphomycosis. [Figure in color on CD-ROM].

INSTRUCTIVE CASE 9

A 34-year-old African American man, who has been followed for approximately 10 years, originally presented with back pain and tenderness over the right sternoclavicular joint. Coccidioidomycosis was suspected and a serology was obtained with an initial complement fixation (CF) titer of 1:256. A whole body bone scan showed focal areas of increased uptake involving the left frontal bone, the right sternoclavicular joint, the left sacroiliac joint, and the cervicothoracic region. These findings were confirmed with plain radiograph and CT scans.

Approximately 1 month after original presentation, an incision and drainage of the proximal clavicle and the posterior superior spine of the iliac crest was performed. Cultures were positive for *Coccidioides immitis*. Three months after presentation, a cervical corpectomy of C5 and C6 with autograft fusion and anterior cervical plating was performed. Five months after presentation, decompression of the spinal cord with corpectomy at T3 and T4 with autologous rib grafting was performed.

Medical therapy initially consisted of amphotericin B, which was infused over a period of approximately 4 months, three times per week. Follow-up therapy with high-dose oral fluconazole (1000 mg daily as a single dose) was administered. As the patient improved clinically, CF titers steadily came down, and the dose was deescalated to 400 mg of fluconazole daily. With approximately 10 years of follow-up, no further evidence of disease has been discerned. Complement fixation titers in the recent past have remained positive at 1:2. It has been recommended that he remain on therapy for life.

INSTRUCTIVE CASE 10

A 68-year-old man with a long standing history of hairy cell leukemia was admitted to receive treatment with the experimental immunotoxin BL-22. He had been pancytopenic for several months and had been receiving antifungal prophylaxis with itraconazole. On admission, antifungal prophylaxis was changed to fluconazole. On day 2 the patient developed fever. At that time, his absolute neutrophil count was 76 cells/μl. Blood cultures recovered a highly susceptible *E. coli* and the patient defervesced promptly on ceftazidime. On day 7 a new fever developed and meropenem, tobramycin, and caspofungin were started. A chest CT was obtained which showed a 3 cm right upper lobe (RUL) nodule (Fig. IC.8). A bronchoalveolar lavage (BAL) was performed, and voriconazole and levofloxacin were added. Bacterial, fungal, and viral cultures, as well as Gram, calcofluor white, acid-fast, modified-acid-fast, and Gomori methenamine silver (GMS) stains were negative. Polymerase chain reaction (PCR) for *Pneumocystis*, *Chlamydophila*, *Mycoplasma*, and *Legionella* was also negative. The patient continued to have fever up to 40°C without new symptoms or hypotension. On day 11 he complained of chest pain and dry cough. A repeat CT showed marked enlargement of the nodule with development of a halo sign and abutting of the fissure (Fig. IC.9). A fine-needle aspirate of the mass showed broad, ribbonlike, nonseptate hyphae (Fig. IC-10). Voriconazole was discontinued and liposomal amphotericin B 7.5 mg/kg per day was started. The patient developed hemoptysis and a repeat CT showed further progression of the mass, but with apparent localization in the RUL

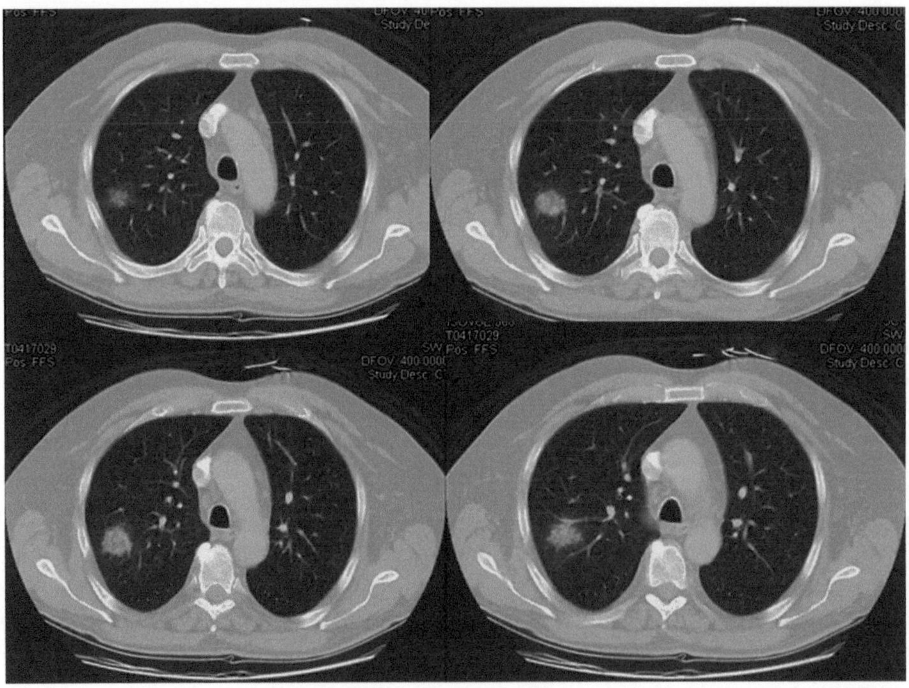

Fig. IC.8. CT scan of chest revealing small pulmonary nodule in the right upper lung.

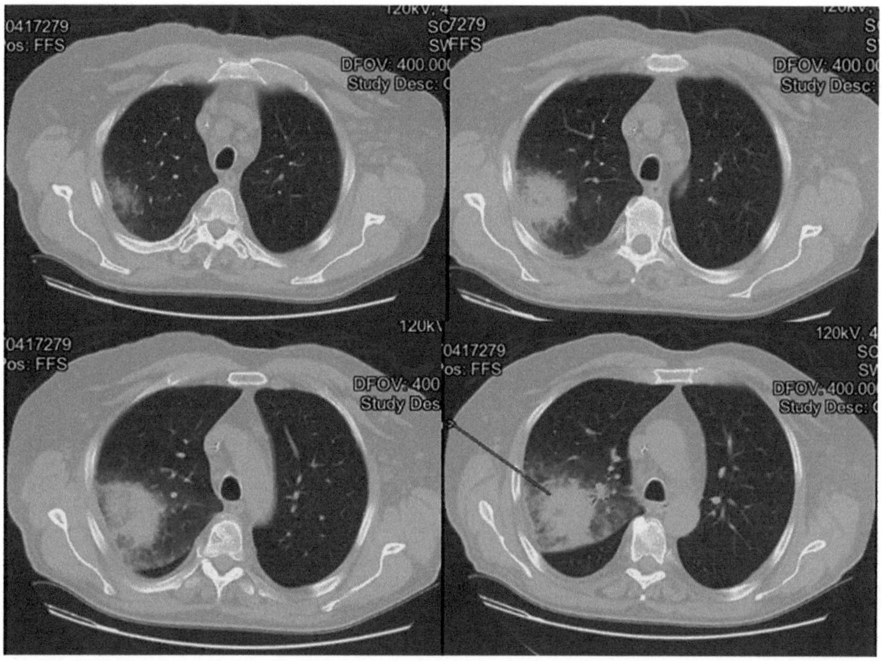

Fig. IC.9. CT scan of chest revealing progression of pulmonary nodule in right upper lung field to involve the right pleural surface.

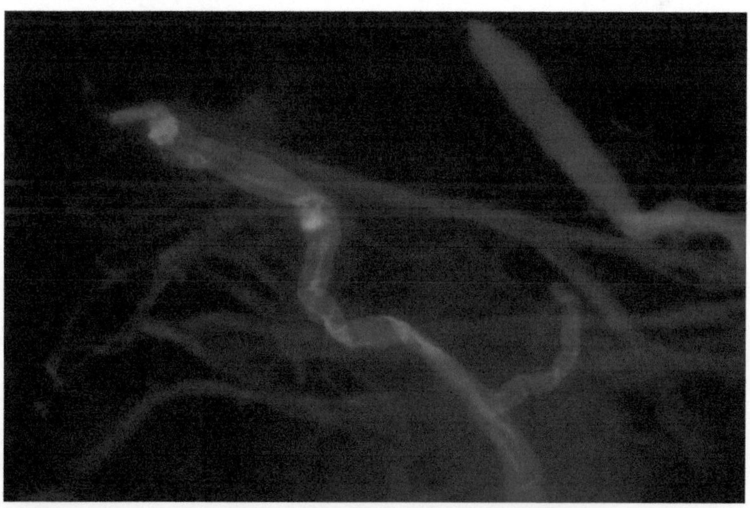

Fig. IC.10. Calcofluor staining of fine-needle aspiration demonstrates broad nonseptate hyphae consistent with zygomycosis. [Figure in color on CD-ROM].

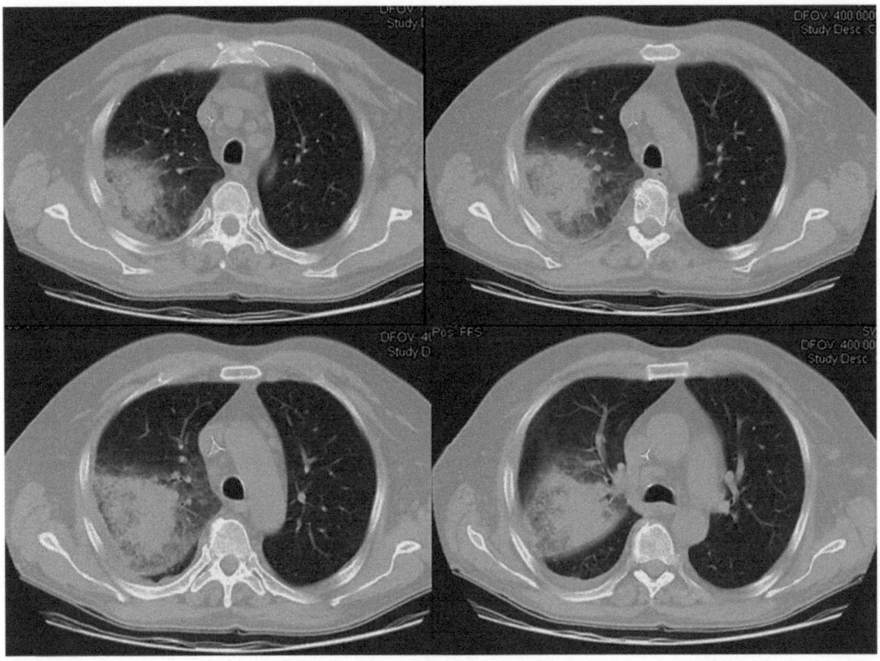

Fig. IC.11. CT scan of chest with severe advancement of locally progressive disease in the right upper lung fields.

(Fig. IC.11). An emergent right upper lobectomy was performed on day 18 (Fig. IC.12). An angioinvasive mould was readily seen on the GMS stain (Fig. IC.13), and was later identified as *Rhizomucor pusillus*. On the day of the surgery, granulocyte transfusions were initiated. Hemoptysis and fever resolved 2 days after the surgery. Despite local control of the fungal disease, the patient never recovered his white blood cell counts and over the next 6 weeks developed several complications in the ICU, including herpes simplex pneumonia. At his own request, care was withdrawn.

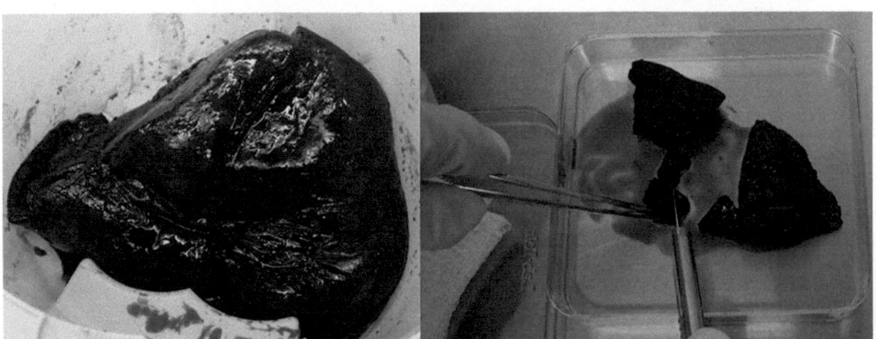

Fig. IC.12. Gross pathology of right upper lobectomy. [Figure in color on CD-ROM].

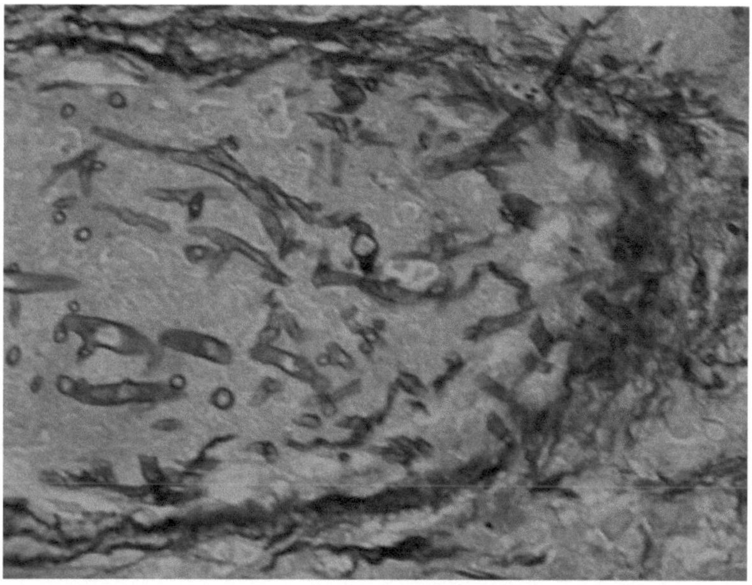

Fig. IC.13. Zygomycosis with hyphae invading blood vessel, infiltrating vascular wall, and causing subsequent thrombosis. GMS. [Figure in color on CD-ROM].

INSTRUCTIVE CASE 11

A 48-year-old male rural worker was referred for consultation to evaluate the presence of painful, ulcerated lesions in the external region of his right foot (Fig. IC.14). This process had gone on for 18 months, and multiple local and systemic treatments had been given without success. The patient looked well and had no other symptoms. Physical examination also revealed the presence of an oral mucosal ulceration and of hypertrophied cervical lymph nodes. Lung auscultation found fine rales and the chest radiograph showed interstitial infiltrates in the central fields with fibrous zones and basal bullae (Fig. IC.15).

Direct KOH examination of ulcer exudate revealed multiple budding yeasts consistent with *Paracoccidioides brasiliensis*; cultures later grew the fungus. The patient's serum gave a band of precipitate and a CF titer of 1:32 with paracoccidioidin.

INSTRUCTIVE CASE 12

A 40-year-female with acute myelogenous leukemia now 115 days following matched allogeneic donor hematopoietic stem cell transplantation complicated by a suspected *Aspergillus* pneumonia presents to the clinic with increasing complaints of nausea, stomach cramping, and rash on the hands spreading up her arms. By laboratory examination, she is noted to have an alanine transaminase (ALT) of 85 units/l, AST 75 units/l, and total bilirubin of 2.1 mg/dl. Her current medications include tacrolimus 5 mg twice daily (recent level 8 ng/ml), voriconazole 200 mg twice daily, levofloxacin 500 mg daily, valacyclovir 500 mg twice daily, metoprolol 25 mg twice daily and benzonatate (tesselon) pearls. She is

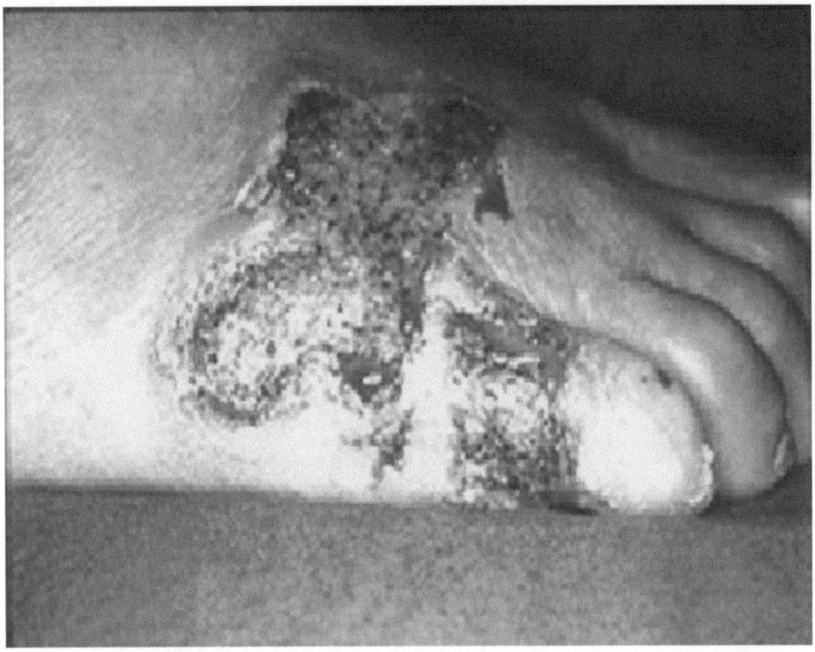

Fig. IC.14. Paracoccidioidomycosis. Multiple ulcerated lesions in the right foot with crusting, exudation, and hemorrhagic dots. The borders are granulomatous and show some scarring. [Figure in color on CD-ROM].

admitted to the hospital for suspected graft versus host disease exacerbation. The primary service wishes to continue voriconazole therapy as this patient has a history of poorly tolerating lipid amphotericin B formulations, but they are concerned about the possibility of drug-induced hepatitis caused by voriconazole.

Questions

1. Which of the following approaches should be recommended to the primary team to manage the suspected drug-induced hepatotoxicity?
   A. Discontinue voriconazole and switch to itraconazole.
   B. Discontinue voriconazole and switch to lipid amphotericin B with premedications.
   C. Continue voriconazole and lower dose by 50%.
   D. Continue voriconazole and closely monitor the patient.

INSTRUCTIVE CASE 13

A 44-year-old male field worker was in his usual state of health until 2 weeks prior to admission, when he developed headache, low-grade fever, nausea, and vomiting. His family noted decreased mentation and brought him to the emergency room. Initial examination revealed a disheveled gentleman with lethargy and disorientation. A CT scan of the head was performed without contrast and was normal. A lumbar puncture revealed 450 white cells/μl, of which 76% were lymphocytes, 10% monocytes, 10% neutrophils, and 4% eosinophils. The protein was 176 mg/dl and the glucose was 27

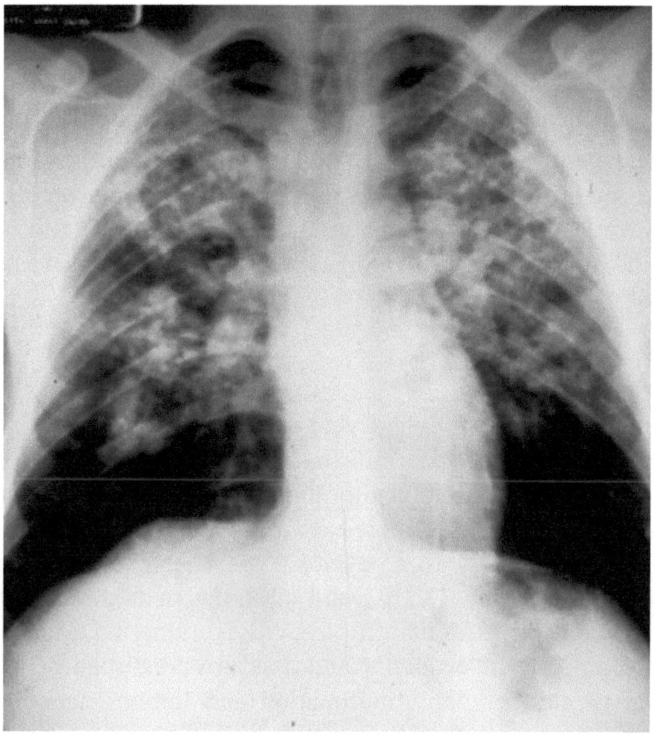

Fig. IC.15. Paracoccidioidomycosis. Bilateral interstitial infiltrates in central fields, basal bullae, and fibrous areas. The apices appear free of disease.

mg/dl. Studies were sent to rule out cryptococcosis, tuberculosis, and coccidioidomycosis. Coccidioidal antibody in the serum was 1:256 and in the cerebrospinal fluid (CSF) was 1:2. Other fungal and mycobacterial laboratory evalutions were negative. Magnetic resonance imaging (MRI) of the brain was done to evaluate for meningeal involvement or vasculitic complications of coccidioidomycosis. This study revealed basilar cisternal enhancement. A bone scan was ordered and was negative for bony involvement. An HIV test was performed and confirmed as positive. The HIV RNA PCR was 330,000 copies/ml with an absolute $CD4^+$ T lymphocyte count of 61 cells/μl. The patient was placed on high-dose oral fluconazole (1000 mg daily as a single dose). Highly active antiretroviral therapy (HAART) was also initiated and patient was discharged to be followed in clinic. Patient and family were counseled regarding strict adherence to fluconazole and HAART therapy, both of which needed to be life-long.

He also underwent lumbar punctures monthly, CSF was sent for cell count, glucose, protein, complement fixation (CF) titers, and fungal culture. Serum for fluconazole level was sent when the possibility of noncompliance was considered. The patient followed up with appointments inconsistently. Four months after admission, he was brought to the Emergency Room with confusion, lethargy, nausea, vomiting, and ataxic gait. Evaluation again showed encephalopathy. CT scan now demonstrated ventriculomegaly. Lumbar puncture revealed an elevated opening pressure of 250 mmH_2O, white cell count 50 cells/μl (85% lymphocytes, 11% neutrophils), protein 153 mg/dl, and glucose of 10 mg/dl. HAART therapy and high dose fluconazole were reinitiated. Neurosurgical consultation was obtained and the patient was taken to the operating room for ventriculoperitoneal shunting. The patient's symptoms improved significantly after shunting, but his clinical course was complicated by hyponatremia secondary to syndrome of inappropriate antidiuretic hormone secretion (SIADH), which was managed with fluid restriction. He gradually improved and was discharged with close follow-up at clinic.

INSTRUCTIVE CASE 14

A 22-year-old female with a failing 4-year-old renal allograft received several doses of OKT3 and high doses of corticosteroids in an attempt to reverse the acute rejection of the transplanted kidney. Three months after this increased immunosuppressive trial and still receiving her normal immunosuppressive regimen of tacrolimus, mycophenolate, and prednisone, she presented with a several week course of headaches, nausea, and vomiting. Her temperature was 37.2°C, and although mental status was normal, she had bilateral clonus and papilledema on physical examination. Her laboratory results showed a normal complete blood count and a serum creatinine of 4 mg/dl. An MRI of her brain demonstrated basilar inflammation and lumbar puncture (LP) revealed a white blood cell count of 100 cells/μl with 80% lymphocytes. CSF glucose was 43 mg/dl and protein 79 mg/dl. India ink was positive for encapsulated yeasts, CSF cryptococcal polysaccharide antigen test was $\geqslant$1:256, and culture grew *Cryptococcus neoformans*. Her opening pressure was 400 mm H_2O. She was started on 5 mg/kg per day of AmBisome for 20 days and flucytosine at 25 mg/kg per day for 14 days, and then placed on 200 mg/day of fluconazole. The patient's symptoms did not worsen and she was reevaluated at 2 weeks with a repeat LP. That LP found an opening pressure of 140 mm H_2O, and India ink and culture were negative. CSF antigen was 1:256 and CSF white cell count was 28 cells/μl.

Case Continued

Patient did relatively well on her suppressive fluconazole therapy at 200 mg/day for 4 months (dosed for reduced renal function), when she developed severe headaches and an MRI scan showed diffuse supra- and infratentorial leptomeningeal enhancement. At that time CSF cryptococcal polysaccharide antigen was 1:16, white blood cell count was 100 cells/μl, and cultures negative. After 2 weeks of AmBisome at 5 mg/kg per day and no improvement, the patient was continued on fluconazole and a 6 week dexamethasone taper was begun with immediate improvement in symptoms. Tacrolimus and mycophenolate were stopped and the patient was started on dialysis. One week after stopping the 6-week taper of corticosteroids, her headaches returned and a 4-month steroid taper was begun. She improved and was eventually weaned off corticosteroids and now has received suppressive fluconazole for 1 to 2 years and is doing well awaiting a new transplant.

INSTRUCTIVE CASE 15

A 47-year-old black man presented to the University Hospital emergency department complaining of pleuritic chest pain for 2 weeks before admission. He subsequently developed severe dyspnea on exertion, fever and chills, and productive cough with hemoptysis. Over the 24 hours preceding admission, pleuritic chest pain, which was initially only on the left side, became bilateral and he presented to the Emergency Department for evaluation. Past medical history was pertinent for hyperthyroidism and cigarette smoking. He denied any risk factors for HIV infection.

In the emergency department, he was in moderate respiratory distress but was afebrile. Chest radiograph revealed diffuse bilateral miliary infiltrates with a masslike lesion in the lung field. White blood count was 14,400 cells/μl with a left shift. Arterial blood gases on room air revealed a pH of 7.41, po_2 of 33 mm Hg, and pco_2 of 46 mm Hg.

The patient was admitted to the hospital and placed in respiratory isolation. Differential diagnosis included severe community-acquired pneumonia, atypical pneumonia, miliary tuberculosis, and fungal disease. He was placed on supplemental oxygen, intravenous azithromycin and ceftriaxone, and a four-drug antituberculous treatment regimen. Multiple sputum samples were remarkable only for many polymorphonuclear leukocytes. Direct fluorescent antibody (DFA) and urinary antigen tests were negative for *Legionella*. Likewise, fungal and acid-fast stains of sputum samples were negative. An ELISA for HIV was also negative.

On hospital day 3 the patient became febrile, a chest radiograph revealed worsening bilateral pulmonary infiltrates, and intravenous trimethoprim–sulfamethoxazole was added to the existing antibacterial regimen as empiric therapy for possible *Pneumocystis* pneumonia. On the fifth hospital day he complained of increasing dyspnea and was noted as having a respiratory rate of 60 breaths per minute. Arterial blood gases on 100% oxygen by face mask revealed a pH of 7.45, po_2 of 102 mm Hg, and pco_2 of 42 mm Hg. The patient was transferred to intensive care unit, where he was intubated and placed on mechanical ventilation. Chest radiographs revealed bilateral pulmonary infiltrates (Fig. IC.16) with acute lung injury. Cytology samples obtained via the endotracheal tube at the time of intubation revealed numerous broad-based budding yeast forms compatible with *Blastomyces* species (Fig. IC.17).

The patient received intravenous amphotericin B immediately at a dose of 0.7 mg/kg per day, but was rapidly increased to 1 mg/kg per day. During the remainder of his hospitalization, the patient became increasingly difficult to oxygenate, developed hypotension requiring pressers, progressed to multiorgan failure, and died with pulseless electrical activity.

INSTRUCTIVE CASE 16

An 18-year-old female presented with chest discomfort. Dilated veins were noted over the chest and upper abdomen. A chest radiograph that showed right hilar enlargement, which was calcified on CT. The right pulmonary artery was narrowed and the superior vena cava was occluded. Ventilation–perfusion lung scan that showed reduced blood flow to the right lung. Pulmonary function tests showed normal air flow and lung capacity. Tuberculin skin test was negative. Histoplasma immunodiffusion

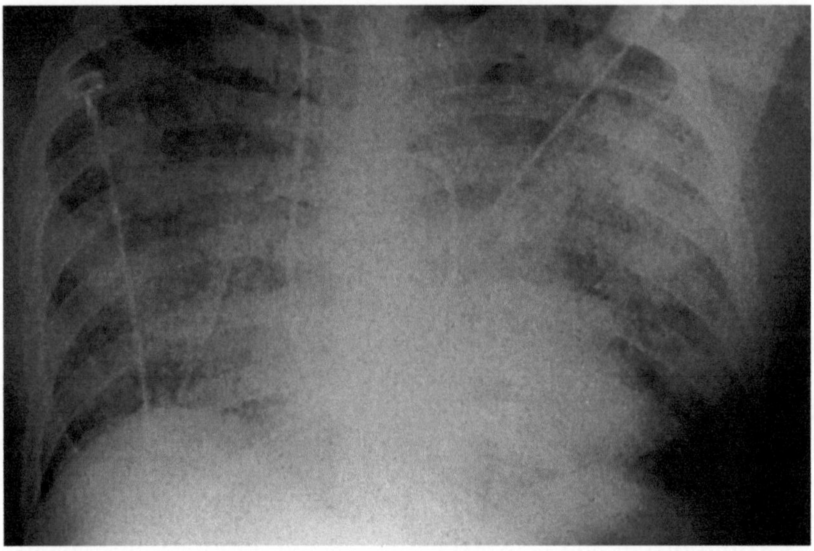

Fig. IC.16. Diffuse pulmonary infiltrates in a patient with ARDS. Patients presenting with this syndrome have a mortality rate greater than 50%.

tests showed an M band and the Histoplasma complement fixation test showed titers of 1:32 to the yeast and 1:16 to the mycelial antigen. Mediastinal biopsy showed chronic inflammatory cells, granuloma, and fibrosis. Culture of the mediastinal biopsy tissue was negative for fungus.

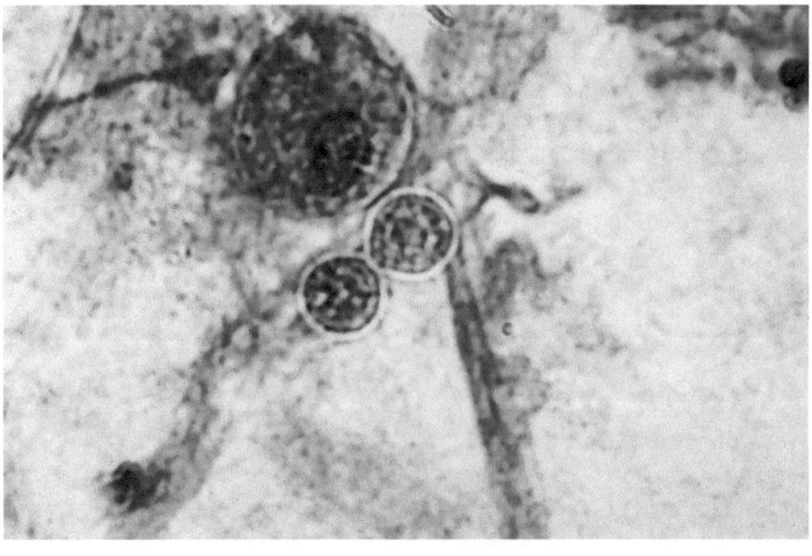

Fig. IC.17. Cytology preparation of endotracheal tube specimen revealing large, thick-walled yeasts consistent with *Blastomyces dermatitidis*. [Figure in color on CD-ROM].

Question

Is surgery indicated to correct the obstruction of the pulmonary artery or of the superior vena cava, and should the patient receive a course of antifungal therapy?

INSTRUCTIVE CASE 17

A 41-year-old male rural worker and heavy smoker consulted because of 3 months of dry cough, severe progressive dyspnea, weight loss, asthenia, adynamia, and anorexia. He looked emaciated and experienced difficulties in breathing even at rest. Respiratory rate was noted to be 36 breaths per minute with accessory muscles utilization. On auscultation rales, rhonchi and hypoventilation were noticed. The chest radiograph (Fig. IC.18) revealed the presence of a diffuse reticulonodular infiltrates predominating in both central fields with fibrous lines. Follow-up CT of chest documented widespread fibrosis (Fig. IC.19). Arterial blood gas analysis revealed pH 7.44, po_2 37 mm Hg, pco_2 23 mm Hg, O_2 saturation 81%, and bicarbonate 16 mEq/l.

A bronchoalveolar lavage fluid sample was examined for acid-fast bacilli with negative results, but multiple budding cells corresponding to*Paracoccidioides brasiliensis* were seen on direct examination and recovered in culture later on. Serologic tests with paracoccidioidin were reactive with one band of precipitate and a titer of 1:1024 in the complement fixation (CF) test.

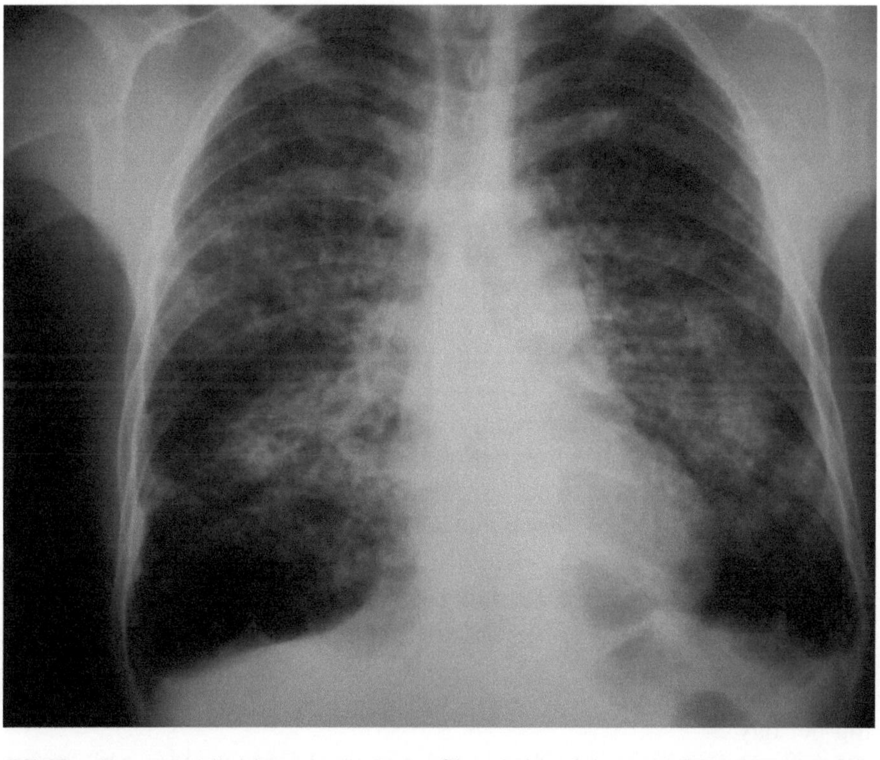

Fig. IC.18. Paracoccidioidomycosis. Lung fibrosis involving specially the central field with apices appearing free. Bilateral basal bullae and pleural adhesions are seen in both lower fields.

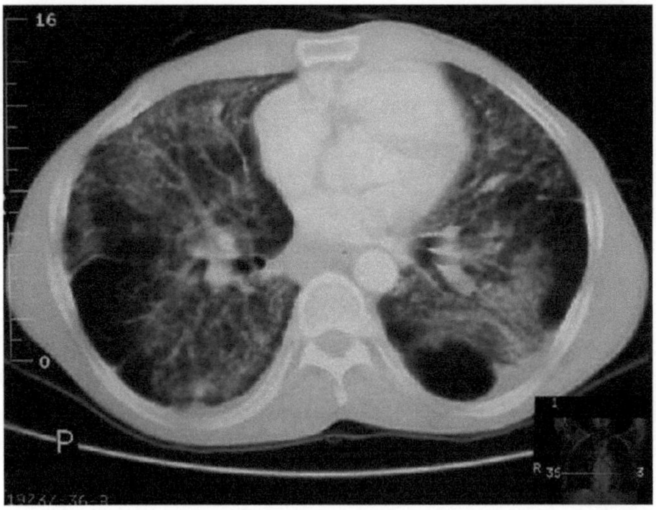

Fig. IC.19. Par acoccidioidomycosis. High-resolution CT showing widespread fibrosis with honeybee aspect, bullae formation. and pleural thickening in both lower lung fields.

INSTRUCTIVE CASE 18

A 51-year-old man was newly assigned to a construction project in Kern County. Two weeks after he began his assignment, he developed cough, shortness of breath, fever, chills, and night sweats. His physician obtained a chest radiograph, which showed consolidation in the anterior left upper lobe and lingula, associated with adenopathy of the lateral aortic, left hilar, and pericarinal nodes. He was diagnosed with community-acquired pneumonia and prescribed antibiotics. One week later, he had not improved and went to the local emergency room, where he was found to be febrile but not hypoxic. His white blood count was 9400 cells/μl, with an absolute eosinophil count of 959 cells/μl. He was prescribed oral levofloxacin 750 mg daily and discharged to home. Serum for *Coccidioides* serology was collected at this visit and reported 5 days later: EIA IgM positive; immunodiffusion (ID) IgG negative, ID IgM positive; and CF titer (IgG) $\leqslant$ 1:2. These results were suggestive of early disease, but were not communicated to the patient and possibly misinterpreted as negative.

Almost 3 weeks after initial presentation, the patient developed increasing shortness of breath, became hypoxic, somewhat confused, with high fevers, and drenching sweats. He presented to our emergency room. His subsequent *Coccidioides* CF titer was 1:64. Since he was hypoxic with a po_2 of less than 70 mm Hg, he was started on a lipid amphotericin preparation at 5 mg/kg daily as well as oral prednisone at a dose of 40 mg twice daily for 5 days, followed by 40 mg once daily for 5 days, then 20 mg once daily for 11 days. He improved and was discharged home with continuation of amphotericin for 6 weeks, three times per week, and then switched to oral fluconazole at 800 mg per day.

He was followed monthly. He developed a painful left shoulder while on therapy. Bone scan was negative and the shoulder pain was considered to be fluconazole shoulder syndrome. Therapy was changed to Itraconazole, 200 mg twice daily. He complained of headache, which eventuated in a lumbar puncture which proved to be unremarkable. He gradually improved clinically and radiologically. His CF titers decreased to 1:2, and remained at this level for three readings, at which point the itraconazole was discontinued almost exactly 1 year from initial presentation. He was followed every 3 months for 1 year with serology after completing treatment with no rise in CF titer or clinical evidence of recurrence.

Instructive Cases Discussion

INSTRUCTIVE CASE 1

Answers: 1. **B**, 2. **C**

Discussion

Question 1

Amphotericin B-induced nephrotoxicity occurs primarily through two mechanisms: (1) constriction of afferent arterioles leading to direct decreases in glomerular filtration rate (GFR; glomerular toxicity) and (2) direct damage to the distal tubules (tubular toxicity; answer B), which in turn can lead to glomerular feedback that further constricts the afferent arterioles. Tubular toxicity of amphotericin B is essentially limited to the distal tubules and most commonly evident as hypokalemia (answer B). It occurs in the majority of patients receiving amphotericin B and may require up to 15 mmol of supplemental potassium per hour. Amphotericin B-induced hypokalemia is not associated with increased plasma aldosterone or renin levels and appears to result from increased permeability of the distal tubular cells due to direct toxic effects of amphotericin B. Although lipid amphotericin B formulations reduce distal tubular toxicity, they do not eliminate this side effect. Distal tubular toxicity (decreases in serum potassium and magnesium) frequently precede decreases in glomerular filtration rate (increases in serum creatinine, BUN) during amphotericin B therapy, particularly in patients receiving lipid amphotericin B formulations. Afferent arteriole constriction (answer A) would be more specifically associated with decreases in glomerular filtration (decrease in serum creatinine). Suppression of erythropoietin synthesis (answer C) is a more chronic effect of amphotericin B and manifests primarily as normochromic, normocytic anemia. Amphotericin B has not been shown to directly damage pancreatic islet cells (answer D).

Question 2

Nephrotoxicity is the dose-limiting toxicity of amphotericin B therapy. Although all of the answers are potential approaches that have been applied to prevent the development of nephrotoxicity during amphotericin B therapy, switching to a lipid amphotericin B formulation (answer C) is advocated by most infectious diseases experts once glomerular toxicity has developed during amphotericin B therapy. Alternative daily dosing of amphotericin B (answer A) is no longer recommended and there is no evidence that this method is less nephrotoxic than daily dosing. Administering amphotericin B by continuous infusion (answer B) has been shown in two small prospective trials to reduce infusion-related and nephrotoxic side effects; however, this dosing method is not practical and the efficacy of amphotericin B administered by continuous infusion has not been well explored. Saline loading (answer D) can reduce tubular-glomerular feedback and delay the onset of glomerular toxicity; however, it will not reverse glomerular toxicity once it has developed.

Instructive case 1 contributed by R. E. Lewis and A. W. Fothergill

INSTRUCTIVE CASE 2

Discussion

This case is somewhat unusual in that the site of inoculation of *Sporothrix schenckii* had received a skin graft, and thus the lesions were atypical. They arose in the grafted area and contributed to loss of portions of the graft. The lack of response to antistaphylococcal antibiotics was a clue that this was not a typical bacterial infection. The possibility of sporotrichosis was raised by the infectious diseases consultant because of the proximal spread of nodules and the exposure to soil during the original accident. Biopsy confirmed this suspicion when the cultures yielded a mould. The fact that no organisms were seen on the biopsy is not unusual.

Fluconazole was used because an experimental protocol was available at the time, and the patient had no insurance and was unable to purchase other antifungal agents. The response to fluconazole was adequate, but slower than usually noted with itraconazole, which is the treatment of choice for sporotrichosis.

Instructive case 2 contributed by C.A. Kauffman

INSTRUCTIVE CASE 3

Discussion

This case demonstrates how an apparently uncomplicated coccidioidal pneumonia can evolve into complex multifocal disseminated disease. Such cases frequently necessitate multiple therapy modalities.

Instructive case 3 contributed by R. H. Johnson and S. Baqi

INSTRUCTIVE CASE 4

Discussion

This is an example of the juvenile type paracoccidioidomycosis.

Instructive case 4 contributed by A. Restrepo, A. M. Tobón, and C. A. Agudelo

INSTRUCTIVE CASE 5

Discussion

This case is instructive for several reasons. The patient's past medical history is significant for a long history of immunosuppression due to long-term corticosteroid use and his diabetes mellitus. Both of these conditions predispose the patient to an increased risk of fungal infections because of alterations in cell-mediated immunity. The case demonstrates the increasing incidence and the capacity of previously nonpathogenic yeast to produce invasive infection. In addition, the presentation of the patient with nonspecific signs and symptoms is not uncommonly seen in many invasive fungal infections. In fact, the problem with the diagnosis of invasive fungal infections is that there are no "classic or pathognomonic manifestations." This makes the diagnosis difficult to establish and creates a delay in the initiation of appropriate antifungal therapy. In this case, the aspiration of the infected knee demonstrated several organisms (gram-negative bacilli and yeast), thus assisting with the diagnosis. However, *Candida*, not *Trichosporon* would have been the more common cause of infection in this patient. It is not until the laboratory identifies the organisms that the true diagnosis is established. Although there are no clinical trials establishing the best antifungal agent for *Trichosporon* species, the azoles (fluconazole, voriconazole) have been shown to have in vitro activity. In this case, in vitro susceptibility results demonstrated that both fluconazole and itraconazole had good activity. Although there are no established breakpoints for the echinocandins, the minimum inhibitory concentration (MIC) of 2.0 μg/ml for caspofungin appears to be within the "standard" ranges described for clinical activity against *Candida* species. Further, although there are some in vitro and animal studies demonstrating additive or synergistic activity with the combination of echinocandins and azoles, the use of combination antifungal therapy has not been demonstrated to be any better than monotherapy.

Instructive case 5 contributed by J. A. Vazquez

INSTRUCTIVE CASE 6

Discussion

Blastomycosis in AIDS

1. Blastomycosis in acquired immunodeficiency syndrome (AIDS) patients is more likely to be multiorgan disease, with CNS involvement being noted in up to 40% of patients. Routine magnetic resonance imaging (MRI) or CT scans should definitely be performed in any patient with severe end-stage AIDS whether or not the patient has neurologic signs or symptoms.
2. Wet preparations of skin lesions allowed a presumptive clinical diagnosis and early initiation of amphotericin B therapy in this patient.
3. Central nervous system disease in end-stage AIDS patients should be treated with a full course of amphotericin B, e.g., 1.5 to 2.5 grams.
4. Fluconazole at high doses (800 mg/day) may be a reasonable substitute in patients intolerant to amphotericin B or as step down therapy in patients who have responded to initial treatment with amphotericin B.
5. In immunosuppressed patients, chronic suppressive therapy with fluconazole should be considered.

Instructive case 6 contributed by S. W. Chapman and D. C. Sullivan

INSTRUCTIVE CASE 7

Discussion

This case represents acute pulmonary histoplasmosis misdiagnosed as sarcoidosis. It illustrates the importance of thorough testing to exclude histoplasmosis before beginning immunosuppressive treatment for sarcoidosis. While there are clinical features that help to distinguish sarcoidosis from histoplasmosis, differentiation requires laboratory testing to exclude histoplasmosis. Administration of corticosteroids resulted in transient clinical improvement, followed by progression with worsening pulmonary disease and progressive dissemination. Failure to demonstrate yeast resembling *H. capsulatum* on the initial bronchoscopy resulted in a mistaken diagnosis of sarcoidosis. Of note is that cytology and culture of respiratory secretions are often negative in acute histoplasmosis, and cannot be used to exclude the diagnosis.

Additional testing should include serology for antibodies to *H. capsulatum*, and tests for *Histoplasma* antigen in urine and respiratory secretions. Serology is often negative during the first month after exposure, but positive thereafter. Antigen may be detected in the urine or bronchoscopy specimen of 75% of cases during the acute illness and before antibodies have appeared. Corticosteroids for sarcoidosis should not be given without thorough evaluation to exclude histoplasmosis. Of note is that fungal cultures require up to 4 weeks of incubation for isolation of *H. capsulatum*, during which corticosteroids should be withheld except in severe cases. Tests for antigen and antibody, and cytology on bronchial washing or bronchoalveolar lavage, should be performed and may provide early evidence for histoplasmosis. Of note, these tests do not exclude the diagnosis. If lung or other tissues are biopsied, they also should be cultured and examined for fungus by histopathology.

If cytology, histopathology, antigen testing, and serology are negative and corticosteroids are required for severe sarcoidosis, itraconazole may be given while waiting for culture results in selected patients in whom the diagnosis of histoplasmosis is suspected based on epidemiologic grounds.

Instructive case 7 contributed by L. J. Wheat and N. G. Conger

INSTRUCTIVE CASE 8

Discussion

Subcutaneous phaeohyphomycosis is among the most common manifestations of disease due to dematiaceous fungi. It is seen in both immunocompetent and immunocompromised individuals and is not usually associated with dissemination, although the risk of dissemination is higher in immunosuppressed patients. Complete excision alone has been reported as a successful therapy, particularly in immunocompetent patients. In immunocompromised patients, antifungal therapy is often given after surgical excision to reduce the risk of dissemination. However, itraconazole and voriconazole both have significant interactions with immunosuppressive agents such as tacrolimus and sirolimus, and combined use of these drugs requires close monitoring and commonly adjustment of the immunosuppressive agents.

Instructive case 8 contributed by S. G. Revankar

INSTRUCTIVE CASE 9

Discussion

This case illustrates the importance of surgery in the management of complex axial and nonaxial osteomyelitis secondary to coccidioidomycosis.

Instructive case 9 contributed by R. H. Johnson and S. Baqi

INSTRUCTIVE CASE 10

Discussion

Nodular infiltrates in the neutropenic patient are often caused by pathogenic fungi. Identification is critical for proper management. This case illustrates that pulmonary zygomycosis in a neutropenic host may be associated with fever but a paucity of other findings on initial presentation. A BAL is often negative and more invasive procedures, such as a fine needle aspiration, may be necessary to establish a diagnosis. During neutropenia, pulmonary zygomycosis may progress rapidly, despite amphotericin B therapy. Surgery has an important role in these patients, as it may be the only way of controlling this angioinvasive infection. Granulocyte transfusions may have a role to gain time until neutropenia resolves. Ultimately, however, recovery from these infections is often contingent on recovery of bone marrow function. In the case presented, control of the pulmonary infection was achieved with combined medical and surgical intervention. Unfortunately, the patient ultimately succumbed to complications of his hairy cell leukemia.

Instructive case 10 contributed by C. Antachopoulos, J. C. Gea-Banacloche, and T. J. Walsh

INSTRUCTIVE CASE 11

Discussion

This patient's case is an example of chronic, adult multifocal paracoccidioidomycosis.

Instructive case 11 contributed by A. Restrepo, A. M. Tobón, and C. A. Agudelo

INSTRUCTIVE CASE 12

Answer: D

Discussion

Unpredictable, low-frequency idiosyncratic liver failure with azoles occurs on a background of a much higher frequency of mild asymptomatic liver injury. Mild liver injury is exacerbated by concomitant medications or dominated by other disease states (as in this case with the graft versus host disease that often affects the liver). Because mild liver injury is generally reversible and transient, immediate discontinuation of voriconazole is not necessary (answer A or B). In clinical trials, voriconazole was continued in the majority of patients with elevated serum transaminases until they reached greater than 3 times the upper limit of normal (which has not been reached in this patient). Because the patient will likely receive corticosteroids for the graft versus host disease reactivation, continuation of voriconazole and monitoring of liver function tests with the initiation of steroid therapy (answer D) would be the most reasonable approach. Although reduction of the voriconazole dose is an option (answer C), reducing antifungal intensity in an immunocompromised patient with active graft versus host disease and receiving steroids is undesirable. Many clinicians would potentially add a second antifungal agent in this patient if she had other signs of infection (i.e., pulmonary nodules in lung).

Instructive case 12 contributed by R. E. Lewis and A. W. Fothergill

INSTRUCTIVE CASE 13

Discussion

This case demonstrates the presentation and evaluation of coccidioidal meningitis and the management of two common complications, hydrocephalus, and SIADH.

Instructive case 13 contributed by R. H. Johnson and S. Baqi

INSTRUCTIVE CASE 14

Discussion

For induction therapy, she had received combination therapy with amphotericin B in a lipid formulation and a reduced dose of flucytosine because of kidney dysfunction. Her clinical response did not require repeated lumbar punctures to control raised intracranial pressure because symptoms did not worsen and actually improved. Her response to antifungal combination therapy was appropriate with a negative CSF culture at the end of 2 weeks of induction therapy.

Discussion

In this case, the patient developed cryptococcal meningitis after receiving severe therapeutic immunosuppression in an attempt to save her renal transplant from rejection. She initially responded to potent antifungal combination therapy, which was adjusted to renal dysfunction. Initially she did well on this suppressive therapy, but as she completely lost kidney function and immunosuppressive therapy was reduced she again developed meningeal symptoms and signs, but the work-up did not reveal evidence of an ongoing viable yeast infection. It was then decided that this may represent immune reconstitution inflammatory syndrome (IRIS) and she was started on corticosteroids, which improved and eventually resolved her symptoms.

This case illustrates the dynamic relationship between the immune system and cryptococcosis. Although there are standardized, well-studied antifungal treatment regimens, there are clearly times when clinical judgment must be used regarding management. Currently management of increased intracranial pressure and IRIS is performed without the luxury of guidance from robust evidence-based studies.

Instructive case 14 contributed by M. Chayakulkeeree and J. R. Perfect

INSTRUCTIVE CASE 15

Discussion

Blastomycosis Presenting with Acute Respiratory Distress Syndrome (ARDS)

1. Patients presenting with severe pulmonary disease, whether miliary or ARDS, have a high rate of mortality ($\geq$ 50%). All patients presenting in this fashion should be initially treated with amphotericin B.
2. Life-threatening pulmonary disease may be seen in nonimmunocompromised patients. Hence, blastomycosis must be considered in any patient living in or with recent travel to the endemic area and who presents with severe or over whelming pneumonia.
3. Most patients who die do so within the first week of therapy, emphasizing that amphotericin B therapy should be initiated as soon as possible after diagnosis.
4. Cytology may have a higher diagnostic yield than expectorated sputum examined under wet preparation.

Instructive case 15 contributed by S. W. Chapman and D. C. Sullivan

INSTRUCTIVE CASE 16

Discussion

Fibrosing mediastinitis (FM) results from excessive scarring around the hilar and mediastinal lymph nodes. This scar tissue extends from the lymph nodes to invade important nearby structures, such as the pulmonary arteries or veins, bronchial arteries, vena cava, trachea, main stem and lobar or segmental bronchi, esophagus, pericardium, and even the heart. FM represents a scarring response to a prior episode of histoplasmosis rather than an active and progressive infection.

The severity of the illness depends on the extent of the scarring, and the specific structures that are involved. In many cases, the consequences are mild and nonprogressive, causing minimal or no limitation to function, and requiring no consideration for therapy. In others, symptoms may be more severe, or even disabling, prompting consideration of the treatment options. In patients with extensive involvement in both lungs, the illness is progressive and eventually fatal in nearly half of cases.

Medical treatment with antifungal drugs that are used for treatment of other types of histoplasmosis is not effective in patients with fibrosing mediastinitis, because the manifestations of FM are caused by the scar tissue, not by active infection, and scar tissue is not affected by any medical treatments.

Minimally invasive procedures to open the blockages are useful in some cases. These procedures are relatively safe and sometimes effective, although the long-term results are not fully understood. The largest experience has been with stenting of the occluded blood vessels. Stenting of obstructed airways is not believed to be as useful, and there is little experience with this procedure. Stenting or dilatation of obstructed vessels is not always successful because the fibrotic tissue may be as hard as stone, preventing passage of a small wire past the blockage. Active bleeding may be stopped by embolization of the involved blood vessel.

Surgical correction of the obstructed blood vessel or airway also is not often possible, and carries a high operative mortality. Thus, surgery should be reserved for severe cases and only then after less risky procedures are tried. The operative mortality is at least 20% overall, but can range from 50% to 75% in patients who undergo total removal of the involved lung (pneumonectomy). Of note is that the operative mortality may be even higher if the surgeon is not experienced with treatment of fibrosing mediastinitis. The reason that the mortality is so high is that the scar tissue is like cement, encasing the blood vessels and airways and obliterating tissue planes. Vital structures are often damaged while attempting to remove the scar tissue, causing bleeding or airway leaks. Death is caused by uncontrollable bleeding, respiratory failure, infection, and other post-operative complications. The indications for surgery are not well described, but at a minimum should include patient limitations severe enough to justify the risk of the known operative mortality. Surgical indications might include severe and recurrent bleeding not responsive to embolization, recurrent pneumonias that are not preventable by antibiotic prophylaxis, or respiratory failure. Surgery should be conducted only by surgeons who are experienced with fibrosing mediastinitis.

Instructive case 16 contributed by L. J. Wheat and N. G. Conger

INSTRUCTIVE CASE 17

Discussion

This patient's case is an example of the chronic unifocal pulmonary paracoccidioidomycosis.

Instructive case 17 contributed by A. Restrepo, A. M. Tobón, and C. A. Agudelo

INSTRUCTIVE CASE 18

Discussion

This case demonstrates the evolution of pneumonia from mild to severe over a time course characteristic of coccidioidomycosis (but not community-acquired pneumonia). The management of coccidioidomycosis with respiratory failure is also noted.

Instructive case 18 contributed by R. H. Johnson and S. Baqi

Index

MIX
Papier aus verantwortungsvollen Quellen
Paper from responsible sources
FSC® C105338

If you have any concerns about our products,
you can contact us on
ProductSafety@springernature.com

In case Publisher is established outside the EU,
the EU authorized representative is:
Springer Nature Customer Service Center GmbH
Europaplatz 3, 69115 Heidelberg, Germany

Printed by Libri Plureos GmbH
in Hamburg, Germany